Cancer Chemotherapy: Basic Science to the Clinic

Cancer Chemotherapy: Basic Science to the Clinic

Editor: Johnny White

AMERICAN
MEDICAL PUBLISHERS
www.americanmedicalpublishers.com

AMERICAN
MEDICAL PUBLISHERS
www.americanmedicalpublishers.com

Cataloging-in-Publication Data

Cancer chemotherapy : basic science to the clinic / edited by Johnny White.
p. cm.
Includes bibliographical references and index.
ISBN 978-1-63927-339-3
1. Cancer--Chemotherapy. 2. Cancer--Treatment. 3. Antineoplastic agents. I. White, Johnny.
RC271.C5 C36 2022
616.994 061--dc23

American Medical Publishers,
41 Flatbush Avenue,
1st Floor, New York,
NY 11217, USA

ISBN 978-1-63927-339-3 (Hardback)

Contents

Preface

Cancer is a collection of related diseases where some cells start to divide rapidly and spread to other parts of the body. The treatment of cancer with one or more anti-cancer drugs is called chemotherapy. It is part of a standardized chemotherapy regimen. It may be given with the intent to cure cancer, or with the aim to prolong life or reduce symptoms. Traditional chemotherapeutic agents act by killing these cells. The dosage as well as the treatment plan of chemotherapy depends on various factors such as the type of cancer, the size and location of tumor, and age of the patient. This book presents the complex subject of chemotherapy in the most comprehensible and easy to understand language. It outlines the processes and applications of chemotherapy in detail. This book, with its detailed analyses and data, will prove immensely beneficial to professionals and students involved in this area at various levels.

Significant researches are present in this book. Intensive efforts have been employed by authors to make this book an outstanding discourse. This book contains the enlightening chapters which have been written on the basis of significant researches done by the experts.

Finally, I would also like to thank all the members involved in this book for being a team and meeting all the deadlines for the submission of their respective works. I would also like to thank my friends and family for being supportive in my efforts.

Editor

1

Hypersensitivity to Carboplatin in Children with Malignancy

Antonio Ruggiero, Daniela Rizzo, Martina Catalano, Giorgio Attinà and Riccardo Riccardi*

Division of Pediatric Oncology, Catholic University of Rome, Rome, Italy

Purpose: Carboplatin-based regimens have proven efficacy in children with cancer. However, the development of hypersensitivity reactions (HSRs) may have a negative impact on treatment intensity and patients' outcome. The aim of this review is to summarize the incidence and the clinical features of HSRs occurring in children with cancer treated with carboplatin and their impact on treatment efficacy.

Methods: Data were collected by searching for relevant studies on the incidence, clinical features and management of possible side effects about the use of carboplatin in children, published from March 1987 to October 2016 in the PubMed database.

Results: Carboplatin HSRs present with mild/moderate to severe clinical patterns. The risk of HSR is related to the cumulative number of infusions. Moreover, a greater risk of developing an HSR has been observed in younger patients than in older age groups of children; risk is also greater in girls and in patients with a prior history of allergy to other drugs. Management options include cessation of carboplatin and switching to another agent, premedication with antihistamines and/or corticosteroids, and carboplatin desensitization. For sensitized patients who have obtained benefits from carboplatin, the continuation of the treatment is desirable and desensitization protocols have showed promising results.

Conclusion: Clinicians must not underestimate the potential risk and occurrence of carboplatin HSRs in the pediatric population in order to outline adequate management strategies. Desensitization protocols should be considered for patients sensitive to carboplatin in order to avoid having to discontinue an effective chemotherapy.

Edited by:
Raquel Abalo,
Universidad Rey Juan Carlos, Spain

Reviewed by:
Lucie Lafay-Cousin,
Alberta Children's Hospital, Canada
Loredana Bergandi,
University of Turin, Italy

***Correspondence:**
Antonio Ruggiero
antonio.ruggiero@unicatt.it

Keywords: hypersensitivity reactions, carboplatin, children, management, desensitization

INTRODUCTION

Carboplatin is a second-generation platinum compound developed to reduce the side effects of cisplatin, particularly neurotoxicity, nephrotoxicity and emesis, while maintaining comparable antitumor activity and effectiveness. Carboplatin is widely used to treat solid tumors in adults, especially for ovarian and lung cancer, and for several types of malignancies in children such as brain tumor, neuroblastoma, retinoblastoma, germ cell tumors, and hepatoblastoma. Moreover, the treatment protocol based upon the combination of carboplatin and vincristine reported by Packer et al. (1997) seems to produce consistent and long-lasting responses in children with low grade glioma (LGG) (Chiaretti et al., 2004; Trisciuzzi et al., 2004). This is the most widely adopted chemotherapy for childhood LGG, offering high objective response rates in relapsed and newly diagnosed patients of 52 and 62%, respectively.

Carboplatin has been used with increasing frequency for the management of childhood cancers, and hypersensitivity reactions (HSRs) have consequently emerged as a significant complication of the therapy. Multiple exposures to this chemotherapeutic agent can cause sometimes life-threatening events, requiring discontinuation of treatment. However, while carboplatin-associated HSRs have been described extensively and analyzed in large cohorts of adult patients, our knowledge of their features in pediatric patients remains limited.

INCIDENCE

Allergic hypersensitivity to carboplatin is frequently reported in children, and the extensive use of carboplatin-based chemotherapy has brought with it an increase in allergic reactions (Allen et al., 1987; Chang et al., 1995; Lazzareschi et al., 2002). Carboplatin HSR has been described mostly in pediatric series of LGG, where the reported incidence is up to 47% depending on the schedules of administration (Lafay-Cousin et al., 2008; Dodgshun et al., 2016).

In the initial reports on the carboplatin-vincristine combination in pediatric LGG, Packer et al. (1997) observed a frequency of 7%. In a cohort of 29 children with LGG, Lazzareschi et al. (2002) reported six patients (20%) who developed HSRs to carboplatin. In the retrospective, cooperative Canadian study 42% of children with LGG who received a carboplatin-based chemotherapy regimen developed HSRs during the course of the treatment (Lafay-Cousin et al., 2008). Genc et al. (2012) observed a frequency of 40% in their study. Recently, carboplatin hypersensitivity was documented in 47% of patients by Dodgshun et al. (2016), and in the study by Shah et al. (2016) of 144 children with LGG treated with carboplatin and vincristine, 56 (39%) experienced an HSR to carboplatin.

CLINICAL FEATURES

Carboplatin can induce mild to moderate and severe HSRs which may develop acutely during infusion or within minutes, hours, or days after the drug has been delivered.

Clinical evidence of HSRs are graded 0 through 5 (grade 5 being death) by using the NCI Common Terminology Criteria for Adverse Events [CTCAE] (2010, CTCAE v. 4.03).

Mild and moderate reactions include all cutaneous reactions (flushing, pruritus, urticaria, angioedema, and maculopapular rash) not associated with symptoms affecting other organ systems. Severe reactions include chest pain, dyspnea, oxygen desaturation, edema/angioedema, changes in blood pressure and cardiovascular collapse.

Urticaria and facial rash may be the first and most common manifestations of hypersensitivity (Lazzareschi et al., 2002) and Markman et al. (1999) reported more than 50% of patients developing at least moderately severe symptoms. Symptoms usually resolved quickly with antihistamines and steroids.

More severe reactions and systemic anaphylaxis may be life-threatening (Cefalo et al., 2010). It is possible that carboplatin HSRs are not always recognized. Often, the early signs are subtle and may include only a mild rash and a mild bronchospasm (Wiesner et al., 2004). Patients should be alerted and appropriately instructed so that symptoms are promptly recognized and the diagnosis of HSR established to prevent potentially dangerous retreatment.

PATHOPHYSIOLOGY

The exact mechanism of carboplatin HSRs remains unclear, but the different clinical patterns of allergic reactions suggest that various immunological and non-immunological mechanisms are involved (Zanotti et al., 2001). Likelihood of type I IgE-mediated hypersensitivity increases with the rising incidence of hypersensitivity with repeated doses and with positive skin prick test reactions to platinum compounds (Leguy-Seguin et al., 2007). Carboplatin can act as a hapten and cause a type I IgE-mediated, histaminergic reaction with release of inflammatory molecules (Navo et al., 2006; Makrilia et al., 2010). Type I IgE-mediated hypersensitivity may be linked to early onset manifestations, such as itching, chest pain, rash, and anaphylactic reactions. An alternative to the type I IgE-mediated mechanism is type IV hypersensitivity, mediated by T cells, a delayed inflammatory reaction occurring hours or days after the infusion.

Some authors have tried to predict HSRs by using skin testing (Zanotti et al., 2001; Cefalo et al., 2010). Zanotti et al. (2001) developed a skin-test protocol for adult patients with gynecological malignancies and first demonstrated that skin testing for carboplatin made it possible to identify patients at risk for HSRs with a 99% negative predictive value. A cohort of 47 patients received a 0.02 ml intradermal injection of an undiluted aliquot of carboplatin 1 h before each course of chemotherapy. A negative skin test accurately predicted the absence of HSRs in 166 out of 168 courses of chemotherapy. Markman et al. (2003) performed skin tests on 126 women with gynecological cancer 30 min before each carboplatin treatment after the sixth cycle. They reported that skin tests had been positive in six out of seven patients who later developed anaphylaxis during carboplatin re-administration, finding a 98.5% negative predictive value. Therefore, a negative carboplatin skin test seems to predict with reasonable reliability the absence of a severe HSR with subsequent infusion of the drug. However, the implications of a positive test remain less certain and the limited experience with continued treatment suggests that this approach must be undertaken with considerable caution. According to Lazzareschi et al. (2002), the lack of sensitivity in skin tests could be explained by the fact that the molecular weight of carboplatin (373.272 g/mol) is low and it is not immunogenic in the native form.

RISK FACTORS

A greater risk of developing an HSR has been observed in younger patients than in older age groups of children (Genc et al., 2012); risk is also greater in girls (Lafay-Cousin et al.,

2008) and in patients with a prior history of allergy to other drugs (Ruggiero et al., 2010). No significant correlation was found between the occurrence of carboplatin HSRs and previous surgery, radiotherapy or tumor location (Genc et al., 2012).

The risk of hypersensitivity is related to the cumulative number of infusions rather than to the cumulative dose of carboplatin (Chang et al., 1995), thus it increases with repeated exposure to carboplatin (Schiavetti et al., 1999; Yu et al., 2001; Lazzareschi et al., 2002; Wiesner et al., 2004). The first HSR generally occurs between the 7th and the 10th carboplatin infusion (Schiavetti et al., 1999; Lazzareschi et al., 2002; Wiesner et al., 2004). Indeed HSRs are uncommon during the first few cycles and the incidence of reactions occurs mainly between the 7th and the 15th carboplatin infusion and may develop acutely during infusion or within minutes, hours, or days after the drug has been delivered (Genc et al., 2012).

Weekly dosing schedules of carboplatin have been identified as a risk factor for HSR in brain tumor patients (Yu et al., 2001). However, in the Canadian study (Lafay-Cousin et al., 2008), patients who received a weekly schedule had an incidence of HSR comparable to that of patients who were treated by monthly dosing, although HSR occurred 3 months earlier in the weekly dosing group.

According to Markman et al. (1999), the threshold for the manifestation of a reaction is expected to drop with each treatment because the patient is sensitized during the first treatment, and retreatment with the same drug provides the additional immunological stimulation necessary for a reaction.

Moreover, an increased severity of HSRs might be linked to re-exposure. Genc et al. (2012) reported seven out of eight patients had worsening hypersensitivity symptoms. Wiesner et al. (2004) observed grade III or IV reactions after re-exposure in five out of nine LGG patients with initial grade II reactions. The Canadian study found that the frequency of grade III and IV reactions rose from 18.2% at the first HSR episode to 41.7% for the second episode (Lafay-Cousin et al., 2008). Dodgshun et al. (2016) reported grade III reactions on rechallenge in two patients who initially experienced grade I and II reactions. In the study by Shah et al. (2016), 19 patients experienced a subsequent high-grade HSR (Grade III or IV) after initiating carboplatin rechallenge. In any case, Chang et al. (1995) did not document any increase in severity of HSR after re-exposure. The main issue is related to the possibility that an increased severity of hypersensitivity after re-exposure might expose the patient to the risk of anaphylaxis (Kook et al., 1998; Yu et al., 2001).

MANAGEMENT

Chemotherapy protocols based on a combination of carboplatin and other drugs produced good results in terms of progression-free survival rate, as in LGG. Thus, when a patient shows a response to a carboplatin-based regimen, strategies that alter the HSRs may be justified as an attempt to salvage an effective therapy.

However, when HSRs occur early in treatment, it may be harder to predict the response to treatment and the benefit of continuing carboplatin may be inferior to the risk of a more severe allergic reaction. Therefore, according to International Society of Pediatric Oncology LGG protocol, in patients developing an allergy to carboplatin during consolidation, therapy shall be continued with alternative drug combinations (cisplatin/vincristine and cyclophosphamide/vincristine) (Azizi, 2010). The substitution of carboplatin with another platinum compound (such as cisplatin) may be limited by cross-reactivity of platinum-specific IgE (Pagani, 2010). The cisplatin and cyclophosphamide combination showed efficacy when alternated with carboplatin in the French "BABY-SFOP" LGG study (Rakotonjanahary et al., 2015). Despite its effectiveness, however, cisplatin is more ototoxic and nephrotoxic than carboplatin (Bertolini et al., 2004). In patients receiving carboplatin, the incidence of ototoxicity is approximately 7% (Dean et al., 2008; Jehanne et al., 2009). In patients receiving cumulative cisplatin doses of $\leq$200 mg/m^2, 200–400 mg/m^2, and $\geq$400 mg/m^2, the incidence increases to 59, 68, and 65%, respectively (Peleva et al., 2014). Moreover, severe nephrotoxicity has not been reported during carboplatin-therapy and reduction of glomerular filtration rate to less than 50% is less frequent than with cisplatin. Moreover, cisplatin combined with cyclophosphamide could further damage renal function, therefore, in order to limit cumulative doses of these agents, no more than five cycles of both combinations shall be given. Therefore, to date the vincristine/carboplatin combination remains the most widely adopted multi-agent chemotherapy for childhood LGG. Of course, in patients sensitive to carboplatin the benefit of continuing this agent must be traded off against the risk of more severe reactions in view of the fact that no precise way to identify patients likely to react or to predict the severity of the reactions has yet been found.

To date, various desensitization and/or premedication protocols have been proposed, in children developing carboplatin HSR as a late event.

Pretreatment with steroids or antihistamines usually fails to prevent IgE-mediated reactions. The effectiveness of oral antihistamines has been found only in mild or moderate cases of carboplatin HSRs (Genc et al., 2012); moreover, the prolonged use of steroids is associated with long-term side effects in children and adolescents, such as mood changes, weight gain, and osteoporosis (Lafay-Cousin et al., 2008). The literature points to a low efficacy of premedication alone in re-exposure to carboplatin in patients with HSR. Aquino et al. (1999) and Heath et al. (2003) have reported complete failure of premedication (100% discontinuation rate). In Chang et al. (1995) and Wiesner et al. (2004) the effectiveness of premedication was 20 and 28.6%, respectively.

To date, several desensitization protocols for re-administering carboplatin have been implemented and have produced promising results (Markman et al., 1999; Lazzareschi et al., 2002; Lee et al., 2009; Castells et al., 2012) (**Table 1**). Drug desensitization is a procedure designed to obtain temporary clinical tolerance, especially in cases where the patient seems to have benefited from the drug (Castells, 2006; Lee et al., 2009; Castells et al., 2012). The complete target dose of the drug is administered in separate incremental steps in order to obtain an

TABLE 1 | Success rate of desensitization in patients with hypersensitivity reactions to carboplatin.

Studies	No. of patients treated with carboplatin	Patients with HSR (No./%)	Patients re-exposed to carboplatin (No./%)	No. of patients re-exposed with desensitization protocol	Success rate of desensitization (%)
Lazzareschi et al., 2002	29	6 (20.6%)	6 (100%)	6	6/6 (100%)
Lafay-Cousin et al., 2008	105	44 (41.9%)	34 (77.2%)	12	1/12 (8.3%)
Genc et al., 2012	50	20 (40%)	19 (95%)	9	6/9 (66.6%)
Dodgshun et al., 2016	59	16 (27.1%)	10 (62.5%)	10	2/10 (20%)
Shah et al., 2016	144	56 (38.9%)	55 (98.2%)	25	19/25(76%)

inhibition of mast-cell activation for the specific drug antigen. Sometimes this procedure is accompanied by a more intense premedication to prevent any risk of reaction (Genc et al., 2012). It is possible that the administration of small, increasing doses of antigen delivered at fixed time intervals may consume IgE antibodies slowly without acute reactions by inducing a prolonged hypo-responsiveness to triggering doses of the desensitizing antigen. Successful re-exposure to carboplatin is defined as the ability to complete the full planned course of treatment. All other cases where carboplatin is discontinued are considered a failure of re-exposure.

In Lazzareschi et al. (2002) described a successfully modified desensitization protocol for carboplatin administration in six children who had an allergic reaction to the drug. The protocol consisted of a standard dose of carboplatin (175 mg/m^2 in 100 ml saline solution) at an increasing infusion rate, without premedication. The drug was administered every 30 min starting with a dose of 0.3 mg/m^2/min and reaching 2.4 mg/m2/min in five steps (Lazzareschi et al., 2002) (**Table 2**). The protocol allowed the patients to receive carboplatin without adverse reactions in all re-treated patients. Genc et al. (2012) (**Table 2**) implemented a seven-step desensitization protocol in nine children affected by LGG, with a success rate of 66.6%. Patients were premedicated with pheniramine maleate (1 mg/kg/dose IV) and dexamethasone (0.3 mg/kg/dose IV) and the drugs were infused progressively every 15 min, beginning with a 0.1 mg/dose bolus, up to a 25 mg/dose. In the study by Shah et al. (2016) patients were re-exposed to therapy with carboplatin using precautionary measures, which included: prolongation of infusion (1–2 h); premedication with H1 antagonists; H2 antagonists, and corticosteroids. In patients with recurrent reactions despite precautionary measures, and in patients in which the first reaction was considered severe, a desensitization scheme was proposed which involved the administration of carboplatin in gradually increasing doses, from as low as 0.01 mg/min up to a maximum of 1.5 mg/min in nine progressive increments (**Table 2**). The success rate was 76%.

However, according to Lafay-Cousin et al. (2008) and Dodgshun et al. (2016), the desensitization protocol demonstrated low efficacy, due to differences in starting dose, infusion rate and number of increments compared with other studies. In the Canadian study, the desensitization protocol consisted of a progressive increase in the rate of carboplatin infusion over various periods (from 1 h to 6 h) according to previously described schedules (doses of 1, 2.5, 5, 10, 25, and 50 mg of carboplatin infused at 1 mg/min every 15 min; the remainder of the dose was infused at the standard rate of 200 mg/h) (Broome et al., 1996; Ogle et al., 2002). Nevertheless, among the 12 patients who underwent desensitization and premedication (antihistamine with or without corticosteroid initiated from 3 days to 1 h before carboplatin infusion), only one patient (8.3%) was able to complete his carboplatin therapy (Lafay-Cousin et al., 2008). In this study the lower success rate of desensitization may be due to the starting dose being higher than in other studies (Lazzareschi et al., 2002; Genc et al., 2012; Shah et al., 2016). Dodgshun et al. (2016) reported a success rate of 20%. All patients received premedication with dexamethasone (between 0.05 and 0.15 mg/kg delivered via IV 1 h prior to carboplatin) and cetirazine (~0.2 mg/kg delivered orally 1 h prior to carboplatin) and all but one, were exposed to the

TABLE 2 | Effective desensitization protocols.

Lazzareschi et al., 2002			Genc et al., 2012			Shah et al., 2016		
Step	Infusion rate (mg/m^2/min)	Time (min)	Step	Infusion rate (mg/m^2/min)	Time (min)	Step	Infusion rate (mg/m^2/min)	Time (min)
1	0.3	30	1	0.1	15	1	0.01	15
2	0.6	30	2	1	15	2	0.1	15
3	1.2	30	3	2.5	15	3	0.5	15
4	1.8	30	4	5	15	4	1	15
5	2.4	30	5	10	15	5	1	15
			6	25	15	6	1	15
			7	Remaining dose	15	7	1	15
						8	1.5	15
						9	1.5	15

desensitization diagram with subsequent infusions of increasing doses of carboplatin according to the scheme described by Confino-Cohen et al. (2005). The protocol consisted of an initial infusion of 1/1000 of the total dose in the first 90 min, followed by 1/100 of the total dose for an additional 90 min, up to 1/10 in 90 min and the remainder of the dose in the last 90 min. Desensitization was not effective in this cohort. It is not clear why the success rate is so different from what was previously reported in adult literature. This may be due to the lack of a gradual increase in the rate of infusion (from 0.6 mg/m^2/min to 5.5 mg/m^2/min in the fourth step), and to the limited number of increments.

CONCLUSION

As carboplatin has been used with increasing frequency for the management of childhood cancers, HSRs have emerged as a significant complication of the therapy although their features involving pediatric patients remain limited. HSRs occur mainly between the 7th and the 15th carboplatin infusion, therefore attention must be paid to the cumulative number of infusions rather than to the cumulative dose.

When a patient shows a response to a carboplatin-based regimen, strategies that alter the HSRs may be justified as an attempt to salvage an effective therapy, although the benefits of continuing the carboplatin chemotherapy should always be carefully weighed against the risks of potential dangerous complications.

Patients with an early onset allergic reaction should switch to alternative chemotherapy regimens that offer a good efficacy rate in order to avoid any risk associated with re-exposure. Thus, the likelihood of completing therapy is higher if restricted to patients with a late onset reaction.

Premedication with anti-histamines and/or corticosteroids is able to prevent an allergic reaction only in a limited number of patients with mild or moderate reactions. Several desensitization protocols have been implemented in order to re-administer carboplatin with various efficacy results. Hypothesis on their effectiveness to be further investigated are based on the potential role of the starting dose, infusion rate and number of increments. A lower starting dose, a slow infusion, and a number of increments greater than or equal to 4 are associated with a greater probability of success.

AUTHOR CONTRIBUTIONS

All authors listed, have made substantial, direct and intellectual contribution to the work, and approved it for publication.

REFERENCES

Allen, J. C., Walker, R., Luks, E., Jennings, M., Barfoot, S., and Tan, C. (1987). Carboplatin and recurrent childhood brain tumors. *J. Clin. Oncol.* 5, 459–463. doi: 10.1200/JCO.1987.5.3.459

Aquino, V. M., Fort, D. W., and Kamen, B. A. (1999). Carboplatin for the treatment of children with newly diagnosed optic chiasm gliomas: a phase II study. *J. Neurooncol.* 41, 255–259. doi: 10.1023/A:1006149809479

Azizi, A. (2010). Current state and therapy strategies in paediatric low grade glioma. *MEMO* 4, 16–18. doi: 10.1007/s11060-013-1284-2

Bertolini, P., Lassalle, M., Mercier, G., Raquin, M. A., Izzi, G., Corradini, N., et al. (2004). Platinum compound-related ototoxicity in children: long-term follow-up reveals continuous worsening of hearing loss. *J. Pediatr. Hematol. Oncol.* 26, 649–655. doi: 10.1097/01.mph.0000141348.62532.73

Broome, C. B., Schiff, R. I., and Friedman, H. S. (1996). Successful desensitization to carboplatin in patients with systemic hypersensitivity reactions. *Med. Pediatr. Oncol.* 26, 105–110. doi: 10.1002/(SICI)1096-911X(199602)26:2<105::AID-MPO7>3.0.CO;2-P

Castells, M. (2006). Rapid desensitization of hypersensitivity reactions to chemotherapy agents. *Curr. Drug Saf.* 1, 243–251. doi: 10.2174/157488606777934413

Castells, M., Sancho-Serra Mdel, C., and Simarro, M. (2012). Hypersensitivity to antineoplastic agents: mechanisms and treatment with rapid desensitization. *Cancer Immunol. Immunother.* 61, 1575–1584. doi: 10.1007/s00262-012-1273-x

Cefalo, M. G., Maurizi, P., Arlotta, A., Scalzone, M., Attinà, G., Ruggiero, A., et al. (2010). Hepatic veno-occlusive disease: a chemotherapy-related toxicity in children with malignancies. *Paediatr. Drugs* 12, 277–284. doi: 10.2165/11531840-000000000-00000

Chang, S. M., Fryberger, S., Crouse, V., Tilford, D., and Prados, M. D. (1995). Carboplatin hypersensitivity in children. A report of five patients with brain tumors. *Cancer* 75, 1171–1175. doi: 10.1002/1097-0142(19950301)75:5<1171::AID-CNCR2820750518>3.0.CO;2-F

Chiaretti, A., Aloe, L., Antonelli, A., Ruggiero, A., Piastra, M., Riccardi, R., et al. (2004). Neurotrophic factor expression in childhood low-grade astrocytomas and ependymomas. *Childs Nerv. Syst.* 20, 412–419. doi: 10.1007/s00381-004-0959-6

Common Terminology Criteria for Adverse Events [CTCAE]. (2010). *CTCAE Version 4. 0.* Bethesda, MD: National Institutes of Health.

Confino-Cohen, R., Fishman, A., Altaras, M., and Goldberg, A. (2005). Successful carboplatin desensitization in patients with proven carboplatin allergy. *Cancer* 104, 640–643. doi: 10.1002/cncr.21168

Dean, J. B., Hayashi, S. S., Albert, C. M., King, A. A., Karzon, R., and Hayashi, R. J. (2008). Hearing loss in pediatric oncology patients receiving carboplatin-containing regimens. *J. Pediatr. Hematol. Oncol.* 30, 130–134. doi: 10.1097/MPH.0b013e31815d1d83

Dodgshun, A. J., Hansford, J. R., Cole, T., Choo, S., and Sullivan, M. J. (2016). Carboplatin hypersensitivity reactions in pediatric low grade glioma are protocol specific and desensitization show poor efficacy. *Pediatr. Blood Cancer* 63, 17–20. doi: 10.1002/pbc.25686

Genc, D. B., Canpolat, C., and Berrak, S. G. (2012). Clinical features and management of carboplatin-related hypersensitivity reactions in pediatric low-grade glioma. *Support. Care Cancer* 20, 385–393. doi: 10.1007/s00520-011-1123-y

Heath, J. A., Turner, C. D., Poussaint, T. Y., Scott, R. M., Goumnerova, L., and Kieran, M. W. (2003). Chemotherapy for progressive low-grade gliomas in children older than ten years: the Dana–Farber experience. *Pediatr. Hematol. Oncol.* 20, 497–504. doi: 10.1080/08880010390232709

Jehanne, M., Lumbroso-Le Rouic, L., Savignoni, A., Aerts, I., Mercier, G., Bours, D., et al. (2009). Analysis of ototoxicity in young children receiving carboplatin in the context of conservative management of unilateral or bilateral retinoblastoma. *Pediatr. Blood Cancer* 52, 637–643. doi: 10.1002/pbc.21898

Kook, H., Kim, K. M., and Choi, S. H. (1998). Life-threatening carboplatin hypersensitivity during conditioning for autologous PBSC transplantation: successful rechallenge after desensitization. *Bone Marrow Transplant.* 21, 727–729. doi: 10.1038/sj.bmt.1701161

Lafay-Cousin, L., Sung, L., Carret, A. S., Hukin, J., Wilson, B., Johnston, D. L., et al. (2008). Carboplatin hypersensitivity reaction in pediatric patients with low-grade glioma: a Canadian Pediatric Brain Tumor Consortium experience. *Cancer* 112, 892–899. doi: 10.1002/cncr.23249

Lazzareschi, I., Ruggiero, A., Riccardi, R., Attinà, G., Colosimo, C., and Lasorella, A. (2002). Hypersensitivity reactions to carboplatin in children. *J. Neurooncol.* 58, 33–37. doi: 10.1023/A:1015853200090

Lee, C., Gianos, M., and Klaustermeyer, W. B. (2009). Diagnosis and management of hypersensitivity reactions related to common cancer chemotherapy agents. *Ann. Allergy Asthma Immunol.* 102, 179–187. doi: 10.1016/S1081-1206(10)60078-6

Leguy-Seguin, V., Jolimoy, G., Coudert, B., Pernot, C., Dalac, S., Vabres, P., et al. (2007). Diagnostic and predictive value of skin testing in platinum salt hypersensitivity. *J. Allergy Clin. Immunol.* 119, 726–730. doi: 10.1016/j.jaci.2006.11.640

Makrilia, N., Syrigou, E., Kaklamanos, I., Manolopoulos, L., and Saif, M. W. (2010). Hypersensitivity reactions associated with platinum antineoplastic agents: a systematic review. *Met. Based Drugs* 2010, 207084. doi: 10.1155/2010/207084

Markman, M., Kennedy, A., Webster, K., Elson, P., Peterson, G., Kulp, B., et al. (1999). Clinical features of hypersensitivity reactions to carboplatin. *J. Clin. Oncol.* 17, 1141–1145. doi: 10.1200/JCO.1999.17.4.1141

Markman, M., Zanotti, K., Peterson, G., Kulp, B., Webster, K., and Belinson, J. (2003). Expanded experience with an intradermal skin test to predict for the presence or absence of carboplatin hypersensitivity. *J. Clin. Oncol.* 15, 4611–4614. doi: 10.1200/JCO.2003.05.539

Navo, M., Kunthur, A., Badell, M. L., Coffer, L. W., Markman, M., Brown, J., et al. (2006). Evaluation of the incidence of carboplatin hypersensitivity reactions in cancer patients. *Gynecol. Oncol.* 103, 608–613. doi: 10.1016/j.ygyno.2006.04.002

Ogle, S. K., Rose, M. M., and Wildes, C. T. (2002). Development and implementation of a carboplatin desensitization protocol for children with neurofibromatosis, type 1 and hypersensitivity reactions in an outpatient oncology clinic. *J. Pediatr. Oncol. Nurs.* 19, 122–126. doi: 10.1177/104345420201900403

Packer, R. J., Ater, J., Allen, J., Phillips, P., Geyer, R., Nicholson, H. S., et al. (1997). Carboplatin and vincristine chemotherapy for children with newly diagnosed progressive low-grade gliomas. *J. Neurosurg.* 86, 747–754. doi: 10.3171/jns.1997.86.5.0747

Pagani, M. (2010). The complex clinical picture of presumably allergic side effects to cytostatic drugs: symptoms, pathomechanism, reexposure, and desensitization. *Med. Clin. North Am.* 94, 835–852. doi: 10.1016/j.mcna.2010.03.002

Peleva, E., Emami, N., Alzahrani, M., Bezdjian, A., Gurberg, J., Carret, A. S., et al. (2014). Incidence of platinum-induced ototoxicity in pediatric patients in Quebec. *Pediatr. Blood Cancer* 61, 2012–2017. doi: 10.1002/pbc.25123

Rakotonjanahary, J., De Carli, E., Delion, M., Kalifa, C., Grill, J., Doz, F., et al. (2015). Brain tumor committee of SFCE.mortality in children with optic pathway glioma treated with up-front BB-SFOP chemotherapy. *PLoS ONE* 10:e0127676. doi: 10.1371/journal.pone.0127676

Ruggiero, A., Rizzo, D., Mastrangelo, S., Battaglia, D., Attinà, G., and Riccardi, R. (2010). Interactions between antiepileptic and chemotherapeutic drugs in children with brain tumors: is it time to change treatment? *Pediatr. Blood Cancer* 54, 193–198. doi: 10.1002/pbc.22276

Schiavetti, A., Varrasso, G., Maurizi, P., and Castello, M. A. (1999). Hypersensitivity to carboplatin in children. *Med. Pediatr. Oncol.* 32, 183–185. doi: 10.1002/(SICI)1096-911X(199903)32:3<183::AID-MPO4>3.0.CO;2-P

Shah, A. C., Minturn, J. E., Li, Y., Belasco, J. B., Phillips, P. C., Kang, T. I., et al. (2016). Carboplatin rechallenge after hypersensitivity reaction in pediatric patient with low grade glioma. *Pediatr. Blood Cancer* 63, 21–26. doi: 10.1002/pbc.25697

Trisciuzzi, M. T., Riccardi, R., Piccardi, M., Iarossi, G., Buzzonetti, L., Dickmann, A., et al. (2004). A fast visual evoked potential method for functional assessment and follow-up of childhood optic gliomas. *Clin. Neurophysiol.* 115, 217–226. doi: 10.1016/S1388-2457(03)00282-7

Wiesner, A., Zucol, F., Roger, P. L., and Grotzer, M. A. (2004). Hypersensitivity reactions to carboplatin in children with low-grade gliomas. *J. Pediatr. Neurol.* 2, 151–155.

Yu, D. Y., Dahl, G. V., Shames, R. S., and Fisher, P. G. (2001). Weekly dosing of carboplatin increases risk of allergy in children. *J. Pediatr. Hematol. Oncol.* 23, 349–352. doi: 10.1097/00043426-200108000-00005

Zanotti, K. M., Rybicki, L. A., Kennedy, A. W., Belinson, J. L., Webster, K. D., Kulp, B., et al. (2001). Carboplatin skin testing: a skin-testing protocol for predicting hypersensitivity to carboplatin chemotherapy. *J. Clin. Oncol.* 19, 3126–3129. doi: 10.1200/JCO.2001.19.12.3126

Conflict of Interest Statement: The authors declare that the research was conducted in the absence of any commercial or financial relationships that could be construed as a potential conflict of interest.

2

Current Diagnosis and Management of Immune Related Adverse Events (irAEs) Induced by Immune Checkpoint Inhibitor Therapy

Vivek Kumar[1], *Neha Chaudhary*[2], *Mohit Garg*[1], *Charalampos S. Floudas*[1], *Parita Soni*[1] *and Abhinav B. Chandra*[3*]

[1] *Department of Medicine, Maimonides Medical Center, Brooklyn, NY, USA,* [2] *Department of Pediatrics, Maimonides Medical Center, Brooklyn, NY, USA,* [3] *Medical Director, Yuma Regional Cancer Center, Yuma, AZ, USA*

Edited by:
Raquel Abalo,
King Juan Carlos University, Spain

Reviewed by:
James M. Rae,
University of Michigan Health System, USA
Robert A. Rollins,
Pfizer Inc., USA

***Correspondence:**
Abhinav B. Chandra
abhinavbck@hotmail.com

The indications of immune checkpoint inhibitors (ICIs) are set to rise further with the approval of newer agent like atezolimumab for use in patients with advanced stage urothelial carcinoma. More frequent use of ICIs has improved our understanding of their unique side effects, which are known as immune-related adverse events (irAEs). The spectrum of irAEs has expanded beyond more common manifestations such as dermatological, gastrointestinal and endocrine effects to rarer presentations involving nervous, hematopoietic and urinary systems. There are new safety data accumulating on ICIs in patients with previously diagnosed autoimmune conditions. It is challenging for clinicians to continuously update their working knowledge to diagnose and manage these events successfully. If diagnosed timely, the majority of events are completely reversible, and temporary immunosuppression with glucocorticoids, infliximab or other agents is warranted only in the most severe grade illnesses. The same principles of management will possibly apply as newer anti- cytotoxic T lymphocytes-associated antigen 4 (CTLA-4) and programmed cell death protein 1 (PD-1/PD-L1) antibodies are introduced. The current focus of research is for prophylaxis and for biomarkers to predict the onset of these toxicities. In this review we summarize the irAEs of ICIs and emphasize their growing spectrum and their management algorithms, to update oncology practitioners.

Keywords: immune related adverse events, checkpoint blockade, irAEs, nivolumab, pembrolizumab, ipilimumab

INTRODUCTION

Recent advances in cancer immunotherapy are notable for the introduction of a novel class of drugs known as immune checkpoint inhibitors (ICIs). These agents inhibit negative regulatory components of the immune response, such as the cytotoxic T lymphocytes-associated antigen 4 (CTLA-4) and the programmed cell death protein-1 and its ligand (PD-1/PD-L1), which lead to enhanced T cell action against the cancer cells (Hodi et al., 2010). Ipilimumab is an anti- CTLA-4 antibody and was the first agent to receive food and drug administration (FDA) approval for use against advanced-stage melanoma[1]. Since then anti- CTLA-4 antibody tremelimumab, anti-PD-1 antibodies pembrolizumab and nivolumab and PD-L1 antibodies, atezolizumab and durvalumab, have shown beneficial effects in several cancers (Wolchok et al., 2010; Topalian et al., 2012, 2014; Ribas et al., 2013b; Larkin et al., 2015; Robert et al., 2015a; Postow et al., 2015; Fehrenbacher et al., 2016; Ferris et al., 2016; Massard et al., 2016; Reck et al., 2016; Rittmeyer et al., 2017) (**Table 1**). In contrast to conventional chemotherapy, boosting the immune system leads to a unique constellation of inflammatory toxicities known as immune-related adverse events (irAEs) that may warrant the discontinuation of therapy and/or the administration of immunosuppressive agents (Gangadhar and Vonderheide, 2014; Cousin and Italiano, 2016). The use of these agents is set to increase due to their dramatic impact on survival in a variety of advanced-stage cancers (Horvat et al., 2015). Thus, it is imperative for personnel involved in the care of oncology patients to be well versed with the heterogeneous presentations of irAEs in terms of recognition and management. Here, we review the current literature on appropriate steps in patient evaluation for the prompt diagnosis of irAEs and describe strategies for optimizing patient outcome with suitable treatment.

Incidence

The incidence of any grade irAEs is reported to range from 15 to 90% (Hodi et al., 2010; Eggermont et al., 2016; Ferris et al., 2016) in single agent trials. The rate of severe irAEs requiring immunosuppression and withdrawal of immunotherapy is estimated to be 0.5–13% (Hodi et al., 2010; Wolchok et al., 2010; Topalian et al., 2012, 2014; Ribas et al., 2013b; Larkin et al., 2015; Postow et al., 2015; Robert et al., 2015a; Ferris et al., 2016; Table S1)[1]. The high incidence reported in a recent study was attributed to subjectivity in toxicity evaluations among investigators and the accumulation of experience leading to early diagnosis (Horvat et al., 2015). The risk of severe grade adverse events increased from 7 to 25% with an increase in the dose of ipilimumab from 3 mg/kg to 10 mg/kg[9]. This was mostly due to increase in the episodes of diarrhea. However, this pattern was not observed when nivolumab dosing was increased from 0.3 mg/kg to 10 mg/kg[10]. Severe grade toxicities with pembrolizumab were also similar at doses of 10 mg/kg every 2 or 3 weeks and its FDA-approved dosage of 2 mg/kg every 3 weeks (Herbst et al., 2016). Thus, it may be argued that toxicities due to anti-CTLA-4 antibodies are dose dependent whereas toxicities with anti-PD-1/anti-PDL-1 antibodies are independent of doses. Ipilimumab, a CTLA-4 inhibitor is associated with higher rates of gastrointestinal (GI) toxicities, pruritus, rash, and hypophysitis whereas use of PD-1/PD-L1 antagonists is associated with higher risk of vitiligo, dysthyroidism, hepatotoxicity, and pneumonitis (Hamid et al., 2013; Weber J. S. et al., 2013; Brahmer et al., 2015; Eggermont et al., 2015, 2016; Herbst et al., 2016; **Table 1** and Table S1). The data on toxicities from newer agents continue to accumulate. The irAEs in select clinical trials have been summarized in Table S1.

[1]*Drugs@FDA: FDA Approved Drug Products*. Available online at www.Accessdata.fda.gov/scripts/cder/drugsatfda/index.cf.

Timing

The majority of toxicities appear temporally, with skin manifestations the earliest to appear at 2–3 weeks after the 1st dose of ipilimumab. Immune-mediated colitis and hepatitis appear approximately 5–10 and 12–16 weeks after the 2nd and 3rd dose, respectively. Endocrine dysfunctions present from the 9th week onwards following the 4th dose (Hodi et al., 2010; Ryder et al., 2014). Immune-mediated pneumonitis is seen 8–14 weeks after treatment initiation (Hodi et al., 2010). Immune-mediated nephritis appears much later, after 14–42 weeks on immunotherapy (Izzedine et al., 2014). However, similar temporal association of the appearance of irAEs has not been described for PD-1/PDL-1 antagonists (Naidoo et al., 2015).

General Principles of Management

Current guidelines are formulated by manufacturers in collaboration with the FDA and are based on the experience from clinical trials examining the efficacy of ICIs and expert consensus. The guidelines are incorporated in the packaging inserts of these agents[2,3,4,5]. Although anti-PD-1/ anti-PDL-1 antibodies may be less toxic than anti-CTLA-4 antibodies, the approach to managing irAEs due to these agents is similar, with slight variations (Postow and Wolchok, 2016). The severity of adverse events is graded using Common Terminology Criteria for Adverse Events (CTCAE) on a scale from 1 to 5 (1 = mild, 2 = moderate, 3 = severe, 4 = life threatening, and 5 = death related to toxicity) (National Cancer Institute, 2009). However, the grading of irAEs may be challenging, due to arbitrary distinctions between grade 2 and 3 toxicities, such as the number of stools in a day, may be affected by recall bias. Thus, this system of grading may not be entirely suitable to grade ICIs toxicities (Horvat et al., 2015). Therefore, it is prudent to use clinical judgment rather than strictly adhering to the guidelines. We have outlined several general principles that should be followed irrespective of affected organs[2,3,4,5].

- The ICIs are interrupted in moderate (grade 2) irAEs and are resumed when symptoms and/or lab values decrease below grade 1. Glucocorticoids (prednisone 0.5–1 mg/kg/day or equivalent) should be started if symptoms persist beyond 1 week.
- For grade 3/4 toxicities, high doses of glucocorticoids (prednisone 1–2 mg/kg/day or equivalent) should be given. The glucocorticoids should be tapered gradually when symptoms subside to grade 1 or less. The eligible patients (those on prednisone 20 mg or equivalent doses for at least 4 weeks) should also receive appropriate prophylaxis against *Pneumocystis jirovecii* as per the established guidelines[6].

[2]http://www.accessdata.fda.gov/drugsatfda_docs/label/2016/761034s000lbl.pdf
[3]Yervoy® [package insert]. Princeton, NJ: Bristol-Myers Squibb Company, 2016. Available online: http://dailymed.nlm.nih.gov/dailymed/drugInfo.cfm?setid=2265ef30-253e-11df-8a39-0800200c9a66
[4]Keytruda® [package insert]. Whitehouse Station, NJ: Merck, and Co., Inc., 2016. Available online: http://dailymed.nlm.nih.gov/dailymed/drugInfo.cfm?setid=9333c79b-d487-4538-a9f0-71b91a02b287
[5]Opdivo® [package insert]. Princeton, NJ: Bristol-Myers Squibb Company, 2016. Available online: http://dailymed.nlm.nih.gov/dailymed/drugInfo.cfm?setid=f570b9c4-6846-4de2-abfa-4d0a4ae4e394
[6]http://www.nccn.org/professionals/physician_gls/pdf/infections.pdf.

TABLE 1 | Mechanism of action of immune checkpoint inhibitors and immune-Related Adverse Events[#].

	Ipilimumab (Hodi et al., 2010; Wolchok et al., 2010; Ibrahim et al., 2011; Eggermont et al., 2015, 2016; Horvat et al., 2015; Larkin et al., 2015; Postow et al., 2015; Robert et al., 2015b)		**Tremelimumab**[@] (Tarhini et al., 2012; Ribas et al., 2013b; Calabro et al., 2015; Kindler et al., 2016)		**Nivolumab** (Topalian et al., 2012, 2014; Weber J. S. et al., 2013; Borghaei et al., 2015; Brahmer et al., 2015; Larkin et al., 2015; Rizvi et al., 2015; Robert et al., 2015a; Ferris et al., 2016)		**Pidilizumab**[&] (Berger et al., 2008; Armand et al., 2013; Westin et al., 2014)		**Pembrolizumab** (Hamid et al., 2013; Garon et al., 2015; Robert et al., 2015b; Herbst et al., 2016; Nanda et al., 2016; Reck et al., 2016; Seiwert et al., 2016)		**Atezolizumab**[^] (Fehrenbacher et al., 2016; Rosenberg et al., 2016; Rittmeyer et al., 2017)		**Durvalumab**[~] (Massard et al., 2016)	
Mechanism of action	CTLA-4 inhibitor		CTLA-4 inhibitor		PD-1 inhibitor		PD-1 inhibitor		PD-L1 inhibitor		PD-L1 inhibitor		PD-L1 inhibitor	
Therapeutic Status	FDA approved to reduce the risk of melanoma recurrence after surgery (2015), and late stage melanoma (2011).		Tremelimumab was granted orphan drug status in 2015 for the treatment of malignant mesothelioma but is not FDA approved yet.		FDA approved in Hodgkin's lymphoma (2016), Head and neck cancer (2016), advanced lung cancer (2015), metastatic renal cell carcinoma (2015), advanced melanoma (2014).		Under trial		FDA approved in recurrent or metastatic head and neck cancer (2016), first-line treatment for metastatic non-small cell lung cancer in selected patients (2016), metastatic non-small cell lung cancer (2015), advanced melanoma (2014).		FDA approved in metastatic non-small cell lung cancer (2016) and urothelial carcinoma (2016).		Under trial	
Adverse Events	All	=III	All	= III	All	=III	All	=III	All	=III	All	=III	All	=III
Grades (%)	55–65	10–18	~14	~5	30–45	3–7	None[$]		40–45	7–12	16–21	~ 5	~23	4–5
SKIN														
Pruritus	25–30*	<1	30–32	1	17	<1			11–21	1	12–14	<1	3–4	0
Rash	33–34*	2–3	32–34	2	15	<1	None		10–21	2	15	<1	NR	NR
Vitiligo	3–4	0	NR	NR	10–11	<1			9*	<1	NR	NR	NR	NR
GASTROINTESTINAL														
Diarrhea	36–38*	6–7	}30–40	5–10	8–16	<1	None		8–20	1	18–20	1–2	9–10	0
Colitis	8–10*	5–6			1–3	1			1–2	1–2	<1	<1	0	0
HEPATIC														
Increased ALT	<1	<1	NR	NR	1–2	<1			2–8*	<1	2–3	0		
Increased AST	1–2	<1	NR	NR	1–2	<1	None		3–10*	1	2–3	0	None	
Hepatitis	<1	<1	1	1	1–2	1			1–2*	<1	1–2	1		
ENDOCRINE														
Hypothyroidism	1–2	<1	}5	1	4–5	<1			8–10*	<1	2–4	<1		
Hyperthyroidism	0–2	<1			0–3	<1	None		3–4*	<1	1	<1	NR	
Hypophysitis	2–3*	2–3	2	1	<1	<1			<1	<1	<1	<1		
Pneumonitis	<1	<1		None	1–5	0–2	None		4–6*	1–2	2.6	<1	0	0

(Continued)

TABLE 1 | Continued

	Ipilimumab (Hodi et al., 2010; Wolchok et al., 2010; Ibrahim et al., 2011; Eggermont et al., 2015, 2016; Horvat et al., 2015; Larkin et al., 2015; Postow et al., 2015; Robert et al., 2015b)		Tremelimumab[@] (Tarhini et al., 2012; Ribas et al., 2013b; Calabro et al., 2015; Kindler et al., 2016)	Nivolumab (Topalian et al., 2012, 2014; Weber J. S. et al., 2013; Borghaei et al., 2015; Brahmer et al., 2015; Larkin et al., 2015; Rizvi et al., 2015; Robert et al., 2015a; Ferris et al., 2016)		Pidilizumab[&] (Berger et al., 2008; Armand et al., 2013; Westin et al., 2014)	Pembrolizumab (Hamid et al., 2013; Garon et al., 2015; Robert et al., 2015b; Herbst et al., 2016; Nanda et al., 2016; Reck et al., 2016; Seiwert et al., 2016)		Atezolizumab[^] (Fehrenbacher et al., 2016; Rosenberg et al., 2016; Rittmeyer et al., 2017)	Durvalumab[~] (Massard et al., 2016)	
Renal Failure	1	<1	None	1–3*	0–2	None	<1	<1	None	1–2	1
Neurological	<1	<1	None	<1	<1	None	<1	<1	None		NR

CTLA-4, cytotoxic T-lymphocyte antigen 4; PD-1, programmed death; PD-L1, programmed death ligand-1; ALT, alanine aminotransferase; AST, aspartate aminotransferase; NR, not reported. Year of FDA approval is written in the bracket.

**Current data suggest that these toxicities are more commonly associated with this particular agent. [$]Event did not occur. [#]Adverse events were included only if they were reported as immune related or adverse events of special interest (AESI). Head to head trials to compare toxicities among different agents have not been conducted yet. [@]Formerly ticilimumab, CP-675, 206.[&]Formerly MDV9300. Has been tested in diffuse large B-cell lymphoma and multiple myeloma. Immune related adverse events did not occur in either study. [^]Formerly MPDL 3280A. [~]Formerly medi4736. Majority of trials on immunotherapy have tested three agents, ipilimumab, nivolumab and pembrolizumab. Data on the toxicities of newer check point inhibitors are still accumulating.*

- ➢ Alternative immunosuppressive agents should be considered (infliximab 5 mg/kg; mycophenolate mofetil in hepatitis) if symptoms continue beyond 3 days on intravenous glucocorticoids. Infliximab 5 mg/kg should be repeated after 2 weeks for persistent symptoms.
- ➢ For grade 4 toxicities, ICIs should be stopped permanently except in endocrinopathies controlled on hormone replacement. Therapy can be resumed in selected patients with grade 3 toxicities, as discussed in the organ-specific toxicities section.

ICIs should also be stopped permanently in the following circumstances[2,3,4,5]:

- ➢ Grade 2 reactions lasting for 6 weeks or longer. However, anti- PD-1/anti-PD-L1 antibodies can be continued in endocrinopathies controlled with hormone replacement.
- ➢ Inability to reduce glucocorticoids dose to 7.5 mg prednisone or equivalent per day for patients treated with anti-CTLA-4 antibodies and less than 10 mg /day within 12 weeks for anti-PD-1 antibodies.
- ➢ Grade 2–4 ocular reactions not improving to grade 1 within 2 weeks after treatment with topical immunosuppression or requiring systemic treatment.

Impact of irAEs and Immunosuppression on Efficacy

The immunosuppressive agents used to treat irAEs do not appear to affect the response to further immunotherapy (Attia et al., 2005). In contrast to previous studies, a recent retrospective analysis reported similar overall survival in patients who received immunosuppression (Horvat et al., 2015). The association between irAEs and the efficacy of ICIs is also controversial (Attia et al., 2005).

Biomarkers

Biomarkers which could predict the development of toxicities have been described in the patients on ipilimumab. An increase from baseline in eosinophils and interleukin 17 (IL-17) after treatment has been shown to be associated with irAEs (Callahan et al., 2011; Schindler et al., 2014). On gene profiling, two markers of neutrophil activation, CD177 and CEACAM1 also show promise as biomarkers of ICIs toxicity. These genes are expressed increasingly in the blood of patients, who developed GI toxicity after treatment with anti-CTLA-4 antibodies (Shahabi et al., 2013). Higher risk of GI toxicity was also seen in patients who exhibited evidence of inflammation on colon biopsies like infiltration of lamina propria by neutrophils and presence of cryptic abscesses, erosions and gland destruction prior to the initiation of treatment (Berman et al., 2010). However, routine testing of these biomarkers is not recommended yet.

Organ-Specific Immune Related Adverse Events

Systemic Adverse Events

Fatigue is the most common symptom reported by up to 40% of patients after treatment with anti-CTLA-4 antibodies (Weber,

2009; Hodi et al., 2010; Ibrahim et al., 2011; Tarhini et al., 2012; Calabro et al., 2015; Larkin et al., 2015; Kindler et al., 2016) and 16–24% of patients treated with anti-PD-1/anti-PD-L1 antibodies in single-agent trials (Borghaei et al., 2015; Garon et al., 2015; Rizvi et al., 2015; Robert et al., 2015a,b; Nanda et al., 2016; Reck et al., 2016; Rosenberg et al., 2016; Seiwert et al., 2016). This fatigue is usually mild, and the presence of severe fatigue should trigger an assessment for underlying disorders such as endocrinopathies[2,3,4,5]. Infusion reactions, including fever and chills, are more common with CTLA-4 inhibitors accounting for AEs in phase III studies (Momtaz et al., 2015). They are rarely high grade and may be managed supportively with antipyretics and antihistamines (Villadolid and Amin, 2015).

Dermatological

Skin manifestations, such as rash/pruritus and mucositis, are the most common irAEs associated with ICIs. Approximately 47–68% of patients treated with anti-CTLA-4 antibodies and 30–40% patients treated with anti-PD-1/anti-PD-L1 antibodies suffer skin toxicities of any grade (Weber, 2009; Hodi et al., 2010; Wolchok et al., 2010; Ibrahim et al., 2011; Tarhini et al., 2012; Topalian et al., 2012; Ribas et al., 2013b; Topalian et al., 2014; Postow et al., 2015; Borghaei et al., 2015; Calabro et al., 2015; Garon et al., 2015; Larkin et al., 2015; Rizvi et al., 2015; Robert et al., 2015a,b; Ferris et al., 2016; Kindler et al., 2016; Nanda et al., 2016; Rosenberg et al., 2016; Seiwert et al., 2016)[1]. The characteristic rash is faintly erythematous and maculopapular, involves the trunk and extremities and may be pruritic (Jaber et al., 2006). Vitiligo is also common and has delayed appearance after several months of treatment with ICIs (Weber, 2012). Histological analysis shows perivascular lymphocytic infiltration deep in the dermis with CD4+ and CD8+ T cells in close proximity with melanocytes (Jaber et al., 2006). The treatment of symptomatic cases with topical glucocorticoids (betamethasone 0.1% cream) or urea-containing creams and oral antipruritic agents (diphenhydramine, hydroxyzine, GABA agonists, or NK-1 receptor antagonists) for troublesome pruritus is usually sufficient (Weber, 2012; Horvat et al., 2015). The majority of skin eruptions are mild, and immunotherapy can be continued in most patients (Weber, 2012). Severe (Grade 3 defined as papules and/or rash covering >30% BSA) cases should be treated with oral glucocorticoids for 3–4 weeks, with temporary discontinuation of ICIs (**Table 2**). Permanent discontinuation should be considered in more severe cases, such as Stevens–Johnson syndrome, but fortunately severe irAEs are rare. Patients who fail to respond to steroids or have bullae formation merit dermatologic evaluation and skin biopsy. Oral mucositis and dryness are seen more frequently with anti-PD-1/anti-PD-L1 antibodies than with anti-CTLA-4 antibodies (Weber, 2009; Ibrahim et al., 2011; Tarhini et al., 2012; Borghaei et al., 2015; Calabro et al., 2015; Garon et al., 2015; Rizvi et al., 2015; Robert et al., 2015b; Kindler et al., 2016; Nanda et al., 2016; Rosenberg et al., 2016; Seiwert et al., 2016). Topical glucocorticoids and lidocaine are used for treatment. These lesions may mimic oral candidiasis, which should be ruled out[2,3,4,5].

Gastrointestinal

Diarrhea and colitis are more common with anti-CTLA-4 antibodies and are reported in 30–40% of patients treated with ipilimumab (Hodi et al., 2010). Grade 3/4 diarrhea is seen in up to 10% of patients on ipilimumab therapy and 1–2% of cases treated with anti-PD-1/anti-PD-L1 antibodies alone (Weber, 2009; Ibrahim et al., 2011; Tarhini et al., 2012; Borghaei et al., 2015; Calabro et al., 2015; Garon et al., 2015; Rizvi et al., 2015; Robert et al., 2015b; Kindler et al., 2016; Nanda et al., 2016; Rosenberg et al., 2016; Seiwert et al., 2016). Enteritis without colonic involvement leading to small bowel obstruction can also be seen. Colitis predominantly affects the descending colon (Oble et al., 2008). Patients with significant diarrhea/colitis during ipilimumab treatment have subsequently been treated with anti-PD-1/anti-PD-L1 antibodies without developing diarrhea/colitis (Naidoo et al., 2015).

Grade 1 gastrointestinal events are classified as increase in stool frequency of less than 4 per day or mildly increased ostomy output from baseline (**Table 2**). Mild cases should be managed symptomatically with loperamide, oral hydration and electrolyte replacement (Weber et al., 2015). Other etiologies such as infection with *Clostridium difficile* or other viral/bacterial pathogens should be excluded (Du-Thanh et al., 2015). The American Dietary Association colitis diet may also be beneficial[2,3,4,5]. Treatment with glucocorticoids is indicated for worsening of symptoms or persistence beyond 3 days. Grade 2 severity events are 4–6 stools per day over baseline or a moderate increase in ostomy output. These events are managed by oral diphenoxylate, atropine or budesonide, in addition to symptomatic treatment. It is important to rule out colitis by performing a colonoscopy in persistent grade 2 or grade 1 diarrhea with hematochezia. Grade 2 diarrhea with bleeding/ulceration should be treated with oral glucocorticoids and interruption of immunotherapy. Grade 3 events include diarrhea with 7 or more stools per day above the baseline, incontinence or severe increase in ostomy limiting self-care activities. Grade 4 is any life-threatening complication, such as bowel perforation, requiring acute intervention. Grade 3 and 4 events should be treated with intravenous glucocorticoids in addition to symptomatic treatment[2,3,4,5].

The symptomatic improvement should be noted in 48–72 h. Hospitalization is warranted for parenteral glucocorticoids with fluid and electrolyte management in cases refractory to oral glucocorticoids (Weber, 2012; Weber et al., 2015). If the symptoms fail to resolve after 3 days on intravenous glucocorticoids (methylprednisolone 2 mg/kg or equivalent), then infliximab should be given at a dose of 5 mg/kg every 2 weeks[2,3,4,5]. The use of infliximab for this indication is based on its efficacy in Crohn's disease (Minor et al., 2009). However, the recommendations are not clear for non-resolving symptoms on infliximab therapy, and prolonged courses of glucocorticoids are preferred. These patients should be cautiously observed for GI complications, including perforation and obstruction. The prompt intervention is mandatory because colitis related mortality has been attributed to delayed reporting and lack of ICI withholding (Naidoo et al., 2015). The efficacy of matrix

TABLE 2 | Summary of management of selected immune related adverse events (irAEs).

S.N.	Organ system	Manifestations	Management
1.	**Dermatological** ❖ Most common manifestation and earliest to occur. ❖ Seen in 2–3 weeks after initiation of treatment with ipilimumab. ❖ Commonly seen after the first dose. ❖ Manifests as maculopapular rash, erythema, pruritus, dry skin, alopecia or hypertrichosis, lichenoid keratosis and vitiligo. More common with CTLA-4 inhibitors. Seen in up to 47–68% patient on anti-CTLA-4 therapy and 30–40% patients on anti-PD-1/anti-PD-L1 therapy. Mucositis and vitiligo are more common in patients receiving anti-PD-1/anti-PD-L1 agents	**Immune mediated dermatitis** **Grade* 1:** Rash affecting <10% BSA. Mostly Asymptomatic	❖ **Diagnosis:** Mucocutaneous examination. ❖ **Treatment: Continue immunotherapy** Symptomatic treatment with oral antihistaminic drugs. Topical steroids.
		Grade 2: Rash affecting 10–30% BSA.	❖ **Diagnosis:** clinical examination and lab testing for LFTs, KFTs, serum tryptase and IgE levels ❖ **Treatment: Withhold immunotherapy****. Resume after toxicity improves to grade 1 or lower[@]. Symptomatic treatment with oral antihistaminic drugs. Oral Prednisone 0.5–1 mg/kg/day or equivalent taper over 4 weeks if symptoms resolve.
		Grade 3/4: Rash covering >30% BSA. Severe life threatening symptoms Generalized exfoliative/ulcerated rash	❖ **Diagnosis:** As in grade 2 plus skin biopsy ❖ **Treatment: Withhold immunotherapy**. Consult Dermatologist. Resume after toxicity improves to grade 1 or lower. Symptomatic treatment with oral antihistaminic drugs. Oral Prednisone[#] 1–2 mg/kg/day or equivalent taper over 4 weeks if symptoms resolve. Consider alternative immunosuppressive agent (Cyclophosphamide, Mycophenolate mofetil, or Infliximab) if symptoms don't improve after 48 h.
2.	**Gastrointestinal** ❖ Seen 5–10 weeks later typically after 2nd dose of ipilimumab. ❖ Manifests as increase in stool frequency, diarrhea or constipation, blood or mucus in stool, abdominal pain/cramping, nausea and vomiting. ❖ More common with anti-CTLA-4 therapy (30–40%). Grade 3 and 4 toxicities 1n 10% patients against 1–2% on anti-PD-1/anti-PD-L1 therapy	**Immune mediated colitis** **Grade 1:** =4 stools/day over baseline. Mild abdominal symptoms	❖ **Diagnosis:** stool microscopic examination for ova, parasites and stool culture. Stool antigen for *c. difficile* if suspected clinically. Lab testing for LFTs and KFTs. ❖ **Treatment: Continue immunotherapy**. Symptomatic treatment and monitor for fluid electrolytes balance. American diet Association (ADA) colitis diet, loperamide or atropine sulfate. Budesonide can be tried if symptoms persist beyond 2–3 days.
		Grade 2: Moderate new symptoms. 4–6 stools/day over baseline.	❖ **Diagnosis:** As above in grade 1. Evaluate for other causes like progression of primary disease. Colonoscopy may be beneficial in selected cases. ❖ **Treatment: withhold immunotherapy**. If symptoms improve to grade I resume immunotherapy. Symptomatic treatment. If symptoms are persistent beyond 5–7 days start oral prednisone 1 mg/kg/day or equivalent. Taper over 4 weeks if symptoms improve. Start Infliximab 5 mg/kg every 2 weeks if symptoms don't improve after 3 days on steroid treatment.
		Grade 3/4: Severe grade. =7 stools/day over baseline. Severe and persistent abdominal pain, fever, ileus. Life threatening complications like intestinal perforation and peritonitis	❖ **Diagnosis:** Rule out infectious and other causes as above. GI consult and endoscopy in selected cases ❖ **Treatment: Discontinue immunotherapy** I.V. Methyl prednisone 2–4 mg/kg/day or equivalent taper over 4 weeks if symptoms resolve. Consider alternative immunosuppressive agent (Cyclophosphamide or mycophenolate mofetil) if symptoms don't improve after 48 h. Monitor for intestinal perforation.

(Continued)

TABLE 2 | Continued

S.N.	Organ system	Manifestations	Management
3.	**Hepatic** ❖ Appears 12–16 weeks after initiation of treatment with ipilimumab. ❖ Typically seen after the 3rd dose of checkpoint inhibitor treatment. ❖ Mostly asymptomatic elevation of liver enzyme. Fever, fatigue and jaundice may be seen in some patients. ❖ Manifests in <10% patients on anti-CTLA-4 therapy but in ~20% patients on combination (anti-CTLA-4 plus anti-PD-1/anti-PD-L1) therapy.	**Immune mediated hepatitis** **Grade 1:** Asymptomatic/mildly symptomatic AST/ALT of 2.5 × ULN Total Bilirubin of 1.5 × ULN	❖ **Diagnosis:** LFTs. ❖ **Treatment: Continue immunotherapy** if asymptomatic. Monitor LFTs until resolution
		Grade 2: Symptomatic. AST/ALT of 2.5–5 × ULN Total Bilirubin of 1.5–3 × ULN	❖ **Diagnosis:** Rule out viral, drug induced or autoimmune causes. Monitor LFTs daily till resolution followed by weekly testing. ❖ **Treatment: Withhold immunotherapy**. Resume after toxicity improves to grade 1 or lower. Oral Prednisone 1 mg/kg/day or equivalent taper over 4 weeks if symptoms resolve. Consider alternative immunosuppressive agent (tacrolimus, cyclophosphamide or mycophenolate mofetil) if symptoms don't improve after 48 h. Infliximab is contraindicated due to potential hepatotoxicity.
		Grade 3/4: Symptoms as above. AST/ALT of 5 × ULN Total Bilirubin of 3 × ULN	❖ **Diagnosis:** As in grade 2 plus imaging to rule out malignant etiology. Monitor LFTs daily till resolution. ❖ **Treatment: Discontinue immunotherapy** I.V. Methyl prednisone 2–4 mg/kg/day or equivalent taper over 4 weeks if symptoms resolve. If no improvement after 5–7 days, add tacrolimus 0.10–0.15 mg/kg/day (trough level 5–20 ng/mL). Consider alternative agents (cyclophosphamide or mycophenolate mofetil), if no response despite therapeutic levels. Infliximab is contraindicated.
4.	**Pulmonary** ❖ Seen after 8–14 weeks of 1st dose of ipilimumab. ❖ Asymptomatic appearance of infiltrates on lung imaging is more common. ❖ Symptomatic pneumonitis is seen in =1%. More common with anti-PD-1/anti-PD-L1 than anti-CTLA-4 therapy	**Immune mediated pneumonitis** **Grade 1:** Asymptomatic, only radiological changes.	❖ **Diagnosis:** Radiological imaging using High resolution computed tomography (HRCT chest). Repeat CT before every cycle ❖ **Treatment: Withhold immunotherapy for 2–4 weeks**. Monitor for symptoms every 3 days. If new symptoms develop, treat as higher grade.
		Grade 2: Mild/Moderate new symptoms limiting instrumental activities of daily living.	❖ **Diagnosis:** As above plus microbiological assessment like sputum examination and cultures. ❖ **Treatment: withhold immunotherapy**. If symptoms improve to grade 1 within 72 h resume immunotherapy otherwise **discontinue immunotherapy**. **Also Discontinue therapy in recurrent grade 2 pneumonitis.** Monitor for symptoms daily. Oral prednisone 1 mg/kg/day or equivalent. Taper over 4 weeks if symptoms improve.
		Grade 3/4: Severe symptoms limiting self-care activities of daily living. Hypoxia or Respiratory failure requiring urgent interventions like endotracheal intubation or tracheostomy.	❖ **Diagnosis:** Rule out infectious and other pulmonary causes. Pulmonary consult and bronchoscopy ❖ **Treatment: Discontinue immunotherapy** I.V. Methyl prednisone 2–4 mg/kg/day or equivalent taper over 4 weeks if symptoms resolve. Consider prophylactic antibiotics. Consider alternative immunosuppressive agent (Cyclophosphamide or Infliximab) if symptoms don't improve after 48 h.

(Continued)

TABLE 2 | Continued

S.N.	Organ system	Manifestations	Management
5.	**Endocrine** ❖ Generally seen 9 weeks after initiation of ipilimumab treatment. ❖ **Immune related thyroiditis** Hypothyroidism/Hyperthyroidism: Fatigue, weakness, asthenia, new onset atrial fibrillation, constipation/diarrhea, cold/heat intolerance, dry skin/excessive diaphoresis, weight gain/weight loss. ❖ **Immune-mediated adrenalitis:** Asthenia, failure to thrive, anorexia, nausea, vomiting, fever, coma, hypotension, hypoglycemia, eosinophilia. ❖ **Immune -mediated hypophysitis:** Headache, visual field defects, blurring of vision, impotence, amenorrhea	**Immune-mediated endocrinopathies** **Grade 1:** Asymptomatic or mild symptoms; clinical or diagnostic observations only; intervention not indicated	❖ **Diagnosis:** Complete blood count, comprehensive metabolic profile. Consult endocrine **Thyroiditis:** TSH. If TSH is below 0.5 × ULN or above 2 × ULN or consistently out of normal range in subsequent cycles consider adding free T3 and T4. **Adrenalitis:** ACTH, Morning serum cortisol-if abnormal Cosyntropin stimulation test. **Hypophysitis:** LH/FSH/Testosterone, Prolactin. MRI brain with pituitary cuts and visual field testing if indicated. ❖ **Treatment: Continue immunotherapy.** Monitor for symptoms. If worsens treat as higher grades. Treat for hyper or hypothyroidism if indicated
	Hypothyroidism is more common with anti-CTLA-4 while hypophysitis and hyperthyroidism is seen more commonly with anti-PD-1/anti-PD-L1 therapy	**Grade 2:** Moderate; minimal, local or noninvasive; intervention indicated; limiting age-appropriate instrumental ADL	❖ **Diagnosis:** As above in grade 1. ❖ **Treatment:** **1. Hyper/Hypothyroidism-continue immunotherapy** **2. Adrenalitis: continue immunotherapy.** **3. Hypophysitis[$]: Withhold immunotherapy.** Prednisone 1–2 mg/kg/day or equivalent. Taper over >4 weeks before resuming immunotherapy. Replace deficient hormone. If patient developed hypophysitis on ipilimumab, it can be replaced with pembrolizumab from next cycle.
		Grade 3: Severe or medically significant but not immediately life-threatening; hospitalization or prolongation of existing hospitalization indicated; disabling; limiting ADL and self-care	❖ **Diagnosis:** As above in grade 1. ❖ **Treatment:** **1. Hyper/Hypothyroidism: continue immunotherapy.** Treatment of hypo/hyperthyroidism as per standard guidelines. **2. Adrenal insufficiency: withhold immunotherapy.** Prednisone 1–2 mg/kg/day or equivalent. Taper over >4 weeks before resuming immunotherapy. **3. Hypophysitis: permanently discontinue immunotherapy.** Prednisone 1–2 mg/kg/day or equivalent. Taper over >4 weeks. Few patients may require hormone replacement therapy for life.
		Grade 4: Life-threatening consequences; urgent intervention indicated	❖ **Diagnosis:** As above in grade 1. ❖ **Treatment:** **1. Hyper/Hypothyroidism: continue immunotherapy.** Treatment of hypo/hyperthyroidism as per standard guidelines. **2. Adrenal insufficiency: Permanently discontinue immunotherapy.** Prednisone 1–2 mg/kg/day or equivalent. Taper over >4 weeks before resuming immunotherapy. If in adrenal crisis stabilize the patient prior to endocrine work-up. Rule out sepsis. If in shock, start with stress dose steroids, antibiotics and iv fluids. **3. Hypophysitis: permanently discontinue immunotherapy.** Prednisone 1–2 mg/kg/day or equivalent. Taper over >4 weeks. Few patients may require hormone replacement therapy for life.

(Continued)

TABLE 2 | Continued

S.N.	Organ system	Manifestations	Management
6.	**Renal** ❖ Seen 14–42 weeks after initiation of treatment. ❖ Rare with both anti-CTLA-4 and anti-PD-1/anti-PD-L1 therapy	**Immune mediated Renal dysfunction** **Grade 1:** ↑ creatinine above the baseline but =1.5 ULN	❖ **Diagnosis:** Kidney Function Tests, Urine analysis ❖ **Treatment: Continue immunotherapy.** Symptomatic treatment and monitor for fluid electrolytes balance.
		Grade 2 and 3: creatinine 1.5–6 mg/dl ULN	❖ **Diagnosis:** As in grade 1. Monitor creatinine every 2–3 days. Consider renal biopsy. ❖ **Treatment: Withhold immunotherapy.** Oral Prednisone 0.5–1 mg/kg/day or equivalent, if no response ↑ to 1–2 mg/kg/day and discontinue immunotherapy permanently. If elevation persists =7 days treat as grade 4.
		Grade 4: creatinine > 6 mg/dl ULN	❖ **Diagnosis:** As in grade 1. Monitor creatinine every day. Consider renal biopsy. Consult nephrology **Treatment: Withhold immunotherapy.** Oral Prednisone 1–2 mg/kg/day. Taper at least over 4 weeks.
7.	**Neurologic** Headache, fever, stiffness, memory problem, confusion, drowsiness, hallucinations, seizures, peripheral neuropathy Rare with both anti-CTLA-4 and anti-PD-1/anti-PD-L1 therapy	**Immune-mediated neurological adverse reactions** **Grade 1:** Asymptomatic or mildly symptomatic	❖ **Diagnosis:** Clinical examination ❖ **Treatment: Continue immunotherapy.** Monitor for progression of disease.
		Grade 2: New onset moderate symptoms limiting instrumental activities of daily living.	❖ **Diagnosis:** Monitor for progression of disease. ❖ **Treatment: Withhold immunotherapy.** Consider consulting neurology. Oral prednisone 0.5–1 mg/kg/day or equivalent. If no response treat as grade 3 and 4.
		Grade 3 and 4: New onset severe symptoms affecting self-care activities of daily living. Life threatening.	❖ **Diagnosis:** MRI brain, lumbar puncture, nerve conduction velocity, electromyography, skin, nerve or muscle biopsy as clinically indicated. ❖ **Treatment: Permanently discontinue immunotherapy.** Consult neurology. Prednisone 1–2 mg/kg/day or equivalent. Taper over at least 4 weeks. If worsens or atypical presentation consider other immunosuppressive agents.

ADL, activities of daily living; ALT, alanine aminotransferase; AST, aspartate aminotransferase; BSA, body surface area; CTLA-4, cytotoxic T-lymphocyte antigen-4; FSH, follicular stimulating hormone; KFT, kidney function test; LFT, liver function tests; LH, luteinizing hormone; MRI, magnetic resonance imaging; PD-1, programmed cell death; PD-L1, programmed cell death ligand-1; TSH, thyroid stimulating hormone; ULN, upper limit of normal.

For References see text.

[*]Common Terminating Criteria for Adverse Events Grading.

[#]Patients receiving prednisone =20 mg/day or equivalent doses for at least 4 weeks are candidates for pneumocystis jirovecii prophylaxis as per National Comprehensive Cancer Network NCCN guidelines.

[**]Treatment with checkpoint inhibitors is permanently discontinued in grade 2 toxicity if it persists beyond 6 weeks. However PD-1 inhibitors can be continued with hormone replacement in endocrinopathies.

[@]Nivolumab is permanently discontinued if prednisone can't be tapered to <7.5 mg/day or equivalent without recurrence of symptoms and ipilimumab is discontinued if prednisone can't be tapered below 10 mg/kg/day or equivalent dose.

[$]Prednisone dose in hypophysitis is controversial. New data suggests that physiological dose is as effective as higher doses advocated previously. See text.

budesonide for prophylaxis against colitis has not been proven and is not recommended (Weber et al., 2009).

Hepatic

Hepatotoxicity can be caused by both anti-CTLA-4 and anti-PD-1/anti-PD-L1 antibodies. Hepatotoxicity occurs in 2–9% of patients (Weber, 2009; Ibrahim et al., 2011; Tarhini et al., 2012; Borghaei et al., 2015; Calabro et al., 2015; Garon et al., 2015; Rizvi et al., 2015; Robert et al., 2015b; Kindler et al., 2016; Nanda et al., 2016; Rosenberg et al., 2016; Seiwert et al., 2016). Liver function should be tested at baseline and prior to each cycle of immunotherapy. The patients should also be monitored regularly during the post-treatment period. An asymptomatic elevation of hepatic transaminases and hyperbilirubinemia is common, and concomitant fever can also occur (Weber, 2012). Liver biopsy is reserved for unclear cases and reveals prominent sinusoidal histiocytic infiltrates and central vein damage with endotheliitis suggestive of ipilimumab-associated hepatitis (Johncilla et al., 2015). Grade 2 reactions require interruption of cancer treatment, with daily or alternate-day monitoring of liver enzymes until they decrease, and then subsequent weekly assessments (**Table 2**). Grade 3 or greater irAEs involve AST/ALT levels >5 times upper limit of normal (ULN) or bilirubin >3 times ULN. Severe hepatotoxicity requires high-dose intravenous glucocorticoids for 24–48 h followed by a slow taper for the next 30 days. The glucocorticoids should be switched to mycophenolate 500 mg every 12 h if the liver enzymes are still elevated after 48 h of treatment[2,3,4,5]. The use of infliximab is contraindicated due its potential hepatotoxicity. The differential diagnoses of immunotherapy-induced liver damage include metastasis to the liver, viral hepatitis and other drug toxicity meriting extensive analysis. Hepatitis persisting for longer periods requires prolonged or repeated glucocorticoids tapering (≥4 weeks) and/or additional immunosuppression[2,3,4,5].

Endocrine

Endocrinopathies can occur secondary to inflammation of the pituitary, thyroid and adrenal glands or may be related to development of type-1 diabetes mellitus. Clinical presentation is confounded by nonspecific symptoms such as behavioral changes, nausea, headache, fatigue and visual complaints (Corsello et al., 2013). Hypophysitis and hypothyroidism are the most common endocrinopathies seen in up to 10% of patients treated with anti-CTLA-4 and anti-PD-1/anti-PD-L1 antibodies (Weber, 2009; Hodi et al., 2010; Wolchok et al., 2010; Ibrahim et al., 2011; Topalian et al., 2012, 2014; Tarhini et al., 2012; Ribas et al., 2013b; Borghaei et al., 2015; Calabro et al., 2015; Garon et al., 2015; Larkin et al., 2015; Postow et al., 2015; Rizvi et al., 2015; Robert et al., 2015a,b; Ferris et al., 2016; Kindler et al., 2016; Nanda et al., 2016; Seiwert et al., 2016; Rosenberg et al., 2016)[1].

Hypophysitis with pituitary dysfunction requires testing for thyroid stimulating hormone (TSH), serum cortisol, adrenocorticotropic hormone (ACTH), growth hormone (GH), prolactin, luteinizing hormone (LH), and follicular stimulating hormone (FSH) in women or testosterone levels in men. Diagnosis is based on clinical symptoms with radiographic abnormalities (pituitary enlargement with enhancement) and biochemical test results (low tropic hormones)[2,3,4,5]. The role of high dose glucocorticoids (1 mg/kg prednisone daily) is controversial in cases with suspected hypophysitis. The use of physiological replacement doses has been suggested, and high doses should be reserved for patients with symptoms related to mass effects such as severe headaches or visual disturbances (Albarel et al., 2015). A recent study reported that TSH and FSH normalized after a follow-up period of 33 months. However, ACTH remained low, with persistent pituitary abnormalities on MRI irrespective of glucocorticoid dose (Albarel et al., 2015; Min et al., 2015).

The routine monitoring of thyroid function is indicated before each dose of ipilimumab. Hypothyroidism is more common than hyperthyroidism. It is important to distinguish primary hypothyroidism (low free T4 with high TSH) from secondary disease (low free T4 with low TSH) caused by hypophysitis. The treatment of hypo and hyperthyroidism should be consistent with standard guidelines (**Table 2**)[2,3,4,5]. Immunotherapy can be continued with hormone replacement.

Hypophysitis[2,3,4,5] with clinically significant adrenal insufficiency (hypotension, dehydration, and dyselectrolytemia) is equivalent to adrenal crisis and is a medical emergency that mandates hospitalization, evaluation by an endocrinologist and treatment with methylprednisolone. It is important to distinguish this condition from sepsis, and prompt testing with cultures is mandatory (**Table 2**).

Pulmonary

Grade 3 or higher pneumonitis has been reported in 5–7% of NSCLC patients treated with nivolumab and pembrolizumab (Langer, 2015; Abdel-Rahman and Fouad, 2016). The incidence of symptomatic pneumonitis is only 1% with ipilimumab (Barjaktarevic et al., 2013). The risk increased in patients with prior thoracic radiation. There have been reported granulomatous reactions similar to sarcoidosis (Berthod et al., 2012). The presence of infiltrates on chest radiographs or CT imaging is more common and resolves rapidly after withholding the drug. Pneumonitis should be excluded by CT imaging in any patient with cough, shortness of breath, and fever[2,3,4,5]. A bronchoscopy may reveal diffuse lymphocytic infiltration and should be performed in moderate to severe cases to exclude infections. Severe cases should be treated with glucocorticoids using 2 mg/kg intravenous methyl prednisolone. Immunotherapy should be permanently discontinued in cases with recurrent grade 2–4 irAEs (**Table 2**)[2,3,4,5].

Rare Events

Ocular

Common ocular manifestations include episcleritis, conjunctivitis and uveitis. The incidence of these events is higher with ipilimumab but remains less than 1% (Huillard et al., 2014; Abu Samra et al., 2016). The patient should be referred to an ophthalmologist and treatment with topical glucocorticoids is required in most cases. The use of oral glucocorticoid therapy is reserved for severe events.

Renal

ICIs can cause acute kidney injury that presents similar to other drug-induced tubulointerstitial nephritis. The median duration for the appearance of the kidney injury is 13 weeks (Cortazar et al., 2016). In addition to nephritis, granulomatous lesions and thrombotic microangiopathy can also be seen on renal biopsy. A previous study demonstrated that renal function partially improved after glucocorticoid treatment, and that one-third of patients required dialysis (Cortazar et al., 2016). Grade 2 or higher toxicity is treated with glucocorticoids (**Table 2**). The immunotherapy should be withheld for Grade 2–3 events and permanently discontinued for Grade 4 events or resistant Grade 2–3 irAEs[2,3,4,5].

Pancreatic

Routine monitoring of amylase/lipase in otherwise asymptomatic individuals is not recommended. Asymptomatic elevation does not require treatment. The significance of elevated amylase and lipase in a large number of patients remains unclear (Ribas et al., 2013b; Postow et al., 2015; Herbst et al., 2016).

Neurological

The reported neurologic complications of immunotherapies include posterior reversible encephalopathy syndrome (Maur et al., 2012), Guillain-Barre Syndrome (Wilgenhof and Neyns, 2011), myasthenia gravis (Liao et al., 2014), transverse myelitis (Liao et al., 2014), and neuropathy (de Maleissye et al., 2016). Serious cases should be treated with glucocorticoids and a neurologist should be consulted for additional therapies such as intravenous immunoglobulin and plasmapheresis. (for detailed management see **Table 2**)

Hematological

Autoimmune anemia (Kong et al., 2016), neutropenia (Akhtari et al., 2009), thrombocytopenia (Ahmad et al., 2012), and acquired hemophilia A have been reported (Delyon et al., 2011). Symptom management is similar to other irAEs and involves the use of glucocorticoids and alternative immunosuppression in refractory cases.

Combination Therapy

The distinct mechanisms of action of anti-CTLA-4 and anti-PD-1/anti-PD-L1 antibodies have led to trials examining combination therapies in a variety of malignancies. The incidence of severe adverse events due to the combination of ipilimumab and nivolumab is reported to be 55%, which is significantly higher than either agent individually and leads to discontinuation of treatment in one-third of patients (Larkin et al., 2015). The toxicity profile of ipilimumab varies with the chemotherapy agent used in combination (Weber J. et al., 2013). The combination with dacarbazine is more hepatotoxic (Robert et al., 2011), and carboplatin and taxanes treatment leads to more cutaneous manifestations (Arriola et al., 2016). There are more nephrotoxic and hepatotoxic events observed when combined with vemurafenib (Ribas et al., 2013a). The combination of ipilimumab (dose 10 mg/kg) with granulocyte-macrophage colony-stimulating factor showed fewer gastrointestinal and pulmonary irAEs than ipilimumab alone (45 vs. 58%)(Hodi et al., 2014). However, the efficacy of this combination is not clear at the FDA-approved dose of 3 mg/kg and requires further confirmation.

Autoimmune Conditions

The safety of ICIs in patients with preexisting autoimmune diseases is not clear, and there is a theoretical concern regarding the exacerbation of preexisting conditions. There have been anecdotal reports of patients with anti-muscle antibodies developing rhabdomyolysis with polymyositis (Bilen et al., 2016), and neurotoxicity has been described in patients with anti-neuronal antibodies (Williams et al., 2016). Ipilimumab treatment led to the exacerbation of previously diagnosed autoimmune conditions in 27% of patients within 6 weeks of treatment, and these conditions were easily managed with steroids (Johnson et al., 2015). Clinicians should engage patients in discussions for trial of these agents due to the significant benefit of these antibodies in life-threatening malignancies. The development of new autoimmune syndromes (30% sicca syndromes, 70% inflammatory arthritis and 40% ANA positivity) have also been reported in patients without any prior history of rheumatic conditions (Cappelli et al., 2017).

CONCLUSION

ICIs targeting CTLA-4 and PD-1/PDL-1 have dramatically changed the outcomes of patients with many advanced-stage malignancies. However, their introduction is associated with unique irAEs that are mostly transient and mild but can occasionally be fatal. Rapid identification and appropriate treatment can improve outcomes without compromising the efficacy of these agents. In the absence of prospective data, these patients should be managed as per established guidelines based upon pooled clinical experience. Additional data on toxicities will enable us to utilize the full therapeutic potential of these novel drugs.

AUTHOR CONTRIBUTIONS

VK: original idea, reviewed literature and manuscript writing and editing. AC: mentored, writing and editing of manuscript. NC: reviewed literature and manuscript writing and editing. MG: writing and editing of manuscript. CF: editing and proofreading. PS: editing and proofreading.

REFERENCES

Abdel-Rahman, O., and Fouad, M. (2016). Risk of pneumonitis in cancer patients treated with immune checkpoint inhibitors: a meta-analysis. *Ther. Adv. Respir. Dis.* 10, 183–193. doi: 10.1177/1753465816636557

Abu Samra, K., Valdes-Navarro, M., Lee, S., Swan, R., Foster, C. S., Anesi, S. D., et al. (2016). A case of bilateral uveitis and papillitis in a patient treated with pembrolizumab. *Eur. J. Ophthalmol.* 26, e46–e48. doi: 10.5301/ejo.5000724

Ahmad, S., Lewis, M., Corrie, P., and Iddawela, M. (2012). Ipilimumab-induced thrombocytopenia in a patient with metastatic melanoma. *J. Oncol. Pharm. Pract.* 18, 287–292. doi: 10.1177/1078155211411001

Akhtari, M., Waller, E. K., Jaye, D. L., Lawson, D. H., Ibrahim, R., Papadopoulos, N. E., et al. (2009). Neutropenia in a patient treated with ipilimumab (anti-CTLA-4 Antibody). *J. Immunother.* 32, 322–324. doi: 10.1097/CJI.0b013e31819aa40b

Albarel, F., Gaudy, C., Castinetti, F., Morange, I., Conte-Devolx, B., Grob, J. J., et al. (2015). Long-term follow-up of ipilimumab-induced hypophysitis, a common adverse event of the anti-CTLA-4 antibody in melanoma. *Eur. J. Endocrinol.* 172, 195–204. doi: 10.1530/EJE-14-0845

Armand, P., Nagler, A., Weller, E. A., Devine, S. M., Avigan, D. E., Chen, Y. B., et al. (2013). Disabling immune tolerance by programmed death-1 blockade with pidilizumab after autologous hematopoietic stem-cell transplantation for diffuse large B-cell lymphoma: results of an international phase II trial. *J. Clin. Oncol.* 31, 4199–4206. doi: 10.1200/JCO.2012.48.3685

Arriola, E., Wheater, M., Galea, I., Cross, N., Maishman, T., Hamid, D., et al. (2016). Outcome and biomarker analysis from a multicenter phase 2 study of ipilimumab in combination with carboplatin and etoposide as first-line therapy for extensive-stage SCLC. *J. Thor. Oncol.* 11, 1511–1521. doi: 10.1016/j.jtho.2016.05.028

Attia, P., Phan, G. Q., Maker, A. V., Robinson, M. R., Quezado, M. M., Yang, J. C., et al. (2005). Autoimmunity correlates with tumor regression in patients with metastatic melanoma treated with anti-cytotoxic T-lymphocyte antigen-4. *J. Clin. Oncol.* 23, 6043–6053. doi: 10.1200/JCO.2005.06.205

Barjaktarevic, I. Z., Qadir, N., Suri, A., Santamauro, J. T., and Stover, D. (2013). Organizing pneumonia as a side effect of ipilimumab treatment of melanoma. *Chest* 143, 858–861. doi: 10.1378/chest.12-1467

Berger, R., Rotem-Yehudar, R., Slama, G., Landes, S., Kneller, A., Leiba, M., et al. (2008). Phase I safety and pharmacokinetic study of CT-011, a humanized antibody interacting with PD-1, in patients with advanced hematologic malignancies. *Clin. Cancer Res.* 14, 3044–3051. doi: 10.1158/1078-0432.CCR-07-4079

Berman, D., Parker, S. M., Siegel, J., Chasalow, S. D., Weber, J., Galbraith, S., et al. (2010). Blockade of cytotoxic T-lymphocyte antigen- 4 by ipilimumab results in dysregulation of gastrointestinal immunity in patients with advanced melanoma. *Cancer Immun.* 10, 11.

Berthod, G., Lazor, R., Letovanec, I., Romano, E., Noirez, L., Mazza Stalder, J., et al. (2012). Pulmonary sarcoid-like granulomatosis induced by ipilimumab. *J. Clin. Oncol.* 30, e156–e159. doi: 10.1200/JCO.2011.39.3298

Bilen, M. A., Subudhi, S. K., Gao, J., Tannir, N. M., Tu, S.-M., and Sharma, P. (2016). Acute rhabdomyolysis with severe polymyositis following ipilimumab-nivolumab treatment in a cancer patient with elevated anti-striated muscle antibody. *J. Immunother Cancer* 4, 36. doi: 10.1186/s40425-016-0139-8

Borghaei, H., Paz-Ares, K. L., Horn, L., Spigel, D. R., Steins, M., Ready, N. E., et al. (2015). Nivolumab versus docetaxel in advanced nonsquamous non–small-cell lung cancer. *N. Engl. J. Med.* 373, 1627–1639. doi: 10.1056/NEJMoa1507643

Brahmer, J., Reckamp, K. L., Baas, P., Crin,ò, L., Eberhardt, W. E., Poddubskaya, E., et al. (2015). Nivolumab versus docetaxel in advanced squamous-cell non-small-cell lung cancer. *N. Engl. J. Med.* 373, 123–135. doi: 10.1056/NEJMoa1504627

Calabro, L., Morra, A., Fonsatti, E., Cutaia, O., Fazio, C., Annesi, D., et al. (2015). Efficacy and safety of an intensified schedule of tremelimumab for chemotherapy-resistant malignant mesothelioma: an open-label, single-arm, phase 2 study. *Lancet Respir Med.* 3, 301–309. doi: 10.1016/S2213-2600(15)00092-2

Callahan, M. K., Yang, A., Tandon, S., Xu, Y., Subudhi, S. K., Roman, R. A., et al. (2011). Evaluation of serum IL-17 levels during ipilimumab therapy: correlation with colitis. *J. Clin. Oncol.* 29s:2505.

Cappelli, L. C., Gutierrez, A. K., Baer, A. N., Albayda, J., Manno, R. L., Haque, U., et al. (2017). Inflammatory arthritis and sicca syndrome induced by nivolumab and ipilimumab. *Ann. Rheum. Dis.* 76, 43–50. doi: 10.1136/annrheumdis-2016-209595

Corsello, S. M., Barnabei, A., Marchetti, P., De Vecchis, L., Salvatori, R., and Torino, F. (2013). Endocrine side effects induced by immune checkpoint inhibitors. *J. Clin. Endocrinol. Metab.* 98, 1361–1375. doi: 10.1210/jc.2012-4075

Cortazar, F. B., Marrone, K. A., Troxell, M. L., Ralto, K. M., Hoenig, M. P., Brahmer, J. R., et al. (2016). Clinicopathological features of acute kidney injury associated with immune checkpoint inhibitors. *Kidney Int.* 90, 638–647. doi: 10.1016/j.kint.2016.04.008

Cousin, S., and Italiano, A. (2016). Molecular Pathways: Immune Checkpoint Antibodies and their Toxicities. *Clin. Cancer Res.* 22, 4550–4555. doi: 10.1158/1078-0432.CCR-15-2569

Delyon, J., Mateus, C., and Lambert, T. (2011). Hemophilia A induced by ipilimumab. *N. Engl. J. Med.* 365, 1747–1748. doi: 10.1056/NEJMc1110923

de Maleissye, M.-F., Nicolas, G., and Saiag, P. (2016). Pembrolizumab-Induced Demyelinating Polyradiculoneuropathy. *N. Engl. J. Med.* 375, 296–297. doi: 10.1056/NEJMc1515584

Du-Thanh, A., Pallure, V., Girard, C., Dereure, O., and Guillot, B. (2015). Clostridium difficile infection may loom behind ipilimumab-induced auto-immune colitis. *Eur. J. Dermatol.* 25, 344. doi: 10.1684/ejd.2015.2561

Eggermont, A. M., Chiarion-Sileni, V., Grob, J. J., Dummer, R., Wolchok, J. D., Schmidt, H., et al. (2016). Prolonged survival in stage III Melanoma with Ipilimumab adjuvant therapy. *N. Engl. J. Med.* 375, 1845–1855. doi: 10.1056/NEJMoa1611299

Eggermont, A. M., Chiarion-Sileni, V., Grob, J.-J., Dummer, R., Wolchok, J. D., Schmidt, H., et al. (2015). Adjuvant ipilimumab versus placebo after complete resection of high-risk stage III melanoma (EORTC 18071): a randomised, double-blind, phase 3 trial. *Lancet Oncol.* 16, 522–530. doi: 10.1016/S1470-2045(15)70122-1

Fehrenbacher, L., Spira, A., Ballinger, M., Kowanetz, M., Vansteenkiste, J., Mazieres, J., et al. (2016). Atezolizumab versus docetaxel for patients with previously treated non-small-cell lung cancer (POPLAR): a multicentre, open-label, phase 2 randomised controlled trial. *Lancet* 2016, 387, 1837–1846. doi: 10.1016/S0140-6736(16)00587

Ferris, R. L., Blumenschein, G. Jr., Fayette, J., Guigay, J., Colevas, A. D., Licitra, L., et al. (2016). Nivolumab for recurrent squamous-cell carcinoma of the head and neck. *N. Engl. J. Med.* 375, 1856–1867. doi: 10.1056/NEJMoa1602252

Gangadhar, T. C., and Vonderheide, R. H. (2014). Mitigating the toxic effects of anticancer immunotherapy. *Nat. Rev. Clin. Oncol.* 11, 91–99. doi: 10.1038/nrclinonc.2013.245

Garon, E. B., Rizvi, N. A., Hui, R., Leighl, N., Balmanoukian, A. S., Eder, J. P., et al. (2015). Pembrolizumab for the treatment of non–small-cell lung cancer. *N. Engl. J. Med.* 372, 2018–2028. doi: 10.1056/NEJMoa1501824

Hamid, O., Robert, C., Daud, A., Hodi, F. S., Hwu, W. J., Kefford, R., et al. (2013). Safety and tumor responses with lambrolizumab (anti-PD-1) in melanoma. *N. Engl. J. Med.* 369, 134–144. doi: 10.1056/NEJMoa1305133

Herbst, R. S., Baas, P., Kim, D., Felip, E., Pérez-Gracia, J. L., Han, J. Y., et al. (2016). Pembrolizumab versus docetaxel for previously treated, PD-L1-positive, advanced non-small-cell lung cancer (KEYNOTE-010): a randomised controlled trial. *Lancet* 387, 1540–1550. doi: 10.1016/S0140-6736(15)01281-7

Hodi, F., Lee, S., McDermott, D. F., Rao, U. N., Butterfield, L. H., Tarhini, A. A., et al. (2014). Ipilimumab plus sargramostim vs ipilimumab alone for treatment of metastatic melanoma: a randomized clinical trial. *JAMA* 312, 1744–1753. doi: 10.1001/jama.2014.13943

Hodi, F. S., O'Day, S. J., McDermott, D. F., Weber, R. W., Sosman, J. A., Haanen, J. B., et al. (2010). Improved survival with ipilimumab in patients with metastatic melanoma. *N. Engl. J. Med.* 363, 711–723. doi: 10.1056/NEJMoa1003466

Horvat, T. Z., Adel, N. G., Dang, T. O., Momtaz, P., Postow, M. A., Callahan, M. K., et al. (2015). Immune-related adverse events, need for systemic immunosuppression, and effects on survival and time to treatment failure in patients with melanoma treated with ipilimumab at memorial sloan kettering cancer center. *J. Clin. Oncol.* 33, 3193. doi: 10.1200/jco.2015.60.8448

Huillard, O., Bakalian, S., Levy, C., Desjardins, L., Lumbroso-Le Rouic, L., Pop, S., et al. (2014). Ocular adverse events of molecularly targeted agents approved in solid tumours: a systematic review. *Eur. Cancer J.* 50, 638–648. doi: 10.1016/j.ejca.2013.10.016

Ibrahim, R., Berman, D., de Pril, V. V., Humphrey, R. W., Chen, T., Messina, M., et al. (2011). Ipilimumab safety profile: summary of findings from completed trials in advanced melanoma. *J. Clin. Oncol.* 29 (abstract).

Izzedine, H., Gueutin, V., Gharbi, C., Mateus, C., Robert, C., Routier, E., et al. (2014). Kidney injuries related to ipilimumab. *Invest. New Drugs* 32, 769. doi: 10.1007/s10637-014-0092-7

Jaber, S. H., Cowen, E. W., Haworth, L. R., Booher, S. L., Berman, D. M., Rosenberg, S. A., et al. (2006). Skin reactions in a subset of patients with stage IV melanoma treated with anti-cytotoxic T-lymphocyte antigen 4 monoclonal antibody as a single agent. *Arch. Dermatol.* 142, 166–172. doi: 10.1001/archderm.142.2.166

Johncilla, M., Misdraji, J., Pratt, D. S., Agoston, A. T., Lauwers, G. Y., Srivastava, A., et al. (2015). Ipilimumab-associated Hepatitis: Clinico pathologic Characterization in a Series of 11 Cases. *Am. J. Surg. Pathol.* 39, 1075–1084. doi: 10.1097/PAS.0000000000000453

Johnson, D. B., Sullivan, R. J., Ott, P. A., Carlino, M. S., Khushalani, N. I., Ye, F., et al. (2015). Ipilimumab therapy in patients with advanced melanoma and preexisting autoimmune. *JAMA Oncol.* 2, 234–240. doi: 10.1001/jamaoncol.2015.4368

Kindler, H. L., Scherpereel, A., Calabrò, L., Aerts, J., Perez, S. C., Bearz, A., et al. (2016). Tremelimumab as second- or third-line treatment of unresectable malignant mesothelioma (MM): Results from the global, double-blind, placebo-controlled DETERMINE study. *J. Clin. Oncol.* 34 (abstract).

Kong, B. Y., Micklethwaite, K. P., Swaminathan, S., Kefford, R. F., and Carlino, M. S. (2016). Autoimmune hemolytic anemia induced by anti-PD-1 therapy in metastatic melanoma. *Melanoma Res.* 26, 202–204. doi: 10.1097/CMR.0000000000000232

Langer, C. J. (2015). Emerging immunotherapies in the treatment of non-small cell lung cancer (NSCLC): the role of immune checkpoint inhibitors. *Am. J. Clin. Oncol.* 38, 422–430. doi: 10.1097/coc.0000000000000059

Larkin, J., Chiarion-Sileni, V., Gonzalez, R., Grob, J. J., Cowey, C. L., Lao, C. D., et al. (2015). Combined nivolumab and ipilimumab or Monotherapy in Untreated Melanoma. *N. Engl. J. Med.* 373, 23–34. doi: 10.1056/NEJMoa1504030

Liao, B., Shroff, S., Kamiya-Matsuoka, C., and Tummala, S. (2014). Atypical neurological complications of ipilimumab therapy in patients with metastatic melanoma. *Neuro-oncology* 16, 589–593. doi: 10.1093/neuonc/nou001

Massard, C., Gordon, M. S., Sharma, S., Rafii, S., Wainberg, Z. A., Luke, J., et al. (2016). Safety and efficacy of durvalumab (MEDI4736), an anti-programmed cell death ligand-1 immune checkpoint inhibitor, in patients with advanced urothelial bladder cancer. *J. Clin. Oncol.* 34, 3119–3125. doi: 10.1200/JCO.2016.67.9761

Maur, M., Tomasello, C., Frassoldati, A., Dieci, M. V., Barbieri, E., Conte, P., et al. (2012). Posterior reversible encephalopathy syndrome during ipilimumab therapy for malignant melanoma. *J. Clin. Oncol.* 30, e76–e78. doi: 10.1200/JCO.2011.38.7886

Min, L., Hodi, F. S., Giobbie-Hurder, A., Ott, P. A., Luke, J. J., Donahue, H., et al. (2015). Systemic high-dose corticosteroid treatment does not improve the outcome of ipilimumab-related hypophysitis: a retrospective cohort study. *Clin. Cancer Res.* 21, 749–755. doi: 10.1158/1078-0432.CCR-14-2353

Minor, D., Chin, K., and Kashani-Sabet, M. (2009). Infliximab in the treatment of anti-CTLA4 antibody (ipilimumab) induced immune-related colitis. *Cancer Biother. Radiopharm.* 24, 321–325. doi: 10.1089/cbr.2008.0607

Momtaz, P., Park, V., Panageas, K. S., Postow, M. A., Callahan, M., Wolchok, J. D., et al. (2015). Safety of Infusing ipilimumab Over 30 Minutes. *J. Clin. Oncol.* 33, 3454–3458. doi: 10.1200/JCO.2015.61.0030

Naidoo, J., Page, D. B., Li, B. T., Connell, L. C., Schindler, K., Lacouture, M. E., et al. (2015). Toxicities of the anti-PD-1 and anti-PD-L1 immune checkpoint antibodies. *Ann. Oncol.* 26, 2375. doi: 10.1093/annonc/mdv383

Nanda, R., Chow, L. Q., Dees, E. C., Berger, R., Gupta, S., Geva, R., et al. (2016). Pembrolizumab in patients with advanced triple-negative breast cancer: phase Ib KEYNOTE-012 study. *J. Clin. Oncol.* 34, 2460–2467. doi: 10.1200/JCO.2015.64.8931

National Cancer Institute (2009). *Common Terminology Criteria for Adverse Events (CTCAE) v4.0.* Available online at: http://evs.nci.nih.gov/ftp1/CTCAE/CTCAE_4.03_2010-06-14_QuickReference_5x7.pdf

Oble, D. A., Mino-Kenudson, M., Goldsmith, J., Hodi, F. S., Seliem, R. M., Dranoff, G., et al. (2008). Alpha-CTLA-4 mAb-associated panenteritis: a histologic and immunohistochemical analysis. *Am. J. Surg. Pathol.* 32, 1130–1137. doi: 10.1097/PAS.0b013e31817150e3

Postow, M. A., Chesney, J., Pavlick, A. C., Robert, C., Grossmann, K., McDermott, D., et al. (2015). Nivolumab and ipilimumab versus ipilimumab in untreated melanoma. *N. Engl. J. Med.* 372, 2006–2017. doi: 10.1056/NEJMoa1414428

Postow, M., and Wolchok, J. (2016). "Toxicities associated with checkpoint inhibitor immunotherapy," in *UpToDate*, ed T. W. Post (Waltham, MA). (Accessed: August 1, 2016).

Reck, M., Rodríguez-Abreu, D., Robinson, A. G., Hui, R., Csőszi,. T., Fülöp, A., et al. (2016). Pembrolizumab versus Chemotherapy for PD-L1–Positive non–small-cell lung cancer. *N. Engl. J. Med.* 375, 1823–1833. doi: 10.1056/NEJMoa1606774

Ribas, A., Hodi, F. S., Callahan, M., Konto, C., and Wolchok, J. (2013a). Hepatotoxicity with combination of vemurafenib and ipilimumab. *N. Engl. J. Med.* 368, 1365–1366. doi: 10.1056/nejmc1302338

Ribas, A., Kefford, R., Marshall, M. A., Punt, C. J., Haanen, J. B., Marmol, M., et al. (2013b). Phase III randomized clinical trial comparing tremelimumab with standard-of-care chemotherapy in patients with advanced melanoma. *J. Clin. Oncol.* 31, 616–622. doi: 10.1200/JCO.2012.44.6112

Rittmeyer, A., Barlesi, F., Waterkamp, D., Park, K., Ciardiello, F., von Pawel, J., et al. (2017). Atezolizumab versus docetaxel in patients with previously treated non-small-cell lung cancer (OAK): a phase 3, open-label, multicentre randomised controlled trial. *Lancet* 389, 255–265. doi: 10.1016/S0140-6736(16)32517-X

Rizvi, N. A., Mazières, J., Planchard, D., Stinchcombe, T. E., Dy, G. K., Antonia, S. J., et al. (2015). Activity and safety of nivolumab, an anti-PD-1 immune checkpoint inhibitor, for patients with advanced, refractory squamous non-small-cell lung cancer (CheckMate 063): a phase 2, single-arm trial. *Lancet Oncol.* 16, 257–265. doi: 10.1016/S1470-2045(15)70054-9

Robert, C., Long, G. V., Brady, B., Dutriaux, C., Maio, M., Mortier, L., et al. (2015a). Nivolumab in previously untreated melanoma without BRAF mutation. *N. Engl. J. Med.* 372, 320–330. doi: 10.1056/NEJMoa1412082

Robert, C., Schachter, J., Long, G. V., Arance, A., Grob, J. J., Mortier, L., et al. (2015b). Pembrolizumab versus ipilimumab in advanced melanoma. *N. Engl. J. Med.* 372, 2521–2532. doi: 10.1056/NEJMoa1503093

Robert, C., Thomas, L., Bondarenko, I., O'Day, S., Weber, J., Garbe, C., et al. (2011). Ipilimumab plus dacarbazine for previously untreated metastatic melanoma. *N. Engl. J. Med.* 364, 2517–2526. doi: 10.1056/NEJMoa1104621

Rosenberg, J. E., Jean, H., Tom, P., van der Heijden, M. S., Balar, A. V., Necchi, A., et al. (2016). Atezolizumab in patients with locally advanced and metastatic urothelial carcinoma who have progressed following treatment with platinum-based chemotherapy: a single-arm, multicentre, phase 2 trial. *Lancet* 387, 1909–1920. doi: 10.1016/S0140-6736(16)00561-4

Ryder, M., Callahan, M., Postow, M., Wolchok, J., and Fagin, J. A. (2014). Endocrine-related adverse events following ipilimumab in patients with advanced melanoma: a comprehensive retrospective review from a single institution. *Endocr. Relat. Cancer* 21, 371–381. doi: 10.1530/ERC-13-0499

Schindler, K., Harmankaya, K., and Kuk, D. (2014). Correlation of absolute and relative eosinophil counts with immune-related adverse events in melanoma patients treated with ipilimumab. *J. Clin. Oncol.* 32:5s (abstract).

Seiwert, T. Y., Burtness, B., Mehra, R., Weiss, J., Berger, R., Eder, J. P., et al. (2016). Safety and clinical activity of pembrolizumab for treatment of recurrent or metastatic squamous cell carcinoma of the head and neck (KEYNOTE-012): an open-label, multicentre, phase 1b trial. *Lancet Oncol.* 17, 956–965. doi: 10.1016/S1470-2045(16)30066-3

Shahabi, V., Berman, D., Chasalow, S. D., Wang, L., Tsuchihashi, Z., Hu, B., et al. (2013). Gene expression profiling of whole blood in ipilimumab-treated patients for identification of potential biomarkers of immune- related gastrointestinal adverse events. *J. Transl. Med.* 11:75. doi: 10.1186/1479-5876-11-75

Tarhini, A. A., Cherian, J., Moschos, S. J., Tawbi, H. A., Shuai, Y., Gooding, W. E., et al. (2012). Safety and efficacy of combination immunotherapy with interferon alfa-2b and tremelimumab in patients with stage IV melanoma. *J. Clin. Oncol.* 30, 322–328. doi: 10.1200/JCO.2011.37.5394

Topalian, S. L., Hodi, F. S., Brahmer, J. R., Gettinger, S. N., Smith, D. C., McDermott, D. F., et al. (2012). Safety, activity, and immune correlates of anti-PD-1 antibody in cancer. *N. Engl. J. Med.* 366, 2443. doi: 10.1056/NEJMoa1200690

Topalian, S. L., Sznol, M., McDermott, D.,Kluger, F. H. M., Carvajal, R. D., Sharfman, W. H., et al. (2014). Survival, durable tumor remission, and long-term safety in patients with advanced melanoma receiving nivolumab. *J. Clin. Oncol.* 32, 1020–1030. doi: 10.1200/JCO.2013.53.0105

Villadolid, J., and Amin, A. (2015). Immune checkpoint inhibitors in clinical practice: update on management of immune-related toxicities. *Transl. Lung Cancer Res.* 4, 560–575. doi: 10.3978/j.issn.2218-6751.2015.06.06

Weber, J. (2009). Ipilimumab: Controversies in its development, utility, and autoimmune adverse events. *Cancer Immunol. Immunother.* 58, 823–830. doi: 10.1007/s00262-008-0653-8

Weber, J., Hamid, O., Amin, A., Masson, E., Goldberg, S. M., Williams, D., et al. (2013). Randomized phase I pharmacokinetic study of ipilimumab with or without one of two different chemotherapy regimens in patients with untreated advanced melanoma. *Cancer Immun.* 13, 7

Weber, J. S. (2012). Practical Management of immune related adverse events from immune checkpoint protein antibodies for the oncologist. *Am. Soc. Clin. Oncol. Educ. Book* 2012, 174–177. doi: 10.14694/EdBook_AM.2012.32.174

Weber, J. S., Kudchadkar, R. R., and Yu, B. (2013). Safety, efficacy, and biomarkers of nivolumab with vaccine in ipilimumab-refractory or -naive melanoma. *J. Clin. Oncol.* 31, 4311. doi: 10.1200/jco.2013.51.4802

Weber, J. S., Yang, J. C., Atkins, M. B., and Disis, M. L. (2015). Toxicities of Immunotherapy for the Practitioner. *J. Clin. Oncol.* doi: 10.1200/jco.2014.60.0379

Weber, J., Thompson, J. A., Hamid, O., Minor, D., Amin, A., Ron, I., et al. (2009). A randomized, double-blind, placebo-controlled, phase II study comparing the tolerability and efficacy of ipilimumab administered with or without prophylactic budesonide in patients with unresectable stage III or IV melanoma. *Clin. Cancer Res.* 15, 5591–5598. doi: 10.1158/1078-0432.CCR-09-1024

Westin, J. R., Chu, F., Zhang, M., Fayad, L. E., Kwak, L. W., Fowler, N., et al. (2014). Safety and activity of PD1 blockade by pidilizumab in combination with rituximab in patients with relapsed follicular lymphoma: a single group, open-label, phase 2 trial. *Lancet Oncol.* 15, 69–77. doi: 10.1016/S1470-2045(13)70551-5

Wilgenhof, S., and Neyns, B. (2011). Anti-CTLA-4 antibody-induced Guillain-Barré syndrome in a melanoma patient. *Ann. Oncol.* 22, 991–993. doi: 10.1093/annonc/mdr028

Williams, T. J., Benavides, D. R., Patrice, K. A., Dalmau, J. O., de Ávila, A. L., Le, D. T., et al. (2016). Association of autoimmune encephalitis with combined immune checkpoint inhibitor treatment for metastatic cancer. *JAMA Neurol.* 73, 928–933. doi: 10.1001/jamaneurol.2016.1399

Wolchok, J. D., Neyns, B., Linette, G., Negrier, S., Lutzky, J., Thomas, L., et al. (2010). Ipilimumab monotherapy in patients with pretreated advanced melanoma: a randomised, double-blind, multicentre, phase 2, dose-ranging study. *Lancet Oncol.* 11, 155–164. doi: 10.1016/S1470-2045(09)70334-1

Conflict of Interest Statement: The authors declare that the research was conducted in the absence of any commercial or financial relationships that could be construed as a potential conflict of interest.

3

Chemotherapy-Induced Constipation and Diarrhea: Pathophysiology, Current and Emerging Treatments

*Rachel M. McQuade[1], Vanesa Stojanovska[1], Raquel Abalo[2,3,4,5], Joel C. Bornstein[6] and Kulmira Nurgali[1]**

[1] Centre for Chronic Disease, College of Health and Biomedicine, Victoria University, Melbourne, VIC, Australia, [2] Área de Farmacología y Nutrición, Universidad Rey Juan Carlos, Madrid, Spain, [3] Grupo de Excelencia Investigadora URJC, Banco de Santander Grupo Multidisciplinar de Investigación y Tratamiento del Dolor, Universidad Rey Juan Carlos, Madrid, Spain, [4] Unidad Asociada al Instituto de Química Médica del Consejo Superior de Investigaciones Científicas, Madrid, Spain, [5] Unidad Asociada al Instituto de Investigación en Ciencias de la Alimentación del Consejo Superior de Investigaciones Científicas, Madrid, Spain, [6] Department of Physiology, University of Melbourne, Melbourne, VIC, Australia

Edited by:
David A. Gewirtz, Virginia Commonwealth University, USA

Reviewed by:
Hamid Akbarali, Virginia Commonwealth University, USA
Liren Qian, Navy General Hospital, China
Chantal Dessy, Université Catholique de Louvain, Belgium

***Correspondence:**
Kulmira Nurgali
kulmira.nurgali@vu.edu.au

Gastrointestinal (GI) side-effects of chemotherapy are a debilitating and often overlooked clinical hurdle in cancer management. Chemotherapy-induced constipation (CIC) and Diarrhea (CID) present a constant challenge in the efficient and tolerable treatment of cancer and are amongst the primary contributors to dose reductions, delays and cessation of treatment. Although prevalence of CIC is hard to estimate, it is believed to affect approximately 16% of cancer patients, whilst incidence of CID has been estimated to be as high as 80%. Despite this, the underlying mechanisms of both CID and CIC remain unclear, but are believed to result from a combination of intersecting mechanisms including inflammation, secretory dysfunctions, GI dysmotility and alterations in GI innervation. Current treatments for CIC and CID aim to reduce the severity of symptoms rather than combating the pathophysiological mechanisms of dysfunction, and often result in worsening of already chronic GI symptoms or trigger the onset of a plethora of other side-effects including respiratory depression, uneven heartbeat, seizures, and neurotoxicity. Emerging treatments including those targeting the enteric nervous system present promising avenues to alleviate CID and CIC. Identification of potential targets for novel therapies to alleviate chemotherapy-induced toxicity is essential to improve clinical outcomes and quality of life amongst cancer sufferers.

Keywords: chemotherapy, chemotherapy-induced constipation, chemotherapy-induced diarrhea, pathophysiology, treatments

INTRODUCTION

Cancer is a leading cause of death worldwide (Jemal et al., 2011; Torre et al., 2015) with approximately 14.1 million new cancer cases and 8.2 million cancer deaths in 2012 alone (Ferlay et al., 2015). Although advances in modern medicine have improved scanning and cancer detection techniques, the burden for global health of cancer is expected to intensify in decades to come particularly in low and middle income families and economically developed countries (Jemal et al., 2010a,b). Population aging and growth coupled with the adoption of high risk lifestyle choices

Abbreviations: CIC, chemotherapy-induced constipation; CID, chemotherapy-induced diarrhea; ENS, enteric nervous system; GI, gastrointestinal.

such as smoking, physical inactivity, and westernization of diets have been identified as underlying factors contributing to the increasing incidence of cancer worldwide (Jemal et al., 2011). It is now anticipated that by 2025 more than 20 million people will be affected by cancer (Ferlay et al., 2015).

Most cancer patients receive curative or palliative chemotherapeutic intervention throughout the course of treatment (Louvet et al., 2002; Benson et al., 2004b; Kaufmann et al., 2006; Wagner et al., 2006; Goffin et al., 2010; Okines et al., 2010). Although chemotherapy has greatly improved overall survival in many types of cancer, cytotoxic side-effects are a significant hurdle greatly impeding the clinical application of otherwise beneficial therapies (Xue et al., 2011; Iwamoto, 2013). GI side-effects such as nausea, vomiting, ulceration, bloating, constipation and, in particular, diarrhea are major obstacles causing delays, adjustments, and discontinuation of treatment whilst greatly impacting quality of life in many cancer patients (Benson et al., 2004a; Stringer et al., 2007, 2009d; Denlinger and Barsevick, 2009; Peterson et al., 2011). Although specific chemotherapeutic agents have been correlated with heightened incidence of GI side-effects (**Table 1**), incidences as high as 40% in patients receiving standard dose chemotherapy and 100% in patients receiving high dose chemotherapy have been reported (McQuade et al., 2014). Furthermore, the incidence of chronic post-treatment constipation and diarrhea amongst cancer survivors has been estimated to be as high as 49% with episodes persisting up to 10 years after the cessation of treatment (Schneider et al., 2007; Denlinger and Barsevick, 2009; Kim et al., 2012). The underlying mechanisms of CIC and diarrhea (CID) remain unclear. Although mucositis presenting as inflammation and ulceration of the intestinal epithelium is a significant contributing factor, the pathophysiology of CID and CIC is likely to be complex, involving several overlapping inflammatory, secretory and neural mechanisms.

CHEMOTHERAPY-INDUCED DIARRHEA

Diarrhea is a frequently under-recognized clinical issue that significantly affects morbidity and mortality of cancer patients worldwide (Maroun et al., 2007). Prevalence and severity of CID vary greatly depending on chemotherapeutic regime administration and dosage. A direct correlation between cumulative dose and severity of CID has been recognized, with high dose regimens associated with heightened incidence of CID (Verstappen et al., 2003). Certain regimens, especially those containing 5-fluorouracil and irinotecan are associated with rates of CID of up to 80% (Benson et al., 2004a; Richardson and Dobish, 2007) with one third of patients experiencing severe (grade 3 or 4) diarrhea (**Table 2**) (Maroun et al., 2007).

Chemotherapy-induced diarrhea severely interferes with anti-cancer treatment, resulting in treatment alterations in approximately 60% of patients, dose reductions in 22% of patients, dose delays in 28% of patients and complete termination of treatment in 15% of patients (Arbuckle et al., 2000; Dranitsaris et al., 2005). Moreover, CID has been reported to last as long as 10 years post-treatment (Denlinger and Barsevick, 2009). Persistent and severe chemotherapy-associated Diarrhea is correlated with significant malnutrition and dehydration resulting in concomitant weight loss (cachexia), fatigue, renal failure, hemorrhoids, and perianal skin breakdown (Mitchell, 2006; Shafi and Bresalier, 2010). CID related dehydration is linked to early death rates in roughly 5% of patients undergoing anti-cancer treatment (Rothenberg et al., 2001). Further to this, chemotherapeutic administration may also prompt severe intestinal inflammation, bowel wall thickening and ulceration (Kuebler et al., 2007) contributing to clinical disruptions with potentially life-threatening ramifications (Rothenberg et al., 2001; Benson et al., 2004a; Stein et al., 2010).

For over 30% of CID sufferers it interferes with their daily activities (Stein et al., 2010), with detrimental effects on the mental and social health of cancer survivors. Persistent and uncontrollable CID has been linked to anxiety, depression, social isolation, and low self-esteem (Viele, 2003), emphasizing the importance of both elucidating the underlying mechanisms of CID and improving treatment efficacy (Carelle et al., 2002).

Pathophysiology of Chemotherapy-Induced Diarrhea

Although several chemotherapy regimens have been associated with Diarrhea to varying degrees (**Table 1**), most basic research into the mechanisms underlying CID has focused on irinotecan and its active metabolite SN38 (Gibson and Keefe, 2006). As diarrhea is a well-recognized side-effect of irinotecan treatment, the histological changes that occur throughout the GI tract in response to irinotecan administration have been examined in several animal studies (Araki et al., 1993; Ikuno et al., 1995; Takasuna et al., 1996; Gibson et al., 2003). Pronounced crypt ablation, villus blunting and epithelial atrophy in the small and large intestines have been reported (Logan et al., 2008), resulting in mucosal damage and degeneration being a major theme throughout the literature surrounding CID. Although patients do not routinely have imaging or endoscopy to diagnose the chemotherapy-induced mucosal inflammation (Touchefeu et al., 2014), CID is still largely believed to be a form, or by-product, of GI mucositis. Mucositis is defined as mucosal injury presenting as inflammation and ulceration, resulting in alterations of intestinal microflora and GI secretion (Stringer, 2009; Stringer et al., 2009a,b). The basic pathophysiology of mucositis can be broken into 5 sequential phases: (i) initiation; (ii) up-regulation; (iii) signaling and amplification; (iv) ulceration and inflammation; and (v) healing (Sonis et al., 2004; Lee et al., 2014).

Initiation of mucositis is believed to result from direct or indirect effects of cytotoxic chemotherapeutics on the rapidly dividing epithelial cells in GI tract, triggering apoptosis. This leads to reductions in crypt length and villus area, coupled with activation of nuclear factor-kappa B (NFκB) and subsequent up-regulation of pro-inflammatory cytokines including interleukin 1 (Lawrence, 2009), which contribute to ulceration and inflammation in the mucosal epithelium (Gibson et al., 2003; Stringer et al., 2007, 2008, 2009a,d; Logan et al., 2008). Intestinal microbiota is known to play an integral role in intestinal homeostasis and are now believed to play a key role in the development of mucositis (van Vliet et al., 2010; Touchefeu et al., 2014). Recent studies have revealed that chemotherapeutic administration has effects on intestinal microbial composition (Stringer et al., 2009a,b), and fecal microbiota (Touchefeu et al., 2014).

Much of the research investigating the effects of chemotherapeutic administration on microbiota has focused primarily on topoisomerase I inhibitor, irinotecan, due to the involvement of microbiota in its metabolism (Stringer, 2013). Upon metabolism in the liver, irinotecan is converted to its active metabolite SN-38 by enzyme carboxylesterase, before being deactivated through glucuronidation by uridine diphosphate glucuronosyltransferase 1A1 (UGT1A1) to form SN38 glucuronide (SN38-G). However, SN38G may be reactivated to SN38 in the presence of enzyme β-glucuronidase, which may be produced by the intestinal microbiome. Several studies have shown a shift in commensal bacteria, in particular *Bifidobacterium* spp. toward *Salmonella* spp. and *Escherichia coli* following irinotecan administration (Stringer et al., 2009b). Of the β-glucuronidase-producing bacteria, *Bacteroides* spp. has been shown to decrease following irinotecan treatment, concurrently *Staphylococcus* spp., *Clostridium* spp. and *E. coli* have been found to be increased, whilst presence of beneficial bacteria, *Lactobacillus* spp. and *Bifidobacterium* spp. was decreased following irinotecan treatment (Stringer et al., 2007). When given in combination with antimetabolite 5-fluorouracil, both *Clostridium cluster XI* and *Enterobacteriaceae* presence was found to be increased, whilst treatment with 5-fluorouracil alone has also been found to increase the presence of *Clostridium* spp. and *Staphylococcus* spp. at 24 h post-treatment (Stringer et al., 2009c).

These changes in microbiota are believed to play an important role not only in maintaining intestinal homeostasis and integrity but in the modulation of inflammatory responses through interaction with Toll-like receptors and the nucleotide

TABLE 1 | Gastrointestinal side-effects of chemotherapy.

Mechanisms	Chemotherapeutic agents	Cancer type	GI side-effects
Alkylating Agents	Cisplatin	Lung, Breast, Stomach, Colorectal, Liver	Nausea, Vomiting, **Diarrhea, Constipation** (Ilson et al., 1999; Ardizzoni et al., 2007)
	Cyclophosphamide	Breast	Nausea, Vomiting, Abdominal Pain, **Diarrhea** (Fraiser et al., 1991; Boussios et al., 2012)
	Oxaliplatin	Colorectal, Breast, Stomach	Nausea, Vomiting, **Diarrhea**, **Constipation** (Extra et al., 1990; Kim et al., 2003)
Antimetabolites	5-Fluorouracil	Breast, Colorectal, Stomach, Liver	Nausea, Vomiting, Abdominal Pain, **Diarrhea** (Douillard et al., 2010; Boussios et al., 2012)
	Capecitabine	Colorectal, Breast, Stomach	Nausea, Vomiting, **Diarrhea** (Walko and Lindley, 2005; Stathopoulos et al., 2007; Boussios et al., 2012)
	Gemcitabine	Lung, Breast	Nausea, Vomiting, Abdominal Pain, **Constipation, Diarrhea** (Wolff et al., 2001; Mutch et al., 2007; Boussios et al., 2012)
	Methotrexate	Breast	Nausea, Vomiting, Abdominal Pain, **Diarrhea** (Boussios et al., 2012)
Anthracycline	Doxorubicin	Breast, Lung, Liver	Nausea, Vomiting, Abdominal pain, GI Ulceration, **Diarrhea** (Boussios et al., 2012; Tacar et al., 2013)
Immunomodulating agent	Thalidomide	Myeloma, Kidney	Nausea, Vomiting, **Diarrhea, Constipation** (Smith et al., 2008)
Mitotic inhibitors	Cabazitaxel	Prostate	Nausea, Vomiting, Abdominal pain, **Diarrhea** (Nightingale and Ryu, 2012; Dieras et al., 2013)
	Docetaxel	Prostate, Breast, Lung, Stomach	Nausea, Vomiting, **Diarrhea** (Boussios et al., 2012)
	Paclitaxel	Lung, Stomach, Prostate, Breast	Nausea, Vomiting, **Diarrhea** (Boussios et al., 2012)
	Vincristine	Breast, Lung	**Constipation**, Abdominal Pain (Holland et al., 1973)
Topoisomerase inhibitor	Irinotecan	Colorectal, Breast, Stomach, Lung	Nausea, Vomiting, Acute and Delayed **Diarrhea** (Hecht, 1998)

TABLE 2 | Common toxicity criteria for diarrhea and constipation grading (adapted from the National Cancer Institute).

Toxicity	Grade 1	Grade 2	Grade 3	Grade 4	Grade 5
Diarrhea	Increase of <4 stools per day over baseline.	Increase of 4–6 stools per day over baseline.	Increase of >7 stools per day over baseline. Incontinence. Hospitalization.	Life threatening consequences. Urgent intervention indicated.	Death
Constipation	Occasional or intermittent symptoms; occasional use of stool softeners, laxatives, dietary modification, or enema.	Persistent symptoms with regular use of laxatives or enemas indicated.	Symptoms interfering with activities of daily living; obstipation with manual evacuation indicated	Life-threatening consequences (e.g., obstruction, toxic megacolon).	Death

oligomerization domain receptors that activate NFκB (van Vliet et al., 2010). In the healing phase, proliferation and differentiation of the GI epithelium return approximately 2 weeks post-chemotherapy (Sonis et al., 2004; Lee et al., 2014), but functional changes persist after recovery of morphological changes (Keefe et al., 2000; Rubenstein et al., 2004). The pathophysiology underlying these persistent changes in GI functions includes several overlapping secretory, osmotic, inflammatory, and neurogenic mechanisms (McQuade et al., 2014).

Disruption to water and electrolyte balance within the GI tract is a key component in the pathophysiology of all types of diarrhea. Direct mucosal damage has been suggested as a major contributor to malabsorption and hypersecretion associated with CID (Richardson and Dobish, 2007; Stringer et al., 2007, 2009b; Stein et al., 2010). Studies using animal models of CID have demonstrated increased apoptosis in the crypts of both the jejunum and colon, resulting in metaplasia of goblet cells and excessive mucous secretion (Ikuno et al., 1995; Gibson et al., 2003). Hyperplasia of the rapidly dividing crypt cells in the epithelium of the gut probably results in heightened proportions of immature secretory cells, leading to increased secretion and decreased absorptive capacity of the villi, thereby contributing to the onset of diarrhea (Castro-Rodríguez et al., 1997). Retention of non-absorbable compounds within the lumen triggers an osmotic shift of water into the lumen (Castro-Rodríguez et al., 1997; Richardson and Dobish, 2007; Stringer et al., 2007). This reduced absorptive capacity and increased secretion in the small intestines results in increased fluid and solutes in the intestinal lumen and overwhelms the absorptive capacity of the colon resulting in diarrhea (Gibson and Keefe, 2006).

Secondary to mucosal damage, CID has been associated with mucosal inflammation throughout the GI tract (Logan et al., 2008). Increased expression of cyclooxygenase (COX)-2, associated with increased release of prostaglandin E2 (PGE2), is seen in rat colon following irinotecan administration (Yang et al., 2005). PGE2 stimulates colonic secretion and hyperperistalsis of the gut, whilst inhibiting sodium, potassium and adenosine triphosphatase, and triggering excessive chloride secretion, all of which further contribute to the onset of diarrhea (Kase et al., 1997a,b; Leahy et al., 2002; Yang et al., 2005). Further, irinotecan stimulates the production of thromboxane A2, a potent physiological stimulant of chloride and water secretion in the colon (Sakai et al., 1997; Suzuki et al., 2000) as well as tumor necrosis factor- α (TNF-α) a pro-inflammatory cytokine and a primary mediator of immune regulation associated with CID (Yang et al., 2005).

Chemotherapy can induce damage to the ENS (Vera et al., 2011; Wafai et al., 2013) which may also underlie GI secretory disturbances involved in pathophysiology of CID. Innervation of the GI tract is primarily from the ENS, sometimes referred to as "the second brain" due to its ability to function autonomously of the central nervous system (Phillips and Powley, 2007). The ENS is comprised of ganglia, primary interganglionic fiber tracts as well as secondary and tertiary fibers which project to many of the effector systems of the gut including muscle cells, glands, and blood vessels (Hansen, 2003). The ENS is divided into two major ganglionated plexi, the myenteric (Auerbach's), and submucosal (Meissner's), which are responsible for controlling gut functions including motility, secretion, absorption and vascular tone. Enteric neuropathy has been linked to a variety of GI pathologies, in part due to its regulation of intestinal epithelial function and colonic motility (De Giorgio et al., 2000, 2004; De Giorgio and Camilleri, 2004; Chandrasekharan et al., 2011; Furness, 2012). However, effects of chemotherapeutics on enteric neurons and GI dysfunction have been largely overlooked until recently. It has been shown that chronic treatment with cisplatin results in myenteric neuronal loss, increase in amplitude of the neurally induced contractions of the gastric fundus strips in mice and occasional diarrhea (Pini et al., 2016). Thus enteric neuropathy may be an underlying cause of chemotherapy-induced GI dysmotility.

Movement of fluid between the lumen of the intestine and the body fluid compartments is a complex and tightly regulated process involving neural, endocrine, paracrine, and autocrine systems that act via the enteric neurons within the submucosal plexus (Lundgren et al., 2000; Johnson et al., 2012). Situated superficially to the mucosa, the submucosal plexus lies between the circular muscle and muscularis mucosa layer of the mucosa and derives innervation from neurons in the myenteric plexus as well as direct innervation from branches of the sympathetic and parasympathetic nervous systems. The submucosal plexus innervates the mucosal epithelium and submucosal arterioles to control and maintain water and electrolyte balance, secretion and vascular tone (Furness, 2012). Fluid is absorbed from the lumen containing nutrients via ion-coupled transporters and returned through secretomotor reflexes. Through activation of secretomotor neurons, water and electrolytes are moved from the interstitium of the lamina propria to the lumen, drawn from both the circulation and the absorbed fluids. Neural control of secretion and absorption of water and electrolytes occurs on multiple interacting levels. While there are secretomotor circuits confined to the submucosal plexus, they can be directly controlled by circuitry within the myenteric plexus. Despite the important role of the ENS in controlling secretory function, very little research has been undertaken to elucidate the relationship between the ENS and CID. Enteric neuropathy and/or neuronal dysfunction may be a contributing factor in chemotherapy-induced secretory dysfunction.

Current Treatments for Chemotherapy-Induced Diarrhea

Chemotherapy-induced diarrhea may be classified as uncomplicated (grade 1–2 with no complications) or complicated (grade 3–4 with one or more complicating signs or symptoms), early onset (<24 h after administration) or late onset (>24 h after administration) and may be categorized as persistent (present for >4 weeks) or non-persistent (present for <4 weeks) according to the National Cancer Institute's Common Terminology Criteria for Adverse Effects grading system (Stein et al., 2010). Although uncomplicated CID may be managed by modification of the diet and administration of standard anti-diarrheal drugs such as loperamide, octreotide and tincture of opium, complicated diarrhea requires aggressive high dose anti-diarrheal administration and hospitalization (McQuade et al., 2014). The recommendations on the management of CID were published in 1998 and updated in 2004 (Wadler et al., 1998; Benson et al., 2004a), providing guidelines for evaluation and management of CID. These guidelines have not been updated since 2004. Currently the only drugs recommended in the updated treatment guidelines are opioid derivatives such as loperamide and deodorized tincture of opium (DTO), and octreotide.

Loperamide

Loperamide is a non-analgesic agonist that acts at μ-opioid receptors at the level of the myenteric plexus to decrease intestinal motility (Regnard et al., 2011). High dose loperamide alleviates diarrhea associated with chemotherapeutic administration (Stein et al., 2010). However, its use leads to a range of side-effects including severe constipation, abdominal pain, dizziness, rashes as well as worsening of already present bloating, nausea and vomiting (Lenfers et al., 1999; Stein et al., 2010). High dose loperamide is reported to increase incidents of paralytic ileus, in association with abdominal distension (Sharma et al., 2005; Richardson and Dobish, 2007). Despite these severe side-effects, loperamide remains the standard first line therapy for CID.

Octreotide

Octreotide is a synthetic somatostatin analog that promotes absorption by inhibiting specific gut hormones to increase intestinal transit time (Högenauer et al., 2002; Mitchell, 2006) as well as hyperpolarizing enteric secretomotor neurons (Högenauer et al., 2002). Octreotide is administered to treat both complicated diarrhea and loperamide-refractory diarrhea and is generally reserved as a second line treatment for patients who are unresponsive to loperamide after 48 h, despite loperamide dose escalation (Regnard et al., 2011). Although octreotide decreases CID effectively, severe side-effects including slow and/or uneven heartbeat, severe constipation, stomach pain, enlarged thyroid, vomiting, nausea, headache and dizziness occur in over 10% of patients (Bhattacharya et al., 2008).

Deodorised Tincture of Opium

Deodorized tincture of opium (DTO) is another widely used antidiarrheal agent, despite the absence of literature to support its use in CID treatment (Stein et al., 2010). Similar to loperamide, DTO activates μ-opioid receptors within the GI tract inhibiting intestinal peristalsis, increasing intestinal transit time and promoting fluid reabsorption (Richardson and Dobish, 2007). The efficacy of DTO in treatment of CID has not been reported, however, it is a commonly used anti-diarrheal drug and may be considered as a second-line therapy for persistent and uncomplicated diarrhea (Richardson and Dobish, 2007). DTO contains 10 mg/ml of morphine and is one of the most potent forms of orally administered morphine available by prescription. DTO induces many side-effects including euphoria, nausea, vomiting, painful/difficult urination, stomach and abdominal pain, seizures and allergic reactions. Further, DTO administration associates with psychological and physical dependence, miosis, respiratory depression (Benson et al., 2004a; Richardson and Dobish, 2007) and constipation, with continued/prolonged opioid use linked to severe constipation (Benyamin et al., 2008).

CHEMOTHERAPY-INDUCED CONSTIPATION

Constipation is a frequent, and underestimated, complication in patients with advanced cancer (Mancini and Bruera, 1998). As constipation is a subjective sensation, there is difficulty surrounding acceptance of a universal definition, although it is broadly recognized clinically as a mixture of reduced frequency of bowel action and increased stool consistency (Connolly and Larkin, 2012). Constipation occurs in 50–87% of advanced cancer patients (Abernethy et al., 2009). Constipation is the third most common symptom in patients receiving cytotoxic chemotherapy with an overall prevalence of 16%, with 5% classified as severe and 11% classified as moderate (Yamagishi et al., 2009; Anthony, 2010).

The mechanisms underlying CIC are poorly defined with minimal clinical studies existing. Distinguishing true CIC from secondary constipation from drugs given to control other chemotherapy or cancer-induced symptoms (such as anti-emetics for nausea and vomiting and opioids for pain) is a major issue hindering investigation (Gibson and Keefe, 2006). Given the scarcity of literature concerning CIC it is hard to estimate accurate incidence and severity among all chemotherapy-treated cancer sufferers, but specific chemotherapeutic agents such as thalidomide, cisplatin and vinca alkaloids such as vincristine, vinblastine, and vinorelbine induce true CIC in up to 80–90% of patients (Ghobrial and Rajkumar, 2003; Pujol et al., 2006; Stojanovska et al., 2015).

Constipation is not deemed to be of clinical importance until it causes physical risks or impairs quality of life. Constipation can cause a number of significant symptoms. Severely constipated patients experience abdominal distension usually accompanied by severe abrupt episodes of abdominal pain (Falcón et al., 2016). Furthermore, rectal tearing, hemorrhoids and rectal fissures caused by passing hard, dry stool are frequent complications of constipation (Leung et al., 2011). Untreated constipation may progress to obstipation, severe persistent constipation, which can have life threatening complications associated with fecal impaction and bowel obstruction (Leung et al., 2011). Fecal impaction, the presence of unpassable masses of stool, and increases intraluminal pressure within the bowel can lead to ischaemic necrosis of the mucosa, pain, bleeding, and perforation. Fecal impaction is also well recognized as a factor in urinary incontinence in the elderly (MacDonald et al., 1991). Constipation can also cause confusion, increase retroperitoneal or liver pain, trigger rapid onset nausea with or without vomiting in the presence of intestinal blockage and lead to inadequate absorption of oral drugs (Mancini and Bruera, 1998), greatly affecting the tolerability and efficacy of chemotherapeutic administration. There is accumulating evidence that self-reported constipation and functional constipation lead to significant impairment of quality of life, with the implication that this is a serious condition in the majority of people afflicted (Talley, 2003;

Dennison et al., 2005), however, little work has been undertaken to elucidate prevalence and mechanisms.

Pathophysiology of Chemotherapy-Induced Constipation

Normal bowel function requires the coordination of motility, mucosal transport, and defecation reflexes (Mancini and Bruera, 1998). Broadly constipation can be classified into three categories: normal-transit constipation, defecatory disorders and slow-transit constipation (Lembo and Camilleri, 2003). Normal-transit constipation is the most common form of constipation, where frequency of colonic evacuation is normal, yet patients believe they are constipated due to a perceived difficulty with evacuation or the presence of hard stools. Symptoms of normal-transit constipation include bloating and abdominal pain or discomfort, as well as increased psychosocial distress (Ashraf et al., 1996). Constipation resulting from defecatory disorders is most commonly due to dysfunction of the pelvic floor or anal sphincter. Defecatory disorders may result from prolonged avoidance of the pain associated with the passage of a large, hard stool or painful, anal fissure or hemorrhoid (Loening-Baucke, 1996). Structural abnormalities, such as rectal intussusception, rectocele, obstructing sigmoidocele, and excessive perineal descent, are less common causes of defecatory disorders (Lembo and Camilleri, 2003). Slow-transit constipation is associated with infrequent urge to defecate, bloating, and abdominal pain or discomfort.

Though little clinical research has been undertaken to elucidate the underlying pathology in CIC, it has been hypothesized that CIC may result from effects of chemotherapy on nerve endings in the gut (Ghobrial and Rajkumar, 2003). The GI tract is innervated by the ENS together with fibers from extrinsic sympathetic, parasympathetic (vagus nerve) and sensory afferent neurons (Phillips and Powley, 2007). Both the extrinsic and intrinsic innervation play an important role in the motor activity of the GI tract. The internal circular smooth muscle layer and the external longitudinal smooth muscle are controlled by two main mechanisms: non-neural pacemaker cells, interstitial cells of Cajal (ICCs), which generate myogenic activity and enteric neurons which provide neurogenic supply. Neuronal terminals are closely associated with ICCs which are linked to smooth muscle cells via gap junctions. Within the ENS, three main neuronal classes of myenteric neurons govern the complex motor reflex pathways: sensory neurons, interneurons, and motor neurons. The integration of inputs from these neurons and ICCs to smooth muscle cells in the colon allows expression of various motor patterns including phasic contractile activity and tonic contractile activity which contribute to colonic motor activity and the peristaltic reflex (Gwynne et al., 2004; Dinning et al., 2009; Huizinga and Lammers, 2009; Kuizenga et al., 2015).

Subtle changes to the ENS, not evident in conventional histological examination, have been suggested as a potential underlying mechanism for abnormal colonic motor function leading to constipation (Bassotti and Villanacci, 2011). For instance, alterations in the number of myenteric neurons expressing the excitatory neurotransmitter substance P, as well as abnormalities in the inhibitory neurotransmitters, vasoactive intestinal peptide and nitric oxide, and a reduction in the number of ICCs (Cortesini et al., 1995; Tzavella et al., 1996; He et al., 2000) have been observed in patients with slow-transit constipation. However, the effects of chemotherapeutics on ENS and GI dysfunction have been largely overlooked until recently. A study investigating the effects of 5-fluorouracil-induced dysmotility in mice uncovered myenteric neuronal loss alongside delayed GI transit and inhibition of propagating colonic contractions (McQuade et al., 2016). Similar results have been demonstrated following oxaliplatin administration in mice, and cisplatin administration in rats, where enteric neuronal loss was associated with a reduction in colonic motor activity and reduced GI transit time, respectively (Vera et al., 2011; Wafai et al., 2013). Loss of enteric neurons following administration of cisplatin and oxaliplatin has been correlated with an increase in a population of the myenteric neurons expressing neuronal nitric oxide synthase (Vera et al., 2011; Wafai et al., 2013) and changes in glial cell populations (Robinson et al., 2016). These studies emphasize the importance of enteric neuronal integrity in GI function whilst suggesting neuroprotection as a potential therapeutic pathway for the treatment of chemotherapy-induced GI disorders.

Opioid-Induced Constipation

As previously mentioned, a major limitation in the estimation and evaluation of true CIC is the onset of secondary constipation, namely opioid-induced constipation produced by opioid analgesia. Whilst opioid analgesics are the gold standard in pain relief for cancer patients, adverse effects such as opioid-induced bowel dysfunction (OIBD) and opioid-induced constipation (OIC) severely compromise their therapeutic potential (Gonzalez and Halm, 2016). Incidence of OIC ranges from 50 to 87% in terminally ill cancer patients and is positively associated with chronic opioid treatment (Abernethy et al., 2009; Abramowitz et al., 2013). Opioid receptors are located throughout the central and peripheral nervous system and are involved in pain transmission (Camilleri, 2011). In the GI tract, μ-receptors are widely distributed throughout the ileum, stomach and proximal colon where they contribute to the control of fluid and electrolyte transport as well as motility (McKay et al., 1981; Fickel et al., 1997; Garg et al., 2016). Opioid analgesics interfere with GI motility by delaying transit, stimulating non-propulsive motility and altering GI segmentation and tone through their effects on enteric neurons (De Schepper et al., 2004; Wood and Galligan, 2004). These changes coupled with activation of mucosal sensory receptors that trigger a reflex arc facilitate excessive fluid reabsorption, resulting in OIC (Panchal et al., 2007; Camilleri, 2011).

Whilst administration of laxatives remains the first-line treatment option for OIC, this intervention alone is frequently ineffective (Gatti and Sabato, 2012). Selective μ-opioid receptor antagonists are emerging as a promising first line treatment for OIC, in particular treatment with methylnaltrexone bromide (methylnaltrexone) has been found to improve GI transit in chronically ill patients and has been recommended for use in cancer patients (Gatti and Sabato, 2012). Methylnaltrexone has demonstrated efficacy in improving opioid-induced delay in the oral–caecal transit time and inducing laxation in both healthy subjects and advanced illness patients (Culpepper-Morgan et al., 1992; Thomas et al., 2005; Thomas et al., 2008). Similarly, treatment with peripheral μ-opioid receptor antagonist Alvimopan has been found to increase the frequency of spontaneous bowel movements in non-cancer patients with opioid induced bowel dysfunction (Webster et al., 2008).

Current Treatments for Chemotherapy-Induced Constipation

The management of constipation can be divided into general interventions and therapeutic measures. The general interventions involve increasing physical exercise, fluid intake and fiber consumption, availability of comfort, privacy and convenience during defecation as well as elimination of medical factors that may be contributing to constipation (Mancini and Bruera, 1998). Therapeutic interventions for the management of constipation, including CIC involve the administration of both oral and/or rectal bulk-forming, emollient, osmotic/saline, stimulant, and lubricant laxatives (Connolly and Larkin, 2012). Laxative compounds may fall into one of several categories depending on their mechanism of action.

Bulk-Forming Laxatives

Bulk-forming laxatives such as methylcellulose, psyllium, and polycarbophil most closely mimic the physiologic mechanisms involved in promoting GI evacuation. Available as natural or semisynthetic hydrophilic polysaccharides, cellulose derivatives, or polyacrylic resins, bulk forming laxatives work by either dissolving or swelling in the intestines to form a viscous liquid that provides mechanical distension. This facilitates the passage of intestinal contents by stimulating peristalsis and reducing GI transit time. Although typically recommended as initial therapy for most forms of mild constipation (Kirschenbaum, 2001), bulk-forming agents can take up to 72 h to exert their effects and therefore are not ideal for the initial management of symptomatic constipation in cancer patients (Avila, 2004; Connolly and Larkin, 2012). Bulk forming laxatives require the patients to drink extra fluids as otherwise a viscous mass may form and aggravate a partial bowel obstruction. In addition, significant allergy to these substances has been reported, and their effectiveness in severe constipation is doubtful (Klaschik et al., 2003). Though they are considered safe, some patients' experience suggests that they may worsen symptoms, causing distension, bloating, and abdominal pain (Costilla and Foxx-Orenstein, 2014).

Osmotic Laxatives

Osmotic laxatives such as lactulose, sorbitol, polyethylene glycol compounds, and saline laxatives (magnesium hydroxide), attract and retain fluid within GI tract (Twycross et al., 2012). Osmotic laxatives include salts of poorly absorbable cations (magnesium), anions (phosphate, sulfate) as well as molecules that are not absorbed in the small bowel but are metabolized in the colon (lactulose and sorbitol) and metabolically inert compounds such as polyethylene glycol. The presence of these molecules in the lumen results in water retention to maintain normal osmolarity of the stool (Costilla and Foxx-Orenstein, 2014). The laxative effect of these agents depends on the extent to which they remain in the lumen with the onset between 24 and 72 h (Xing and Soffer, 2001). Adverse effects such as abdominal pain, flatulence, cramping and distension can arise shortly after ingestion, although side-effects may subside after several days of treatment, higher lactulose doses can induce bloating and colic (Ford and Suares, 2011; Costilla and Foxx-Orenstein, 2014). Excessive use of osmotic laxatives may result in hypermagnesemia, hyperphosphatemia, hypercalcemia, hypernatremia, hypokalemia, and hypoalbuminemia (Xing and Soffer, 2001; Kurniawan and Simadibrata, 2011).

Emollient (Stool Softener) Laxatives

Emollient laxatives, also known as stool softeners, are anionic surfactants increasing efficiency of intestinal fluids and facilitating the mixing of aqueous and fatty substances within the feces; this softens the feces allowing them to move more easily through the GI tract (Avila, 2004). Stool softeners are of little value when administered unaccompanied in the treatment of long-term constipation as they do not stimulate peristalsis and evacuation, but concurrent administration with bulk-forming agents and dietary fiber provides beneficial effect reducing straining (O'Mahony et al., 2001; Avila, 2004). Increased fluid intake essential during treatment with emollient laxatives to facilitate stool softening and so are not ideal for chronic constipation in cancer patients. Docusate is the most widely used emollient laxative produced as docusate calcium, docusate sodium, and docusate potassium. The onset of action is 1–2 days after administration but might be up to 5 days. However, docusates have been found to enhance GI or hepatic uptake of other drugs, increasing the risk of hepatotoxicity (Xing and Soffer, 2001). There is also some evidence that docusates cause significant neuronal loss in the myenteric plexus (Fox et al., 1983) and cause structural changes in the gut mucosa of humans (Xing and Soffer, 2001), but the clinical significance of this remains unclear.

Stimulant Laxatives

Stimulant laxatives such as diphenylmethane derivatives (phenolphthalein, sodium picosulfate, anthranoids (senna and cascara), ricinoleic acid (castor oil), and surface-acting agents directly stimulate myenteric neurons to increase peristalsis resulting in reduced net absorption of water and electrolytes from the intraluminal contents (Twycross et al., 2012). Stimulant laxatives are more potent than bulk-forming and osmotic laxatives and appear to be more effective than enemas (Dosh, 2002; Scarlett, 2004). They are amongst the most commonly administered laxatives for opioid-induced constipation (Ruston et al., 2013). Although short-term use is safe, overuse can cause dehydration and long-term ingestion may result in laxative dependence. This dependence also known as 'laxative bowel' is thought to result from damage to the myenteric plexus and smooth muscles cells in the colon (Xing and Soffer, 2001; Kurniawan and Simadibrata, 2011).

Lubricant Laxatives

Lubricant laxatives emulsify themselves into the fecal mass, coating the feces and rectum for easier passage whilst retarding colonic water absorption to simultaneously soften stool (Avila, 2004). Liquid paraffin, also known as mineral oil, is the major lubricant laxative in use although seed oils from croton and arachis are also available (Xing and Soffer, 2001). These laxatives can be administered orally or rectally and are useful for patients who complain of excess straining, but long-term use is associated with malabsorption of fat soluble vitamins and minerals, as well as anal leakage (Costilla and Foxx-Orenstein, 2014). Lubricant laxatives are not routinely recommended for long-term use due to possible inflammatory conditions such as lipoid pneumonia (Schiller, 1999).

Rectal Laxatives

Rectal laxatives such as bisacodyl (stimulant), sodium phosphate (saline), glycerin (osmotic), and mineral oil (lubricant) (Avila, 2004) generally accepted not to be regularly used for CIC treatment (Fallon and O'Neill, 1997), but may be necessary alongside digital stimulation for treating fecal impaction or constipation associated with neurogenic bowel dysfunction. Rectal suppository of bisacodyl (stimulant) is most commonly utilized when evacuation of soft stools is needed, while glycerin suppositories are more appropriate when a hard stool needs to be softened (Fallon and O'Neill, 1997). Acute severe constipation might require an administration of rectal laxatives by enema, however, rectal suppositories or enemas cannot be used in patients with neutropenia and thrombocytopenia (O'Mahony et al., 2001).

EMERGING AND POTENTIAL TREATMENTS FOR CID AND CIC

As current therapies for CID and CIC have limited efficacy and a plethora of adverse effects, a search for and use of novel anti-diarrheal and laxative agents is essential to improve quality of life and chemotherapeutic efficacy for cancer patients. Several emerging and already existing therapies used for treatment of other conditions such as diarrhea predominant irritable bowel syndrome (IBS-D), constipation predominant irritable bowel syndrome (IBS-C) and chronic idiopathic diarrhea and constipation could be employed for the treatment of CID and CIC.

Chloride Channel Inhibition and Activation

Chloride is an essential ion in intestinal secretion and absorption. Secretory diarrhea, such as that experienced in irinotecan-treated patients, results from a combination of excessive secretion and reduced absorption in the intestinal lumen (Thiagarajah and Verkman, 2012). Excessive fluid secretion is driven by active chloride secretion, followed by secondary movement of water and sodium into the intestine. Although there is a lack of selective potent inhibitors of voltage gated chloride channels, inhibition of calcium-activated chloride channels throughout the intestines successfully reduced secretion of chloride into the intestinal lumen (Thiagarajah and Verkman, 2013; Thiagarajah et al., 2015). In a mouse model of rotavirus-induced severe secretory diarrhea, inhibition of calcium-activated chloride channels with a red wine extract reduced intestinal fluid secretion, diminishing the symptoms of diarrhea (Ko et al., 2014).

Conversely, chloride channel activation has been used in the management of chronic idiopathic constipation and constipation related to irritable bowel syndrome (IBS-C). Lubiprostone is a bicyclic fatty acid derived from prostaglandin E1 that specifically activates chloride channels in the intestine, whilst having no effect on smooth muscle contraction (Jun, 2013). The underlying mechanism of lubiprostone involves stimulation of electrogenic chloride secretion though activation of chloride channel type-2 (Lacy and Levy, 2007) and cystic fibrosis transmembrane conductance regulator chloride channels (Bijvelds et al., 2009) in the apical membrane of intestinal epithelial cells. Activation of these epithelial channels results in active secretion of chloride into the intestinal lumen followed by a passive secretion of electrolytes and water increasing the liquidity of the luminal contents (June, 2013). Resulting luminal distension from increased intestinal fluid content promotes GI motility and increases intestinal and colonic transit. In healthy volunteers, daily lubiprostone delays gastric emptying, increases fasting gastric volume, reduces maximum tolerated gastric volume, and accelerates small bowel and colon transit (Camilleri et al., 2006). In randomized trials involving patients with IBS-C, lubiprostone twice daily reduced abdominal pain and increased complete spontaneous bowel movement and improved stool consistency, straining, and bloating (Schey and Rao, 2011). Currently, oral lubiprostone is approved for IBS-C at 8 μg twice daily and CIC at doses of 24 μg twice daily, but approval for CIC is limited to only women who have not responded to laxatives (Davis and Gamier, 2015). At present there are no studies investigating the efficacy of lubiprostone for CID.

Cannabinoid Receptor Inhibition and Activation

Cannabinoids mediate their effects via binding to two main G-protein coupled receptors, CB_1 and CB_2, widely expressed in the GI tract (Abalo et al., 2012). Although the activity of the endocannabinoid system varies between species and different regions of the GI tract within the same species, activation of CB_1 receptors coupled to cholinergic motor neurons has been found to inhibit excitatory neuromuscular transmission in human colonic circular muscle (Hinds et al., 2006) and inhibit colonic propulsion in mice and rat (Pinto et al., 2002; Abalo et al., 2015). In recent human trials, dronabinol, a non-selective cannabinoid receptor agonist, was found to inhibit colonic motility in both healthy subjects (Esfandyari et al., 2006, 2007) and patients with IBS-related diarrhea (IBS-D) (Wong et al., 2011). Conversely, a CB_1 receptor inverse agonist, taranabant, has been shown to improve symptoms related to slow GI motility and abdominal pain when administered *in vivo* in mice (Fichna et al., 2013). Taranabant increased the number of bowel movements after systemic and oral administration and significantly increased fecal pellet output in mice with constipation induced by ipratropium

(Fichna et al., 2013). It has been demonstrated that a low dose of a non-selective cannabinoid agonist WIN55,212-2 reduced the severity of 5-fluorouracil-induced diarrhea in rats (Abalo et al., 2016).

Guanylate Cyclase C Activation

Guanylate cyclase C is the principal receptor for heat-stable enterotoxins and plays a major role in *E. coli*-induced secretory diarrhea (Camilleri, 2010). Enterotoxins and endogenous peptides bind to guanylate cyclase C and stimulate the production of intracellular cyclic guanosine monophosphate (cGMP). Increased levels of cGMP activate the secretion of chloride ions through the cystic fibrosis transmembrane conductance regulator. Linaclotide is a minimally absorbed 14-aminoacid peptide that selectively stimulates intestinal epithelial cell guanylate cyclase C receptors, resulting in increased intracellular and extracellular cGMP leading to accelerated stool transit and laxation (Harris and Crowell, 2007). In phase II and III placebo-controlled studies in chronically constipated and IBS-C patients, linaclotide was found to accelerate colonic transit and improve abdominal pain and symptoms of constipation (Andresen et al., 2007; Johnston et al., 2009, 2010; Lembo et al., 2010). Linaclotide is particularly interesting in that it is both a laxative and analgesic, reducing visceral hypersensitivity with very few drug interactions, it is presently licensed for chronic idiopathic constipation and IBS-C in the USA (Davis and Gamier, 2015), but no trials on CIC have been reported to date.

Probiotics, Antibiotics, and β-glucuronidase Inhibitors

With the recognition that intestinal microbiota play key roles in the pathophysiology of mucositis and development of CID/CIC, both antibiotics and probiotics have emerged as promising therapeutic options. Administration of probiotics have been shown to prevent CID in both 5-fluorouracil and irinotecan-treated animals (Bültzingslöwen et al., 2003; Bowen et al., 2007). Similarly, a combination of *Lactobacillus rhamnosus* and fiber has been found to reduce the severity of grade 3/4 5-fluorouracil/leucovorin-induced diarrhea by 15% in a randomized study of patients treated for colorectal cancer (Österlund et al., 2007). Administration of oral antibiotics, such as fluoroquinolone, has also been recommended for aggressive treatment of CID (Benson et al., 2004a; Maroun et al., 2007).

The selective inhibition of bacterial β-glucuronidase has recently been shown to alleviate drug-induced GI toxicity in mice (Wallace et al., 2015). A low-potency β-glucuronidase inhibitor showed promise in reducing the GI toxicity associated with irinotecan in rats (Fittkau et al., 2004). Similarly, oral administration of potent bacterial β-glucuronidase inhibitors has been found to reduce the severity of irinotecan-induced toxicity (Wallace et al., 2010). In clinical trials, Kampo medicine Hangeshashinto (TJ-14) which contains baicalin, a β-glucuronidase inhibitor, has been found to successfully reduce both the incidence and duration of chemotherapy-induced oral mucositis in colorectal cancer patients when compared to placebo patients (Matsuda et al., 2015). In non-small-cell lung cancer patients TJ-14 alleviated irinotecan-induced diarrhea (Mori et al., 2003). Compared with control patients, the TJ-14-treated patients showed a significant improvement in both diarrhea grade, as well as a reduced frequency of grade 3 and 4 diarrhea (Mori et al., 2003).

CONCLUSION

Chemotherapy-induced diarrhea and CIC are amongst the most common chemotherapy-induced GI toxicities, heavily contributing to treatment delays, dose reductions and in some cases cessation of anti-cancer treatment, greatly effecting management and clinical outcomes. Current treatments for CID and CIC are limited and come with a profuse amount of concomitant symptoms; however, novel therapies present a promising avenue of treatment for CID and CIC. Identification of potential targets and the development of novel treatments alleviating chemotherapy-induced toxicity are essential to improve clinical outcomes and quality of life amongst cancer sufferers.

AUTHOR CONTRIBUTIONS

RM: conception and manuscript writing; VS, RA, JB, and KN: critical revision of the manuscript. All authors approved final version of the manuscript to be published and agreed to be accountable for all aspects of the work in ensuring that questions related to the accuracy or integrity of any part of the work are appropriately investigated and resolved.

FUNDING

This study is funded by the Victoria University (Australia) Research Support Fund.

REFERENCES

Abalo, R., Chen, C., Vera, G., Fichna, J., Thakur, G., López-Pérez, A., et al. (2015). In vitro and non-invasive in vivo effects of the cannabinoid-1 receptor agonist AM841 on gastrointestinal motor function in the rat. *Neurogastroenterol. Motil.* 27, 1721–1735. doi: 10.1111/nmo.12668

Abalo, R., Uranga, J. A., Pérez-García, I., De Andrés, R., Girón, R., Vera, G., et al. (2016). May cannabinoids prevent the development of chemotherapy-induced diarrhea and intestinal mucositis? Experimental study in the rat. *Neurogastroenterol. Motil.* doi: 10.1111/nmo.12952 [Epub ahead of print],

Abalo, R., Vera, G., López-Pérez, A. E., Martínez-Villaluenga, M., and Martín-Fontelles, M. I. (2012). The gastrointestinal pharmacology of cannabinoids: focus on motility. *Pharmacology* 90, 1–10. doi: 10.1159/000339072

Abernethy, A. P., Wheeler, J. L., and Zafar, S. Y. (2009). Detailing of gastrointestinal symptoms in cancer patients with advanced disease: new methodologies, new insights, and a proposed approach. *Curr. Opin. Support. Palliat. Care* 3, 41–49. doi: 10.1097/SPC.0b013e32832531ce

Abramowitz, L., Béziaud, N., Labreze, L., Giardina, V., Caussé, C., Chuberre, B., et al. (2013). Prevalence and impact of constipation and bowel dysfunction induced by strong opioids: a cross-sectional survey of 520 patients with cancer pain: DYONISOS study. *J. Med. Econ.* 16, 1423–1433. doi: 10.3111/13696998.2013.851082

Andresen, V., Camilleri, M., Busciglio, I. A., Grudell, A., Burton, D., Mckinzie, S., et al. (2007). Effect of 5 days linaclotide on transit and bowel function in females with constipation-predominant irritable bowel syndrome. *Gastroenterology* 133, 761–768. doi: 10.1053/j.gastro.2007.06.067

Anthony, L. B. (2010). "Diarrhea, constipation, and obstruction in cancer management," in *The MASCC Textbook of Cancer Supportive Care and Survivorship*, ed. N. Ian Olver (Berlin: Springer), 249–260.

Araki, E., Ishikawa, M., Iigo, M., Koide, T., Itabashi, M., and Hoshi, A. (1993). Relationship between development of diarrhea and the concentration of SN-38, an active metabolite of CPT-11, in the intestine and the blood plasma of athymic mice following intraperitoneal administration of CPT-11. *Cancer Sci.* 84, 697–702.

Arbuckle, R., Huber, S., and Zacker, C. (2000). The consequences of diarrhea occurring during chemotherapy for colorectal cancer: a retrospective study. *Oncologist* 5, 250–259. doi: 10.1634/theoncologist.5-3-250

Ardizzoni, A., Boni, L., Tiseo, M., Fossella, F. V., Schiller, J. H., Paesmans, M., et al. (2007). Cisplatin- versus carboplatin-based chemotherapy in first-line treatment of advanced non–small-cell lung cancer: an individual patient data meta-analysis. *J. Natl. Cancer Inst.* 99, 847–857. doi: 10.1093/jnci/djk196

Ashraf, W., Park, F., Lof, J., and Quigley, E. M. (1996). An examination of the reliability of reported stool frequency in the diagnosis of idiopathic constipation. *Am. J. Gastroenterol.* 91, 26–32.

Avila, J. G. (2004). Pharmacologic treatment of constipation in cancer patients. *Cancer Control* 11, 10–18.

Bassotti, G., and Villanacci, V. (2011). Can "functional" constipation be considered as a form of enteric neuro-gliopathy? *Glia* 59, 345–350. doi: 10.1002/glia.21115

Benson, A. B., Ajani, J. A., Catalano, R. B., Engelking, C., Kornblau, S. M., Martenson, J. A., et al. (2004a). Recommended guidelines for the treatment of cancer treatment-induced diarrhea. *J. Clin. Oncol.* 22, 2918–2926. doi: 10.1200/JCO.2004.04.132

Benson, A. B., Schrag, D., Somerfield, M. R., Cohen, A. M., Figueredo, A. T., Flynn, P. J., et al. (2004b). American Society of Clinical Oncology recommendations on adjuvant chemotherapy for stage II colon cancer. *J. Clin. Oncol.* 22, 3408–3419. doi: 10.1200/JCO.2004.05.063

Benyamin, R., Trescot, A. M., Datta, S., Buenaventura, R., Adlaka, R., Sehgal, N., et al. (2008). Opioid complications and side effects. *Pain Physician* 11, S105–S120.

Bhattacharya, S., Vijayasekar, C., Worlding, J., and Mathew, G. (2008). Octreotide in chemotherapy induced diarrhoea in colorectal cancer: a review article. *Acta Gastroenterol. Belg.* 72, 289–295.

Bijvelds, M. J., Bot, A. G., Escher, J. C., and De Jonge, H. R. (2009). Activation of intestinal Cl-secretion by lubiprostone requires the cystic fibrosis transmembrane conductance regulator. *Gastroenterology* 137, 976–985. doi: 10.1053/j.gastro.2009.05.037

Boussios, S., Pentheroudakis, G., Katsanos, K., and Pavlidis, N. (2012). Systemic treatment-induced gastrointestinal toxicity: incidence, clinical presentation and management. *Ann. Gastroenterol.* 25, 106–118.

Bowen, J. M., Stringer, A. M., Gibson, R. J., Yeoh, A. S., Hannam, S., and Keefe, D. M. (2007). VSL# 3 probiotic treatment reduces chemotherapy-induced diarrhoea and weight loss. *Cancer Biol. Ther.* 6, 1445–1450. doi: 10.4161/cbt.6.9.4622

Bültzingslöwen, I., Adlerberth, I., Wold, A., Dahlén, G., and Jontell, M. (2003). Oral and intestinal microflora in 5-fluorouracil treated rats, translocation to cervical and mesenteric lymph nodes and effects of probiotic bacteria. *Oral Microbiol. Immunol.* 18, 278–284. doi: 10.1034/j.1399-302X.2003.00075.x

Camilleri, M. (2010). Review article: new receptor targets for medical therapy in irritable bowel syndrome. *Aliment. Pharmacol. Ther.* 31, 35–46. doi: 10.1111/j.1365-2036.2009.04153.x

Camilleri, M. (2011). Opioid-induced constipation: challenges and therapeutic opportunities. *Am. J. Gastroenterol.* 106, 835–842. doi: 10.1038/ajg.2011.30

Camilleri, M., Bharucha, A. E., Ueno, R., Burton, D., Thomforde, G. M., Baxter, K., et al. (2006). Effect of a selective chloride channel activator, lubiprostone, on gastrointestinal transit, gastric sensory, and motor functions in healthy volunteers. *Am. J. Physiol.Gastrointest. Liver Physiol.* 290, G942–G947. doi: 10.1152/ajpgi.00264.2005

Carelle, N., Piotto, E., Bellanger, A., Germanaud, J., Thuillier, A., and Khayat, D. (2002). Changing patient perceptions of the side effects of cancer chemotherapy. *Cancer* 95, 155–163. doi: 10.1002/cncr.10630

Castro-Rodríguez, J. A., Salazar-Lindo, E., and León-Barúa, R. (1997). Differentiation of osmotic and secretory diarrhoea by stool carbohydrate and osmolar gap measurements. *Arch. Dis. Child.* 77, 201–205. doi: 10.1136/adc.77.3.201

Chandrasekharan, B., Anitha, M., Blatt, R., Shahnavaz, N., Kooby, D., Staley, C., et al. (2011). Colonic motor dysfunction in human diabetes is associated with enteric neuronal loss and increased oxidative stress. *Neurogastroenterol. Motil.* 23, 131–138. doi: 10.1111/j.1365-2982.2010.01611.x

Connolly, M., and Larkin, P. (2012). Managing constipation: a focus on care and treatment in the palliative setting. *Br. J. Community Nurs.* 17, 60–67. doi: 10.12968/bjcn.2012.17.2.60

Cortesini, C., Cianchi, F., Infantino, A., and Lise, M. (1995). Nitric oxide synthase and VIP distribution in enteric nervous system in idiopathic chronic constipation. *Dig. Dis. Sci.* 40, 2450–2455. doi: 10.1007/BF02063253

Costilla, V. C., and Foxx-Orenstein, A. E. (2014). Constipation: understanding mechanisms and management. *Clin. Geriatr. Med.* 30, 107–115. doi: 10.1016/j.cger.2013.10.001

Culpepper-Morgan, J. A., Inturrisi, C. E., Portenoy, R. K., Foley, K., Houde, R. W., Marsh, F., et al. (1992). Treatment of opioid-induced constipation with oral naloxone: a pilot study. *Clin. Pharmacol. Ther.* 52, 90–95. doi: 10.1038/clpt.1992.106

Davis, M., and Gamier, P. (2015). New options in constipation management. *Curr. Oncol. Rep.* 17, 1–11. doi: 10.1007/s11912-015-0481-x

De Giorgio, R., and Camilleri, M. (2004). Human enteric neuropathies: morphology and molecular pathology. *Neurogastroenterol. Motil.* 16, 515–531. doi: 10.1111/j.1365-2982.2004.00538.x

De Giorgio, R., Guerrini, S., Barbara, G., Cremon, C., Stanghellini, V., and Corinaldesi, R. (2004). New insights into human enteric neuropathies. *Neurogastroenterol. Motil.* 16, 143–147. doi: 10.1111/j.1743-3150.2004.00491.x

De Giorgio, R., Stanghellini, V., Barbara, G., Corinaldesi, R., De Ponti, F., Tonini, M., et al. (2000). Primary enteric neuropathies underlying gastrointestinal motor dysfunction. *Scand. J. Gastroenterol.* 35, 114–122. doi: 10.1080/003655200750024263

Denlinger, C. S., and Barsevick, A. M. (2009). The challenges of colorectal cancer survivorship. *J. Natl. Compr. Canc. Netw.* 7, 883–894.

Dennison, C., Prasad, M., Lloyd, A., Bhattacharyya, S. K., Dhawan, R., and Coyne, K. (2005). The health-related quality of life and economic burden of constipation. *Pharmacoeconomics* 23, 461–476. doi: 10.2165/00019053-200523050-00006

De Schepper, H. U., Cremonini, F., Park, M. I., and Camilleri, M. (2004). Opioids and the gut: pharmacology and current clinical experience. *Neurogastroenterol. Motil.* 16, 383–394. doi: 10.1111/j.1365-2982.2004.00513.x

Dieras, V., Lortholary, A., Laurence, V., Delva, R., Girre, V., Livartowski, A., et al. (2013). Cabazitaxel in patients with advanced solid tumours: results of a phase I and pharmacokinetic study. *Eur. J. Cancer* 49, 25–34. doi: 10.1016/j.ejca.2012.07.008

Dinning, P., Smith, T., and Scott, S. (2009). Pathophysiology of colonic causes of chronic constipation. *Neurogastroenterol. Motil.* 21, 20–30. doi: 10.3748/wjg.v19.i26.4099

Dosh, S. A. (2002). Evaluation and treatment of constipation (Clinical Update). *J. Fam. Pract.* 51, 555–560.

Douillard, J.-Y., Siena, S., Cassidy, J., Tabernero, J., Burkes, R., Barugel, M., et al. (2010). Randomized, phase III trial of panitumumab with infusional fluorouracil, leucovorin, and oxaliplatin (FOLFOX4) versus FOLFOX4 alone as first-line treatment in patients with previously untreated metastatic colorectal cancer: the PRIME study. *J. Clin. Oncol.* 28, 4697–4705. doi: 10.1200/JCO.2009.27.4860

Dranitsaris, G., Maroun, J., and Shah, A. (2005). Estimating the cost of illness in colorectal cancer patients who were hospitalized for severe chemotherapy-induced diarrhea. *Can. J. Gastroenterol.* 19, 83–87. doi: 10.1155/2005/618504

Esfandyari, T., Camilleri, M., Busciglio, I., Burton, D., Baxter, K., and Zinsmeister, A. R. (2007). Effects of a cannabinoid receptor agonist on colonic motor and sensory functions in humans: a randomized, placebo-controlled study. *Am. J. Physiol. Gastrointest. Liver Physiol.* 293, G137–G145. doi: 10.1152/ajpgi.00565.2006

Esfandyari, T., Camilleri, M., Ferber, I., Burton, D., Baxter, K., and Zinsmeister, A. (2006). Effect of a cannabinoid agonist on gastrointestinal transit and postprandial satiation in healthy human subjects: a randomized, placebo-controlled study. *Neurogastroenterol. Motil.* 18, 831–838. doi: 10.1111/j.1365-2982.2006.00834.x

Extra, J. M., Espie, M., Calvo, F., Ferme, C., Mignot, L., and Marty, M. (1990). Phase I study of oxaliplatin in patients with advanced cancer. *Cancer Chemother. Pharmacol.* 25, 299–303. doi: 10.1007/BF00684890

Falcón, B. S., López, M. B., Muñoz, B. M., Sánchez, A. Á, and Rey, E. (2016). Fecal impaction: a systematic review of its medical complications. *BMC Geriatrics* 16:4. doi: 10.1186/s12877-015-0162-5

Fallon, M., and O'Neill, B. (1997). ABC of palliative care. Constipation and diarrhoea. *BMJ: Br. Med. J.* 315, 1293–1296. doi: 10.1136/bmj.315.7118.1293

Ferlay, J., Soerjomataram, I., Dikshit, R., Eser, S., Mathers, C., Rebelo, M., et al. (2015). Cancer incidence and mortality worldwide: sources, methods and major patterns in GLOBOCAN 2012. *Int. J. Cancer* 136, E359–E386. doi: 10.1002/ijc.29210

Fichna, J., Sibaev, A., Sałaga, M., Sobczak, M., and Storr, M. (2013). The cannabinoid-1 receptor inverse agonist taranabant reduces abdominal pain and increases intestinal transit in mice. *Neurogastroenterol. Motil.* 25, e550–e559. doi: 10.1111/nmo.12158

Fickel, J., Bagnol, D., Watson, S. J., and Akil, H. (1997). Opioid receptor expression in the rat gastrointestinal tract: a quantitative study with comparison to the brain. *Brain Res. Mol. Brain Res.* 46, 1–8. doi: 10.1016/S0169-328X(96)00266-5

Fittkau, M., Voigt, W., Holzhausen, H.-J., and Schmoll, H.-J. (2004). Saccharic acid 1.4-lactone protects against CPT-11-induced mucosa damage in rats. *J. Cancer Res. Clin. Oncol.* 130, 388–394. doi: 10.1007/s00432-004-0557-8

Ford, A. C., and Suares, N. C. (2011). Effect of laxatives and pharmacological therapies in chronic idiopathic constipation: systematic review and meta-analysis. *Gut* 60, 209–218. doi: 10.1136/gut.2010.227132

Fox, D. A., Epstein, M. L., and Bass, P. (1983). Surfactants selectively ablate enteric neurons of the rat jejunum. *J. Pharmacol. Exp. Ther.* 227, 538–544.

Fraiser, L. H., Kanekal, S., and Kehrer, J. P. (1991). Cyclophosphamide toxicity. *Drugs* 42, 781–795. doi: 10.2165/00003495-199142050-00005

Furness, J. B. (2012). The enteric nervous system and neurogastroenterology. *Nat. Rev. Gastroenterol. Hepatol.* 9, 286–294. doi: 10.1038/nrgastro.2012.32

Garg, S., Nurgali, K., and Mishra, V. K. (2016). Food proteins as source of opioid peptides-a review. *Curr. Med. Chem.* 23, 893–910. doi: 10.2174/0929867323666160219115226

Gatti, A., and Sabato, A. F. (2012). Management of opioid-induced constipation in cancer patients. *Clin. Drug Investig.* 32, 293–301. doi: 10.2165/11598000-000000000-00000

Ghobrial, I. M., and Rajkumar, V. S. (2003). Management of thalidomide toxicity. *J. Support. Oncol.* 1, 194–213.

Gibson, R. J., Bowen, J. M., Inglis, M. R., Cummins, A. G., and Keefe, D. M. (2003). Irinotecan causes severe small intestinal damage, as well as colonic damage, in the rat with implanted breast cancer. *J. Gastroenterol. Hepatol.* 18, 1095–1100. doi: 10.1046/j.1440-1746.2003.03136.x

Gibson, R. J., and Keefe, D. M. (2006). Cancer chemotherapy-induced diarrhoea and constipation: mechanisms of damage and prevention strategies. *Support. Care Cancer* 14, 890–900. doi: 10.1007/s00520-006-0040-y

Goffin, J., Lacchetti, C., Ellis, P. M., Ung, Y. C., and Evans, W. K. (2010). First-line systemic chemotherapy in the treatment of advanced non-small cell lung cancer: a systematic review. *J. Thorac. Oncol.* 5, 260–274. doi: 10.1097/JTO.0b013e3181c6f035

Gonzalez, C. E., and Halm, J. K. (2016). "Constipation in cancer patients," in *Oncologic Emergency Medicine*, eds K. H. Todd, C. R. Jr. Thomas (Switzerland: Springer International Publishing), 327–332. doi: 10.1007/978-3-319-26387-8_28

Gwynne, R. M., Thomas, E., Goh, S., Sjövall, H., and Bornstein, J. (2004). Segmentation induced by intraluminal fatty acid in isolated guinea-pig duodenum and jejunum. *J. Physiol.* 556, 557–569. doi: 10.1113/jphysiol.2003.057182

Hansen, M. B. (2003). The enteric nervous system II: gastrointestinal functions. *Pharmacol. Toxicol.* 92, 249–257. doi: 10.1034/j.1600-0773.2003.920601.x

Harris, L. A., and Crowell, M. D. (2007). Linaclotide, a new direction in the treatment of irritable bowel syndrome and chronic constipation. *Curr. Opin. Mol. Ther.* 9, 403–410.

He, C. L., Burgart, L., Wang, L., Pemberton, J., Young-Fadok, T., Szurszewski, J., et al. (2000). Decreased interstitial cell of Cajal volume in patients with slow-transit constipation. *Gastroenterology* 118, 14–21. doi: 10.1016/S0016-5085(00)70409-4

Hecht, J. R. (1998). Gastrointestinal toxicity or irinotecan. *Oncology (Williston Park)* 12, 72–78.

Hinds, N. M., Ullrich, K., and Smid, S. D. (2006). Cannabinoid 1 (CB1) receptors coupled to cholinergic motorneurones inhibit neurogenic circular muscle contractility in the human colon. *Br. J. Pharmacol.* 148, 191–199. doi: 10.1038/sj.bjp.0706710

Högenauer, C., Aichbichler, B., Santa Ana, C., Porter, J., and Fordtran, J. (2002). Effect of octreotide on fluid absorption and secretion by the normal human jejunum and ileum in vivo. *Aliment. Pharmacol. Ther.* 16, 769–777. doi: 10.1046/j.1365-2036.2002.01228.x

Holland, J. F., Scharlau, C., Gailani, S., Krant, M. J., Olson, K. B., Horton, J., et al. (1973). Vincristine treatment of advanced cancer: a cooperative study of 392 cases. *Cancer Res.* 33, 1258–1264.

Huizinga, J. D., and Lammers, W. J. (2009). Gut peristalsis is governed by a multitude of cooperating mechanisms. *Am. J. Physiol.Gastrointest. Liver Physiol.* 296, G1–G8. doi: 10.1152/ajpgi.90380.2008

Ikuno, N., Soda, H., Watanabe, M., and Oka, M. (1995). Irinotecan (CPT-11) and characteristic mucosal changes in the mouse ileum and cecum. *J. Natl. Cancer Inst.* 87, 1876–1883. doi: 10.1093/jnci/87.24.1876

Ilson, D. H., Saltz, L., Enzinger, P., Huang, Y., Kornblith, A., Gollub, M., et al. (1999). Phase II trial of weekly irinotecan plus cisplatin in advanced esophageal cancer. *J. Clin. Oncol.* 17, 3270–3275.

Iwamoto, T. (2013). Clinical application of drug delivery systems in cancer chemotherapy: review of the efficacy and side effects of approved drugs. *Biol. Pharm. Bull.* 36, 715–718. doi: 10.1248/bpb.b12-01102

Jemal, A., Bray, F., Center, M. M., Ferlay, J., Ward, E., and Forman, D. (2011). Global cancer statistics. *CA Cancer J. Clin.* 61, 69–90. doi: 10.3322/caac.20107

Jemal, A., Center, M. M., Desantis, C., and Ward, E. M. (2010a). Global patterns of cancer incidence and mortality rates and trends. *Cancer Epidemiol. Biomarkers Prev.* 19, 1893–1907. doi: 10.1158/1055-9965.EPI-10-0437

Jemal, A., Siegel, R., Xu, J., and Ward, E. (2010b). Cancer statistics, 2010. *CA Cancer J. Clin.* 60, 277–300. doi: 10.3322/caac.20073

Johnson, L., Ghishan, F. K., Kaunitz, J., Merchant, J., Said, H., and Wood, J. (2012). *Physiology of the Gastrointestinal Tract.* Amsterdam: Elsevier Inc.

Johnston, J. M., Kurtz, C. B., Drossman, D. A., Lembo, A. J., Jeglinski, B. I., Macdougall, J. E., et al. (2009). Pilot study on the effect of linaclotide in patients with chronic constipation. *Am. J. Gastroenterol.* 104, 125–132. doi: 10.1038/ajg.2008.59

Johnston, J. M., Kurtz, C. B., Macdougall, J. E., Lavins, B. J., Currie, M. G., Fitch, D. A., et al. (2010). Linaclotide improves abdominal pain and bowel habits in a phase IIb study of patients with irritable bowel syndrome with constipation. *Gastroenterology* 139, 1877–1886. doi: 10.1053/j.gastro.2010.08.041

Jun, J. Y. (2013). Role of lubiprostone on gastrointestinal motility. *J Neurogastroenterol. Motil.* 19, 277–278. doi: 10.5056/jnm.2013.19.3.277

Kase, Y., Hayakawa, T., Aburada, M., Komatsu, Y., and Kamataki, T. (1997a). Preventive effects of Hange-shashin-to on irinotecan hydrochloride-caused diarrhea and its relevance to the colonic prostaglandin E2 and water absorption in the rat. *Jpn. J. Pharmacol.* 75, 407–413. doi: 10.1254/jjp.75.407

Kase, Y., Hayakawa, T., Togashi, Y., and Kamataki, T. (1997b). Relevance of irinotecan hydrochloride-induced diarrhea to the level of prostaglandin E2 and water absorption of large intestine in rats. *Jpn. J. Pharmacol.* 75, 399–405. doi: 10.1254/jjp.75.407

Kaufmann, M., Hortobagyi, G. N., Goldhirsch, A., Scholl, S., Makris, A., Valagussa, P., et al. (2006). Recommendations from an international expert panel on the use of neoadjuvant (primary) systemic treatment of operable breast cancer: an update. *J. Clin. Oncol.* 24, 1940–1949. doi: 10.1200/JCO.2005.02.6187

Keefe, D., Brealey, J., Goland, G., and Cummins, A. (2000). Chemotherapy for cancer causes apoptosis that precedes hypoplasia in crypts of the small intestine in humans. *Gut* 47, 632–637. doi: 10.1136/gut.47.5.632

Kim, A. R., Cho, J., Hsu, Y.-J., Choi, M. G., Noh, J. H., Sohn, T. S., et al. (2012). Changes of quality of life in gastric cancer patients after curative resection: a longitudinal cohort study in Korea. *Ann. Surg.* 256, 1008–1013. doi: 10.1097/SLA.0b013e31827661c9

Kim, D., Kim, J., Lee, S.-H., Kim, T., Heo, D., Bang, Y.-J., et al. (2003). Phase II study of oxaliplatin, 5-fluorouracil and leucovorin in previously platinum-treated patients with advanced gastric cancer. *Ann. Oncol.* 14, 383–387. doi: 10.1093/annonc/mdg106

Kirschenbaum, H. L. (2001). Handbook of nonprescription drugs. *Am. J. Pharm. Educ.* 65, 100.

Klaschik, E., Nauck, F., and Ostgathe, C. (2003). Constipation—modern laxative therapy. *Support. Care Cancer* 11, 679–685. doi: 10.1007/s00520-003-0525-x

Ko, E.-A., Jin, B.-J., Namkung, W., Ma, T., Thiagarajah, J. R., and Verkman, A. (2014). Chloride channel inhibition by a red wine extract and a synthetic small molecule prevents rotaviral secretory diarrhoea in neonatal mice. *Gut* 63, 1120–1129. doi: 10.1136/gutjnl-2013-305663

Kuebler, P. J., Colangelo, L., O'connell, M. J., Smith, R. E., Yothers, G., Begovic, M., et al. (2007). Severe enteropathy among patients with stage II/III colon cancer treated on a randomized trial of bolus 5-fluorouracil/leucovorin plus or minus oxaliplatin. *Cancer* 110, 1945–1950. doi: 10.1002/cncr.23013

Kuizenga, M. H., Sia, T. C., Dodds, K. N., Wiklendt, L., Arkwright, J. W., Thomas, A., et al. (2015). Neurally mediated propagating discrete clustered contractions superimposed on myogenic ripples in ex vivo segments of human ileum. *American Journal of Physiology-Gastrointestinal and Liver Physiology* 308, G1–G11. doi: 10.1152/ajpgi.00230.2014

Kurniawan, I., and Simadibrata, M. (2011). Management of chronic constipation in the elderly. *Acta Med Indones* 43, 195–205.

Lacy, B. E., and Levy, L. C. (2007). Lubiprostone: a chloride channel activator. *J. Clin. Gastroenterol.* 41, 345–351. doi: 10.1097/01.mcg.0000225665.68920.df

Lawrence, T. (2009). The nuclear factor NF-κB pathway in inflammation. *Cold Spring Harb. Perspect. Biol.* 1, a001651. doi: 10.1101/cshperspect.a001651

Leahy, K. M., Ornberg, R. L., Wang, Y., Zweifel, B. S., Koki, A. T., and Masferrer, J. L. (2002). Cyclooxygenase-2 inhibition by celecoxib reduces proliferation and induces apoptosis in angiogenic endothelial cells in vivo. *Cancer Res.* 62, 625–631.

Lee, C. S., Ryan, E. J., and Doherty, G. A. (2014). Gastro-intestinal toxicity of chemotherapeutics in colorectal cancer: the role of inflammation. *World J. Gastroenterol.* 20, 3751–3761. doi: 10.3748/wjg.v20.i14.3751

Lembo, A., and Camilleri, M. (2003). Chronic constipation. *N. Engl. J. Med.* 349, 1360–1368. doi: 10.1056/NEJMra020995

Lembo, A. J., Kurtz, C. B., Macdougall, J. E., Lavins, B., Currie, M. G., Fitch, D. A., et al. (2010). Efficacy of linaclotide for patients with chronic constipation. *Gastroenterology* 138, 886–895. doi: 10.1053/j.gastro.2009.12.050

Lenfers, B., Loeffler, T., Droege, C., and Hausamen, T. (1999). Substantial activity of budesonide in patients with irinotecan (CPT-11) and 5-fluorouracil induced diarrhea and failure of loperamide treatment. *Ann. Oncol.* 10, 1251–1253. doi: 10.1023/A:1008390308416

Leung, L., Riutta, T., Kotecha, J., and Rosser, W. (2011). Chronic constipation: an evidence-based review. *J. Am. Board Fam. Med.* 24, 436–451. doi: 10.3122/jabfm.2011.04.100272

Loening-Baucke, V. (1996). Encopresis and soiling. *Pediatr. Clin. North Am.* 43, 279–298. doi: 10.1016/S0031-3955(05)70406-5

Logan, R. M., Gibson, R. J., Bowen, J. M., Stringer, A. M., Sonis, S. T., and Keefe, D. M. (2008). Characterisation of mucosal changes in the alimentary tract following administration of irinotecan: implications for the pathobiology of mucositis. *Cancer Chemother. Pharmacol.* 62, 33–41. doi: 10.1007/s00280-007-0570-0

Louvet, C., Andre, T., Tigaud, J., Gamelin, E., Douillard, J., Brunet, R., et al. (2002). Phase II study of oxaliplatin, fluorouracil, and folinic acid in locally advanced or metastatic gastric cancer patients. *J. Clin. Oncol.* 20, 4543–4548. doi: 10.1200/JCO.2002.02.021

Lundgren, O., Peregrin, A. T., Persson, K., Kordasti, S., Uhnoo, I., and Svensson, L. (2000). Role of the enteric nervous system in the fluid and electrolyte secretion of rotavirus diarrhea. *Science* 287, 491–495. doi: 10.1126/science.287.5452.491

MacDonald, A., Shearer, M., Paterson, P., and Finlay, I. (1991). Relationship between outlet obstruction constipation and obstructed urinary flow. *Br. J. Surg.* 78, 693–695. doi: 10.1002/bjs.1800780620

Mancini, I., and Bruera, E. (1998). Constipation in advanced cancer patients. *Support. Care Cancer* 6, 356–364. doi: 10.1007/s005200050177

Maroun, J. A., Anthony, L. B., Blais, N., Burkes, R., Dowden, S. D., Dranitsaris, G., et al. (2007). Prevention and management of chemotherapy-induced diarrhea in patients with colorectal cancer: a consensus statement by the canadian working group on chemotherapy-induced diarrhea. *Curr. Oncol.* 14, 13–20. doi: 10.3747/co.2007.96

Matsuda, C., Munemoto, Y., Mishima, H., Nagata, N., Oshiro, M., Kataoka, M., et al. (2015). Double-blind, placebo-controlled, randomized phase II study of TJ-14 (Hangeshashinto) for infusional fluorinated-pyrimidine-based colorectal cancer chemotherapy-induced oral mucositis. *Cancer Chemother. Pharmacol.* 76, 97–103. doi: 10.1007/s00280-015-2767-y

McKay, J. S., Linaker, B. D., and Turnberg, L. A. (1981). Influence of opiates on ion transport across rabbit ileal mucosa. *Gastroenterology* 80, 279–284.

McQuade, R., Stojanovska, V., Donald, E., Abalo, R., Bornstein, J., and Nurgali, K. (2016). Gastrointestinal dysfunction and enteric neurotoxicity following treatment with anticancer chemotherapeutic agent 5-fluorouracil. *Neurogastroenterol. Motil.* doi: 10.1111/nmo.12890 [Epub ahead of print],

McQuade, R. M., Bornstein, J. C., and Nurgali, K. (2014). Anti-colorectal cancer chemotherapy-induced diarrhoea: current treatments and side-effects. *Int. J. Clin. Med.* 5, 393–406. doi: 10.4236/ijcm.2014.57054

Mitchell, E. P. (2006). Gastrointestinal toxicity of chemotherapeutic agents. *Semin. Oncol.* 33, 106–120. doi: 10.1053/j.seminoncol.2005.12.001

Mori, K., Kondo, T., Kamiyama, Y., Kano, Y., and Tominaga, K. (2003). Preventive effect of Kampo medicine (Hangeshashin-to) against irinotecan-induced diarrhea in advanced non-small-cell lung cancer. *Cancer Chemother. Pharmacol.* 51, 403–406.

Mutch, D. G., Orlando, M., Goss, T., Teneriello, M. G., Gordon, A. N., Mcmeekin, S. D., et al. (2007). Randomized phase III trial of gemcitabine compared with pegylated liposomal doxorubicin in patients with platinum-resistant ovarian cancer. *J. Clin. Oncol.* 25, 2811–2818. doi: 10.1200/JCO.2006.09.6735

Nightingale, G., and Ryu, J. (2012). Cabazitaxel (jevtana): a novel agent for metastatic castration-resistant prostate cancer. *Pharm. Ther.* 37, 440–448.

Okines, A., Verheij, M., Allum, W., Cunningham, D., Cervantes, A., and Group, E. G. W. (2010). Gastric cancer: ESMO clinical practice guidelines for diagnosis, treatment and follow-up. *Ann. Oncol.* 21, v50–v54. doi: 10.1093/annonc/mdq164

O'Mahony, S., Coyle, N., and Payne, R. (2001). Current management of opioid-related side effects. *Oncology (Williston Park)* 15, 61–82.

Österlund, P., Ruotsalainen, T., Korpela, R., Saxelin, M., Ollus, A., Valta, P., et al. (2007). Lactobacillus supplementation for diarrhoea related to chemotherapy of colorectal cancer: a randomised study. *Br. J. Cancer* 97, 1028–1034. doi: 10.1038/sj.bjc.6603990

Panchal, S. J., Müller-Schwefe, P., and Wurzelmann, J. I. (2007). Opioid-induced bowel dysfunction: prevalence, pathophysiology and burden. *Int. J. Clin. Pract.* 61, 1181–1187. doi: 10.1111/j.1742-1241.2007.01415.x

Peterson, D., Bensadoun, R.-J., Roila, F., and Group, E. G. W. (2011). Management of oral and gastrointestinal mucositis: ESMO clinical practice guidelines. *Ann. Oncol.* 22, vi78–vi84. doi: 10.1093/annonc/mdr391

Phillips, R. J., and Powley, T. L. (2007). Innervation of the gastrointestinal tract: patterns of aging. *Auton. Neurosci.* 136, 1–19. doi: 10.1016/j.autneu.2007.04.005

Pini, A., Garella, R., Idrizaj, E., Calosi, L., Baccari, M., and Vannucchi, M. (2016). Glucagon-like peptide 2 counteracts the mucosal damage and the neuropathy induced by chronic treatment with cisplatin in the mouse gastric fundus. *Neurogastroenterol. Motil.* 28, 206–216. doi: 10.1111/nmo.12712

Pinto, L., Izzo, A. A., Mascolo, N., Capasso, F., Cascio, M. G., Bisogno, T., et al. (2002). Endocannabinoids as physiological regulators of colonic propulsion in mice. *Gastroenterology* 123, 227–234. doi: 10.1053/gast.2002.34242

Pujol, J. L., Viens, P., Rebattu, P., Laurie, S. A., Feld, R., Deneulin, A., et al. (2006). Gefitinib (IRESSA) with vinorelbine or vinorelbine/cisplatin for chemotherapy-naive non-small cell lung cancer patients. *J. Thorac. Oncol.* 1, 417–424. doi: 10.1097/01243894-200606000-00007

Regnard, C., Twycross, R., Mihalyo, M., and Wilcock, A. (2011). Loperamide. *J. Pain Symptom Manage.* 42, 319–323. doi: 10.1016/j.jpainsymman.2011.06.001

Richardson, G., and Dobish, R. (2007). Chemotherapy induced diarrhea. *J. Oncol. Pharm. Pract.* 13, 181–198. doi: 10.1177/1078155207077335

Robinson, A. M., Stojanovska, V., Rahman, A. A., McQuade, R. M., Senior, P. V., and Nurgali, K. (2016). Effects of oxaliplatin treatment on the enteric glial cells and neurons in the mouse ileum. *J. Histochem. Cytochem.* 64, 530–545. doi: 10.1369/0022155416656842

Rothenberg, M. L., Meropol, N. J., Poplin, E. A., Van Cutsem, E., and Wadler, S. (2001). Mortality associated with irinotecan plus bolus fluorouracil/leucovorin: summary findings of an independent panel. *J. Clin. Oncol.* 19, 3801–3807.

Rubenstein, E. B., Peterson, D. E., Schubert, M., Keefe, D., Mcguire, D., Epstein, J., et al. (2004). Clinical practice guidelines for the prevention and treatment of cancer therapy-induced oral and gastrointestinal mucositis. *Cancer* 100, 2026–2046. doi: 10.1002/cncr.20163

Ruston, T., Hunter, K., Cummings, G., and Lazarescu, A. (2013). Efficacy and side-effect profiles of lactulose, docusate sodium, and sennosides compared to PEG in opioid-induced constipation: a systematic review. *Can. Oncol. Nurs. J.* 23, 236–240. doi: 10.5737/1181912x234236240

Sakai, H., Sato, T., Hamada, N., Yasue, M., Ikari, A., Kakinoki, B., et al. (1997). Thromboxane A2, released by the anti-tumour drug irinotecan, is a novel stimulator of Cl- secretion in isolated rat colon. *J. Physiol.* 505, 133–144. doi: 10.1111/j.1469-7793.1997.133bc.x

Scarlett, Y. (2004). Medical management of fecal incontinence. *Gastroenterology* 126, S55–S63. doi: 10.1053/j.gastro.2003.10.007

Schey, R., and Rao, S. S. (2011). Lubiprostone for the treatment of adults with constipation and irritable bowel syndrome. *Dig. Dis. Sci.* 56, 1619–1625. doi: 10.1007/s10620-011-1702-2

Schiller, L. R. (1999). Clinical pharmacology and use of laxatives and lavage solutions. *J. Clin. Gastroenterol.* 28, 11–18. doi: 10.1097/00004836-199901000-00003

Schneider, E. C., Malin, J. L., Kahn, K. L., Ko, C. Y., Adams, J., and Epstein, A. M. (2007). Surviving colorectal cancer. *Cancer* 110, 2075–2082. doi: 10.1002/cncr.23021

Shafi, M. A., and Bresalier, R. S. (2010). The gastrointestinal complications of oncologic therapy. *Gastroenterol. Clin. North Am.* 39, 629–647. doi: 10.1016/j.gtc.2010.08.004

Sharma, R., Tobin, P., and Clarke, S. J. (2005). Management of chemotherapy-induced nausea, vomiting, oral mucositis, and diarrhoea. *Lancet Oncol.* 6, 93–102. doi: 10.1016/S1470-2045(05)01735-3

Smith, L. C., Bertolotti, P., Curran, K., and Jenkins, B. (2008). Gastrointestinal side effects associated with novel therapies in patients with multiple myeloma: consensus statement of the IMF nurse leadership board. *Clin. J. Oncol. Nurs.* 12, 37–52. doi: 10.1188/08.CJON.S1.37-51

Sonis, S. T., Elting, L. S., Keefe, D., Peterson, D. E., Schubert, M., Hauer-Jensen, M., et al. (2004). Perspectives on cancer therapy-induced mucosal injury. *Cancer* 100, 1995–2025. doi: 10.1002/cncr.20162

Stathopoulos, G., Koutantos, J., Lazaki, H., Rigatos, S., Stathopoulos, J., and Deliconstantinos, G. (2007). Capecitabine (Xeloda) as monotherapy in advanced breast and colorectal cancer: effectiveness and side-effects. *Anticancer Res.* 27, 1653–1656.

Stein, A., Voigt, W., and Jordan, K. (2010). Review: chemotherapy-induced diarrhea: pathophysiology, frequency and guideline-based management. *Ther Adv. Med. Oncol.* 2, 51–63. doi: 10.1177/1758834009355164

Stojanovska, V., Sakkal, S., and Nurgali, K. (2015). Platinum-based chemotherapy: gastrointestinal immunomodulation and enteric nervous system toxicity. *Am. J. Physiol.Gastrointest. Liver Physiol.* 308, G223–G232. doi: 10.1152/ajpgi.00212.2014

Stringer, A. M. (2009). Chemotherapy-induced mucositis: the role of gastrointestinal microflora and mucins in the luminal environment. *J. Support Oncol.* 5, 259–267.

Stringer, A. M. (2013). Interaction between host cells and microbes in chemotherapy-induced mucositis. *Nutrients* 5, 1488–1499. doi: 10.3390/nu5051488

Stringer, A. M., Gibson, R. J., Bowen, J. M., and Keefe, D. M. (2009a). Chemotherapy-induced modifications to gastrointestinal microflora: evidence and implications of change. *Curr. Drug Metab.* 10, 79–83. doi: 10.2174/138920009787048419

Stringer, A. M., Gibson, R. J., Bowen, J. M., Logan, R. M., Ashton, K., Yeoh, A. S., et al. (2009b). Irinotecan-induced mucositis manifesting as diarrhoea corresponds with an amended intestinal flora and mucin profile. *Int. J. Exp. Pathol.* 90, 489–499. doi: 10.1111/j.1365-2613.2009.00671.x

Stringer, A. M., Gibson, R. J., Logan, R. M., Bowen, J. M., Yeoh, A. S., Hamilton, J., et al. (2009c). Gastrointestinal microflora and mucins may play a critical role in the development of 5-fluorouracil-induced gastrointestinal mucositis. *Exp. Biol. Med.* 234, 430–441. doi: 10.3181/0810-RM-301

Stringer, A. M., Gibson, R. J., Logan, R. M., Bowen, J. M., Yeoh, A. S., Laurence, J., et al. (2009d). Irinotecan-induced mucositis is associated with changes in intestinal mucins. *Cancer Chemother. Pharmacol.* 64, 123–132. doi: 10.1007/s00280-008-0855-y

Stringer, A. M., Gibson, R. J., Logan, R. M., Bowen, J. M., Yeoh, A. S., Burns, J., et al. (2007). Chemotherapy-induced diarrhea is associated with changes in the luminal environment in the DA rat. *Exp. Biol. Med.* 232, 96–106.

Stringer, A. M., Gibson, R. J., Logan, R. M., Bowen, J. M., Yeoh, A. S., and Keefe, D. M. (2008). Faecal microflora and β-glucuronidase expression are altered in an irinotecan-induced diarrhea model in rats. *Cancer Biol. Ther.* 7, 1919–1925. doi: 10.4161/cbt.7.12.6940

Suzuki, T., Sakai, H., Ikari, A., and Takeguchi, N. (2000). Inhibition of thromboxane A2-induced Cl- secretion by antidiarrhea drug loperamide in isolated rat colon. *J. Pharmacol. Exp. Ther.* 295, 233–238.

Tacar, O., Sriamornsak, P., and Dass, C. R. (2013). Doxorubicin: an update on anticancer molecular action, toxicity and novel drug delivery systems. *J. Pharm. Pharmacol.* 65, 157–170. doi: 10.1111/j.2042-7158.2012.01567.x

Takasuna, K., Hagiwara, T., Hirohashi, M., Kato, M., Nomura, M., Nagai, E., et al. (1996). Involvement of β-glucuronidase in intestinal microflora in the intestinal toxicity of the antitumor camptothecin derivative irinotecan hydrochloride (CPT-11) in rats. *Cancer Res.* 56, 3752–3757.

Talley, N. J. (2003). Definitions, epidemiology, and impact of chronic constipation. *Rev. Gastroenterol. Disord.* 4, S3–S10.

Thiagarajah, J., Donowitz, M., and Verkman, A. (2015). Secretory diarrhoea: mechanisms and emerging therapies. *Nat. Rev. Gastroenterol. Hepatol.* 12, 446–457. doi: 10.1038/nrgastro.2015.111

Thiagarajah, J., and Verkman, A. (2012). CFTR inhibitors for treating diarrheal disease. *Clin. Pharmacol. Ther.* 92, 287–290. doi: 10.1016/j.cgh.2013.12.001

Thiagarajah, J., and Verkman, A. (2013). Chloride channel-targeted therapy for secretory diarrheas. *Curr. Opin. Pharmacol.* 13, 888–894. doi: 10.1016/j.coph.2013.08.005

Thomas, J., Karver, S., Cooney, G. A., Chamberlain, B. H., Watt, C. K., Slatkin, N. E., et al. (2008). Methylnaltrexone for opioid-induced constipation in advanced illness. *N. Engl. J. Med.* 358, 2332–2343. doi: 10.1056/NEJMoa0707377

Thomas, J., Lipman, A., Slatkin, N., Wilson, G., Moehl, M., Wellman, C., et al. (2005). A phase III double-blind placebo-controlled trial of methylnaltrexone (MNTX) for opioid-induced constipation (OIC) in advanced medical illness (AMI). *Proc. Am. Soc. Clin. Oncol.* 25:8003.

Torre, L. A., Bray, F., Siegel, R. L., Ferlay, J., Lortet-Tieulent, J., and Jemal, A. (2015). Global cancer statistics, 2012. *CA Cancer J. Clin.* 65, 87–108. doi: 10.3322/caac.21262

Touchefeu, Y., Montassier, E., Nieman, K., Gastinne, T., Potel, G., Bruley Des Varannes, S., et al. (2014). Systematic review: the role of the gut microbiota in chemotherapy-or radiation-induced gastrointestinal mucositis–current evidence and potential clinical applications. *Aliment. Pharmacol. Ther.* 40, 409–421.

Twycross, R., Sykes, N., Mihalyo, M., and Wilcock, A. (2012). Stimulant laxatives and opioid-induced constipation. *J. Pain Symptom Manage.* 43, 306–313. doi: 10.1016/j.jpainsymman.2011.12.002

Tzavella, K., Riepl, R. L., Klauser, A. G., Voderholzer, W. A., Schindlbeck, N. E., and Müller-Lissner, S. A. (1996). Decreased substance P levels in rectal biopsies from patients with slow transit constipation. *Eur. J. Gastroenterol. Hepatol.* 8, 1207–1211. doi: 10.1097/00042737-199612000-00014

van Vliet, M. J., Harmsen, H. J., De Bont, E. S., and Tissing, W. J. (2010). The role of intestinal microbiota in the development and severity of chemotherapy-induced mucositis. *PLoS Pathogens* 6:e1000879. doi: 10.1371/journal.ppat.1000879

Vera, G., Castillo, M., Cabezos, P., Chiarlone, A., Martín, M., Gori, A., et al. (2011). Enteric neuropathy evoked by repeated cisplatin in the rat. *Neurogastroenterol. Motil.* 23, 370–378. doi: 10.1111/j.1365-2982.2011.01674.x

Verstappen, C. C., Heimans, J. J., Hoekman, K., and Postma, T. J. (2003). Neurotoxic complications of chemotherapy in patients with cancer. *Drugs* 63, 1549–1563. doi: 10.2165/00003495-200363150-00003

Viele, C. S. (2003). Overview of chemotherapy-induced diarrhea. *Semin. Oncol. Nurs.* 19, 2–5. doi: 10.1053/j.soncn.2003.09.007

Wadler, S., Benson, A., Engelking, C., Catalano, R., Field, M., Kornblau, S. M., et al. (1998). Recommended guidelines for the treatment of chemotherapy-induced diarrhea. *J. Clin. Oncol.* 16, 3169–3178.

Wafai, L., Taher, M., Jovanovska, V., Bornstein, J. C., Dass, C. R., and Nurgali, K. (2013). Effects of oxaliplatin on mouse myenteric neurons and colonic motility. *Front. Neurosci.* 7:30. doi: 10.3389/fnins.2013.00030

Wagner, A. D., Grothe, W., Haerting, J., Kleber, G., Grothey, A., and Fleig, W. E. (2006). Chemotherapy in advanced gastric cancer: a systematic review and meta-analysis based on aggregate data. *J. Clin. Oncol.* 24, 2903–2909. doi: 10.1200/JCO.2005.05.0245

Walko, C. M., and Lindley, C. (2005). Capecitabine: a review. *Clin. Ther.* 27, 23–44. doi: 10.1016/j.clinthera.2005.01.005

Wallace, B. D., Roberts, A. B., Pollet, R. M., Ingle, J. D., Biernat, K. A., Pellock, S. J., et al. (2015). Structure and inhibition of microbiome β-glucuronidases essential to the alleviation of cancer drug toxicity. *Chem. Biol.* 22, 1238–1249. doi: 10.1016/j.chembiol.2015.08.005

Wallace, B. D., Wang, H., Lane, K. T., Scott, J. E., Orans, J., Koo, J. S., et al. (2010). Alleviating cancer drug toxicity by inhibiting a bacterial enzyme. *Science* 330, 831–835. doi: 10.1126/science.1191175

Webster, L., Jansen, J. P., Peppin, J., Lasko, B., Irving, G., Morlion, B., et al. (2008). Alvimopan, a peripherally acting mu-opioid receptor (PAM-OR) antagonist for the treatment of opioid-induced bowel dysfunction: results from a randomized, double-blind, placebo-controlled, dose-finding study in subjects taking opioids for chronic non-cancer pain. *Pain* 137, 428–440. doi: 10.1016/j.pain.2007.11.008

Wolff, R. A., Evans, D. B., Gravel, D. M., Lenzi, R., Pisters, P. W., Lee, J. E., et al. (2001). Phase I trial of gemcitabine combined with radiation for the treatment of locally advanced pancreatic adenocarcinoma. *Clin. Cancer Res* 7, 2246–2253.

Wong, B. S., Camilleri, M., Busciglio, I., Carlson, P., Szarka, L. A., Burton, D., et al. (2011). Pharmacogenetic trial of a cannabinoid agonist shows reduced fasting colonic motility in patients with nonconstipated irritable bowel syndrome. *Gastroenterology* 141, 1638–1647. doi: 10.1053/j.gastro.2011.07.036

Wood, J. D., and Galligan, J. J. (2004). Function of opioids in the enteric nervous system. *Neurogastroenterol. Motil.* 16, 17–28. doi: 10.1111/j.1743-3150.2004.00554.x

Xing, J. H., and Soffer, E. E. (2001). Adverse effects of laxatives. *Dis. Colon Rectum* 44, 1201–1209. doi: 10.1007/BF02234645

Xue, H., Sawyer, M. B., Wischmeyer, P. E., and Baracos, V. E. (2011). Nutrition modulation of gastrointestinal toxicity related to cancer chemotherapy from preclinical findings to clinical strategy. *J. Parenter. Enteral Nutr.* 35, 74–90. doi: 10.1177/0148607110377338

Yamagishi, A., Morita, T., Miyashita, M., and Kimura, F. (2009). Symptom prevalence and longitudinal follow-up in cancer outpatients receiving chemotherapy. *J. Pain Symptom Manage.* 37, 823–830. doi: 10.1016/j.jpainsymman.2008.04.015

Yang, X., Hu, Z., Chan, S. Y., Chan, E., Goh, B. C., Duan, W., et al. (2005). Novel agents that potentially inhibit irinotecan-induced diarrhea. *Curr. Med. Chem.* 12, 1343–1358. doi: 10.2174/0929867054020972

Conflict of Interest Statement: The authors declare that the research was conducted in the absence of any commercial or financial relationships that could be construed as a potential conflict of interest.

4

Fatal Liver and Bone Marrow Toxicity by Combination Treatment of Dichloroacetate and Artesunate in a Glioblastoma Multiforme Patient

Martin Uhl[1], *Stefan Schwab*[1] *and Thomas Efferth*[2*]

[1] *Department of Neurology, University of Erlangen-Nuremberg, Erlangen, Germany,* [2] *Institute of Pharmacy and Biochemistry, Johannes Gutenberg University, Mainz, Germany*

Edited by:
Raquel Abalo,
King Juan Carlos University, Spain

Reviewed by:
Janet K. Coller,
University of Adelaide, Australia
Ursula Gundert-Remy,
Charité – Universitätsmedizin Berlin, Germany

***Correspondence:**
Thomas Efferth
efferth@uni-mainz.de

A 52-year-old male patient was treated with standard radiochemotherapy with temozolomide for glioblastoma multiforme (GBM). After worsening of his clinical condition, further tumor-specific treatment was unlikely to be successful, and the patient seeked help from an alternative practitioner, who administered a combination of dichloroacetate (DCA) and artesunate (ART). A few days later, the patient showed clinical and laboratory signs of liver damage and bone marrow toxicity (leukopenia, thrombocytopenia). Despite successful restoration of laboratory parameters upon symptomatic treatment, the patient died 10 days after the infusion. DCA bears a well-documented hepatotoxic risk, while ART can be considered as safe concerning hepatotoxicity. Bone marrow toxicity can appear upon ART application as reduced reticulocyte counts and disturbed erythropoiesis. It can be assumed that the simultaneous use of both drugs caused liver injury and bone marrow toxicity. The compassionate use of DCA/ART combination therapy outside of clinical trials cannot be recommended for GBM treatment.

Keywords: adverse side effects, cancer, chemotherapy, toxicology

INTRODUCTION

Glioblastoma multiforme (GBM) is an aggressive brain tumor that is currently treated with a combination of radiotherapy and temozolomide (TMZ) chemotherapy. The prognosis is unfavorable with an average survival of 15 months (1–3). In this desperate situation, it is not uncommon for patients to seek help outside standard medicine from alternative practitioners and healers. Often, non-approved remedies or unproven combination of drugs are prescribed, which occasionally may lead to undesired side effects or even life-threatening toxicities.

Dichloroacetate (DCA) is generated as by-product of chlorination of drinking water and by metabolitzation of drugs and chemicals (4). DCA accumulation in groundwater is considered as

Abbreviations: ARS, artemisinin; ART, artesunate; DCA, dichloroacetate; GBM, glioblastoma multiforme; TMZ, temozolomide; VA, valproic acid.

potential health hazard. *In vitro* and *in vivo* investigations showed that DCA inhibits tumor growth by redirecting glycolysis to oxidative phosphorylation and oxidative removal of lactate *via* pyruvate (5). Although five GBM patients have been previously treated with DCA (6), there is only limited knowledge about the efficacy or toxicity of DCA in cancer therapy.

In addition to their antimalarial activity, the artemisinin (ARS) derivatives [artesunate (ART), artemether, dehydroartemisinin] also exert anticancer activity *in vitro* and *in vivo* (7–13), including some brain tumor models (14–18). Compassionate use of ARS-type drugs encouraged the initiation of phase I/II trials in cancer patients (19–27). Most of these studies report are case reports or consist of only small numbers of patients. Therefore, there is still limited evidence regarding the safe use of ARS in cancer patients.

In the present case report, we describe a patient, who died with severe liver and bone marrow toxicity after intake of combined DCA and ART.

CASE REPORT

A 52-year-old male patient was diagnosed with GBM after suffering for several weeks from cognitive decline, headaches, gait ataxia, and a series of epileptic seizures. The initiation of adjuvant therapy was delayed by complicated wound healing, but finally – 53 days after surgery – radiotherapy up to 60 Gy of the tumor region was initiated with simultaneous TMZ chemotherapy (75 mg/m^2) according to local guidelines (28).

The general state of health was unfavorable (Karnofsky score: 50). The patient suffered from right-side hemiparesis and

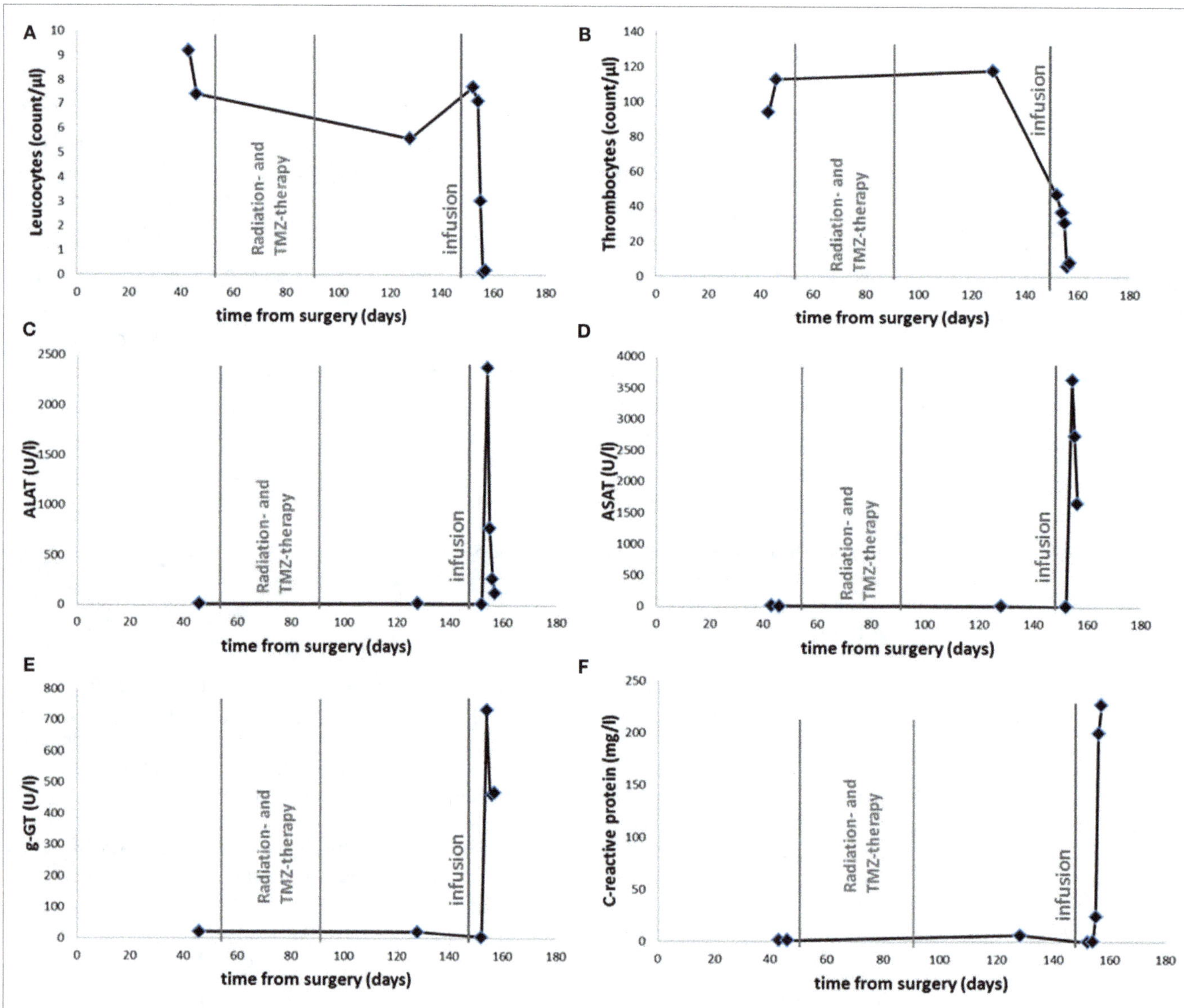

FIGURE 1 | Time course of leukocyte (A), thrombocyte (B) count, serum levels of ALAT (C), ASAT (D), g-GT (E), and CRP (F). Radiotherapy with Temozolomide as indicated between 53 and 92 days after surgery. Infusion with ART and DCA is labeled 148 days after surgery.

required considerable help and medical assistance. Therefore, adjuvant TMZ chemotherapy was ruled out, and rehabilitation actions were initiated. Rehabilitation had to be discontinued 128 days after surgery, because of another series of epileptic seizures. Antiepileptic treatment was escalated to 1800 mg valproic acid (VA), 3000 mg levetiracetam, 200 mg lacosamide, and 20 mg clobazam. Progressive intracranial tumor burden by CT and Fet-PET scan diagnosis was considered as non-suitable for tumor-specific treatment, and steroid medication was escalated.

At that point, the patient and his family were seeking help from an alternative practitioner. An unknown amount of DCA was administered and ART (2.5 mg/kg bodyweight) was intravenously infused 148 days after surgery. At that time, the patient had a stable/unchanged concomitant medication. The patient's cognitive condition declined during the following days with adynamia, severe headaches, and psychomotoric retardation in rapid change with signs of delusions. After admission to the hospital, epileptic activity was not found by EEG and CT scanning did not show relevant changes concerning mass effect or edema. However, blood examinations showed signs of exsiccosis, pancytopenia, and markedly increased hepatic enzyme activities (**Figure 1**). Upon fluid substitution, laboratory parameter stabilized. However, two days after hospitalization, the state of the patient suddenly deteriorated with hypotension, systemic signs of infection, and a series of epileptic seizures. Discussing the need for intensified medical intervention and possible mechanical ventilation, the family did not wish these the actions to be undertaken according to the patient's provision. The patient died during the course of the following night and 157 days after surgery.

The timing of events can be summarized as follows:

- Surgery at day 0
- Start of radiotherapy 53 days after surgery
- End of radiotherapy 92 days after surgery
- Infusion of ART and DCA 148 days after surgery
- First signs of toxicity 154 days after surgery (elevated liver enzymes and hematotoxicity)
- Death of the patient 157 days after surgery

A valuable measure for the causality of adverse reactions of drugs in patients with liver injury is the Roussel Uclaf Causality Assessment Method (RUCAM) (29, 30). RUCAM considers all relevant criteria for liver injury by drugs. We applied the RUCAM scoring system to the patient presented here and found an overall quantitative grading of causality of 6, which indicates reasonable probability that the combinational administration of DCA and ART caused liver injury (**Table 1**).

DISCUSSION

The severity and outcome of this case of compassionate use of alternative medication is remarkable. While the hepatotoxic potential of DCA is well documented, ART is actually considered a rather safe antimalarial drug. It can be speculated that the specific combination of both drugs provoked fatal liver and bone marrow toxicity in the patient.

At the day of hospitalization, prior alternative medication had not been declared by the patient. Therefore, liver toxicity by VA or TMZ has been suspected. In the past, severe and even fatal toxicity were reported for both for VA (31–36) and for TMZ (37–40). Taking into account the additional sudden decline in leukocyte and thrombocyte counts during the next days and considering the prior normal values made this possibility, however, rather unlikely. The dynamics of TMZ- or VA-caused liver damage usually represent more continuous processes. The nadir of TMZ is expected after 21 days. Even delayed forms of bone marrow toxicity are not comparable to the dramatic decline observed here.

The cause of death remains speculative, since an autopsy was not performed in accordance to the patient's provision and family wishes. We consider aspiration pneumonia or spontaneous internal bleeding as possible causes for the sudden decline of blood pressure.

As shown in **Table 2**, DCA administration in animal experiments induced hepatotoxicity and hepatocarcinogenesis. DCA increased hepatic oxidative stress and disturbed liver metabolism. Although treatment of five GBM patients with DCA did not reveal hepatotoxicity (6), there is evidence from preclinical *in vivo* experiments that DCA affects the liver (**Table 2**) (4, 41). However, a straightforward conclusion to the observed hepatotoxicity in the present case is difficult, because the dose of applied DCA to the patient was not disclosed by the alternative practitioner.

The clinical safety of ART is well documented. Large clinical trials and meta-analyses of clinical trials dealing with many thousands of malaria patients did not unravel serious adverse effects (59, 60). Preclinical toxicity studies gave some hints for neurotoxicity, embryotoxicity, genotoxicity, hematotoxicity, cardiotoxicity, nephrotoxicity, and allergic reaction (61). Long-term application of low ARS concentrations may be more toxic than short-term application of high doses. This may explain, why toxicities can

TABLE 1 | Causality assessment of adverse reactions to the DCA/ART combination treatment according to RUCAM (29, 30).

Criterion	Observation	Given score	Score range
1. Time to onset of the reaction	Toxic reaction 6 days after treatment	2	(+1 to +2)
2. Course of the reaction	Decrease <50% within 30 days	3	(−2 to +3)
3. Risk factors for drug reaction	Age of patient ≥55 years	0	(0 to +1)
4. Concomitant drugs	No information	0	(−3 to 0)
5. Non-drug-related causes	HAV, HBV, and HCV serology missing, no biliary obstruction, no alcoholism, no hypotension	0	(−3 to +2)
6. Previous information on the drug	Hepatotoxicity published, but unlabeled	1	(0 to +2)
7. Response to readministration	Not possible, because patient died	0	(−2 to +3)
Total		6	

Quantitative grading of causality: ≤0, excluded; 1–2, unlikely; 3–5, possible; 6–8 probable; ≥9, highly probable.

TABLE 2 | Literature survey on hepatotoxicity by DCA *in vivo*.

Experimental model	Treatment dose	Route of administration	Duration of treatment	Effect	Reference
Dogs	300 mg/kg	Intravenously	1 h	Decrease of tissue lactate levels in liver	(42)
B6C3F1 mice	1–2 g/L	Drinking water	52 weeks	Enlarged livers, cytomegaly, and glycogen accumulation	(43)
B6C3F1 and Swiss-Webster mice	300–2000 mg/L	Drinking water	14 days	Tumorigenesis is influenced by necrosis and reparative hyperplasia, increased ^{3}H-thymidine labeling index	(44)
B6C3F1 mice	200–600 mg/L	Drinking water	72 h	Markedly enlarged liver, cytomegaly, glycogen accumulation, recurrent liver necrosis with high proliferation rates, peroxisome induction, and lipofuscin accumulation	(45)
B6C3F1 mice	2.0 g/L	Drinking water	38 or 50 weeks	Induction of hepatocellular lesions with increased cell divisions; increased c-Jun/c-Fos expression	(46)
B6C3F1 mice	0.5 g/L	Drinking water	2 weeks	4-fold increase of *in vitro* colony formation of hepatocytes suggesting promotion of clonal expansion of anchorage-independent hepatocytes *in vivo*	(47)
B6C3F1 mice	2 g/L	Drinking water	48 weeks	Increase of tumor growth rates	(48)
B6C3F1 mice	0.2–3 g/L	Drinking water	4–12 weeks	Increase of glycogen concentration in liver	(49)
B6C3F1 mice	0.1–2 g/L	Drinking water	2–10 weeks	Reduction of serum insulin, downregulation of insulin receptor, and increased MAP kinase phosphorylation	(50)
B6C3F1 mice	0.5 or 2 g/L	Drinking water	35–52 weeks	Induction of liver tumors, which were c-Jun-positive	(51)
Fischer-344 rats	0.05–20 mg/kg	Intravenously or by gavage	7 days	Oral bioavailability was 0–13% in control rats and 14–75% in GSTZ-depleted rats	(52)
Sprague-Dawley rats	2.5 μg–50 mg/kg/day	Drinking water	12 weeks	GSTZ1-1 activity and expression decreased to 95–100% and recovered 8 weeks after cessation	(53)
B6C3F1 mice	300 mg/kg	By gavage	6 or 12 h	Increased production of superoxide anion, lipid peroxidation, and DNA-single strand breaks	(54)
B6C3F1 male mice	7.7–410 mg/kg/day	By gavage	4 or 13 weeks	Hepatomegaly at 410 mg/kg/day. Dose-dependent increase of SOD activity, lipid peroxidation, and DNA-single strand breaks	(55)
Sprague-Dawley rats	500 mg/kg/day	By gavage	8 weeks	Dechlorination of DCA was higher in cytosol than in mitochondria by GSTZ1	(56)
PKD rats	75 mg/L	Drinking water	8 weeks	Only male rats with polycystic kidney disease (PKD) showed increased disease severity (cystic enlargement and proteinuria)	(57)
B6C3F1 mice	7.5–30 mg/kg/day	By gavage	13 weeks	Dose-dependent increase of SOD production, lipid peroxidation and DNA-single strand breaks	(58)

be observed in animal experiments, but not in human studies. A large meta-analysis with 5000 malaria patients revealed that hepatotoxicity was a rare event, and elevated liver enzymes have been found in 0.9% of all cases (59). Although most papers on clinical safety were published in the context of malaria treatment, there are also some reports on the use of ARS-derivatives in cancer patients. Case reports on the compassionate use of ART or artemether in patients, with laryngeal squamous cell carcinoma, uveal melanoma, pituitary macroadenoma, and prostate carcinoma, reported that the ARSs were well tolerated with no additional side effects in addition to those caused by standard chemotherapy. A randomized controlled trial with 120 advanced non-small cell lung cancer patients on vinorelbine alone versus vinorelbine plus ART did not find significant differences in toxicity between the two treatment groups (23). In a pilot phase I/II trial in 10 patients suffering from cervical carcinoma, artenimol reduced clinical symptoms, vaginal discharge, and pain, and no adverse events of grade 3 and 4 were observed (24). Another phase I/II pilot study in veterinary cancers was conducted in 23 dogs with non-resectable tumors. No neurological or cardiac toxicity was observed, and seven dogs exhibited no adverse effects at all. Fever and hematological or gastrointestinal toxicity, mostly transient, occurred in 16 dogs. One dog died from treatment-unrelated pneumonia (25). As reported from a randomized, double-blind placebo-controlled pilot study in 23 colorectal cancer patients, oral ART therapy was well tolerated without signs of hepatotoxicity (26). Another recent phase I trial on 23 metastasized breast cancer patients reported that four patients had adverse events of the auditory system possibly related to the intake of ART. However, none of these side effects were severe adverse events. Four patients had adverse events concerning the vestibular system, one of which was severe, but fully reversible after discontinuation of ART treatment (27). In summary, hepatotoxicity has not been found in any of these patients.

Hematotoxicity is worth mentioning in this context, because the patient suffered from reduced leukocyte and thrombocyte counts. The toxicity of ARS-type drugs on leukopoiesis is controversially discussed, and both enhanced and inhibited leukocyte functions have been observed (61). Dihydroartemisinin ameliorated inflammatory disease (62). However, ARS-derivatives exhibited higher cytotoxicity *in vitro* toward hematopoietic progenitor cells of the granulocyte-monocyte lineage (CFU-GM) than toward cancer cells (63), indicating that myelosuppression might be an issue in cancer therapy. While thrombocytopenia was apparently not relevant, damage of erythrocytes occurred in animal experiments (61). A sensitive measure for erythropoiesis is the blood count of reticulocytes in peripheral blood. Reduced reticulocyte counts (as erythrocyte precursors) have not only been observed *in vitro* and in animals, but also in human patients upon treatment with ARS-type drugs (59, 61, 64, 65).

In conclusion, the presented case illustrates the possible consequences of compassionate use of non-approved drugs or unproven drug combinations. Drug therapy should always be in accordance to the guidelines of good clinical practice.

AUTHOR CONTRIBUTIONS

MU and SS: treated the patient. TE: wrote the paper.

REFERENCES

1. Stupp R, Hegi ME, Mason WP, van den Bent MJ, Taphoorn MJ, Janzer RC, et al. Effects of radiotherapy with concomitant and adjuvant temozolomide versus radiotherapy alone on survival in glioblastoma in a randomised phase III study: 5-year analysis of the EORTC-NCIC trial. *Lancet Oncol* (2009) 10(5):459–66. doi:10.1016/S1470-2045(09)70025-7
2. Woehrer A, Bauchet L, Barnholtz-Sloan JS. Glioblastoma survival: has it improved? Evidence from population-based studies. *Curr Opin Neurol* (2014) 27(6):666–74. doi:10.1097/WCO.0000000000000144
3. Yang LJ, Zhou CF, Lin ZX. Temozolomide and radiotherapy for newly diagnosed glioblastoma multiforme: a systematic review. *Cancer Invest* (2014) 32(2):31–6. doi:10.3109/07357907.2013.861474
4. Stacpoole PW, Henderson GN, Yan Z, James MO. Clinical pharmacology and toxicology of dichloroacetate. *Environ Health Perspect* (1998) 106(Suppl 4):989–94. doi:10.1289/ehp.98106s4989
5. Kankotia S, Stacpoole PW. Dichloroacetate and cancer: new home for an orphan drug? *Biochim Biophys Acta* (2014) 1846(2):617–29. doi:10.1016/j.bbcan.2014.08.005
6. Michelakis ED, Sutendra G, Dromparis P, Webster L, Haromy A, Niven E, et al. Metabolic modulation of glioblastoma with dichloroacetate. *Sci Transl Med* (2010) 2(31):31ra34. doi:10.1126/scitranslmed.3000677
7. Moore JC, Lai H, Li JR, Ren RL, McDougall JA, Singh NP, et al. Oral administration of dihydroartemisinin and ferrous sulfate retarded implanted fibrosarcoma growth in the rat. *Cancer Lett* (1995) 98(1):83–7. doi:10.1016/0304-3835(95)03999-D
8. Efferth T, Rücker G, Falkenberg M, Manns D, Olbrich A, Fabry U, et al. Detection of apoptosis in KG-1a leukemic cells treated with investigational drugs. *Arzneimittelforschung* (1996) 46(2):196–200.
9. Efferth T, Dunstan H, Sauerbrey A, Miyachi H, Chitambar CR. The anti-malarial artesunate is also active against cancer. *Int J Oncol* (2001) 18(4):767–73.
10. Efferth T, Olbrich A, Bauer R. mRNA expression profiles for the response of human tumor cell lines to the antimalarial drugs artesunate, arteether, and artemether. *Biochem Pharmacol* (2002) 64(4):617–23. doi:10.1016/S0006-2952(02)01221-2
11. Efferth T, Sauerbrey A, Olbrich A, Gebhart E, Rauch P, Weber HO, et al. Molecular modes of action of artesunate in tumor cell lines. *Mol Pharmacol* (2003) 64(2):382–94. doi:10.1124/mol.64.2.382
12. Dell'Eva R, Pfeffer U, Vene R, Anfosso L, Forlani A, Albini A, et al. Inhibition of angiogenesis in vivo and growth of Kaposi's sarcoma xenograft tumors by the anti-malarial artesunate. *Biochem Pharmacol* (2004) 68(12):2359–66. doi:10.1016/j.bcp.2004.08.021
13. Disbrow GL, Baege AC, Kierpiec KA, Yuan H, Centeno JA, Thibodeaux CA, et al. Dihydroartemisinin is cytotoxic to papillomavirus-expressing epithelial cells in vitro and in vivo. *Cancer Res* (2005) 65(23):10854–61. doi:10.1158/0008-5472.CAN-05-1216
14. Efferth T, Ramirez T, Gebhart E, Halatsch ME. Combination treatment of glioblastoma multiforme cell lines with the anti-malarial artesunate and the epidermal growth factor receptor tyrosine kinase inhibitor OSI-774. *Biochem Pharmacol* (2004) 67(9):1689–700. doi:10.1016/j.bcp.2003.12.035
15. Huang XJ, Ma ZQ, Zhang WP, Lu YB, Wei EQ. Dihydroartemisinin exerts cytotoxic effects and inhibits hypoxia inducible factor-1alpha activation in C6 glioma cells. *J Pharm Pharmacol* (2007) 59(6):849–56. doi:10.1211/jpp.59.6.0011
16. Wu ZP, Gao CW, Wu YG, Zhu QS, Yan C, Xin L, et al. Inhibitive effect of artemether on tumor growth and angiogenesis in the rat C6 orthotopic brain gliomas model. *Integr Cancer Ther* (2009) 8(1):88–92. doi:10.1177/1534735408330714
17. Berdelle N, Nikolova T, Quiros S, Efferth T, Kaina B. Artesunate induces oxidative DNA damage, sustained DNA double-strand breaks, and the ATM/ATR damage response in cancer cells. *Mol Cancer Ther* (2011) 10(12):2224–33. doi:10.1158/1535-7163.MCT-11-0534
18. Chen J, Chen X, Wang F, Gao H, Hu W. Dihydroartemisinin suppresses glioma proliferation and invasion via inhibition of the ADAM17 pathway. *Neurol Sci* (2015) 36(3):435–40. doi:10.1007/s10072-014-1963-6
19. Singh NP, Verma KB. Case report of a laryngeal squamous cell carcinoma treated with artesunate. *Arch Oncol* (2002) 10:279–80. doi:10.2298/AOO0204279S
20. Berger TG, Dieckmann D, Efferth T, Schultz ES, Funk JO, Baur A, et al. Artesunate in the treatment of metastatic uveal melanoma – first experiences. *Oncol Rep* (2005) 14(6):1599–603.
21. Singh NP, Panwar VK. Case report of a pituitary macroadenoma treated with artemether. *Integr Cancer Ther* (2006) 5:391–4. doi:10.1177/1534735406295311
22. Michaelsen FW, Saeed ME, Schwarzkopf J, Efferth T. Activity of Artemisia annua and artemisinin derivatives, in prostate carcinoma. *Phytomedicine* (2015) 22(14):1223–31. doi:10.1016/j.phymed.2015.11.001
23. Zhang ZY, Yu SQ, Miao LY, Huang XY, Zhang XP, Zhu YP, et al. [Artesunate combined with vinorelbine plus cisplatin in treatment of advanced non-small cell lung cancer: a randomized controlled trial]. *Zhong Xi Yi Jie He Xue Bao* (2008) 6(2):134–8. doi:10.3736/jcim20080206
24. Jansen FH, Adoubi I, Kouassi JC, DE C, Jansen N, Tschulakow A, et al. First study of oral Artenimol-R in advanced cervical cancer: clinical benefit, tolerability and tumor markers. *Anticancer Res* (2011) 31(12):4417–22.
25. Rutteman GR, Erich SA, Mol JA, Spee B, Grinwis GC, Fleckenstein L, et al. Safety and efficacy field study of artesunate for dogs with non-resectable tumours. *Anticancer Res* (2013) 33(5):1819–27.
26. Krishna S, Ganapathi S, Ster IC, Saeed ME, Cowan M, Finlayson C, et al. A randomised, double blind, placebo-controlled pilot study of oral artesunate therapy for colorectal cancer. *EBioMedicine* (2015) 2(1):82–90. doi:10.1016/j.ebiom.2014.11.010
27. Konig M, von Hagens C, Hoth S, Baumann I, Walter-Sack I, Edler L, et al. Investigation of ototoxicity of artesunate as add-on therapy in patients with metastatic or locally advanced breast cancer: new audiological results from a prospective, open, uncontrolled, monocentric phase I study. *Cancer Chemother Pharmacol* (2016) 77(2):413–27. doi:10.1007/s00280-016-2960-7
28. Weller M, van den Bent M, Hopkins K, Tonn JC, Stupp R, Falini A, et al. EANO guideline for the diagnosis and treatment of anaplastic gliomas and glioblastoma. *Lancet Oncol* (2014) 15(9):e395–403. doi:10.1016/S1470-2045(14)70011-7
29. Danan G, Benichou C. Causality assessment of adverse reactions to drugs – I. A novel method based on the conclusions of international consensus meetings: application to drug-induced liver injuries. *J Clin Epidemiol* (1993) 46(11):1323–30. doi:10.1016/0895-4356(93)90101-6
30. Teschke RLD, Melchart D, Danan G. Traditional Chinese Medicine (TCM) and herbal hepatotoxicity: RUCAM and the role of novel diagnostic biomarkers such as MicroRNAs. *Medicines* (2016) 3(3):18. doi:10.3390/medicines3030018
31. Hjelm M, de Silva LV, Seakins JW, Oberholzer VG, Rolles CJ. Evidence of inherited urea cycle defect in a case of fatal valproate toxicity. *Br Med J (Clin Res Ed)* (1986) 292(6512):23–4. doi:10.1136/bmj.292.6512.23

32. Evans RJ, Miranda RN, Jordan J, Krolikowski FJ. Fatal acute pancreatitis caused by valproic acid. *Am J Forensic Med Pathol* (1995) 16(1):62–5. doi:10.1097/00000433-199503000-00014
33. Pinkston R, Walker LA. Multiorgan system failure caused by valproic acid toxicity. *Am J Emerg Med* (1997) 15(5):504–6. doi:10.1016/S0735-6757(97)90195-9
34. Acharya S, Bussel JB. Hematologic toxicity of sodium valproate. *J Pediatr Hematol Oncol* (2000) 22(1):62–5. doi:10.1097/00043426-200001000-00012
35. Pronicka E, Weglewska-Jurkiewicz A, Pronicki M, Sykut-Cegielska J, Kowalski P, Pajdowska M, et al. Drug-resistant epilepsia and fulminant valproate liver toxicity. Alpers-Huttenlocher syndrome in two children confirmed post mortem by identification of p.W748S mutation in POLG gene. *Med Sci Monit* (2011) 17(4):CR203–9. doi:10.12659/MSM.881716
36. Star K, Edwards IR, Choonara I. Valproic acid and fatalities in children: a review of individual case safety reports in VigiBase. *PLoS One* (2014) 9(10):e108970. doi:10.1371/journal.pone.0108970
37. Su YW, Chang MC, Chiang MF, Hsieh RK. Treatment-related myelodysplastic syndrome after temozolomide for recurrent high-grade glioma. *J Neurooncol* (2005) 71(3):315–8. doi:10.1007/s11060-004-2028-0
38. George BJ, Eichinger JB, Richard TJ. A rare case of aplastic anemia caused by temozolomide. *South Med J* (2009) 102(9):974–6. doi:10.1097/SMJ.0b013e3181b1d2fa
39. Letarte N, Gabay MP, Bressler LR, Long KE, Stachnik JM, Villano JL. Analyzing temozolomide medication errors: potentially fatal. *J Neurooncol* (2014) 120(1):111–5. doi:10.1007/s11060-014-1523-1
40. Grieco A, Tafuri MA, Biolato M, Diletto B, Di Napoli N, Balducci N, et al. Severe cholestatic hepatitis due to temozolomide: an adverse drug effect to keep in mind. Case report and review of literature. *Medicine (Baltimore)* (2015) 94(12):e476. doi:10.1097/MD.0000000000000476
41. Bull RJ. Mode of action of liver tumor induction by trichloroethylene and its metabolites, trichloroacetate and dichloroacetate. *Environ Health Perspect* (2000) 108(Suppl 2):241–59. doi:10.1289/ehp.00108s2241
42. Graf H, Leach W, Arieff AI. Effects of dichloroacetate in the treatment of hypoxic lactic acidosis in dogs. *J Clin Invest* (1985) 76(3):919–23. doi:10.1172/JCI112090
43. Bull RJ, Sanchez IM, Nelson MA, Larson JL, Lansing AJ. Liver tumor induction in B6C3F1 mice by dichloroacetate and trichloroacetate. *Toxicology* (1990) 63(3):341–59. doi:10.1016/0300-483X(90)90195-M
44. Sanchez IM, Bull RJ. Early induction of reparative hyperplasia in the liver of B6C3F1 mice treated with dichloroacetate and trichloroacetate. *Toxicology* (1990) 64(1):33–46. doi:10.1016/0300-483X(90)90097-Z
45. Bull RJ, Templin M, Larson JL, Stevens DK. The role of dichloroacetate in the hepatocarcinogenicity of trichloroethylene. *Toxicol Lett* (1993) 68(1–2):203–11. doi:10.1016/0378-4274(93)90131-G
46. Stauber AJ, Bull RJ. Differences in phenotype and cell replicative behavior of hepatic tumors induced by dichloroacetate (DCA) and trichloroacetate (TCA). *Toxicol Appl Pharmacol* (1997) 144(2):235–46. doi:10.1006/taap.1997.8159
47. Stauber AJ, Bull RJ, Thrall BD. Dichloroacetate and trichloroacetate promote clonal expansion of anchorage-independent hepatocytes in vivo and in vitro. *Toxicol Appl Pharmacol* (1998) 150(2):287–94. doi:10.1006/taap.1998.8417
48. Miller JH, Minard K, Wind RA, Orner GA, Sasser LB, Bull RJ. In vivo MRI measurements of tumor growth induced by dichloroacetate: implications for mode of action. *Toxicology* (2000) 145(2–3):115–25. doi:10.1016/S0300-483X(00)00148-7
49. Kato-Weinstein J, Stauber AJ, Orner GA, Thrall BD, Bull RJ. Differential effects of dihalogenated and trihalogenated acetates in the liver of B6C3F1 mice. *J Appl Toxicol* (2001) 21(2):81–9. doi:10.1002/jat.717
50. Lingohr MK, Thrall BD, Bull RJ. Effects of dichloroacetate (DCA) on serum insulin levels and insulin-controlled signaling proteins in livers of male B6C3F1 mice. *Toxicol Sci* (2001) 59(1):178–84. doi:10.1093/toxsci/59.1.178
51. Bull RJ, Orner GA, Cheng RS, Stillwell L, Stauber AJ, Sasser LB, et al. Contribution of dichloroacetate and trichloroacetate to liver tumor induction in mice by trichloroethylene. *Toxicol Appl Pharmacol* (2002) 182(1):55–65. doi:10.1006/taap.2002.9427
52. Saghir SA, Schultz IR. Low-dose pharmacokinetics and oral bioavailability of dichloroacetate in naive and GST-zeta-depleted rats. *Environ Health Perspect* (2002) 110(8):757–63. doi:10.1289/ehp.02110757
53. Guo X, Dixit V, Liu H, Shroads AL, Henderson GN, James MO, et al. Inhibition and recovery of rat hepatic glutathione S-transferase zeta and alteration of tyrosine metabolism following dichloroacetate exposure and withdrawal. *Drug Metab Dispos* (2006) 34(1):36–42. doi:10.1124/dmd.105.003996
54. Hassoun EA, Dey S. Dichloroacetate- and trichloroacetate-induced phagocytic activation and production of oxidative stress in the hepatic tissues of mice after acute exposure. *J Biochem Mol Toxicol* (2008) 22(1):27–34. doi:10.1002/jbt.20210
55. Hassoun EA, Cearfoss J, Spildener J. Dichloroacetate- and trichloroacetate-induced oxidative stress in the hepatic tissues of mice after long-term exposure. *J Appl Toxicol* (2010) 30(5):450–6. doi:10.1002/jat.1516
56. Li W, James MO, McKenzie SC, Calcutt NA, Liu C, Stacpoole PW. Mitochondrion as a novel site of dichloroacetate biotransformation by glutathione transferase zeta 1. *J Pharmacol Exp Ther* (2011) 336(1):87–94. doi:10.1124/jpet.110.173195
57. Gattone VH II, Bacallao RL. Dichloroacetate treatment accelerates the development of pathology in rodent autosomal recessive polycystic kidney disease. *Am J Physiol Renal Physiol* (2014) 307(10):F1144–8. doi:10.1152/ajprenal.00009.2014
58. Hassoun E, Cearfoss J, Mamada S, Al-Hassan N, Brown M, Heimberger K, et al. The effects of mixtures of dichloroacetate and trichloroacetate on induction of oxidative stress in livers of mice after subchronic exposure. *J Toxicol Environ Health A* (2014) 77(6):313–23. doi:10.1080/15287394.2013.864576
59. Ribeiro IR, Olliaro P. Safety of artemisinin and its derivatives. A review of published and unpublished clinical trials. *Med Trop (Mars)* (1998) 58(3 Suppl):50–3.
60. Adjuik M, Babiker A, Garner P, Olliaro P, Taylor W, White N. Artesunate combinations for treatment of malaria: meta-analysis. *Lancet* (2004) 363(9402):9–17. doi:10.1016/S0140-6736(03)15162-8
61. Efferth T, Kaina B. Toxicity of the antimalarial artemisinin and its dervatives. *Crit Rev Toxicol* (2010) 40(5):405–21. doi:10.3109/10408441003610571
62. Zhao YG, Wang Y, Guo Z, Gu AD, Dan HC, Baldwin AS, et al. Dihydroartemisinin ameliorates inflammatory disease by its reciprocal effects on Th and regulatory T cell function via modulating the mammalian target of rapamycin pathway. *J Immunol* (2012) 189(9):4417–25. doi:10.4049/jimmunol.1200919
63. Beekman AC, Wierenga PK, Woerdenbag HJ, Van Uden W, Pras N, Konings AW, et al. Artemisinin-derived sesquiterpene lactones as potential antitumour compounds: cytotoxic action against bone marrow and tumour cells. *Planta Med* (1998) 64(7):615–9. doi:10.1055/s-2006-957533
64. Wootton DG, Opara H, Biagini GA, Kanjala MK, Duparc S, Kirby PL, et al. Open-label comparative clinical study of chlorproguanil-dapsone fixed dose combination (Lapdap) alone or with three different doses of artesunate for uncomplicated *Plasmodium falciparum* malaria. *PLoS One* (2008) 3(3):e1779. doi:10.1371/journal.pone.0001779
65. Clark RL. Effects of artemisinins on reticulocyte count and relationship to possible embryotoxicity in confirmed and unconfirmed malarial patients. *Birth Defects Res A Clin Mol Teratol* (2012) 94(2):61–75. doi:10.1002/bdra.22868

Conflict of Interest Statement: The authors declare that the research was conducted in the absence of any commercial or financial relationships that could be construed as a potential conflict of interest.

5

Delayed Chemotherapy-Induced Nausea and Vomiting: Pathogenesis, Incidence, and Current Management

*Bernardo L. Rapoport**

The Medical Oncology Centre of Rosebank, Johannesburg, South Africa

Even when chemotherapy-induced nausea and vomiting (CINV) can be effectively controlled in the acute phase, it may still occur in the delayed phase. Identifying at-risk patients is complex and requires consideration of clinical, personal, demographic, and behavioral factors. Delayed CINV has a significant detrimental effect on patients' daily life and is responsible for significant healthcare resource utilization. Patients who do not experience acute CINV are not necessarily exempt from delayed CINV, and healthcare professionals have been shown to underestimate the incidence of delayed CINV. Failure to protect against CINV during the first cycle of chemotherapy is the most significant independent risk factor for delayed CINV during subsequent cycles. Addition of a neurokinin-1 receptor antagonist to antiemetic prophylactic regimens involving a 5-hydroxytryptamine type 3 receptor antagonist and a corticosteroid helps to ameliorate delayed CINV, particularly vomiting. Netupitant and rolapitant are second-generation neurokinin-1 receptor antagonists that provide effective prophylaxis against delayed chemotherapy-induced vomiting and also have an antinausea benefit. All of the neurokinin-1 receptor antagonists with the exception of rolapitant inhibit or induce cytochrome P450 3A4 (CYP3A4), and a reduced dose of dexamethasone (a CYP3A4 substrate) should be administered with aprepitant or netupitant; by contrast, this is not necessary with rolapitant. Here we review specific challenges associated with delayed CINV, its pathophysiology, epidemiology, treatment, and outcomes relative to acute CINV, and its management within the larger context of overall CINV.

Edited by:
Raquel Abalo,
King Juan Carlos University, Spain

Reviewed by:
Andrea Lapucci,
University of Florence, Italy
Pere N/a Gascon,
University Hospital Clínic de Barcelona, Spain

***Correspondence:**
Bernardo L. Rapoport
brapoport@rosebankoncology.co.za

Keywords: antiemetics, delayed chemotherapy-induced nausea and vomiting, emesis, highly emetogenic chemotherapy, moderately emetogenic chemotherapy, nausea, neurokinin-1 receptor antagonists, vomiting

INTRODUCTION

Nausea and vomiting are the most feared side effects of cytotoxic chemotherapy (de Boer-Dennert et al., 1997; Sun et al., 2005) and can have a deleterious effect on health-related quality of life (Bloechl-Daum et al., 2006; Hilarius et al., 2012), compromise treatment outcomes (Vidall et al., 2011; Jordan et al., 2015; Van Laar et al., 2015; National Comprehensive Cancer Network, 2016; Navari, 2016), and increase healthcare resource utilization (Schwartzberg L. et al., 2015). Chemotherapy-induced nausea and vomiting (CINV) typically presents in two phases, the acute phase and the delayed phase, over a 5-day period (Navari and Aapro, 2016). Acute CINV occurs within 1–2 h of chemotherapy administration and can last for up to 24 h; delayed CINV presents more than 24 h after chemotherapy administration, and it is most frequently reported with the agents cisplatin, carboplatin, cyclophosphamide, and doxorubicin (National Comprehensive Cancer Network, 2016).

While acute CINV is reasonably well managed with serotonin (5-hydroxytryptamine) type 3 (5-HT_3) receptor antagonists in the majority of patients (Jordan et al., 2007), delayed CINV continues to present a treatment challenge (Grunberg et al., 2004; Hsieh et al., 2015; Baba et al., 2016). This review discusses the pathophysiology, burden of illness, and treatment outcomes associated with delayed CINV, together with advances and future directions for management.

The Pathophysiology of Delayed CINV

Chemotherapy-induced nausea and vomiting is a highly complex reflex that involves contributory pathways from both the central and peripheral nervous systems. While the pathophysiology of emesis is not completely understood, it is currently thought that chemotherapy-induced release of neurotransmitters stimulates receptors on the terminals of afferent nerves in various locations, including the gastrointestinal tract, cerebral cortex and thalamus, vestibular region, and area postrema, which project to the nucleus tractus solitarius (NTS) located in the brain stem (Aapro et al., 2014a; Babic and Browning, 2014; National Comprehensive Cancer Network, 2016; Navari and Aapro, 2016). The NTS plays a dominant role in coordinating the autonomic processes involved in vomiting, such as swallowing, salivation, respiration, abdominal muscle contraction and relaxation, and intestinal contraction and relaxation (Babic and Browning, 2014). In addition, neurotransmitters may directly stimulate receptors located in the area postrema of the brain (known as the chemoreceptor trigger zone), which also activates the NTS (Aapro et al., 2014a). Neurotransmitters that have been identified as important mediators of CINV include serotonin and substance P (Navari and Aapro, 2016).

The typical pattern of CINV is shown in **Figure 1**. The acute phase occurs within the first 24 h after chemotherapy and is largely mediated by 5-HT_3 receptors in the intestine (Navari, 2016). In this phase, free radicals generated after administration of chemotherapy induce the release of serotonin from enterochromaffin cells located in the intestinal mucosa (Aapro et al., 2014a; Navari, 2016). Serotonin then interacts with 5-HT_3 receptors located on vagal afferent nerves in the intestinal wall, which project to the area postrema and NTS, stimulating the vomiting reflex (Aapro et al., 2014a). Serotonin may also directly interact with 5-HT_3 receptors on the area postrema (Aapro et al., 2014a). Acute CINV is therefore particularly sensitive to 5-HT_3 receptor antagonists (Aapro, 2005) (**Figure 1**); however, these agents have little impact on delayed CINV (Aapro, 2005), suggesting that different pathophysiologic mechanisms may be at play during the second emetic phase.

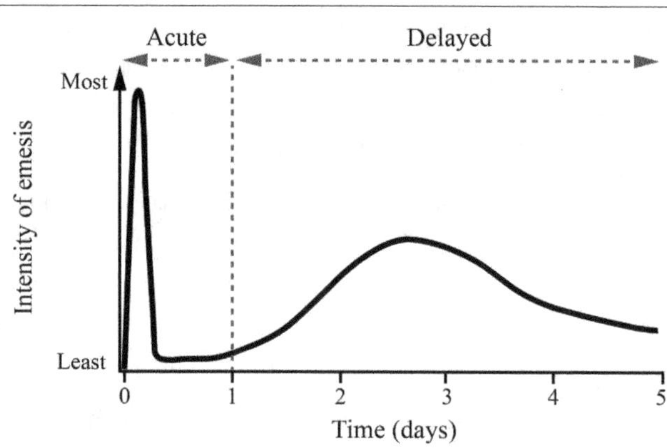

FIGURE 1 | Pattern of cisplatin-induced delayed emesis. This illustrates the biphasic pattern of emesis after the administration of high-dose cisplatin, with the maximum intensity seen with the initial 24 h, followed by a second peak of less intense nausea and emesis on days 2 and 3. Reprinted from *Springer Drugs* 1996 Nov; 52 (5): 639–648, Tavorath R and Hesketh PJ (© Adis International Limited. All rights reserved). With permission of Springer.

The delayed phase of CINV starts on day 2 after chemotherapy and can last up to day 5. Delayed CINV is predominantly driven by a central pathway involving the neurotransmitter/neuromodulator substance P, which is a member of the mammalian tachykinin family of peptides (Garcia-Recio and Gascon, 2015). Substance P is released from neurons in response to chemotherapy and binds to neurokinin-1 (NK-1) receptors in the area postrema and NTS, thereby mediating the induction of vomiting (Armstrong et al., 1981; Aapro et al., 2014a). The dominant role of substance P in delayed CINV is demonstrated by the effectiveness of NK-1 receptor antagonists in preventing CINV during this phase (Navari, 2016) (**Figure 1**). NK-1 receptors are also located on vagal afferent terminals in the gastrointestinal tract, suggesting that substance P released from enterochromaffin cells in response to chemotherapy may also play an auxiliary role in the acute phase of CINV (Hesketh, 2008).

Classification of Emetic Agents

The emetogenicity of chemotherapy refers to its capacity to induce nausea and vomiting when administered without adequate antiemetic prophylaxis. One of the most commonly used schemes divides chemotherapeutic agents into four categories (high, moderate, low, and minimal), depending on the percentage of patients who would experience emesis in the acute phase while receiving the agent without adequate antiemetic prophylaxis (Hesketh et al., 1997). In the absence of such prophylaxis, it is estimated that over 90% of patients exposed to highly emetogenic chemotherapy (HEC) and between 30 and 90% of patients exposed to moderately emetogenic chemotherapy (MEC) will experience acute-phase CINV (**Table 1**). Emetogenic categories are regularly updated by guidelines groups to incorporate new agents or new data from existing agents (Basch et al., 2011; Hesketh et al., 2016a; National Comprehensive Cancer Network, 2016). One particularly significant change for CINV was the reclassification of anthracycline-cyclophosphamide (AC)–based chemotherapy from the moderately emetogenic category to the highly emetogenic category in 2011. In addition, while carboplatin-based chemotherapy is defined as MEC, the Multinational Association of Supportive Care in Cancer (MASCC) and European Society for Medical Oncology (ESMO) guidelines were recently updated to recommend that CINV associated with carboplatin therapy be treated in the same way as HEC, with an

TABLE 1 | Emetogenic risk categories for antineoplastic agents (based on acute emetogenicity) (Hesketh et al., 1997).

Emetogenic risk	Frequency of emesis in the absence of effective antiemetic prophylaxis	Intravenous antineoplastic agents
High	>90%	• AC combination: doxorubicin or epirubicin + cyclophosphamide • Carmustine >250 mg/m^2 • Cisplatin • Cyclophosphamide >1,500 mg/m^2 • Dacarbazine • Doxorubicin ≥60 mg/m^2 • Epirubicin ≥90 mg/m^2 • Ifosfamide ≥2 g/m^2 per dose • Mechlorethamine • Streptozocin
Moderate	30–90%	• Aldesleukin >12–15 million IU/m^2 • Amifostine >300 mg/m^2 • Arsenic trioxide • Bendamustine • Busulfan • Carboplatin[a] • Carmustine[a] ≤250 mg/m^2 • Cloforabine • Cyclophosphamide <1,500 mg/m^2 • Cytarabine >200 mg/m^2 • Dactinomycin[a] • Daunorubicin[a] • Dinutuximab • Doxorubicin[a] <60 mg/m^2 • Epirubicin[a] <90 mg/m^2 • Idarubicin • Ifosfamide[a] <2 g/m^2 per dose • Interferon-alfa ≥10 million IU/m^2 • Irinotecan[a] • Melphalan • Methotrexate[a] ≥250 mg/m^2 • Oxaliplatin • Temozolomide • Trabectedin

[a]*May be highly emetogenic in some patients.*

NK-1 receptor antagonist as well as a 5-HT$_3$ receptor antagonist and dexamethasone (MASCC/ESMO, 2016).

It should be noted that emetogenic categories are based only on the incidence of acute CINV, rather than delayed or overall CINV. Indeed, one recent study found that the chemotherapy regimen is an inconsistent predictor of CINV in the delayed phase (Jordan et al., 2014). This suggests that emetogenic classifications may not be the most appropriate determinant of prophylactic antiemetic regimen for delayed CINV and may contribute to undertreatment of delayed CINV due to a lack of appreciation of the true emetogenic risk of particular types of chemotherapy.

Epidemiology and Risk Factors for Delayed CINV

Chemotherapy-induced nausea and vomiting may be more problematic during the delayed phase than the acute phase in patients receiving HEC and MEC (Grunberg et al., 2004; Escobar et al., 2015; Hsieh et al., 2015; Baba et al., 2016). For example, in an international, prospective observational study of 298 adult patients receiving chemotherapy for the first time, delayed nausea and vomiting were observed in 60 and 50% of HEC patients, respectively, and in 52 and 28% of MEC patients, respectively (Grunberg et al., 2004), whereas acute nausea and vomiting were seen in 12 and 33% of HEC patients, respectively, and in 13 and 37% of MEC patients, respectively. The majority of patients were receiving antiemetic prophylaxis according to then-current guidelines, with 97% receiving a 5-HT$_3$ receptor antagonist and 78% a corticosteroid. The study concluded that patients who do not experience acute CINV are not necessarily protected from delayed CINV: 24 and 23% of patients reported delayed nausea and emesis, respectively, even in the absence of these events in the acute phase. Similar patterns were observed among patients assigned to HEC and MEC. In another study in 240 chemotherapy-naive patients in Spain who received MEC with a 5-HT$_3$ receptor antagonist plus corticosteroid antiemetic prophylaxis, the incidence of CINV was higher in the delayed phase than in the acute phase (Escobar et al., 2015). This difference was statistically significant for the endpoints of vomiting, nausea, and significant nausea, with rates increasing from 9.2 to 16.5% ($p = 0.0112$), from 23.3 to 38.5% ($p < 0.0001$), and from 9.4 to 21.7% ($p = 0.0002$), respectively. Twice as many patients required rescue antiemetics (metoclopramide or ondansetron) during the delayed phase (14.5%) as during the acute phase (7.2%).

More recent observational studies continue to show that delayed CINV may be incompletely controlled even if acute CINV is adequately managed (Molassiotis et al., 2014; Hsieh et al., 2015). In a large, heterogeneous group of European cancer patients ($n = 991$) receiving their first cycle of routine HEC or MEC, complete response (CR) rates (the proportion of patients without vomiting or significant nausea) were 72% in the acute phase and 62% in the delayed phase (Jordan et al., 2014). The delayed-phase CR rate increased to 67% by cycle 3 ($p = 0.0144$ compared with cycle 1); this improvement seemed to be driven by patients reporting no vomiting (71% in cycle 1 and 78% in cycle 3; $p < 0.0001$) rather than those reporting no significant nausea (81% in cycle 1 and 81% in cycle 3).

Survey data indicates that oncologists and oncology nurses can accurately predict the incidence of acute CINV after HEC; however, the incidence of delayed CINV after HEC is often underestimated. In one study, the predicted incidence of delayed nausea was 39% (95% confidence interval [CI] 30–48%), whereas the observed incidence was 60% (95% CI 48–72%), and the predicted incidence of delayed vomiting was 22% (95% CI 12–31%), whereas the observed incidence was 50% (95% CI 37–63%) (Grunberg et al., 2004). Delayed CINV has also been underestimated in patients receiving MEC (Grunberg et al., 2004; Escobar et al., 2015). Misperceptions regarding the incidence of delayed CINV may have implications for treatment. For example, in a hospital-based study in Spain, patients who experienced acute vomiting in cycle 1 were significantly more likely to have a change in antiemetic therapy in subsequent cycles; by contrast, delayed vomiting or nausea at any stage did not lead to changes in subsequent antiemetic regimens (Molassiotis et al., 2008).

Identifying which patients are at greatest risk for CINV is a complex analysis combining clinical, personal, demographic, and behavioral characteristics. A number of factors have been identified that increase susceptibility to CINV, including female sex, age <55 years, a history of nausea/vomiting, anxiety, fatigue or motion sickness, impaired quality of life, and limited alcohol use (Dranitsaris et al., 2013; Jordan et al., 2014). One study evaluated independent risk factors for the development of delayed CINV during cycle 1 of chemotherapy, identifying guideline-inconsistent CINV prophylaxis, no use of secondary antiemetics for delayed CINV, a history of nausea/vomiting, and prechemotherapy (anticipatory) nausea (Jordan et al., 2014). Other factors that have been associated with delayed CINV include a history of motion sickness, acute CINV, and the use of cisplatin (Kottschade et al., 2016). A small prospective study of 56 cancer patients (Higgins et al., 2007) also noted a significant relationship between pretreatment distress and the severity of subsequent delayed nausea but not acute nausea.

Studies evaluating multiple cycles of chemotherapy have revealed that an important predictor of CINV in a given cycle is whether CINV occurred in a previous cycle. A study of patients from Italian oncology centers receiving ondansetron or metoclopramide for cisplatin-associated CINV found that protection from emesis during the first cycle of cisplatin-based chemotherapy was an important predictor of protection in subsequent cycles (Italian Group for Antiemetic Research, 1994). Jordan et al. (2014) showed that the most significant independent risk factor for delayed CINV during cycles 2 and 3 was not achieving a CR in the previous cycle: patients without a CR in the earlier cycle were 5.7–7.3 times more likely to have no CR during the delayed phase in the subsequent cycle. Furthermore, the failure to protect against delayed CINV in the first cycle of chemotherapy can impair protection against acute CINV in subsequent cycles (Ellebaek and Herrstedt, 2008). These findings underscore the importance of effective management of delayed CINV during the first cycle of chemotherapy.

Clinical Implications of Delayed CINV

Delayed CINV has a significant detrimental effect on a patient's daily life (Bloechl-Daum et al., 2006; Hilarius et al., 2012; Grassi et al., 2015), even in the absence of acute CINV. In a representative sample of 298 treatment-naive patients receiving HEC or MEC and given CINV prophylaxis under then-current patterns of clinical practice, the impact of CINV on daily life was assessed using the Functional Living Index–Emesis questionnaire on day 6 of cycle 1 (Bloechl-Daum et al., 2006). Only 32% of patients who experienced delayed vomiting without acute vomiting reported that CINV had no or minimal impact on daily life, similar to the proportion of patients who experienced only acute vomiting (30%). In the same study, 80% of patients who experienced acute nausea without delayed nausea reported that emesis did not affect their daily life; by contrast, only 56% of those who experienced delayed nausea without acute nausea reported no or minimal impact.

Delayed CINV is also responsible for significant healthcare resource utilization (Ihbe-Heffinger et al., 2004; Burke et al., 2011). In a United States–based retrospective cohort study that included 19,139 patients receiving HEC or MEC, 13.7% of patients had a delayed CINV-associated hospital visit and 0.2% had an acute CINV-associated hospital visit (Burke et al., 2011). CINV-associated visits included inpatient (64%), outpatient (26%), and emergency room (<1%) visits.

PREVENTION OF DELAYED EMESIS

NK-1 Receptor Antagonists

The growing understanding of the role of substance P in emesis led to the development of NK-1 receptor antagonists for the treatment of delayed CINV. The first oral NK-1 receptor antagonist, aprepitant, was approved in 2003, followed by fosaprepitant (a prodrug of aprepitant that is administered intravenously), netupitant (administered as a fixed oral combination with the 5-HT$_3$ receptor antagonist palonosetron), and rolapitant. The efficacy and tolerability of NK-1 receptor antagonists for prevention of delayed CINV when used in combination with a 5-HT$_3$ receptor antagonist and a corticosteroid has been established in a number of randomized controlled trials, as described below. The findings of these trials, along with the demonstrated inability of 5-HT$_3$ receptor antagonists to prevent delayed CINV (Aapro, 2005), show the need to incorporate NK-1 receptor antagonists in the treatment of delayed CINV.

The addition of aprepitant to ondansetron plus dexamethasone was shown to increase protection against delayed CINV in patients receiving HEC (Hesketh et al., 2003; Poli-Bigelli et al., 2003) and MEC (Rapoport et al., 2010). In a phase 3, randomized, double-blind study in patients scheduled to receive treatment with high-dose cisplatin, CR rates during the delayed phase were 68% in the aprepitant group and 47% in the standard-therapy group ($p < 0.001$) (Poli-Bigelli et al., 2003). While aprepitant was associated with a significant improvement in the proportion of patients who did not experience delayed vomiting (72 vs. 48%; $p < 0.01$), between-treatment differences in rates of no significant nausea (73 vs. 65%) were not statistically significant. In a similar study, CR rates during the delayed phase were 66% in the aprepitant group and 52% in the standard-therapy group ($p < 0.001$) (Hesketh et al., 2003). As in the previous study, aprepitant had a significant benefit with respect to rates of emesis but not nausea. Benefits on delayed CINV were also reported in patients treated with MEC (including AC regimens) (Rapoport et al., 2010).

Single-dose fosaprepitant was approved for use in delayed CINV based on the results of a phase 3 non-inferiority trial versus aprepitant (administered once daily for 3 days) in patients receiving HEC and treated with background ondansetron and dexamethasone (Grunberg et al., 2011). No significant difference was reported between the fosaprepitant and aprepitant arms with regard to CR rate in the delayed phase (74.3 vs. 76.8%). A recent phase 3 study evaluated the addition of fosaprepitant to ondansetron and dexamethasone in patients receiving non-AC MEC (Weinstein et al., 2016). In this randomized, double-blind, placebo-controlled study, fosaprepitant significantly improved rates of delayed CR (79 vs. 69%; $p < 0.001$) and no emesis (84 vs. 75%; $p < 0.001$). The impact of fosaprepitant on nausea in the delayed phase of this study was not described.

In 2014, netupitant was approved for prevention of CINV. Netupitant is administered as a fixed oral combination with palonosetron (NEPA), and this formulation has been evaluated in phase 3 randomized controlled trials in patients receiving HEC (Hesketh et al., 2014) and AC (considered MEC at the time of the study) (Aapro et al., 2014c). In the HEC population, a CR during the delayed phase was reported in 92% of the NEPA plus dexamethasone group compared with 80% of the control group receiving palonosetron plus dexamethasone ($p \leq 0.01$), with significant benefits reported in terms of both vomiting and nausea (Hesketh et al., 2014). In the AC study, the percentage of patients with a CR during the delayed phase was significantly higher with NEPA plus dexamethasone than with palonosetron plus dexamethasone (76.9 vs. 69.5%; $p = 0.0001$) (Aapro et al., 2014c). Likewise, NEPA plus dexamethasone was associated with significantly higher rates of no emesis (81.8 vs. 75.6%; $p = 0.004$) and no significant nausea (defined as a reading of <25 mm on a 100-mm horizontal visual analog scale) (76.9 vs. 71.3%; $p = 0.014$).

Rolapitant is the most recent NK-1 receptor antagonist to be approved, and it is licensed for the treatment of delayed CINV associated with initial and repeat courses of emetogenic chemotherapy including, but not limited to, HEC (Varubi, 2015). The efficacy of rolapitant in preventing CINV when added to granisetron plus dexamethasone has been evaluated in two phase 3 clinical trials in patients receiving HEC (Rapoport B.L. et al., 2015) and one phase 3 clinical trial in patients receiving MEC or AC-based chemotherapy (Schwartzberg L.S. et al., 2015). In a pooled analysis of the HEC studies, the addition of rolapitant to active therapy resulted in a 60% improvement in the likelihood of achieving a CR in the delayed phase (71% of rolapitant recipients vs. 60% of active-control recipients; odds ratio 1.6; 95% CI 1.3–2.1; $p = 0.0001$) (Rapoport B.L. et al., 2015). The addition of rolapitant to active therapy also produced a significantly higher rate of no emesis and no clinically significant nausea in the delayed phase.

In the MEC study, rolapitant recipients had a higher rate of CR in the delayed phase than active-control recipients (71 vs. 62%; OR 1.6; 95% CI 1.2–2.0; $p = 0.0002$), and rolapitant was associated with significant benefits in the prevention of vomiting but not of nausea. A prespecified analysis found that the benefit of rolapitant on CR in the delayed phase was maintained irrespective of whether patients were treated with AC. A further analysis in the subgroup of patients treated with carboplatin-based chemotherapy found that the absolute benefit observed with rolapitant (the absolute difference between the proportion of rolapitant and active-control respondents) was 16.7 percentage points for CR in the delayed phase (Hesketh et al., 2016b). Interestingly, in the study mentioned above that showed improved rates of delayed-phase CR and delayed-phase emesis with fosaprepitant in patients receiving non-AC MEC, approximately 53% of these patients were receiving a carboplatin-based chemotherapy regimen (Weinstein et al., 2016). While this study did not stratify efficacy findings by individual MEC agent, it does support the use of NK-1–receptor antagonists in patients receiving carboplatin. This is borne out in the recent update to the MASCC/ESMO guidelines, in which an NK-1 receptor antagonist is recommended in addition to a 5-HT_3 receptor antagonist and dexamethasone for patients receiving carboplatin (MASCC/ESMO, 2016).

In the trials of rolapitant for the treatment of CINV associated with HEC, more patients receiving rolapitant than active control reported no nausea (≤5 mm on a 100-mm horizontal visual analog scale) in both the overall phase (52 vs. 42%, $p = 0.0004$) and the delayed phase (56 vs. 44%; $p = 0.0002$) (Rapoport B.L. et al., 2015). In one of the trials of aprepitant in patients receiving cisplatin, a greater proportion of patients in the aprepitant group than in the active-control group reported no nausea in the overall phase (49 vs. 39%; $p < 0.005$) and the delayed phase (53 vs. 40%, $p < 0.05$) (Poli-Bigelli et al., 2003), but these effects were not replicated in the second concurrent aprepitant trial in cisplatin-treated patients (Hesketh et al., 2003). Neither rolapitant, aprepitant, nor fosaprepitant significantly increased the number of patients reporting no nausea after treatment with MEC (Rapoport et al., 2010; Schwartzberg L.S. et al., 2015; Weinstein et al., 2016). Trials of NEPA did not include no nausea as an endpoint measure (Aapro et al., 2014c; Hesketh et al., 2014).

Three studies have been published describing the efficacy and safety of aprepitant over multiple cycles of chemotherapy. The first assessed the use of aprepitant over six cycles of cisplatin treatment, using transitional probability models to estimate response rates; it showed that the probability of a CR (no emesis and no significant nausea) was greater in patients receiving aprepitant than active control in the first, fifth, and sixth cisplatin treatment cycles ($p < 0.05$) (de Wit et al., 2003), with drug-related adverse events (AEs) reported in 34% of patients receiving aprepitant versus 25% of those receiving standard therapy. A much larger pooled analysis of the two aforementioned phase 3 trials (Hesketh et al., 2003; Poli-Bigelli et al., 2003), also using transitional probability analyses, found that aprepitant-treated patients were more likely than those receiving standard therapy to exhibit a CR over all six cycles of cisplatin-based therapy (de Wit et al., 2004), with similar rates of drug-related AEs (6 and 4%, respectively). Aprepitant treatment was also associated with a greater probability of CR in each treatment cycle in patients receiving four cycles of MEC (Herrstedt et al., 2005); overall rates of drug-related AEs were not reported.

In a multiple-cycle extension of the phase 3 trial reported by Aapro et al. (2014c), NEPA was associated with superior CR rates compared with palonosetron over four cycles of AC-based chemotherapy ($p < 0.001$ in cycles 2–4), with a similar incidence of AEs observed in each treatment arm (Aapro et al., 2014b). The efficacy and safety of NEPA versus aprepitant over six cycles of chemotherapy in patients receiving MEC or HEC was evaluated in a phase 3 clinical trial (Gralla et al., 2014); overall rates of CR in each cycle were similar for the two treatments (81–91% and

76–88%, respectively), and rates of drug-related AEs were also similar over all cycles (10 and 6%, respectively).

To determine the efficacy and safety of rolapitant over multiple cycles of chemotherapy, a post hoc analysis was carried out on pooled safety and efficacy data from four rolapitant clinical studies (Rapoport et al., 2016): the phase 2 dose-determining study of rolapitant in patients receiving HEC (Rapoport B. et al., 2015) and the three previously mentioned phase 3 trials (Rapoport B.L. et al., 2015; Schwartzberg L.S. et al., 2015). Rates of emesis were lower in the pooled population of patients receiving rolapitant than in those receiving placebo in all chemotherapy cycles after the first (cycles 2–6), and a higher proportion of patients in the pooled rolapitant group reported no nausea interfering with daily life and the combined measure of no emesis or interfering nausea over cycles 2–5 (Rapoport et al., 2016). The incidence of treatment-emergent AEs was low and was similar in both groups after cycle 1 (rolapitant, 5.5%; control, 6.8%), and it did not increase with each subsequent cycle.

NK-1 receptor antagonists are generally well tolerated; the most commonly reported treatment-emergent AEs with NK-1 receptor antagonists in clinical trials included headache, constipation, fatigue, and hiccups, which appeared with a similar frequency as in active-control groups (Navari, 2016).

Differences in pharmacokinetic properties between NK-1 receptor antagonists may affect their dosing (**Table 2**). Aprepitant has a relatively short half-life of 9–13 h, requiring daily dosing across days 1–3 of each cycle (Emend, 2015), whereas the half-lives for NEPA and rolapitant are approximately 80 and 180 h, respectively, and each agent is administered as a single dose 1–2 h prior to chemotherapy (Akynzeo, 2015; Varubi, 2015). All of the NK-1 receptor antagonists, with the exception of rolapitant, inhibit or induce CYP3A4. A reduced dose of dexamethasone (a CYP3A4 substrate) should be administered with aprepitant and NEPA, but it is not required with rolapitant. Rolapitant does not inhibit or induce CYP3A4, with no effect shown on the pharmacokinetics of the sensitive CYP3A4 substrate midazolam (Poma et al., 2013). Rolapitant is a moderate inhibitor of CYP2D6 and an inhibitor of breast cancer resistance protein (BCRP) and P-glycoprotein, and its concomitant use with substrates of these enzymes that have a narrow therapeutic index should be avoided.

TABLE 2 | Recommended dosing of NK-1 receptor antagonists.

NK-1 receptor antagonist	Day 1	Days 2–3
Aprepitant	Single oral 125-mg dose prior to chemotherapy	Oral dose of 80 mg once daily on days 2 and 3
Fosaprepitant	Single intravenous 150-mg dose prior to chemotherapy	–
Netupitant	Single oral 300 mg netupitant/0.5-mg palonosetron dose prior to chemotherapy	–
Rolapitant	Single oral 180-mg dose prior to chemotherapy	–

However, in an integrated safety analysis of randomized trials, the incidence of treatment-emergent AEs was similar in the rolapitant and control arms in patients who used concomitant CYP2D6, BCRP, or CYP3A4 substrate drugs (Barbour et al., 2015).

Other Antiemetics for Delayed Emesis

Corticosteroids have been used as prophylaxis against CINV, particularly delayed CINV, for many years, although their exact mechanism of action is unknown. The antiemetic efficacy of 5-HT_3 receptor antagonists (or dopamine antagonists) increases when they are used in combination with corticosteroids (Grunberg, 2007); therefore, these agents are typically administered concurrently.

Olanzapine, an atypical antipsychotic drug that blocks dopaminergic, serotonergic, adrenergic, and histamine receptors, has been evaluated in combination with 5-HT_3 receptor antagonist and corticosteroid for delayed CINV prophylaxis (Tan et al., 2009; Navari et al., 2011). Benefits with this agent have been reported for both acute and delayed nausea control (Abe et al., 2016; Chiu et al., 2016; Navari et al., 2016). The National Comprehensive Cancer Network (2016) guidelines include olanzapine with a 5-HT_3 antagonist and corticosteroid as a treatment option for prevention of both HEC- and MEC-associated CINV. The recommendations also include consideration of replacing NK-1 receptor antagonist–containing regimens with an olanzapine-containing regimen for management of breakthrough emesis.

CURRENT CINV PROPHYLAXIS GUIDELINES

Several evidence-based guidelines for the prevention of CINV have been developed by international professional societies (Hesketh et al., 2016b; MASCC/ESMO, 2016; National Comprehensive Cancer Network, 2016), which are relatively consistent in their key recommendations (summarized in **Table 3**). In general, the guidelines recommend prescribing a NK-1 receptor antagonist along with a 5-HT_3 receptor antagonist and dexamethasone for prevention of CINV in patients receiving HEC, and a 5-HT_3 receptor antagonist and dexamethasone in patients receiving MEC (Hesketh et al., 2016b; MASCC/ESMO, 2016; National Comprehensive Cancer Network, 2016). The National Comprehensive Cancer Network and the American Society of Clinical Oncology also recommend that an NK-1 receptor antagonist be considered for patients treated with MEC, particularly those with additional risk factors for CINV (Hesketh et al., 2016b; National Comprehensive Cancer Network, 2016). The authors of these guidelines have made a concerted effort to define antiemetic regimens that cover both the acute and delayed phases of CINV.

Adherence to antiemetic guidelines improves the control of acute and delayed CINV (Aapro et al., 2012); however, such adherence is suboptimal across a range of settings (Aapro et al., 2012; Burmeister et al., 2012; Gomez et al., 2013; Gilmore

TABLE 3 | Summary of evidence-based guidelines for chemotherapy-induced nausea and vomiting (CINV) prophylaxis with intravenous chemotherapy.

Emetic risk category	Guideline recommendation
High (including AC combinations)	NK-1 receptor antagonist + 5-HT_3 receptor antagonist + dexamethasone (Hesketh et al., 2016b; MASCC/ESMO, 2016; National Comprehensive Cancer Network, 2016) *or* Olanzapine + 5-HT_3 receptor antagonist + dexamethasone (National Comprehensive Cancer Network, 2016)
Moderate	5-HT_3 receptor antagonist + dexamethasone (± NK-1 receptor antagonist[a]) (Basch et al., 2011; National Comprehensive Cancer Network, 2016) *or* Olanzapine + 5-HT_3 receptor antagonist + dexamethasone (National Comprehensive Cancer Network, 2016) *or* 5-HT_3 receptor antagonist + dexamethasone (MASCC/ESMO, 2016)
Low	Dexamethasone (Basch et al., 2011; MASCC/ESMO, 2016; National Comprehensive Cancer Network, 2016) *or* Dopamine receptor antagonist OR 5-HT_3 receptor antagonist (MASCC/ESMO, 2016; National Comprehensive Cancer Network, 2016)
Minimal	No prophylactic antiemetic (Basch et al., 2011; MASCC/ESMO, 2016; National Comprehensive Cancer Network, 2016)

[a]An NK-1 receptor antagonist should be added for patients with additional risk factors or who are failing 5-HT_3 receptor antagonist + dexamethasone (National Comprehensive Cancer Network, 2016). The NK-1 receptor antagonist recommended in the ASCO guidelines is aprepitant (Basch et al., 2011). 5-HT_3, 5-hydroxytryptamine type 3; AC, anthracycline–cyclophosphamide; CINV, chemotherapy-induced nausea and vomiting; NK-1, neurokinin-1.

et al., 2014; Jordan et al., 2014; Yu et al., 2015). Nonadherence to guidelines may include the failure to use NK-1 receptor antagonists as part of the antiemetic regimen (Gomez et al., 2013; Gilmore et al., 2014) and the overuse of 5-HT_3 receptor antagonists for prevention of delayed CINV (Burmeister et al., 2012).

CONCLUSION AND FUTURE DIRECTIONS

At present, antiemetic therapy recommendations are based largely on the emetogenic potential of the chemotherapy regimen, with less consideration of individual risk factors. Incorporation of personal risk factors may allow better prediction of CINV and improve personalized management of CINV. Indices that can discriminate between patients at high and low risk of both acute and delayed CINV are currently in development (Dranitsaris et al., 2013) and are being validated in randomized controlled trials. For example, patients with early-stage breast cancer receiving AC were randomized to risk-model guided (RMG) antiemetic prophylaxis or physician's choice of therapy. Benefits were seen in both the acute and delayed phase with RMG therapy: specifically, significantly more patients in the RMG group than the physician's choice group reported no delayed nausea (39.6 vs. 30.7%; $p = 0.01$) and no delayed vomiting (87.1 vs. 78.0%; $p < 0.001$) (Clemons et al., 2016). The development of algorithms with high sensitivity and specificity to aid clinical decision making may improve CINV prophylaxis, particularly in the delayed phase.

There are several possible explanations for the persistence of delayed CINV even in the absence of acute CINV. The delayed phase may be inherently resistant to treatment, appropriate prophylactic antiemetics may be inadequately prescribed because of underestimation of delayed CINV control, or patients may be nonadherent to prescribing instructions when pills need to be taken at home. Whatever the case, delayed CINV continues to be a treatment challenge. Effective treatment of nausea over both the acute and delayed phases also remains an unmet clinical need in both patients receiving HEC and those receiving MEC (Ng et al., 2015), although the addition of olanzapine to standard triple therapy of an NK-1 receptor antagonist, a 5-HT_3 receptor antagonist, and dexamethasone has shown benefit in patients receiving cisplatin- or cyclophosphamide-doxorubicin–based HEC (Abe et al., 2016; Chiu et al., 2016; Navari et al., 2016). Identifying patients at risk of delayed CINV and initiating prophylaxis with triple therapy before administration of chemotherapy is likely to improve clinical outcomes and patients' daily lives.

AUTHOR CONTRIBUTIONS

BLR developed the concept of this work, critically revised all drafts, gave final approval for submission of the final version for publication, and is accountable for all aspects of the work.

FUNDING

Analysis, writing, and editorial support for this work were fully funded by Tesaro.

ACKNOWLEDGMENTS

Hannah Mace, MPharmacol, and Jeremy Kennard, PhD (Ashfield Healthcare Communications, Middletown, CT, USA), drafted and revised the manuscript based on input from the author, and Joshua Safran (Ashfield Healthcare Communications) copyedited and styled the manuscript per journal requirements.

REFERENCES

Aapro, M. (2005). 5-HT(3)-receptor antagonists in the management of nausea and vomiting in cancer and cancer treatment. *Oncology* 69, 97–109. doi: 10.1159/000087979

Aapro, M., Jordan, K., and Feyer, P. (2014a). *Prevention of Nausea and Vomiting in Adult Cancer Patients Receiving Tumour-Directed Therapy.* Amsterdam: Elsevier.

Aapro, M., Karthaus, M., Schwartzberg, L., Rossi, G., Rizzi, G., Borroni, M. E., et al. (2014b). Phase 3 study of NEPA, a fixed-dose combination of netupitant and palonosetron, for prevention of chemotherapy-induced nausea and vomiting during repeated moderately emetogenic chemotherapy (MEC) cycles. *J. Clin. Oncol.* 32, 5s.

Aapro, M., Molassiotis, A., Dicato, M., Pelaez, I., Rodriguez-Lescure, A., Pastorelli, D., et al. (2012). The effect of guideline-consistent antiemetic therapy on chemotherapy-induced nausea and vomiting (CINV): the Pan European Emesis Registry (PEER). *Ann. Oncol.* 23, 1986–1992. doi: 10.1093/annonc/mds021

Aapro, M., Rugo, H., Rossi, G., Rizzi, G., Borroni, M. E., Bondarenko, I., et al. (2014c). A randomized phase III study evaluating the efficacy and safety of NEPA, a fixed-dose combination of netupitant and palonosetron, for prevention of chemotherapy-induced nausea and vomiting following moderately emetogenic chemotherapy. *Ann. Oncol.* 25, 1328–1333. doi: 10.1093/annonc/mdu101

Abe, M., Hirashima, Y., Kasamatsu, Y., Kado, N., Komeda, S., Kuji, S., et al. (2016). Efficacy and safety of olanzapine combined with aprepitant, palonosetron, and dexamethasone for preventing nausea and vomiting induced by cisplatin-based chemotherapy in gynecological cancer: KCOG-G1301 phase II trial. *Support Care Cancer* 24, 675–682. doi: 10.1007/s00520-015-2829-z

Akynzeo (2015). Woodcliff Lake, NJ: Eisai Inc. Available at: https://www.akynzeo.com/assets/pdf/Prescribing_Information.pdf [Accessed 25th October, 2016].

Armstrong, D. M., Pickel, V. M., Joh, T. H., Reis, D. J., and Miller, R. J. (1981). Immunocytochemical localization of catecholamine synthesizing enzymes and neuropeptides in area postrema and medial nucleus tractus solitarius of rat brain. *J. Comp. Neurol.* 196, 505–517. doi: 10.1002/cne.901960312

Baba, Y., Baba, H., Yamamoto, S., Shimada, H., Shibata, T., Miyazaki, T., et al. (2016). Chemotherapy-induced nausea and vomiting is less controlled at delayed phase in patients with esophageal cancer: a prospective registration study by the CINV Study Group of Japan. *Dis. Esophagus* doi: 10.1111/dote.12482 [Epub ahead of print].

Babic, T., and Browning, K. N. (2014). The role of vagal neurocircuits in the regulation of nausea and vomiting. *Eur. J. Pharmacol* 722, 38–47. doi: 10.1016/j.ejphar.2013.08.047

Barbour, S., Wang, X., Poma, A., Arora, S., Aapro, M., and Herrstedt, J. (2015). 1529 Low risk of drug interactions when rolapitant is coadministered with CYP2D6 or BCRP substrates: Integrated safety results. *Eur. J. Cancer* 51(Suppl. 3), S214. doi: 10.1016/S0959-8049(16)30619-0

Basch, E., Prestrud, A. A., Hesketh, P. J., Kris, M. G., Feyer, P. C., Somerfield, M. R., et al. (2011). Antiemetics: American Society of Clinical Oncology clinical practice guideline update. *J. Clin. Oncol.* 29, 4189–4198. doi: 10.1200/JCO.2010.34.4614

Bloechl-Daum, B., Deuson, R. R., Mavros, P., Hansen, M., and Herrstedt, J. (2006). Delayed nausea and vomiting continue to reduce patients' quality of life after highly and moderately emetogenic chemotherapy despite antiemetic treatment. *J. Clin. Oncol.* 24, 4472–4478. doi: 10.1200/JCO.2006.05.6382

Burke, T. A., Wisniewski, T., and Ernst, F. R. (2011). Resource utilization and costs associated with chemotherapy-induced nausea and vomiting (CINV) following highly or moderately emetogenic chemotherapy administered in the US outpatient hospital setting. *Support Care Cancer* 19, 131–140. doi: 10.1007/s00520-009-0797-x

Burmeister, H., Aebi, S., Studer, C., Fey, M. F., and Gautschi, O. (2012). Adherence to ESMO clinical recommendations for prophylaxis of chemotherapy-induced nausea and vomiting. *Support Care Cancer* 20, 141–147. doi: 10.1007/s00520-010-1079-3

Chiu, L., Chow, R., Popovic, M., Navari, R. M., Shumway, N. M., Chiu, N., et al. (2016). Efficacy of olanzapine for the prophylaxis and rescue of chemotherapy-induced nausea and vomiting (CINV): a systematic review and meta-analysis. *Support Care Cancer* 24, 2381–2392. doi: 10.1007/s00520-016-3075-8

Clemons, M., Bouganim, N., Smith, S., Mazzarello, S., Vandermeer, L., Segal, R., et al. (2016). Risk model-guided antiemetic prophylaxis vs physician's choice in patients receiving chemotherapy for early-stage breast cancer: a randomized clinical trial. *JAMA Oncol.* 2, 225–231. doi: 10.1001/jamaoncol.2015.3730

de Boer-Dennert, M., De Wit, R., Schmitz, P. I, Djontono, J. V., Beurden, V., Stoter, G., et al. (1997). Patient perceptions of the side-effects of chemotherapy: the influence of 5HT3 antagonists. *Br. J. Cancer* 76, 1055–1061. doi: 10.1038/bjc.1997.507

de Wit, R., Herrstedt, J., Rapoport, B., Carides, A. D., Carides, G., Elmer, M., et al. (2003). Addition of the oral NK1 antagonist aprepitant to standard antiemetics provides protection against nausea and vomiting during multiple cycles of cisplatin-based chemotherapy. *J. Clin. Oncol.* 21, 4105–4111. doi: 10.1200/JCO.2003.10.128

de Wit, R., Herrstedt, J., Rapoport, B., Carides, A. D., Guoguang-Ma, J., Elmer, M., et al. (2004). The oral NK(1) antagonist, aprepitant, given with standard antiemetics provides protection against nausea and vomiting over multiple cycles of cisplatin-based chemotherapy: a combined analysis of two randomised, placebo-controlled phase III clinical trials. *Eur. J. Cancer* 40, 403–410. doi: 10.1016/S0959-8049(03)00931-6

Dranitsaris, G., Bouganim, N., Milano, C., Vandermeer, L., Dent, S., Wheatley-Price, P., et al. (2013). Prospective validation of a prediction tool for identifying patients at high risk for chemotherapy-induced nausea and vomiting. *J. Support Oncol.* 11, 14–21.

Ellebaek, E., and Herrstedt, J. (2008). Optimizing antiemetic therapy in multiple-day and multiple cycles of chemotherapy. *Curr. Opin. Support Palliat Care* 2, 28–34. doi: 10.1097/SPC.0b013e3282f44a75

Emend (2015). Whitehouse, NJ: Merck Sharp & Dohme Corp. Available at: https://www.merck.com/product/usa/pi_circulars/e/emend/emend_pi.pdf [Accessed 25th October, 2016].

Escobar, Y., Cajaraville, G., Virizuela, J. A., Alvarez, R., Munoz, A., Olariaga, O., et al. (2015). Incidence of chemotherapy-induced nausea and vomiting with moderately emetogenic chemotherapy: ADVICE (Actual Data of Vomiting Incidence by Chemotherapy Evaluation) study. *Support Care Cancer* 23, 2833–2840. doi: 10.1007/s00520-015-2809-3

Garcia-Recio, S., and Gascon, P. (2015). Biological and pharmacological aspects of the NK1-receptor. *Biomed. Res. Int.* 2015, 495704. doi: 10.1155/2015/495704

Gilmore, J. W., Peacock, N. W., Gu, A., Szabo, S., Rammage, M., Sharpe, J., et al. (2014). Antiemetic guideline consistency and incidence of chemotherapy-induced nausea and vomiting in US community oncology practice: INSPIRE Study. *J. Oncol. Pract.* 10, 68–74. doi: 10.1200/JOP.2012.000816

Gomez, D. R., Liao, K. P., Giordano, S., Nguyen, H., Smith, B. D., and Elting, L. S. (2013). Adherence to national guidelines for antiemesis prophylaxis in patients undergoing chemotherapy for lung cancer: a population-based study. *Cancer* 119, 1428–1436. doi: 10.1002/cncr.27899

Gralla, R. J., Bosnjak, S. M., Hontsa, A., Balser, C., Rizzi, G., Rossi, G., et al. (2014). A phase III study evaluating the safety and efficacy of NEPA, a fixed-dose combination of netupitant and palonosetron, for prevention of chemotherapy-induced nausea and vomiting over repeated cycles of chemotherapy. *Ann. Oncol.* 25, 1333–1339. doi: 10.1093/annonc/mdu096

Grassi, L., Berardi, M. A., Ruffilli, F., Meggiolaro, E., Andritsch, E., Sirgo, A., et al. (2015). Role of psychosocial variables on chemotherapy-induced nausea and vomiting and health-related quality of life among cancer patients: a European study. *Psychother. Psychosom.* 84, 339–347. doi: 10.1159/000431256

Grunberg, S., Chua, D., Maru, A., Dinis, J., Devandry, S., Boice, J. A., et al. (2011). Single-dose fosaprepitant for the prevention of chemotherapy-induced nausea and vomiting associated with cisplatin therapy: randomized, double-blind study protocol–EASE. *J. Clin. Oncol.* 29, 1495–1501. doi: 10.1200/JCO.2010.31.7859

Grunberg, S. M. (2007). Antiemetic activity of corticosteroids in patients receiving cancer chemotherapy: dosing, efficacy, and tolerability analysis. *Ann. Oncol.* 18, 233–240. doi: 10.1093/annonc/mdl347

Grunberg, S. M., Deuson, R. R., Mavros, P., Geling, O., Hansen, M., Cruciani, G., et al. (2004). Incidence of chemotherapy-induced nausea and emesis after modern antiemetics. *Cancer* 100, 2261–2268. doi: 10.1002/cncr.20230

Herrstedt, J., Muss, H. B., Warr, D. G., Hesketh, P. J., Eisenberg, P. D., Raftopoulos, H., et al. (2005). Efficacy and tolerability of aprepitant for the prevention of chemotherapy-induced nausea and emesis over multiple cycles of moderately emetogenic chemotherapy. *Cancer* 104, 1548–1555. doi: 10.1002/cncr.21343

Hesketh, P. J. (2008). Chemotherapy-induced nausea and vomiting. *N. Engl. J. Med.* 358, 2482–2494. doi: 10.1056/NEJMra0706547

Hesketh, P. J., Bohlke, K., Lyman, G. H., Basch, E., Chesney, M., Clark-Snow, R. A., et al. (2016a). Antiemetics: American Society of Clinical Oncology focused guideline update. *J. Clin. Oncol.* 34, 381–386. doi: 10.1200/JCO.2015.64.3635

Hesketh, P. J., Grunberg, S. M., Gralla, R. J., Warr, D. G., Roila, F., De Wit, R., et al. (2003). The oral neurokinin-1 antagonist aprepitant for the prevention of chemotherapy-induced nausea and vomiting: a multinational, randomized, double-blind, placebo-controlled trial in patients receiving high-dose cisplatin–the Aprepitant Protocol 052 Study Group. *J. Clin. Oncol.* 21, 4112–4119.

Hesketh, P. J., Kris, M. G., Grunberg, S. M., Beck, T., Hainsworth, J. D., Harker, G., et al. (1997). Proposal for classifying the acute emetogenicity of cancer chemotherapy. *J. Clin. Oncol.* 15, 103–109.

Hesketh, P. J., Rossi, G., Rizzi, G., Palmas, M., Alyasova, A., Bondarenko, I., et al. (2014). Efficacy and safety of NEPA, an oral combination of netupitant and palonosetron, for prevention of chemotherapy-induced nausea and vomiting following highly emetogenic chemotherapy: a randomized dose-ranging pivotal study. *Ann. Oncol.* 25, 1340–1346. doi: 10.1093/annonc/mdu110

Hesketh, P. J., Schnadig, I. D., Schwartzberg, L. S., Modiano, M. R., Jordan, K., Arora, S., et al. (2016b). Efficacy of the neurokinin-1 receptor antagonist rolapitant in preventing nausea and vomiting in patients receiving carboplatin-based chemotherapy. *Cancer* 122, 2418–2425. doi: 10.1002/cncr.30054

Higgins, S. C., Montgomery, G. H., and Bovbjerg, D. H. (2007). Distress before chemotherapy predicts delayed but not acute nausea. *Support Care Cancer* 15, 171–177. doi: 10.1007/s00520-006-0113-y

Hilarius, D. L., Kloeg, P. H., Van Der Wall, E., Van Den Heuvel, J. J., Gundy, C. M., and Aaronson, N. K. (2012). Chemotherapy-induced nausea and vomiting in daily clinical practice: a community hospital-based study. *Support Care Cancer* 20, 107–117. doi: 10.1007/s00520-010-1073-9

Hsieh, R. K., Chan, A., Kim, H. K., Yu, S., Kim, J. G., Lee, M. A., et al. (2015). Baseline patient characteristics, incidence of CINV, and physician perception of CINV incidence following moderately and highly emetogenic chemotherapy in Asia Pacific countries. *Support Care Cancer* 23, 263–272. doi: 10.1007/s00520-014-2373-2

Ihbe-Heffinger, A., Ehlken, B., Bernard, R., Berger, K., Peschel, C., Eichler, H. G., et al. (2004). The impact of delayed chemotherapy-induced nausea and vomiting on patients, health resource utilization and costs in German cancer centers. *Ann. Oncol.* 15, 526–536. doi: 10.1093/annonc/mdh110

Italian Group for Antiemetic Research. (1994). Cisplatin-induced delayed emesis: pattern and prognostic factors during three subsequent cycles. Italian Group for Antiemetic Research. *Ann. Oncol.* 5, 585–589.

Jordan, K., Gralla, R., Jahn, F., and Molassiotis, A. (2014). International antiemetic guidelines on chemotherapy induced nausea and vomiting (CINV): content and implementation in daily routine practice. *Eur. J. Pharmacol.* 722, 197–202. doi: 10.1016/j.ejphar.2013.09.073

Jordan, K., Hinke, A., Grothey, A., Voigt, W., Arnold, D., Wolf, H. H., et al. (2007). A meta-analysis comparing the efficacy of four 5-HT3-receptor antagonists for acute chemotherapy-induced emesis. *Support Care Cancer* 15, 1023–1033. doi: 10.1007/s00520-006-0186-7

Jordan, K., Jahn, F., and Aapro, M. (2015). Recent developments in the prevention of chemotherapy-induced nausea and vomiting (CINV): a comprehensive review. *Ann. Oncol.* 26, 1081–1090. doi: 10.1093/annonc/mdv138

Kottschade, L., Novotny, P., Lyss, A., Mazurczak, M., Loprinzi, C., and Barton, D. (2016). Chemotherapy-induced nausea and vomiting: incidence and characteristics of persistent symptoms and future directions NCCTG N08C3 (Alliance). *Support Care Cancer* 24, 2661–2667. doi: 10.1007/s00520-016-3080-y

MASCC/ESMO (2016). *Antiemetic Guideline 2016.* Version 1.2. Available at: http://www.mascc.org/assets/Guidelines_Tools/mascc_antiemetic_guidelines_english_2016_v.1.2.pdf

Molassiotis, A., Aapro, M., Dicato, M., Gascon, P., Novoa, S. A., Isambert, N., et al. (2014). Evaluation of risk factors predicting chemotherapy-related nausea and vomiting: results from a European prospective observational study. *J. Pain Symptom Manage.* 47:e834. doi: 10.1016/j.jpainsymman.2013.06.012

Molassiotis, A., Saunders, M. P., Valle, J., Wilson, G., Lorigan, P., Wardley, A., et al. (2008). A prospective observational study of chemotherapy-related nausea and vomiting in routine practice in a UK cancer centre. *Support Care Cancer* 16, 201–208. doi: 10.1007/s00520-007-0343-7

National Comprehensive Cancer Network (2016). *NCCN Clinical Practice Guidelines in Oncology: Antiemesis.* Version 1. 2016. Available at: www.nccn.org

Navari, R. M. (2016). The safety of antiemetic medications for the prevention of chemotherapy-induced nausea and vomiting. *Exp. Opin. Drug Saf.* 15, 343–356. doi: 10.1517/14740338.2016.1135899

Navari, R. M., and Aapro, M. (2016). Antiemetic prophylaxis for chemotherapy-induced nausea and vomiting. *N. Engl. J. Med.* 374, 1356–1367. doi: 10.1056/NEJMra1515442

Navari, R. M., Gray, S. E., and Kerr, A. C. (2011). Olanzapine versus aprepitant for the prevention of chemotherapy-induced nausea and vomiting: a randomized phase III trial. *J. Support. Oncol.* 9, 188–195. doi: 10.1016/j.suponc.2011.05.002

Navari, R. M., Qin, R., Ruddy, K. J., Liu, H., Powell, S. F., Bajaj, M., et al. (2016). Olanzapine for the prevention of chemotherapy-induced nausea and vomiting. *N. Engl. J. Med.* 375, 134–142. doi: 10.1056/NEJMoa1515725

Ng, T. L., Hutton, B., and Clemons, M. (2015). Chemotherapy-induced nausea and vomiting: time for more emphasis on nausea? *Oncologist* 20, 576–583. doi: 10.1634/theoncologist.2014-0438

Poli-Bigelli, S., Rodrigues-Pereira, J., Carides, A. D., Julie Ma, G., Eldridge, K., Hipple, A., et al. (2003). Addition of the neurokinin 1 receptor antagonist aprepitant to standard antiemetic therapy improves control of chemotherapy-induced nausea and vomiting. Results from a randomized, double-blind, placebo-controlled trial in Latin America. *Cancer* 97, 3090–3098. doi: 10.1002/cncr.11433

Poma, A., Christensen, J., Pertikis, H., Arora, S., and Hedley, M. (2013). Rolapitant and its major metabolite do not affect the pharmacokinetics of midazolam, a sensitive cytochrome P450 3A4 substrate. *Support Care Cancer* 21:S154.

Rapoport, B., Chua, D., Poma, A., Arora, S., Wang, Y., and Fein, L. E. (2015). Study of rolapitant, a novel, long-acting, NK-1 receptor antagonist, for the prevention of chemotherapy-induced nausea and vomiting (CINV) due to highly emetogenic chemotherapy (HEC). *Support Care Cancer* 23, 3281–3288. doi: 10.1007/s00520-015-2738-1

Rapoport, B., Schwartzberg, L., Chasen, M., Powers, D., Arora, S., Navari, R., et al. (2016). Efficacy and safety of rolapitant for prevention of chemotherapy-induced nausea and vomiting over multiple cycles of moderately or highly emetogenic chemotherapy. *Eur. J. Cancer* 57, 23–30. doi: 10.1016/j.ejca.2015.12.023

Rapoport, B. L., Chasen, M. R., Gridelli, C., Urban, L., Modiano, M. R., Schnadig, I. D., et al. (2015). Safety and efficacy of rolapitant for prevention of chemotherapy-induced nausea and vomiting after administration of cisplatin-based highly emetogenic chemotherapy in patients with cancer: two randomised, active-controlled, double-blind, phase 3 trials. *Lancet Oncol.* 16, 1079–1089. doi: 10.1016/S1470-2045(15)00035-2

Rapoport, B. L., Jordan, K., Boice, J. A., Taylor, A., Brown, C., Hardwick, J. S., et al. (2010). Aprepitant for the prevention of chemotherapy-induced nausea and vomiting associated with a broad range of moderately emetogenic chemotherapies and tumor types: a randomized, double-blind study. *Support Care Cancer* 18, 423–431. doi: 10.1007/s00520-009-0680-9

Schwartzberg, L., Harrow, B., Lal, L. S., Radtchenko, J., and Lyman, G. H. (2015). Resource utilization for chemotherapy-induced nausea and vomiting events in patients with solid tumors treated with antiemetic regimens. *Am. Health Drug Benefits* 8, 273–282.

Schwartzberg, L. S., Modiano, M. R., Rapoport, B. L., Chasen, M. R., Gridelli, C., Urban, L., et al. (2015). Safety and efficacy of rolapitant for prevention of chemotherapy-induced nausea and vomiting after administration of moderately emetogenic chemotherapy or anthracycline and cyclophosphamide regimens in patients with cancer: a randomised, active-controlled, double-blind, phase 3 trial. *Lancet Oncol.* 16, 1071–1078. doi: 10.1016/S1470-2045(15)00034-0

Sun, C. C., Bodurka, D. C., Weaver, C. B., Rasu, R., Wolf, J. K., Bevers, M. W., et al. (2005). Rankings and symptom assessments of side effects from chemotherapy: insights from experienced patients with ovarian cancer. *Support Care Cancer* 13, 219–227. doi: 10.1007/s00520-004-0710-6

Tan, L., Liu, J., Liu, X., Chen, J., Yan, Z., Yang, H., et al. (2009). Clinical research of Olanzapine for prevention of chemotherapy-induced nausea and vomiting. *J. Exp. Clin. Cancer Res.* 28, 131. doi: 10.1186/1756-9966-28-131

Van Laar, E. S., Desai, J. M., and Jatoi, A. (2015). Professional educational needs for chemotherapy-induced nausea and vomiting (CINV): multinational survey results from 2388 health care providers. *Support Care Cancer* 23, 151–157. doi: 10.1007/s00520-014-2325-x

Varubi (2015). Waltham, MA: Tesaro. Available at: http://varubirx.com/downloads/VARUBI_(rolapitant)_Full_Prescribing_Information.pdf [Accessed 25th October, 2016].

Vidall, C., Dielenseger, P., Farrell, C., Lennan, E., Muxagata, P., Fernandez-Ortega, P., et al. (2011). Evidence-based management of chemotherapy-induced nausea and vomiting: a position statement from a European cancer nursing forum. *Ecancermedicalscience* 5:211. doi: 10.3332/ecancer.2011.211

Weinstein, C., Jordan, K., Green, S. A., Camacho, E., Khanani, S., Beckford-Brathwaite, E., et al. (2016). Single-dose fosaprepitant for the prevention of chemotherapy-induced nausea and vomiting associated with moderately emetogenic chemotherapy: results of a randomized, double-blind phase III trial. *Ann. Oncol.* 27, 172–178. doi: 10.1093/annonc/mdv482

Yu, S., Burke, T. A., Chan, A., Kim, H. K., Hsieh, R. K., Hu, X., et al. (2015). Antiemetic therapy in Asia Pacific countries for patients receiving moderately and highly emetogenic chemotherapy–a descriptive analysis of practice patterns, antiemetic quality of care, and use of antiemetic guidelines. *Support Care Cancer* 23, 273–282. doi: 10.1007/s00520-014-2372-3

Conflict of Interest Statement: BLR has received honoraria and expenses from Herron, Merck and Co. and Tesaro, has sat on advisory boards for Herron, Merck and Co. and Tesaro and has received research funding from Merck and Co. and Tesaro.

6

New Frontiers in the Pathobiology and Treatment of Cancer Regimen-Related Mucosal Injury

*Marika Cinausero[1], Giuseppe Aprile[1,2], Paola Ermacora[1], Debora Basile[1], Maria G. Vitale[1], Valentina Fanotto[1], Giuseppe Parisi[1], Lorenzo Calvetti[2] and Stephen T. Sonis[3,4,5]**

[1] Department of Oncology, University and General Hospital, Udine, Italy, [2] Department of Oncology, San Bortolo General Hospital, Vicenza, Italy, [3] Divisions of Oral Medicine, Brigham and Women's Hospital, Boston, MA, United States, [4] Dana-Farber Cancer Institute, Boston, MA, United States, [5] Biomodels LLC, Watertown, MA, United States

Edited by:
Kulmira Nurgali,
Victoria University, Australia

Reviewed by:
Loredana Bergandi,
University of Turin, Italy
Hu Liu,
Anhui Medical University, China

***Correspondence:**
Stephen T. Sonis
ssonis@partners.org

Mucositis is a common complication of chemotherapy, radiotherapy and targeted agents. It often affects compliance to anticancer therapies as it frequently causes schedule delays, interruptions or discontinuations of treatment. Moreover, the economic impact related to the management of mucositis is topical and several estimations of additional hospital costs due to this clinical condition have been recently reported. The ability to determine risk factors for mucositis, to early detect its onset, to assess correctly the degree of this toxicity and to plan its multidisciplinary management are all key elements to guarantee the quality of life of patients and to avoid useless dose reduction or interruption of treatment. The pathogenesis of mucositis is multifactorial and it is classily subdivided into oral and gastrointestinal mucositis according to its anatomic presentation. Treatment and patients' related factors might help in predicting the frequency and the potential degree of symptoms onset. Here we discuss about clinical presentation and pathogenesis of mucositis in relation to different kinds of treatments. Moreover, we focus on therapeutic and prevention strategies, describing past and present management according to international guidelines and the most promising new data about agents potentially able to further improve the treatment of mucositis in the next future.

Keywords: gastrointestinal mucositis, oral mucositis, pathobiology, anticancer treatment, management

INTRODUCTION

Mucositis is a common and clinically significant side effect of both anticancer chemotherapy (CT) and radiation therapy (RT) that can affect any portion of the gastrointestinal (GI) tract. Not only it is associated with an adverse symptom profile, but also it may limit patients' ability to tolerate treatment if not adequately prevented and managed. Moreover, it may be associated with secondary local and systemic infection and poor health outcomes, and generates additional use of healthcare resources resulting in additional costs (Villa and Sonis, 2015).

Historically, mucositis has been described by its anatomical distribution: oral mucositis (OM) for involvement of the tissues of the upper aerodigestive tract, gastrointestinal mucositis (GIM) for lesions dominantly in the small intestine, and proctitis for injury of the rectal mucosa. The incidence and course of mucositis is site-dependent and related to the cancer treatment regimen.

OM has been the most studied, probably as a consequence of its frequency, ease of access and its course and symptom impact (Sonis et al., 2004). Nonetheless, all forms of mucositis (as well as other epithelially based toxicities) share common features in a complex scheme of pathogenesis. While the historical paradigm suggested that mucosal injury was solely the consequence of damaging effects of CT or RT on rapidly dividing normal cells of the GI tract, more current research has demonstrated that tissue damage occurs as a manifestation of a sequence of biological events that ultimately target epithelial stem cells. Experimental evidence has accumulated to validate mucositis' pathogenesis as a multi-stage process (Sonis, 1998, 2004).

EPIDEMIOLOGY

Like most other toxicities, the incidence of mucositis is likely to be under-reported by clinicians. The incidence of clinically significant mucositis has been reported to range from 15% among patients receiving low-risk treatments up to 60–100% among patients being treated with high-dose CT, radiotherapy and bone marrow transplantation. Nonetheless, this percentage is estimated to be about 40% in patients undergoing standard dose, cycled CT (Kwon, 2016). The incidence range of oral and non-oral mucositis at fixed doses of CT ranges from the single digits to well over 50% (i.e., TPF induction regimens for the treatment of HN cancer). Antimetabolites, anthracyclines, and taxanes are chemotherapeutic drugs frequently associated with the development of mucositis (Pico et al., 1998).

Chemotherapy-induced diarrhea, the key clinical sign of GIM, was reported to occur in 89% of patients treated with FOLFIRI and 50% of patients treated with FOLFOX for colorectal cancer (Keefe et al., 2014). Concomitant use of total body RT in hematopoietic stem cell transplant (HSCT) conditioning regimens markedly increased mucositis throughout the GI tract. RT-induced diarrhea in patients being treated for HN or lung cancers was noted in 29% of patients treated with radiation alone and 42% of patients treated with concomitant CT-RT.

Overall, almost a half million patients will suffer from mucositis this year in the U.S. with a likely similar number in Europe (Sonis et al., 2015).

Both OM and GIM can adversely impact on patients' quality of life and may cause treatment delays, unplanned interruptions or even premature discontinuation of anticancer therapies, resulting in prolonged hospital stays, increased re-admission rates, more complications and economic burden. It has been reported an estimated incremental cost of hospitalization that may exceed 3,500 USD per cycle with mucositis (Elting et al., 2003) and an incremental cost of about 18,000 USD in HN cancer patients undergoing CT-RT (Nonzee et al., 2008).

PATHOBIOLOGY OF MUCOSITIS

The pathogenesis of mucositis is multifaceted and involves not only the epithelium, but also the cells and tissues within the submucosa (**Figure 1**). Signaling from damaged endothelium, fibroblasts and infiltrating leukocyte cells contributes to apoptosis, loss of renewal, atrophy and ulceration. Whereas these changes occur more slowly in stratified mucosa, they are abrupt in the single layers of the small intestine (Chaveli-López, 2014; Villa and Sonis, 2015).

A five-phase sequence has been used to describe the biological phases of mucositis: initiation, up-regulation and activation leading to generation of messengers, signal amplification, ulceration with inflammation, and healing. For the most part, this order is independent of the insult (RT and CT) or the target tissue involved. Importantly, the elements driving each phase represent potential interventional targets (Sonis et al., 2004).

The initiation of mucositis is triggered by oxidative stress and the generation of reactive oxygen species (ROS), direct DNA and non-DNA damage, and activation of the innate immune response. These events follow the release of endogenous damage-associated molecular pattern molecules from injured cells of the basal epithelial layers, submucosa, and endothelium. Based on the trajectory of gene activation and pathway analysis, it is clear that the initiating biological cascade happens within seconds of the stimulating insult.

Following initiation, ROS and the innate immune response further damage cell membranes, stimulate macrophages and activate several transcription factors of which nuclear factor NF-κB plays a prominent role. Once activated, NF-κB-mediated gene expression results in a surge of many pro-inflammatory cytokines such as tumor necrosis factor-α (TNF-α), interleukin (IL)-6 and IL-1β and cyclooxygenase-2 (COX-2). The up-regulation of other genes causes the expression of adhesion molecules and angiogenesis (Sonis, 2002; Rm et al., 2007).

More in depth, TNF-α up-regulation may activate caspase pathways and generate a feedback on NF-κB to amplify its response and initiate mitogen-activated protein kinase (MAPK) pathway, leading to activation of c-Jun N-terminal kinase (JNK) signaling; fibronectin breakdown leads to macrophage activation. NF-κB independent pathways such as ceramide pathway may also play a role, resulting in apoptosis of submucosal and basal epithelial cells leading to mucosal ulceration (ulcerative phase) and atrophic changes. Recent studies confirmed the involvement of deregulated expression of metalloproteinases (MMPs) in the pathobiology of mucositis (Al-Dasooqi et al., 2010).

The first three phases rapidly lead to apoptosis of epithelial stem cells. In the case of stratified epithelium (i.e., the upper aerodigestive tract and rectal mucosa), loss of renewal leads to atrophy and then ulceration. From the clinical point of view, the overlying mucosa appears initially normal despite the biological havoc taking placing beneath it. In the case of bolus CT, the time between initial basal cell injury and clinical notable mucosal changes (erythema and thinning) takes about 4 days with ulceration occurring shortly thereafter. In contrast, the consequences of cellular damage in the intestinal villi are almost immediate with clinical evidence of enteritis becoming apparent within 24–48 h of CT.

Bacterial colonization of non-intestinal lesions lags slightly behind ulcer development. However, at that time, a large increase in the bacterial load is seen. In the case of patients receiving CT, this occurs at the time that the patient is least capable of dealing

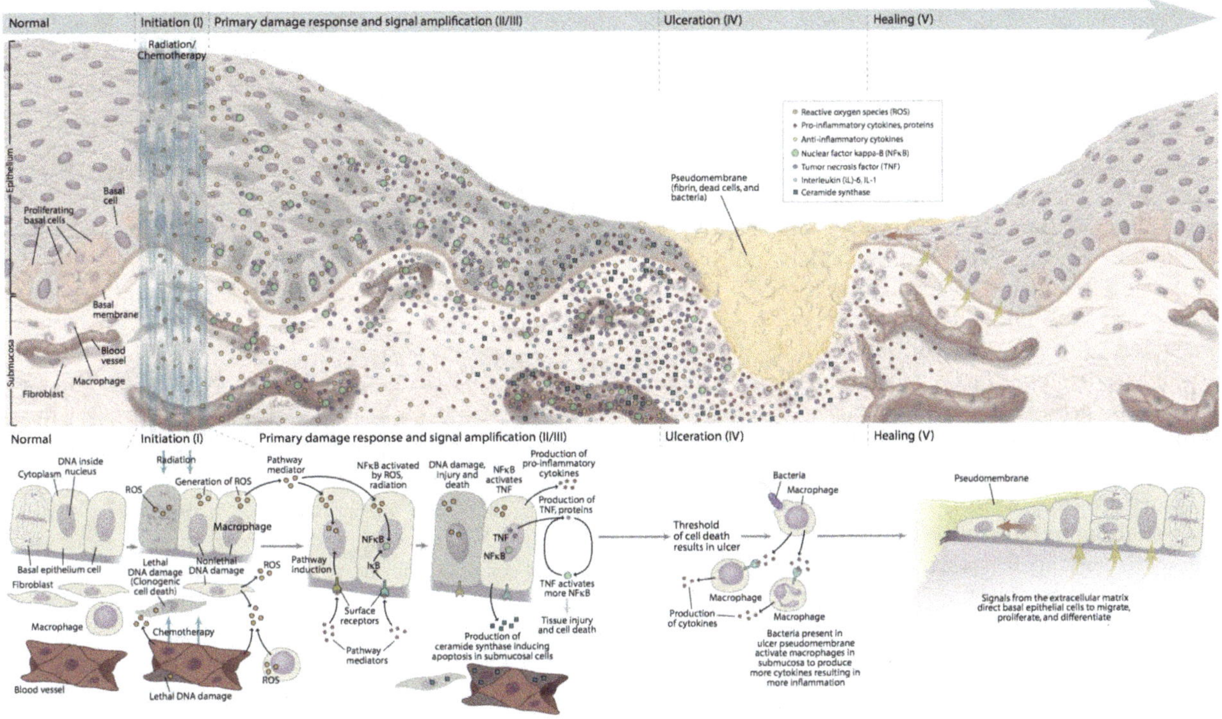

FIGURE 1 | Pathobiology of mucositis. With permission of Sonis (2007). "Reprinted with permission from Frontline Medical Communications, Inc."

with potential infection as it roughly inversely parallels the course of the leukopenia. Ulcer colonization also results in the release of bacterial cell wall products and cytokine production. Healing generally occurs spontaneously and is characterized by epithelial proliferation, migration, and differentiation stimulated by the extracellular matrix (Blijlevens and Sonis, 2007; Al-Ansari et al., 2015). After the healing phase, the oral mucosa returns normal, although the patient have an increased risk of future episodes of mucositis due to residual angiogenesis.

The Role of Microbiota

An active role for the oral and intestinal microbiome in the course of mucositis has not been conclusively established. Antimicrobial strategies aimed at mitigating mucositis have been unsuccessful; moreover, the kinetics of the bacterial load seem to follow, rather than lead ulceration development. Nonetheless, it would be naïve to believe that bacteria are simply inert once lesions are colonized. Certainly, we know that cell wall products that easily penetrate disrupted mucosa have the ability to stimulate macrophages to produce pro-inflammatory cytokines (Stringer and Logan, 2015).

In the GI tract, cancer treatments may affect the composition of luminal microbiota. Generally, they cause a decrease in *Lactobacillus* and other protective bacterial species and an increase in specific pathogenic species (Stringer et al., 2013).

Probiotic bacteria may activate cytoprotective pathways in epithelial cells, counteract ROS, displace pathogenic bacteria and interact with tight junctions to enhance mucosal integrity (Ciorba, 2012). Determining a role for bacteria in intestinal mucositis is further complicated by the observation that GIM is most often manifest in the small intestine, an area of the GI tract in which bacteria are markedly less dense than in the colon (Ciorba et al., 2015). Nonetheless, bacterial transmigration across disrupted epithelium provides an opportunity for bacteremia or systemic infection.

A role for oral viruses, particularly herpes simplex, in the patho-etiology of mucositis, especially in myeloablated patients has been considered for years. Likewise, the potential role for *Candida albicans* in the mucositis development has also been considered (Chen et al., 2011). Based on clinical presentation, cellular data around pathogenesis, and the consistent observed failure of anti-viral or anti-fungal prophylaxis to mitigate mucositis, attribution of mucositis to an infectious etiology is highly unlikely.

Chemotherapy-Induced Mucositis

Although different CT drugs may target different parts of the cell cycle or metabolism, their effect on intestinal morphology is consistent and characterized by decreased crypt length, blunting and fusion of villi, enterocytes hyperplasia and increased apoptosis. The small intestine is most often affected. Commonality of aspects of mucositis pathogenesis is also noted, although the lack of uniform study endpoints hinders some comparisons across different classes and specific agents. A role for pro-inflammatory cytokines has been suggested by a number of studies of both 5-FU, methotrexate and irinotecan (Logan et al., 2008, pp. 1139–1145) in which TNF, IL-1β, and IL-6 levels were all elevated prior to tissue changes (Logan et al., 2008). Likewise, proteins associated with apoptosis (i.e., Bcl-2) regulation are impacted by a range of cytotoxic agents (Ribeiro et al., 2016).

Irinotecan, a topoisomerase I inhibitor, has been broadly studied relative to mucositis pathogenesis. Results of an extensive series of animal studies confirm similarities of cancer regimen-related GI injury pathobiology with that suggested for OM including roles for tight junction disruption and matrix metalloproteinase-mediated connective tissue damage (Wardill et al., 2014; Chen et al., 2016). Likewise, irinotecan-induced mucositis is associated with the activation of caspases, p53 and downregulation of the PI3K/Akt pathway (Mayo et al., 2017), activation of the MAPK and PKC pathways.

The specific anatomy of the small and large intestine contribute to the establishment of mucositis as a 'downstream event.' For example, reduction in goblet cells number and mucin hypersecretion likely contribute to the development of diarrhea.

Some evidences suggest that GIM may manifest in two different ways during irinotecan treatment. Early-onset diarrhea is due to the activation of parasympathetic system leading to cholinergic syndrome by the inhibition of acetylcholinesterase or the release of large quantities of acetylcholine. On the other hand, late-onset diarrhea appears to be multifactorial with both cytokines and direct toxic inflammatory-mediated effects on the mucosa as well as motility alteration (Ribeiro et al., 2016).

Likewise, the development of mucosal injury in platinum-based CT is associated to the mucin reduction.

Radiotherapy-Induced Mucositis

In the case of radiation, damage signaling at the cellular and tissue level happens within seconds of exposure. While the biological sequence is similar to that described above, the fractionated schedule of radiation dosing insures continuing and overlapping damage signals and tissue change. In the case of the upper GI tract and rectal mucosa, symptoms associated with atrophic changes (burning and modest pain) begin as soon as the end of the first week of dosing when patients have typically received 10 Gy of radiation. Ulceration is noted between the second and third week of treatment and becomes contiguous and extremely painful (so as to limit function) at cumulative radiation doses of 30–40 Gy. Lesions persist for up to 6 weeks following the completion of RT (Villa and Sonis, 2015).

Some authors have examined the role of p16 on mucositis and dysphagia incidence rate and duration in HN cancer patients undergoing RT plus cetuximab or RT alone. They have demonstrated that the addition of cetuximab is not related to higher incidence or duration of grade 3 or 4 mucositis compared to RT alone. Finally, they have also seen that patients with p16 negative seem to develop more frequently grade 3 or 4 mucositis (Bonner et al., 2016).

Interestingly, Bossi et al. (2016) found that baseline salivary cytokines levels in HN cancer patients undergoing CT-RT were not associated with severity of OM. However, the salivary concentration of IL-6, TNF-α, IL-10, and IL-1β tend to increase because of anticancer treatment especially during the third week, and it seems to be associated with mucositis severity. Particularly, higher IL-6 and IL-1β levels predicted the development of severe oral toxicity. On the other hand, osteopontin is very high at baseline and decreases after CT-RT (Bossi et al., 2016).

Meirovitz et al. (2010) previously showed that high levels of IL-6 and low levels of IL-8 were associated with percutaneous endoscopic gastrostomy (PEG) placement.

Targeted Therapies-Induced Stomatitis

Among the targeted therapies currently used in oncologic practice, the mTOR-inhibitors produce the most consistent mucosal toxicity. While other sites in the GI tract may also be affected, the severity and impact of mTOR-inhibitor-associated stomatitis (mIAS) is most profound.

Because of its role as a central modulator of extracellular and intracellular signaling of mediators and growth factors associated with negative tumor behaviors, the mTOR pathway has become an attractive target for a class of targeted anti-tumor agents. mTOR-inhibitors, such as everolimus, are currently being used in the management of a number of solid tumors including breast, neuroendocrine of the GI tract and renal cell cancers. Of patients receiving these agents, about 40% develop severe ulcerative stomatitis, termed mIAS which is phenotypically similar to aphthous stomatitis (Peterson et al., 2015). Clinically, mIAS differs from conventional mucositis. mIAS lesions are seen on the movable oral mucosa appearing as relatively shallow, disproportionately painful, ulcers surrounded by an erythematous halo. The central portion of the ulcers is grayish reflecting an area of necrosis. Pseudomembranes are atypical and histologically lesions present as non-specific ulcers. The course of the mIAS is unpredictable, but ulcers can be manifest as soon as 5 days after the start of treatment (Sonis et al., 2010; Elting et al., 2013; Bossi et al., 2015). It appears that the pathogenesis of mIAS is associated with direct epithelial injury followed by a second inflammatory phase. In a recent study using an organotypic model of oral mucosa, histologic changes of mIAS were noted in the absence of any microorganisms. Increases in apoptosis and a reduction in cell proliferation based on immunohistochemical outcomes were seen as were changes in keratinocyte-derived pro-inflammatory cytokines. *In vivo* it is likely that the latter act to attract and facilitate the infusion of inflammatory cells (Sonis et al., 2016).

RISK FACTORS FOR MUCOSITIS

It is clear to anyone treating cancer patients that the risk of any toxicity, including mucositis, is not consistent. While some patients sail through treatment, others suffer immensely, despite having similar tumors and equivalent treatment. Given the imperatives of the Precision Medicine Initiative and the Cancer Moon Shot, prospective identification of patients at risk for mucositis is an important ongoing research objective. Understanding the mechanisms and incidence rates of GIM is essential to set an effective treatment avoiding treatment discontinuation that could negatively influence patients' outcome. In general, risk factors may be associated with the treatment regimen and/or the patient (Villa and Sonis, 2015).

Treatment's Related Variables

Treatment's related factors are linked to the type of anticancer treatment (CT, RT, targeted therapy, etc.), the agent used, the dose and schedule of the anticancer drug, agent or radiation (Sonis, 2010; Villa and Sonis, 2015, 2016).

Chemotherapy

The rates of onset and severity of mucosal injury depend on the type of CT used (Shi et al., 2016).

Chemotherapeutic agents vary in their mucotoxicity. For example, the antimetabolites, i.e., 5-FU (Schwab et al., 2008; Abdel-Rahman et al., 2016) and methotrexate, irinotecan (Stein et al., 2010; Mayo et al., 2017), alkylating agents like cyclophosphamide, and cisplatin (Villa and Sonis, 2015), and anthracyclines and taxanes (Kwon, 2016) all tend to be more consistently associated with mucosal toxicities than bleomycin, hydroxyurea, or etoposide. Moreover, bolus infusion tends to be more toxic.

Recently, a meta-analysis by Abdel-Rahman et al. (2016) has shown that the fluoropyrimidine S-1 induced lower risk of mucositis compared to 5-FU. Instead, patients treated with capecitabine had the same toxicity profile of S-1. The combination of fluoropyrimidines and irinotecan is associated with increased risk of GIM (Abdel-Rahman et al., 2016), especially when capecitabine is used. In the BICC study (Skof et al., 2009) patients who received XELIRI reported higher rates of severe diarrhea (~50%) compared to patients exposed to FOLFIRI.

Moreover, some preclinical studies have found that ileal mucosa is more sensitive to the cisplatin than the remaining GI tract (Yamamoto et al., 2013). Despite this, patients with lung and GI cancer receiving platinum salts and 5-FU have a low risk of platinum-associated severe mucositis (Al-Ansari et al., 2015). Notably, GI toxicity induced by oxaliplatin and carboplatin tend to have a lower grade compared to that of cisplatin (Hartmann and Lipp, 2003).

Patients treated with taxanes experience mucositis in approximately 29–63% of cases. Interestingly, taxanes-associated mucosal damages usually are mild or moderate. Grades 3 and 4 occur only in a few percentage of patients. Furthermore, mucositis occurs more often in patients who receive docetaxel than paclitaxel.

In general, if a patient develops mucositis in the first cycle of treatment, the probability of the condition recurring in a subsequent cycle is high in the absence of dose de-escalation. Mucosal toxicities also arise due to an physiologically driven "overdosing." Patients with hepatic and renal impairment may have a reduced clearance of antineoplastic drugs, which could potentially lead to a greater exposure to these agents.

Radiotherapy

Not surprisingly, patients being radiated for treatment of HN cancers are at high risk for OM (Trotti et al., 2003; Sonis, 2013). In fact, about two-thirds will develop severe forms of the condition. The incidence jumps to close to 100% for cancers located in the mouth or oropharynx.

The addition of concomitant CT, most typically cisplatin, is associated with an increased mucositis risk (Trotti et al., 2003). Sanguineti et al. (2012) showed that HN cancer patients receiving CT-RT had a 4.1-fold and a 5.1-fold increased risk of mucositis development when using IMRT and conventional RT fractions, respectively. It appears that both the incidence and duration of OM is increased with the addition of cetuximab to a standard regimen of RT when compared to CT-RT ($p = 0.014$) (De Sanctis et al., 2016).

Since radiation induces both direct and indirect injury, the observation that patients being treated for HN cancer also manifest damage to lower portions of the GI tract is not unexpected. The consequences of such lesions are impressive. Noteworthy, RT is often associated with the development of esophagitis. High-dose RT and concurrent CT results in significantly increased risk of severe esophagitis. Some patients may require a feeding tube and/or treatment interruptions. Furthermore, damage at this level may lead to superinfection and dysphagia or odynophagia, lower dietary intake, cachexia and consequently to worse prognosis (Adebahr et al., 2016). Radiation on pelvic or abdominal site leads to enteritis, which prevalence ranges from 0.5 to 50% (Abayomi et al., 2009; Theis et al., 2010; Webb et al., 2013). Small bowel-related complications are proportional to the volume of small intestine in the radiation field. Usually, this side effect was delayed, graded 1 or 2, with low rate of hospitalization. Obviously, toxicity was increased by the CT-RT combination therapy (Hernández-Moreno et al., 2015).

Finally, regimens using accelerated dosing schedules in which the daily cumulative dose exceeds 2 Gy are associated with an increased incidence and severity of mucositis.

Targeted Agents

As noted above, some forms of targeted therapy are associated with increased risk of mucosal injury. Since most of these agents, especially the biologicals such as cetuximab are given in conjunction with radiation, their specific mucotoxicity is difficult to assess. The combination of EGFR-I with RT or CT may further increase the toxicity. Notably, in the CRYSTAL trial, colorectal cancer patients randomized to receive FOLFIRI plus cetuximab showed higher frequency of grades 3 and 4 GIM than patients receiving FOLFIRI alone (Van Cutsem et al., 2009, 2011). The PRIME trial, randomizing patients to FOLFOX and panitumumab or FOLFOX alone, showed similar results (Douillard et al., 2014). Furthermore, FIRE-3 (Heinemann et al., 2014) and CALG-B (Venook et al., 2014) trials demonstrated that CT plus cetuximab induced more GI toxicities than CT plus bevacizumab (Aprile et al., 2015).

mTOR-inhibitors produce the most consistent stomatotoxicity of targeted agents and their incidence approaches or exceeds that observed with conventional cytotoxic agents (Elting et al., 2013; Rugo et al., 2014; Sonis et al., 2017). The related frequency and gravity depends on drugs doses and treatment duration, but mIAS is a common cause of dose-de-escalation or termination of treatment. Nonetheless, mIAS usually resolves spontaneously without treatment discontinuation (Boers-Doets et al., 2012).

A meta-analysis (Abdel-Rahman and Fouad, 2015) evaluating the risk of oral stomatitis and enteritis in patients treated with everolimus, temsirolimus, and ridaforolimus showed an increased risk of toxicities compared to the control group. Median time of dose interruption was 7 days.

In the meta-analysis by Shameem et al. (2015), toxicities incidence and grade depended on cancer types independent of dose ($p = 0.004$). Particularly, renal cell carcinoma (RCC) were associated with fewer rate of mucositis (RR 1) than astrocytoma (RR 5.29), gastric cancer or breast cancer, regardless the combination of mTOR-inhibitors with other drugs. Furthermore, everolimus was associated with the highest risk of stomatitis (RR 4.5).

Mucosal damage caused by TKIs is associated with hypersensitivity and dysgeusia. OM occurs in 26% of sunitinib-treated patients and in 36% of patients receiving sorafenib (Lee et al., 2009). A meta-analysis on metastatic RCC showed that 81% of patients treated with sunitinib and 90% of those treated with sorafenib experienced AEs after 4 week of treatment. Dose reduction was required in 26% and in 18%, respectively (Boers-Doets et al., 2012).

In the CORRECT trial, regorafenib induced GI toxicity of any grade, among which diarrhea (34% vs. 8% in placebo arm) and OM (27% vs. 4%) were frequently reported (Grothey et al., 2013).

Patient-Related Risk Factors

While a range of descriptive parameters have been indicated as predictors of mucositis risk including poor oral health, low body mass index, younger or older age, and female sex, none have been consistent and accurate. (Sonis et al., 2004; Chansky et al., 2005; Schwab et al., 2008; Sonis, 2010; Krishna et al., 2011; Chaveli-López and Bagán-Sebastián, 2016; Vasconcelos et al., 2016; Villa and Sonis, 2016). However, it now appears that identification of genomic drivers of pharmacokinetic and radio/pharmacodynamic factors which impact mucositis risk is possible through assessment of germline mutations, associated with those pathways affecting mucositis development or drug metabolism

The first genomic tests for toxicities were associated with the identification of mutations that impacted enzymes associated with drug metabolism.

For example, patients with deletion polymorphism of the thymidylate synthase (TYMS) gene (Cho et al., 2007) or dihydropyrimidine dehydrogenase (DPD) deficiency (Meulendijks et al., 2015) tend to have increased toxicity from 5-FU. However, the percentage of patients having even partial mutations of these genes is relatively small (<5% of the at risk population). Consequently, the impact of genomics on toxicity risk had to be more broadly based and associated with genes effecting those pathways involved in pathogenesis. This hypothesis has been confirmed for a number of regimen-related toxicities induced by both RT and CT. However, additional studies are mandatory to produce a working clinically applicable tool that can be routinely applied. The recent application of machine learning algorithms to this issue has accelerated the process.

CLINICAL PRESENTATION

Gastrointestinal mucositis can affect any site of the alimentary tract and it may present with a large spectrum of clinical manifestations according to the involved area (Al-Dasooqi et al., 2013).

The first clinical manifestation of OM is erythema of one or more sites of the movable mucosa (i.e., buccal or labial mucosa, ventral tongue, floor of the mouth or soft palate). Lesions typically progress to form painful ulcerations often covered by a pseudomembrane and accompanied by odynophagia, dysphagia, malnutrition, and weight loss (Peterson et al., 2012; Chaveli-López and Bagán-Sebastián, 2016). Disruption of the intact mucosa may be associated with microbial colonization that may remain localized or become disseminated, especially in patients with severe neutropenia (Chaveli-López, 2014; Chaveli-López and Bagán-Sebastián, 2016). OM is usually self-limiting and its course depends on the anticancer treatment. Among patients receiving CT, first signs appear shortly after administration and usually peak at about days 7–14 to completely recover within the following week (Al-Ansari et al., 2015; Villa and Sonis, 2015). On the other hand, RT-induced mucositis usually develops during the second or third week of treatment and often persist until 2–4 weeks after the last dose (Villa and Sonis, 2015).

Little data exist to accurately characterize the course of esophageal or gastric mucositis. Consequently, symptoms such as pain, dysphagia, dyspepsia, nausea, and vomiting are often attributed to gastroesophageal reflux or candidosis, leading to underestimate mucositis in this tract (Squier and Kremer, 2001; Aprile et al., 2015).

The onset of CT-associated intestinal mucositis (enteritis) tends to be acute (usually within 24–48 h after treatment) and may present with diarrhea, constipation, abdominal pain, nausea, vomiting, and anorexia. In some cases malnutrition, dehydration, infections, and sepsis may also occur (Al-Dasooqi et al., 2013; Ribeiro et al., 2016). Typhlitis, otherwise known as neutropenic enterocolitis, is a mucositis of ileo-cecal region with high mortality risk, typically affecting patients with neutropenic fever. Its clinical manifestation ranges from abdominal pain, bloating and diarrhea to acute abdomen (Davila, 2006). This severe form of enteritis may complicate treatments for hematologic tumors but it is observed also in patients undergoing cytotoxic drugs for solid malignancies (Sachak et al., 2015).

Proctitis usually occurs in patients undergoing chemoradiation for rectal, prostate or other pelvic cancers; symptoms include painful tenesmus with mucus discharge and rectal bleeding. Onset may be acute and/or not develop until several weeks after starting treatment. While these conditions are usually transient and resolve within a few weeks following the completion of RT, chronicity is not rare.

Moreover, both OM and GIM may cause systemic clinical manifestation such as anorexia, malabsorption, weight loss, anemia, fatigue, and sepsis (Al-Dasooqi et al., 2013).

In this landscape, targeted therapies-induced mucositis, such as mIAS, deserves a special mention and represents an emerging issue with different characteristics (Peterson et al., 2015; Kwon, 2016). According to ESMO guidelines (Peterson et al., 2015), the term stomatitis is more appropriate and should be used to indicate the mucosal inflammation related to these novel drugs.

ASSESSMENT SCALES

Assessment scales provide the basis of objective comparisons of regimen-related toxicities or efficacy of toxicity treatment intervention. Currently, there is not a single instrument which is used universally. Rather, a range of scoring instruments are used with each depending on somewhat different subjective and/or objective criteria to define the severity of GIM (Villa and Sonis, 2016). One of the most commonly used is the National Cancer Institute-Common Terminology Criteria for Adverse Events (NCI-CTCAE, most recent version 4.03), which grades mucositis severity 0–5, based primarily upon symptom severity, functional alteration and intervention requirements. NCI-CTC criteria for mucositis vary by anatomic site. The changing nature of NCI-CTC benchmarks, which has been a feature of each new iteration of the scale, has hindered longitudinal regimen-related toxicity comparisons (United States Department of Health and Human Services, 2010; Peterson et al., 2015). The World Health Organization (WHO) scale is widely used for grading OM and incorporates both objective and functional (ability to eat) assessments (Peterson et al., 2015; Villa and Sonis, 2015). Independently, the Radiation Therapy Oncology Group (RTOG) has developed Cooperative Group Common Toxicity Criteria which are, in some ways, a hybrid of those described by the NCI-CTC and WHO scores (Sonis, 2011).

Over the years, other scales designed primarily for use in clinical trials have been developed, such as the Oral Mucositis Assessment Scale (OMAS) (Sonis et al., 1999). However, measures developed for CT or RT-induced mucositis may not apply to patients treated with targeted agents. Thus, *ad hoc* scales have been designed for this population, such as the mIAS scale to assess mIAS (Boers-Doets and Lalla, 2013). Moreover, the integration with patient-reported outcome (PRO) becomes critical to improving the accuracy of clinical evaluation (Sonis, 2010; Bossi et al., 2015). Indeed, clinicians may underestimate the real burden of mucositis. Furthermore, the inter-observer variability can lead to discrepant scoring. Examples of PRO instruments are represented by the Oral Mucositis Daily Questionnaire (OMDQ) (Stiff et al., 2006b), the abovementioned OMAS and the Patient-Reported Oral Mucositis Symptom (PROMS) scale (Kushner et al., 2008).

It would be worthy to have a single standardized scale that incorporated clinicians and patients' measures to describe GIM severity and to compare different prevention modalities and treatment regimens.

MANAGEMENT OF GASTROINTESTINAL MUCOSITIS: CURRENT AND INVESTIGATIONAL APPROACHES

Although the quality of evidence derived from clinical studies is somewhat limited (Worthington et al., 2011), MASCC and ESMO have developed guidelines which offer potential strategies for managing mucositis (Lalla et al., 2014). It should be noted that the guidelines themselves are not definitive and represent the synthesis of a consensus of opinions of their authors. The guidelines should be viewed as fluid and will likely undergo changes as higher levels of evidence which support or refute treatment develop.

Notably, given the relatively recent development of new drugs, only expert opinions on the management of targeted therapies-induced mucositis are available (Peterson et al., 2015).

Prevention and treatment strategies for OM and GIM are listed in **Tables 1, 2**, respectively.

Basic Oral Hygiene

Oral health at the start of and during cancer therapy appears to impact the course of OM. Consequently, oral care protocols which include pre-treatment comprehensive oral examination and elimination of sources of mucosal irritation and infection are crucial to prevent and reduce oral injury across all cancer treatment strategies (Peterson et al., 2015). Oral hygiene helps to reduce the bacterial load and, consequently, the infection risk (Rubenstein et al., 2004; Campos et al., 2014). It includes general hygiene standards, dental care, normal saline and baking soda mouthwashes, dietary and behavioral measures (Peterson et al., 2015; Mallick et al., 2016).

Antioxidant Agents

Reactive oxygen species play a significant role in the pathogenesis of OM. Consequently, reducing their production or scavenging them from tissue is a potential interventional strategy. Antioxidant drugs may have a role in reducing mucositis through the suppression of ROS or the increasing of endogenous production of antioxidative enzymes (Ozben, 2015; Kwon, 2016).

Amifostine

It is a pro-drug of phosphorylated aminothiol and presents a cytoprotective action on salivary gland, decreasing Il-6 and TNF-α, protecting normal endothelium, connective tissue and gland tissue. The mechanism of action of this agent may be related to the recruitment of ROS scavengers, the protection of DNA and the induction of cellular hypoxia (Koukourakis and Maltezos, 2006). The use of this agent may have utility in preventing RT-induced proctitis, esophagitis, and OM (Lalla et al., 2014). With respect to OM, amifostine's favorable effect on salivary gland function could also be beneficial in depressing OM course. However, intravenous administration and its unfavorable toxicity profile have limited amifostine's utilization in routine clinical practice (Yuan and Sonis, 2014).

Glutamine

It is an amino-acid involving in glutathione synthesis. It acts across exhibiting antioxidant properties, particularly by accelerating mucosal remodeling (Tsujimoto et al., 2015). Results of studies assessing the efficacy of topical or systemic formulations of glutamine, a precursor of nucleotide synthesis, on the development and course of mucositis have been inconsistent.

TABLE 1 | Prevention and treatment strategies for oral mucositis.

Intervention	Aim	Clinical setting	Authors' comment	Guidelines (grade of evidence)
Oral care protocols	Prevention	All cancer patients	General agreement on the value of oral care protocols	MASCC/ESMO (III) NCCN
Oral cryotherapy	Prevention	Bolus 5-FU chemotherapy	Safe, low cost, with some positive results	MASCC/ESMO (II) NCCN
		High-dose melphalan +/− TB-RT for HSCT	As above	MASCC/ESMO (III) NCCN
Palifermin	Prevention	High-dose CT and TB-RT for HSCT	Only approved agent for OM mitigation in a narrow patient population	MASCC/ESMO (II) NCCN ASCO
Low-laser therapy	Prevention	High-dose CT +/− TB-RT for HSCT	Data suggesting possible benefit	MASCC/ESMO (II)
		HN cancer patients receiving RT alone	Data suggests possible benefit, but potential tumor impact unresolved	MASCC/ESMO (III)
Benzydamine mouthwash	Prevention	HN cancer patients receiving moderate dose RT alone	Anti-inflammatory rinse with some data supporting its use in patients receiving radiation only	MASCC/ESMO (I)
0.2% morphine mouthwash	Pain treatment	HN cancer patients receiving CT-RT	Data suggests effective adjunct for topical pain control	MASCC/ESMO (III)
Doxepin mouthwash	Pain treatment	All cancer patients	Data suggests effective adjunct for topical pain control	MASCC/ESMO (IV)

CT, chemotherapy; RT, radiotherapy; TB-RT, total-body radiotherapy, HN, head and neck; HSCT, hematopoietic stem cell transplantation; MASCC, Multinational Association of Supportive Care in Cancer; ESMO, European Society for Medical Oncology.

Oral Zinc Supplement

This drug acts as an antioxidant through several functions, including epithelial proliferation, extracellular matrix synthesis and wound healing in damage tissue. Although the evidence supporting its use are relatively sparse (Arbabi-kalati et al., 2012; Van Sebille et al., 2015) and a mechanism of action is not completely clear, systemic zinc could be beneficial in the prevention of OM in oral cancer patients undergoing CT or CT-RT (Lalla et al., 2014).

Vitamin E

The efficacy of vitamin E as a mucositis intervention has been explored in animals and humans using different formulations. It is a α-tocopherol, that can limit tissue damage caused by therelease of ROS. The results of these studies has been inconsistent (Uçüncü et al., 2006; El-Housseiny et al., 2007; Ghoreishi et al., 2007; Azizi et al., 2015).

N-Acetyl-Cysteine (NAC)

This compound contains thiol groups. It is involved in antioxidant process by reducing the production of ROS, myeloperoxidase activity, as well as xanthine dehydrogenase and xanthine oxidase activity. Moreover, it participates in inflammation response, by activating of NF-kB. Moslehi et al. (2014) evaluated the efficacy of this glutathione precursor in a double-blind, randomized study in leukemic patients, showing a significantly lower OM rate in patients receiving NAC than patients receiving placebo. A rinse formulation of NAC was also shown to be effective in mitigating radiation-induced OM. In addition to its antioxidant properties, NAC's mechanism also includes modulation of a variety of pathways known to important in mucositis pathogenesis including NF-κB.

Superoxide Dismutase Mimetics

Superoxide dismutase has been recognized as a potential interventional target. A phase 2 trial (NCT02508389) testing a superoxide dismutase mimetic is currently ongoing (ClinicalTrials. gov, 2017a).

Inflammation and Cytokines Production-Inhibitors

Benzydamine

Benzydamine HCl is a non-steroidal anti-inflammatory agent in an oral rinse formulation. This anti-inflammatory effect is possible by inhibiting the production and the effect of pro-inflammatory cytokines, such as TNF-α. In addition, it has been shown that it has anesthetic, analgesic, and antimicrobial properties (Rubenstein et al., 2004). While it has demonstrated modest efficacy in patients with HN cancer being treated with RT in the absence of concomitant CT, it has been ineffective in attenuating OM in patients receiving standard combined regimens of cisplatin and radiation (Epstein et al., 2001; Kazemian et al., 2009; Sheibani et al., 2015).

Pentoxifylline

Pentoxifylline's rationale as a mucositis intervention is based on its anti-TNF activity. It plays an important role in modulating inflammation, by inhibiting pro-inflammatory cytokines such as IL-1-β, TNF-α, and NF-kB. There is no evidence to support its use in clinical practice, although NCT02397486 trial is ongoing to

TABLE 2 | Prevention and treatment strategies for gastrointestinal mucositis.

Intervention	Aim	Clinical setting	Guidelines (grade of evidence)
Intravenous amifostine	Prevention of RT-induced proctitis	Patients receiving RT	MASCC/ESMO (II)
	Prevention of CT-RT-induced esophagitis	NSCLC patients	MASCC/ESMO (II) ASCO with reserve
Octreotide	Treatment of diarrhea	Standard or high-dose CT for HSCT	MASCC/ESMO (II)
Sucralfate enemas	Treatment of chronic RT-induced proctitis	Patients receiving RT with rectal bleeding	MASCC/ESMO (III)
Oral sulfasalazine	Prevention of RT-induced enteropathy	Patients receiving RT to the pelvis	MASCC/ESMO (II)
Lactobacillus probiotics	Prevention of diarrhea	Patients receiving CT +/− RT to the pelvis	MASCC/ESMO (III)
Hyperbaric oxygen	Treatment of RT-induced proctitis	Patients receiving RT for solid tumors	MASCC/ESMO (III)

CT, chemotherapy; RT, radiotherapy; NSCLC, Non-small cell lung cancer; HSCT, hematopoietic stem cell transplantation; ASA, acetylsalicylic acid; MASCC, Multinational Association of Supportive Care in Cancer; ESMO, European Society for Medical Oncology.

evaluate the impact of pentoxifylline and vitamin E on mucositis in HN cancer patients receiving RT (ClinicalTrials. gov, 2016g).

Salicylates

A role for salicylates in the management of GIM is questionable. While sulfasalazine has been suggested to efficacious in attenuating RT-induced enteropathy in patients receiving pelvic RT, curiously acetylsalicylic acid, mesalazine or olsalazine are ineffective in preventing RT-induced diarrhea.

Interleukin Inhibitors

While pro-inflammatory cytokines appear to be a desirable target for mucositis prevention and treatment, clinical data assessing their use are sparse. A phase 2 trial (NCT01403064) failed to demonstrated efficacy of anti-IL-6 monoclonal antibody as an OM intervention (ClinicalTrials. gov, 2016f).

Other Biological Modifiers in Development

Given its complex pathogenesis, a number of mechanistically targeted agents are in various phases of development. Smad7, a TGFβ and NF-κB inhibitor has demonstrated interesting outcomes in animal models. Likewise, Antrum Mucosal Protein (AMP), which targets cell junctions and blocks endothelial and epithelial apoptosis effectively mitigated OM in an orthotopic mouse model (Chen et al., 2016). Favorable results of a Phase 2 study of an innate immune inhibitor (dusquetide) were recently reported (Kudrimoti et al., 2016). A proprietary topical formulation of clonidine successfully reduced the duration of OM in patients receiving concomitant CT-RT for HN cancer (Onxeo press release). Trefoil factor 1 released by genetically modified *Lactococcus lactis* bacteria was effective in decreasing the duration of OM in patients receiving induction CT as part of treatment regimen for HN cancer (Limaye et al., 2013). A phase 2 trial evaluating the defensin mimetic brilacidin is ongoing (ClinicalTrials. gov, 2017b).

Cytoprotective Agents

Prostaglandin Analogs

Prostaglandin analogs have a cytoprotective action on mucosal tissue. More in depth, it stimulates the production of bicarbonate, mucous, blood flow with subsequently endothelial and epithelial cellular protection. Despite this background, it has not proved to be effective as a mucositis intervention (Lalla et al., 2012, 2014).

Sucralfate

Sucralfate is a basic albumin salt. It binds to proteins exposed by ulceration, providing a protective coat against the action of pepsin and gastric acid. Moreover, it stimulates the production of local prostaglandins, angiogenesis, and fibroblast proliferation. On the other hand, it inhibits the release of cytokines and it has antimicrobial activity. Therefore, it has thus been suggested to be potentially of value in palliating mucosal injury, particularly by generating granulation tissue and wound-healing process (Ala et al., 2016). However, clinical trial results using the compound have been conflicting (Lalla et al., 2014).

Growth Factors

Palifermin

It is the recombinant human keratinocyte growth factor-1 (KGF-1) which belongs to fibroblast growth factors' (FGF's) family. It stimulates the proliferation and the differentiation of epithelials cells, but it has more stability than the analogous native protein, due to its particular structure (Rubin et al., 1989). In preclinical setting palifermin has showed defensive role in several epithelial tissues (Farrell et al., 1998).

This drug has also has pleotropic, antiapoptotic, antioxidant and anti-pro-inflammatory activity (Villa and Sonis, 2015). Intravenous infusion of KGF-1 successfully impacted the course of severity of OM in patients receiving aggressive stomatotoxic conditioning regimens prior to HSCT (Spielberger et al., 2004; Stiff et al., 2006a) and was subsequently approved by Food and Drug Administration (FDA) and European Medical Agency (EMA) for use restricted to this patient population. The efficacy of palifermin in other patient populations has not been sufficiently studied and its use in patients bearing tumors which themselves have KGF receptors has limited its more broad application.

Other Growth Factors

There is no consistent or compelling evidence to support the use of granulocyte-macrophage colony-stimulating factor (GM-CSF), granulocyte colony-stimulating factors (G-CSF, e.g., filgrastim) or FGF (Yuan and Sonis, 2014; Chaveli-López and Bagán-Sebastián, 2016; Mallick et al., 2016) as an OM mitigator. (Lalla et al., 2014).

Antiapoptotic Agents

Apoptosis has been demonstrated to be critical for the development of OM (Kwon, 2016) so it is not unexpected that therapeutic antiapoptotic strategies have been considered. The finding that chemokine ligand 9 (CXCL9) exacerbated intestinal injury in a 5-FU animal model suggests that it might represent a viable therapeutic target (Han et al., 2011). Similarly, specific caspase-3 inhibition was protective in an animal model of RT-induced OM.

Physical Strategies

Oral Cryotherapy

Several controlled trials provide evidence for the benefit of cryotherapy (ice chips) in modulating OM (Cascinu et al., 1994; Baydar et al., 2005; Sorensen et al., 2008; Riley et al., 2016). A recent Cochrane review concluded that oral cryotherapy probably reduces the severity of OM (RR 0.61, 95% CI 0.52–0.72) and the incidence of severe OM (RR 0.4, 95% CI 0.27–0.61) in patients undergoing FU-based treatment (Riley et al., 2015). It was hypothesized that cryotherapy's benefit was derived from local vasoconstriction, leading to reduced exposure of the mucosa to FU (Chaveli-López and Bagán-Sebastián, 2016). A randomized-controlled, open-label, phase 1–2 NCT02326675 trial is ongoing to evaluate cryotherapy in the prevention of CT-induced mucositis in stem cell transplant (ClinicalTrials. gov, 2016b).

Laser Therapy (Photobiomodulation)

Several trials suggest that mucosal treatment with a low level helium-neon laser (LLLT) reduces the severity of mucositis and promotes healing in patients undergoing conditioning therapy for HSCT (Barasch et al., 1995; Cowen et al., 1997; Schubert et al., 2007; Ferreira et al., 2016). Similar trials have been performed in patients receiving RT alone for HN cancer (Lalla et al., 2014; Peterson et al., 2015). A significant amount of data exists documenting the robust biological activities of LLLT. As has been recently pointed out, many of the biological pathways activated by LLLT have been associated with poor tumor outcomes and/or resistance to treatment. Until there is definitive data establishing that LLLT is inert relative to tumor response and behavior the use of such therapy in areas of tumor is to be approached with caution (Sonis et al., 2016; Zecha et al., 2016).

Pain Management

Pain management plays a crucial role in improving patient's quality of life. To date, patient-controlled analgesia with morphine is recommended only in the treatment of OM-related pain in hematologic patients (Lalla et al., 2014). Transdermal fentanyl, morphine mouthwashes, and doxepin rinse are other possible options in various clinical settings (Lalla et al., 2014; Van Sebille et al., 2015). Tapentadol, gabapentin, and pregabalin are under investigation.

To date, magic or miracle mouthwash are also available; this term applies to a variety of rinses typically based on institution-specific formulations and folklore. They include various compounds of topical anesthetic (e.g., lidocaine), a muco-adherent vehicle and other agents such as antimicotics, steroids or antibiotics. Their efficacy is unproven (Chaveli-López and Bagán-Sebastián, 2016).

Moreover, a number of topical coating agents are currently available including GelClair®, Episil®, and MuGard®. Of these, the only MuGard® has been evaluated in a prospective, randomized, placebo-controlled, blinded, multi-institutional trial and has shown palliative benefit (Allison et al., 2014). Nonetheless, there are reports of symptomatic benefits for the other agents (Yuan and Sonis, 2014; Villa and Sonis, 2016). Caphosol, a remineralizing solution, has been tested in multiple, randomized, blinded trials of which the results do not generally support its efficacy for an OM indication (Rao et al., 2014; Svanberg et al., 2015; Wong et al., 2016; Treister et al., 2017).

A recent exploratory study investigated the role of methylene blue, a type A inhibitor of monoamine oxidase acting on microglial cells that seem to be involved in neuroinflammation and pain control (Roldan et al., 2017).

Other Management Approaches

Probiotics and Antimicrobial Agents

Lactobacillus species-containing probiotics may be of value in preventing diarrhea in patients undergoing CT and/or RT for pelvic tumors. Even if the mechanism remain unclear, in preclinical models probiotics seem to improve the crypts of small intestinal, preserving architecture and preventing some alterations of the goblet cell, such as the decrease of acidic mucin, after CT (Prisciandaro et al., 2011). NCT01707641 (ClinicalTrials. gov, 2016c) is an ongoing trial evaluating the preventive effect of *Lactobacillus* on RT-CT-induced OM in HN cancer patients, while NCT02819960 trial is investigating the role of probiotics in preventing irinotecan-induced diarrhea (Mego et al., 2015).

Antibiotic strategies using conventional or investigational agents have not proven to be efficacious in favorably impacting mucositis. Conflicting data exist about the use of chlorhexidine rinse (Dodd et al., 2000; Campos et al., 2014).

Dexamethasone Mouthwash

The preliminary results of the multicenter phase II SWISH trial suggest a benefit in managing mIAS (Rugo et al., 2016). If true, such an approach most likely targets the secondary inflammatory phase of these lesions, but a properly performed, randomize, placebo-controlled trial is currently lacking.

Glucagon-Like Peptide-2 (GLP-2) analogs

Several studies have suggested a potential role of these agents in treating irinotecan-induced mucositis and diarrhea. GLP-2 analogs have been demonstrated to limit and improve this toxicity in animal models.

Natural Remedies

A number of organic agents are under investigation to determine potential preventive or therapeutic effect. Vitamin A, ascorbic acid (ClinicalTrials. gov, 2016d), manuka honey, aloe vera, chamomile, curcumin (ClinicalTrials. gov, 2016e), and other plant extracts (ClinicalTrials. gov, 2016a) are just some examples of an emerging approach (Yuan and Sonis, 2014; Van Sebille et al., 2015).

CONCLUSION

Gastrointestinal mucositis remains a significant, common unmet clinical need in cancer patients. Although frequently reported, the real rate and impact of this worrisome toxicity may be underestimated, and it consistently contributes to burden in terms of negative impact on quality of life, outcome and healthcare costs. The baseline risk-assessment is crucial to identify patients more likely to develop severe GIM in order to provide the best possible preventive and therapeutic approaches, with the aim of preserving optimal treatment intensity and maximize patients' safety.

To date, most of the literature reports refer to OM, while the management of GIM remains a major challenge. In recent years, the increasing knowledge on the mucositis pathobiology has provided opportunities for the development of new approaches based upon the underlying molecular pathways. Although an increasing number of possible treatments have emerged, no standard measures have been established. A future, biologically based strategy may consist in combining interventions acting on the different phases of mucositis' pathogenesis.

More research efforts are needed to better understand the underpinning biological processes in order to develop new effective treatments. Investigations should be performed to further characterize the role of the oral environment, including studies on the potential contribution of the oral/periodontal microbiome in the pathobiology of mucositis associated with targeted agents. Similarly, studies on changes in salivary output and proteome induced by anticancer therapies may contribute to a scientific base for OM risk prediction, early diagnosis and interventions (Al-Ansari et al., 2015).

Despite its longstanding recognition, frequency, clinical impact and cost, the treatment options for mucositis are disappointingly sparse. Only one agent, palifermin, has been approved for mitigation of OM in the U.S. - and only for a very limited segment of the at-risk population. GI mucositis suffers a similar fate. Its management is reliant on symptom control.

Next year will mark two decades since the recognition that the biological basis for mucositis' pathogenesis is far more complex than simply being ascribed solely to non-specific clonogenic cell death of epithelial stem cells. The presentation of that concept and data from the subsequent studies that have followed, provided a plethora of information which have had tremendous potential translational value in identifying druggable targets for the enablement of new drugs and biologicals. Consequently, as discussed above, we are seeing a broad range of mechanistically based compounds in all phases of pre-clinical and clinical development. Preventing or limiting CT- or RT-induced normal tissue injury, while not interfering with a desired anti-tumor effect is not easy. The development of animal models to both study the pathobiology of mucositis and to serve as pre-clinical development platforms has been critical. For the most part, animal models for mucositis have been rodent (mouse, rat, and hamster) based. While no model is perfect, the predictive value of these ones relative to assessing a compounds behavior in humans has been unquestionably valuable. For example, the efficacy outcomes of a number of compounds that were observed in hamster models has been replicated in human studies. Likewise, although accumulating data highlight the differences between normal and tumor cells behavior, assessing that medications for supportive care do nothing to hinder the effectiveness of cancer therapy or induce negative tumor behaviors is critical. Animal models have been conducted for this purpose prior to the start of clinical trials.

However, animal models are characterized by several limitations and some successes which may be present in pre-clinical setting are not always evident in the clinical one. First of all, few animal studies focus on GIM, with most of the evidence deriving from trials on OM (Bowen et al., 2005; Viet et al., 2014). Moreover, in some animal models mucosal ulceration requires mechanical injury (Sonis et al., 1990), while in human patients the development of mucositis is independent of mechanical irritation. Another issue of pre-clinical models is represented by doses and scheduling; indeed, the susceptibility to a particular chemotherapic or radiotherapic regimen may be different between species. In addition, some animal models are characterized by the need of higher doses of CT than humans to induce the same grade of mucositis, due to the different keratinization of the epithelium. Moreover, such models sometimes require a route of drug administration not translatable to human patients. A further issue derives from the use of fully humanized monoclonal antibodies, which may not be active in animal setting (Bowen et al., 2011). Finally, few pre-clinical trials exist in order to investigate the molecular pathways of mucosal pain and most of the evidence is derived from animal models of pain related to oral cavity tumors or temporomandibular disorders (Viet et al., 2014).

Continued development of models and robust analyses of how animal results compare with those in humans will provide the information needed to help optimize the pre-clinical pathway for the development of new therapies.

All of this is taking place in an environment which increasingly recognizes that patients differ in their individual risk for mucositis (and other toxicities) and in how they might respond to one treatment or another. As a result, the literature reflects studies which now embed concepts of precision medicine in clinical trial design for mucositis interventions.

Given the impact of the above on the trajectory and enthusiasm for developing effective preventive and treatment options for mucositis, it is hard not to be optimistic that the current pipeline will result in effective therapies for mucositis in the relatively near future.

AUTHOR CONTRIBUTIONS

Manuscript writing: MC, GA, PE, DB, MV, and SS. Final approval of manuscript: MC, GA, PE, DB, MV, VF, GP, LC, and SS.

REFERENCES

Abayomi, J., Kirwan, J., and Hackett, A. (2009). The prevalence of chronic radiation enteritis following radiotherapy for cervical or endometrial cancer and its impact on quality of life. *Eur. J. Oncol. Nurs.* 13, 262–267. doi: 10.1016/j.ejon.2009.02.007

Abdel-Rahman, O., ElHalawani, H., and Essam-Eldin, S. (2016). S-1-based regimens and the risk of oral and gastrointestinal mucosal injury: a meta-analysis with comparison to other fluoropyrimidines. *Expert Opin. Drug Saf.* 15, 5–20. doi: 10.1517/14740338.2016.1105959

Abdel-Rahman, O., and Fouad, M. (2015). Risk of oral and gastrointestinal mucosal injury in patients with solid tumors treated with everolimus, temsirolimus or ridaforolimus: a comparative systematic review and meta-analysis. *Expert Rev. Anticancer Ther.* 15, 847–858. doi: 10.1586/14737140.2015.1047350

Adebahr, S., Schimek-Jasch, T., Nestle, U., and Brunner, T. B. (2016). Oesophagus side effects related to the treatment of oesophageal cancer or radiotherapy of other thoracic malignancies. *Best Pract. Res. Clin. Gastroenterol.* 30, 565–580. doi: 10.1016/j.bpg.2016.07.003

Ala, S., Saeedi, M., Janbabai, G., Ganji, R., Azhdari, E., and Shiva, A. (2016). Efficacy of sucralfate mouth wash in prevention of 5-fluorouracil induced oral mucositis: a prospective, randomized, double-blind, controlled trial. *Nutr. Cancer* 68, 456–463. doi: 10.1080/01635581.2016.1153666

Al-Ansari, S., Zecha, J. A. E. M., Barasch, A., de Lange, J., Rozema, F. R., and Raber-Durlacher, J. E. (2015). Oral mucositis induced by anticancer therapies. *Curr. Oral Health Rep.* 2, 202–211. doi: 10.1007/s40496-015-0069-4

Al-Dasooqi, N., Gibson, R. J., Bowen, J. M., Logan, R. M., Stringer, A. M., and Keefe, D. M. (2010). Matrix metalloproteinases are possible mediators for the development of alimentary tract mucositis in the dark agouti rat. *Exp. Biol. Med.* 235, 1244–1256. doi: 10.1258/ebm.2010.010082

Al-Dasooqi, N., Sonis, S. T., Bowen, J. M., Bateman, E., Blijlevens, N., Gibson, R. J., et al. (2013). Emerging evidence on the pathobiology of mucositis. *Support. Care Cancer* 21, 2075–2083. doi: 10.1007/s00520-013-1810-y

Allison, R. R., Ambrad, A. A., Arshoun, Y., Carmel, R. J., Ciuba, D. F., Feldman, E., et al. (2014). Multi-institutional, randomized, double-blind, placebo-controlled trial to assess the efficacy of a mucoadhesive hydrogel (MuGard) in mitigating oral mucositis symptoms in patients being treated with chemoradiation therapy for cancers of the head and neck. *Cancer* 120, 1433–1440. doi: 10.1002/cncr.28553

Aprile, G., Rihawi, K., De Carlo, E., and Sonis, S. T. (2015). Treatment-related gastrointestinal toxicities and advanced colorectal or pancreatic cancer: a critical update. *World J. Gastroenterol.* 21, 11793–11803. doi: 10.3748/wjg.v21.i41.11793

Arbabi-kalati, F., Arbabi-kalati, F., Deghatipour, M., and Ansari Moghadam, A. (2012). Evaluation of the efficacy of zinc sulfate in the prevention of chemotherapy-induced mucositis: a double-blind randomized clinical trial. *Arch. Iran. Med.* 15, 413–417.

Azizi, A., Alirezaei, S., Pedram, P., and Mafi, A. R. (2015). Efficacy of topical and systemic vitamin e in preventing chemotherapy-induced oral mucositis. *Rep. Radiother. Oncol.* 2:e796. doi: 10.5812/rro.2(1)2015.796

Barasch, A., Peterson, D. E., Tanzer, J. M., D'Ambrosio, J. A., Nuki, K., Schubert, M. M., et al. (1995). Helium-neon laser effects on conditioning-induced oral mucositis in bone marrow transplantation patients. *Cancer* 76, 2550–2556. doi: 10.1002/1097-0142(19951215)76:12<2550::AID-CNCR2820761222>3.0.CO;2-X

Baydar, M., Dikilitas, M., Sevinc, A., and Aydogdu, I. (2005). Prevention of oral mucositis due to 5-fluorouracil treatment with oral cryotherapy. *J. Natl. Med. Assoc.* 97, 1161–1164.

Blijlevens, N., and Sonis, S. (2007). Palifermin (recombinant keratinocyte growth factor-1): a pleiotropic growth factor with multiple biological activities in preventing chemotherapy- and radiotherapy-induced mucositis. *Ann. Oncol.* 18, 817–826. doi: 10.1093/annonc/mdl332

Boers-Doets, C. B., Epstein, J. B., Raber-Durlacher, J. E., Ouwerkerk, J., Logan, R. M., Brakenhoff, J. A., et al. (2012). Oral adverse events associated with tyrosine kinase and mammalian target of rapamycin inhibitors in renal cell carcinoma: a structured literature review. *Oncologist* 17, 135–144. doi: 10.1634/theoncologist.2011-0111

Boers-Doets, C. B., and Lalla, R. V. (2013). The mIAS scale: a scale to measure mTOR inhibitor-associated stomatitis. *Supp. Care Cancer* 21(Suppl. 1), S140.

Bonner, J. A., Giralt, J., Harari, P. M., Baselga, J., Spencer, S., Bell, D., et al. (2016). Association of human papillomavirus and p16 status with mucositis and dysphagia for head and neck cancer patients treated with radiotherapy with or without cetuximab: assessment from a phase 3 registration trial. *Eur. J. Cancer* 64, 1–11. doi: 10.1016/j.ejca.2016.05.008

Bossi, P., Bergamini, C., Miceli, R., Cova, A., Orlandi, E., Resteghini, C., et al. (2016). Salivary cytokine levels and oral mucositis in head and neck cancer patients treated with chemotherapy and radiation therapy. *Int. J. Radiat. Oncol. Biol. Phys.* 96, 959–966. doi: 10.1016/j.ijrobp.2016.08.047

Bossi, P., Lucchesi, M., and Antonuzzo, A. (2015). Gastrointestinal toxicities from targeted therapies: measurement, duration and impact. *Curr. Opin. Support. Palliat. Care* 9, 163–167. doi: 10.1097/SPC.0000000000000128

Bowen, J. M., Gibson, R. J., Keefe, D. M., and Cummins, A. G. (2005). Cytotoxic chemotherapy upregulates pro-apoptotic Bax and Bak in the small intestine of rats and humans. *Pathology* 37, 56–62. doi: 10.1080/00313020400023461

Bowen, J. M., Gibson, R. J., and Keefe, D. M. K. (2011). Animal models of mucositis: implications for therapy. *J. Support. Oncol.* 9, 161–168. doi: 10.1016/j.suponc.2011.04.009

Campos, M. I. D. C., Campos, C. N., Aarestrup, F. M., and Aarestrup, B. J. V. (2014). Oral mucositis in cancer treatment: natural history, prevention and treatment. *Mol. Clin. Oncol.* 2, 337–340. doi: 10.3892/mco.2014.253

Cascinu, S., Fedeli, A., Fedeli, S. L., and Catalano, G. (1994). Oral cooling (cryotherapy), an effective treatment for the prevention of 5-fluorouracil-induced stomatitis. *Eur. J. Cancer. B. Oral Oncol.* 30B, 234–236. doi: 10.1016/0964-1955(94)90003-5

Chansky, K., Benedetti, J., and Macdonald, J. S. (2005). Differences in toxicity between men and women treated with 5-fluorouracil therapy for colorectal carcinoma. *Cancer* 103, 1165–1171. doi: 10.1002/cncr.20878

Chaveli-López, B. (2014). Oral toxicity produced by chemotherapy: a systematic review. *J. Clin. Exp. Dent.* 6, e81–e90. doi: 10.4317/jced.51337

Chaveli-López, B., and Bagán-Sebastián, J. V. (2016). Treatment of oral mucositis due to chemotherapy. *J. Clin. Exp. Dent.* 8, e201–e209. doi: 10.4317/jced.52917

Chen, P., Mancini, M., Sonis, S. T., Fernandez-Martinez, J., Liu, J., Cohen, E. E. W., et al. (2016). A novel peptide for simultaneously enhanced treatment of head and neck cancer and mitigation of oral mucositis. *PLoS ONE* 11:e0152995. doi: 10.1371/journal.pone.0152995

Chen, Y.-K., Hou, H.-A., Chow, J.-M., Chen, Y.-C., Hsueh, P.-R., and Tien, H.-F. (2011). The impact of oral herpes simplex virus infection and candidiasis on chemotherapy-induced oral mucositis among patients with hematological malignancies. *Eur. J. Clin. Microbiol. Infect. Dis.* 30, 753–759. doi: 10.1007/s10096-010-1148-z

Cho, H.-J., Park, Y. S., Kang, W. K., Kim, J.-W., and Lee, S.-Y. (2007). Thymidylate synthase (TYMS) and dihydropyrimidine dehydrogenase (DPYD) polymorphisms in the Korean population for prediction of 5-fluorouracil-associated toxicity. *Ther. Drug Monit.* 29, 190–196. doi: 10.1097/FTD.0b013e318040b1fe

Ciorba, M. A. (2012). A gastroenterologist's guide to probiotics. *Clin. Gastroenterol. Hepatol.* 10, 960–968. doi: 10.1016/j.cgh.2012.03.024

Ciorba, M. A., Hallemeier, C. L., Stenson, W. F., and Parikh, P. J. (2015). Probiotics to prevent gastrointestinal toxicity from cancer therapy: an interpretive review and call to action. *Curr. Opin. Support. Palliat. Care* 9, 157–162. doi: 10.1097/SPC.0000000000000134

ClinicalTrials. gov (2016a). *A Mouth Rinse Containing East Indian Sandalwood Oil (EISO) for the Prevention and Treatment of Oral Mucositis.* Available at: https://clinicaltrials.gov/ct2/show/NCT02399228?term=NCT02399228&rank=1 [accessed December 9, 2016].

ClinicalTrials. gov (2016b). *Cryotherapy in the Prevention of Chemotherapy-Induced Mucositis in Stem Cell Transplant.* Available at: https://clinicaltrials.gov/ct2/show/record/NCT02326675 [accessed December 13, 2016].

ClinicalTrials. gov (2016c). *Effect of Lactobacillus Brevis CD2 in Prevention of Radio-chemotherapy Induced Oral Mucositis in Head and Neck Cancer.* Available at: https://clinicaltrials.gov/ct2/show/NCT01707641?term=NCT01707641&rank=1 [accessed December 9, 2016].

ClinicalTrials. gov (2016d). *Effect of Oral Vitamin C in Assessing the Severity of Oral Mucositis in Chemoradiation of Head and Neck Cancers.* Available at: https://clinicaltrials.gov/ct2/show/NCT02868151?term=NCT02868151&rank=1 [accessed December 9, 2016].

ClinicalTrials. gov (2016e). *Study to See How Safe Curcumin is and How Well it Works When Used to Treat Mucositis in Patients Getting Chemotherapy*. Available at: https://clinicaltrials.gov/ct2/show/NCT02300727?term=NCT02300727&rank=1 [accessed December 9, 2016].

ClinicalTrials. gov (2016f). *Safety and Efficacy of ALD518 for Reducing Oral Mucositis in Head and Neck Cancer Subjects*. Available at: https://clinicaltrials.gov/ct2/show/NCT01403064 [accessed December 7, 2016].

ClinicalTrials. gov (2016g). *The Impact of Pentoxifylline and Vitamin E on Radiotherapy-Induced Toxicity in Head & Neck Cancer Patients*. Available at: https://clinicaltrials.gov/ct2/show/record/NCT02397486 [accessed December 9, 2016].

ClinicalTrials. gov (2017a). *A Study of the Effects of GC4419 on Radiation Induced Oral Mucositis in Patients With Head/Neck Cancer*. Available at: https://clinicaltrials.gov/ct2/show/NCT02508389 [accessed January 30, 2017].

ClinicalTrials. gov (2017b). *Phase 2 Study to Evaluate the Safety & Efficacy of Brilacidin Oral Rinse in Patients With Head and Neck Cancer*. Available at: https://clinicaltrials.gov/ct2/show/NCT02324335?term=brilacidin&rank=1 [accessed January 30, 2017].

Cowen, D., Tardieu, C., Schubert, M., Peterson, D., Resbeut, M., Faucher, C., et al. (1997). Low energy Helium-Neon laser in the prevention of oral mucositis in patients undergoing bone marrow transplant: results of a double blind randomized trial. *Int. J. Radiat. Oncol. Biol. Phys.* 38, 697–703. doi: 10.1016/S0360-3016(97)00076-X

Davila, M. L. (2006). Neutropenic enterocolitis. *Curr. Opin. Gastroenterol.* 22, 44–47.

De Sanctis, V., Bossi, P., Sanguineti, G., Trippa, F., Ferrari, D., Bacigalupo, A., et al. (2016). Mucositis in head and neck cancer patients treated with radiotherapy and systemic therapies: literature review and consensus statements. *Crit. Rev. Oncol. Hematol.* 100, 147–166. doi: 10.1016/j.critrevonc.2016.01.010

Dodd, M. J., Dibble, S. L., Miaskowski, C., MacPhail, L., Greenspan, D., Paul, S. M., et al. (2000). Randomized clinical trial of the effectiveness of 3 commonly used mouthwashes to treat chemotherapy-induced mucositis. *Oral Surg. Oral Med. Oral Pathol. Oral Radiol. Endod.* 90, 39–47. doi: 10.1067/moe.2000.105713

Douillard, J. Y., Siena, S., Cassidy, J., Tabernero, J., Burkes, R., Barugel, M., et al. (2014). Final results from PRIME: randomized phase III study of panitumumab with FOLFOX4 for first-line treatment of metastatic colorectal cancer. *Ann. Oncol. Off. J. Eur. Soc. Med. Oncol.* 25, 1346–1355. doi: 10.1093/annonc/mdu141

El-Housseiny, A. A., Saleh, S. M., El-Masry, A. A., and Allam, A. A. (2007). The effectiveness of vitamin "E" in the treatment of oral mucositis in children receiving chemotherapy. *J. Clin. Pediatr. Dent.* 31, 167–170. doi: 10.17796/jcpd.31.3.r8371x45m42l10j7

Elting, L. S., Chang, Y.-C., Parelkar, P., Boers-Doets, C. B., Michelet, M., Hita, G., et al. (2013). Risk of oral and gastrointestinal mucosal injury among patients receiving selected targeted agents: a meta-analysis. *Support. Care Cancer Off. J. Multinatl. Assoc. Support. Care Cancer* 21, 3243–3254. doi: 10.1007/s00520-013-1821-8

Elting, L. S., Cooksley, C., Chambers, M., Cantor, S. B., Manzullo, E., and Rubenstein, E. B. (2003). The burdens of cancer therapy. Clinical and economic outcomes of chemotherapy-induced mucositis. *Cancer* 98, 1531–1539. doi: 10.1002/cncr.11671

Epstein, J. B., Silverman, S., Paggiarino, D. A., Crockett, S., Schubert, M. M., Senzer, N. N., et al. (2001). Benzydamine HCl for prophylaxis of radiation-induced oral mucositis: results from a multicenter, randomized, double-blind, placebo-controlled clinical trial. *Cancer* 92, 875–885. doi: 10.1002/1097-0142(20010815)92:4<875::AID-CNCR1396>3.0.CO;2-1

Farrell, C. L., Bready, J. V., Rex, K. L., Chen, J. N., DiPalma, C. R., Whitcomb, K. L., et al. (1998). Keratinocyte growth factor protects mice from chemotherapy and radiation-induced gastrointestinal injury and mortality. *Cancer Res.* 58, 933–939.

Ferreira, B., da Motta Silveira, F. M., and de Orange, F. A. (2016). Low-level laser therapy prevents severe oral mucositis in patients submitted to hematopoietic stem cell transplantation: a randomized clinical trial. *Support. Care Cancer* 24, 1035–1042. doi: 10.1007/s00520-015-2881-8

Ghoreishi, Z., Shidfar, F., Iravani, M., Esfahani, A., and Ghavamzadeh, A. (2007). Effect of vitamin E on chemotherapy-induced mucositis and neutropenia in leukemic patients undergoing bone marrow transplantation. *Asia Pac. J. Clin. Oncol.* 3, 113–118. doi: 10.1111/j.1743-7563.2007.00111.x

Grothey, A., Van Cutsem, E., Sobrero, A., Siena, S., Falcone, A., Ychou, M., et al. (2013). Regorafenib monotherapy for previously treated metastatic colorectal cancer (CORRECT): an international, multicentre, randomised, placebo-controlled, phase 3 trial. *Lancet Lond. Engl.* 381, 303–312. doi: 10.1016/S0140-6736(12)61900-X

Han, X., Wu, Z., Di, J., Pan, Y., Zhang, H., Du, Y., et al. (2011). CXCL9 attenuated chemotherapy-induced intestinal mucositis by inhibiting proliferation and reducing apoptosis. *Biomed. Pharmacother. Biomedecine Pharmacother.* 65, 547–554. doi: 10.1016/j.biopha.2011.03.008

Hartmann, J. T., and Lipp, H.-P. (2003). Toxicity of platinum compounds. *Expert Opin. Pharmacother.* 4, 889–901. doi: 10.1517/14656566.4.6.889

Heinemann, V., Weikersthal, L. F., von Decker, T., Kiani, A., Vehling-Kaiser, U., Al-Batran, S.-E., et al. (2014). FOLFIRI plus cetuximab versus FOLFIRI plus bevacizumab as first-line treatment for patients with metastatic colorectal cancer (FIRE-3): a randomised, open-label, phase 3 trial. *Lancet Oncol.* 15, 1065–1075. doi: 10.1016/S1470-2045(14)70330-4

Hernández-Moreno, A., Vidal-Casariego, A., Calleja-Fernández, A., Kyriakos, G., Villar-Taibo, R., Urioste-Fondo, A., et al. (2015). Chronic enteritis in patients undergoing pelvic radiotherapy: prevalence, risk factors and associated complications. *Nutr. Hosp.* 32, 2178–2183. doi: 10.3305/nh.2015.32.5.9562

Kazemian, A., Kamian, S., Aghili, M., Hashemi, F. A., and Haddad, P. (2009). Benzydamine for prophylaxis of radiation-induced oral mucositis in head and neck cancers: a double-blind placebo-controlled randomized clinical trial. *Eur. J. Cancer Care* 18, 174–178. doi: 10.1111/j.1365-2354.2008.00943.x

Keefe, D. M., Elting, L. S., Nguyen, H. T., Grunberg, S. M., Aprile, G., Bonaventura, A., et al. (2014). Risk and outcomes of chemotherapy-induced diarrhea (CID) among patients with colorectal cancer receiving multi-cycle chemotherapy. *Cancer Chemother. Pharmacol.* 74, 675–680. doi: 10.1007/s00280-014-2526-5

Koukourakis, M. I., and Maltezos, E. (2006). Amifostine administration during radiotherapy for cancer patients with genetic, autoimmune, metabolic and other diseases. *Anticancer. Drugs* 17, 133–138. doi: 10.1097/00001813-200602000-00003

Krishna, S. G., Zhao, W., Grazziutti, M. L., Sanathkumar, N., Barlogie, B., and Anaissie, E. J. (2011). Incidence and risk factors for lower alimentary tract mucositis after 1529 courses of chemotherapy in a homogenous population of oncology patients: clinical and research implications. *Cancer* 117, 648–655. doi: 10.1002/cncr.25633

Kudrimoti, M., Curtis, A., Azawi, S., Worden, F., Katz, S., Adkins, D., et al. (2016). Dusquetide: a novel innate defense regulator demonstrating a significant and consistent reduction in the duration of oral mucositis in preclinical data and a randomized, placebo-controlled phase 2a clinical study. *J. Biotechnol.* 239, 115–125. doi: 10.1016/j.jbiotec.2016.10.010

Kushner, J. A., Lawrence, H. P., Shoval, I., Kiss, T. L., Devins, G. M., Lee, L., et al. (2008). Development and validation of a Patient-Reported Oral Mucositis Symptom (PROMS) scale. *J. Can. Dent. Assoc.* 74, 59.

Kwon, Y. (2016). Mechanism-based management for mucositis: option for treating side effects without compromising the efficacy of cancer therapy. *OncoTargets Ther.* 9, 2007–2016. doi: 10.2147/OTT.S96899

Lalla, R. V., Bowen, J., Barasch, A., Elting, L., Epstein, J., Keefe, D. M., et al. (2014). MASCC/ISOO clinical practice guidelines for the management of mucositis secondary to cancer therapy. *Cancer* 120, 1453–1461. doi: 10.1002/cncr.28592

Lalla, R. V., Gordon, G. B., Schubert, M., Silverman, S., Hutten, M., Sonis, S. T., et al. (2012). A randomized, double-blind, placebo-controlled trial of misoprostol for oral mucositis secondary to high-dose chemotherapy. *Support. Care Cancer* 20, 1797–1804. doi: 10.1007/s00520-011-1277-7

Lee, W. J., Lee, J. L., Chang, S. E., Lee, M. W., Kang, Y. K., Choi, J. H., et al. (2009). Cutaneous adverse effects in patients treated with the multitargeted kinase inhibitors sorafenib and sunitinib. *Br. J. Dermatol.* 161, 1045–1051. doi: 10.1111/j.1365-2133.2009.09290.x

Limaye, S. A., Haddad, R. I., Cilli, F., Sonis, S. T., Colevas, A. D., Brennan, M. T., et al. (2013). Phase 1b, multicenter, single blinded, placebo-controlled, sequential dose escalation study to assess the safety and tolerability of topically applied AG013 in subjects with locally advanced head and neck cancer receiving induction chemotherapy. *Cancer* 119, 4268–4276. doi: 10.1002/cncr.28365

Logan, R. M., Stringer, A. M., Bowen, J. M., Gibson, R. J., Sonis, S. T., and Keefe, D. M. K. (2008). Serum levels of NFkappaB and pro-inflammatory cytokines following administration of mucotoxic drugs. *Cancer Biol. Ther.* 7, 1139–1145. doi: 10.4161/cbt.7.7.6207

Mallick, S., Benson, R., and Rath, G. K. (2016). Radiation induced oral mucositis: a review of current literature on prevention and management. *Eur. Arch. Otorhinolaryngol.* 273, 2285–2293. doi: 10.1007/s00405-015-3694-6

Mayo, B. J., Stringer, A. M., Bowen, J. M., Bateman, E. H., and Keefe, D. M. (2017). Irinotecan-induced mucositis: the interactions and potential role of GLP-2 analogues. *Cancer Chemother. Pharmacol.* 79, 233–249. doi: 10.1007/s00280-016-3165-9

Mego, M., Chovanec, J., Vochyanova-Andrezalova, I., Konkolovsky, P., Mikulova, M., Reckova, M., et al. (2015). Prevention of irinotecan induced diarrhea by probiotics: a randomized double blind, placebo controlled pilot study. *Complement. Ther. Med.* 23, 356–362. doi: 10.1016/j.ctim.2015.03.008

Meirovitz, A., Kuten, M., Billan, S., Abdah-Bortnyak, R., Sharon, A., Peretz, T., et al. (2010). Cytokines levels, severity of acute mucositis and the need of PEG tube installation during chemo-radiation for head and neck cancer - a prospective pilot study. *Radiat. Oncol. Lond. Engl.* 5:16. doi: 10.1186/1748-717X-5-16

Meulendijks, D., Henricks, L. M., Sonke, G. S., Deenen, M. J., Froehlich, T. K., Amstutz, U., et al. (2015). Clinical relevance of DPYD variants c.1679T > G, c.1236G > A/HapB3, and c.1601G > A as predictors of severe fluoropyrimidine-associated toxicity: a systematic review and meta-analysis of individual patient data. *Lancet Oncol.* 16, 1639–1650. doi: 10.1016/S1470-2045(15)00286-7

Moslehi, A., Taghizadeh-Ghehi, M., Gholami, K., Hadjibabaie, M., Jahangard-Rafsanjani, Z., Sarayani, A., et al. (2014). N-acetyl cysteine for prevention of oral mucositis in hematopoietic SCT: a double-blind, randomized, placebo-controlled trial. *Bone Marrow Transplant.* 49, 818–823. doi: 10.1038/bmt.2014.34

Nonzee, N. J., Dandade, N. A., Patel, U., Markossian, T., Agulnik, M., Argiris, A., et al. (2008). Evaluating the supportive care costs of severe radiochemotherapy-induced mucositis and pharyngitis?: results from a Northwestern University Costs of Cancer Program pilot study with head and neck and nonsmall cell lung cancer patients who received care at a county hospital, a Veterans Administration hospital, or a comprehensive cancer care center. *Cancer* 113, 1446–1452. doi: 10.1002/cncr.23714

Ozben, T. (2015). Antioxidant supplementation on cancer risk and concurrent use of antioxidants during cancer therapy: an update. *Curr. Top. Med. Chem.* 15, 170–178. doi: 10.2174/1568026615666141209160918

Peterson, D. E., Boers-Doets, C. B., Bensadoun, R. J., Herrstedt, J., and Esmo Guidelines Committee. (2015). Management of oral and gastrointestinal mucosal injury: ESMO clinical practice guidelines for diagnosis, treatment, and follow-up. *Ann. Oncol.* 26(Suppl. 5), v139–v151. doi: 10.1093/annonc/mdv202

Peterson, D. E., Keefe, D. M., and Sonis, S. T. (2012). New frontiers in mucositis. *Am. Soc. Clin. Oncol. Educ. Book* 2012, 545–551. doi: 10.14694/EdBook_AM.2012.32.545

Pico, J., Avila-Garavito, A., and Naccache, P. (1998). Mucositis: its occurrence, consequences, and treatment in the oncology setting. *Oncologist* 3, 446–451.

Prisciandaro, L. D., Geier, M. S., Butler, R. N., Cummins, A. G., and Howarth, G. S. (2011). Probiotic factors partially improve parameters of 5-fluorouracil-induced intestinal mucositis in rats. *Cancer Biol. Ther.* 11, 671–677. doi: 10.4161/cbt.11.7.14896

Rao, N. G., Trotti, A., Kim, J., Schell, M. J., Zhao, X., Amdur, R. J., et al. (2014). Phase II multicenter trial of Caphosol for the reduction of mucositis in patients receiving radiation therapy for head and neck cancer. *Oral Oncol.* 50, 765–769. doi: 10.1016/j.oraloncology.2014.06.001

Ribeiro, R. A., Wanderley, C. W. S., Wong, D. V. T., Mota, J. M. S. C., Leite, C. A. V. G., Souza, M. H. L. P., et al. (2016). Irinotecan- and 5-fluorouracil-induced intestinal mucositis: insights into pathogenesis and therapeutic perspectives. *Cancer Chemother. Pharmacol.* 78, 881–893. doi: 10.1007/s00280-016-3139-y

Riley, P., Glenny, A.-M., Worthington, H. V., Littlewood, A., Clarkson, J. E., and McCabe, M. G. (2015). Interventions for preventing oral mucositis in patients with cancer receiving treatment: oral cryotherapy. *Cochrane Database Syst. Rev.* 23:CD011552. doi: 10.1002/14651858.CD011552.pub2

Riley, P., McCabe, M. G., and Glenny, A.-M. (2016). Oral cryotherapy for preventing oral mucositis in patients receiving cancer treatment. *JAMA Oncol.* 2, 1365–1366. doi: 10.1001/jamaoncol.2016.2680

Rm, L., Rj, G., St, S., and Dm, K. (2007). Nuclear factor-kappaB (NF-kappaB) and cyclooxygenase-2 (COX-2) expression in the oral mucosa following cancer chemotherapy. *Oral Oncol.* 43, 395–401. doi: 10.1016/j.oraloncology.2006.04.011

Roldan, C. J., Nouri, K., Chai, T., and Huh, B. (2017). Methylene blue for the treatment of intractable pain associated with oral mucositis. *Pain Pract.* doi: 10.1111/papr.12566 [Epub ahead of print].

Rubenstein, E. B., Peterson, D. E., Schubert, M., Keefe, D., McGuire, D., Epstein, J., et al. (2004). Clinical practice guidelines for the prevention and treatment of cancer therapy-induced oral and gastrointestinal mucositis. *Cancer* 100, 2026–2046. doi: 10.1002/cncr.20163

Rubin, J. S., Osada, H., Finch, P. W., Taylor, W. G., Rudikoff, S., and Aaronson, S. A. (1989). Purification and characterization of a newly identified growth factor specific for epithelial cells. *Proc. Natl. Acad. Sci. U.S.A.* 86, 802–806. doi: 10.1073/pnas.86.3.802

Rugo, H. S., Pritchard, K. I., Gnant, M., Noguchi, S., Piccart, M., Hortobagyi, G., et al. (2014). Incidence and time course of everolimus-related adverse events in postmenopausal women with hormone receptor-positive advanced breast cancer: insights from BOLERO-2. *Ann. Oncol.* 25, 808–815. doi: 10.1093/annonc/mdu009

Rugo, H. S., Seneviratne, L., Beck, J. T., Glaspy, J. A., Peguero, J. A., Pluard, T. J., et al. (2016). Prevention of everolimus/exemestane (EVE/EXE) stomatitis in postmenopausal (PM) women with hormone receptor-positive (HR+) metastatic breast cancer (MBC) using a dexamethasone-based mouthwash (MW): results of the SWISH trial. *J. Clin. Oncol.* 34:189. doi: 10.1200/jco.2016.34.26_suppl.189

Sachak, T., Arnold, M. A., Naini, B. V., Graham, R. P., Shah, S. S., Cruise, M., et al. (2015). Neutropenic enterocolitis: new insights into a deadly entity. *Am. J. Surg. Pathol.* 39, 1635–1642. doi: 10.1097/PAS.0000000000000517

Sanguineti, G., Sormani, M. P., Marur, S., Gunn, G. B., Rao, N., Cianchetti, M., et al. (2012). Effect of radiotherapy and chemotherapy on the risk of mucositis during intensity-modulated radiation therapy for oropharyngeal cancer. *Int. J. Radiat. Oncol. Biol. Phys.* 83, 235–242. doi: 10.1016/j.ijrobp.2011.06.2000

Schubert, M. M., Eduardo, F. P., Guthrie, K. A., Franquin, J.-C., Bensadoun, R.-J. J., Migliorati, C. A., et al. (2007). A phase III randomized double-blind placebo-controlled clinical trial to determine the efficacy of low level laser therapy for the prevention of oral mucositis in patients undergoing hematopoietic cell transplantation. *Support. Care Cancer* 15, 1145–1154. doi: 10.1007/s00520-007-0238-7

Schwab, M., Zanger, U. M., Marx, C., Schaeffeler, E., Klein, K., Dippon, J., et al. (2008). Role of genetic and nongenetic factors for fluorouracil treatment-related severe toxicity: a prospective clinical trial by the German 5-FU Toxicity Study Group. *J. Clin. Oncol.* 26, 2131–2138. doi: 10.1200/JCO.2006.10.4182

Shameem, R., Lacouture, M., and Wu, S. (2015). Incidence and risk of high-grade stomatitis with mTOR inhibitors in cancer patients. *Cancer Invest.* 33, 70–77. doi: 10.3109/07357907.2014.1001893

Sheibani, K. M., Mafi, A. R., Moghaddam, S., Taslimi, F., Amiran, A., and Ameri, A. (2015). Efficacy of benzydamine oral rinse in prevention and management of radiation-induced oral mucositis: a double-blind placebo-controlled randomized clinical trial. *Asia Pac. J. Clin. Oncol.* 11, 22–27. doi: 10.1111/ajco.12288

Shi, V. J., Levy, L. L., and Choi, J. N. (2016). Cutaneous manifestations of nontargeted and targeted chemotherapies. *Semin. Oncol.* 43, 419–425. doi: 10.1053/j.seminoncol.2016.02.018

Skof, E., Rebersek, M., Hlebanja, Z., and Ocvirk, J. (2009). Capecitabine plus Irinotecan (XELIRI regimen) compared to 5-FU/LV plus Irinotecan (FOLFIRI regimen) as neoadjuvant treatment for patients with unresectable liver-only metastases of metastatic colorectal cancer: a randomised prospective phase II trial. *BMC Cancer* 9:120. doi: 10.1186/1471-2407-9-120

Sonis, S., Andreotta, P. W., and Lyng, G. (2017). On the pathogenesis of mTOR-associated stomatitis (mIAS) - studies using an organotypic model of the oral mucosa. *Oral Dis.* 23, 347–352. doi: 10.1111/odi.12616

Sonis, S., Elting, L., Keefe, D., Nguyen, H., Grunberg, S., Randolph-Jackson, P., et al. (2015). Unanticipated frequency and consequences of regimen-related diarrhea in patients being treated with radiation or chemoradiation regimens for cancers of the head and neck or lung. *Support. Care Cancer* 23, 433–439. doi: 10.1007/s00520-014-2395-9

Sonis, S., Treister, N., Chawla, S., Demetri, G., and Haluska, F. (2010). Preliminary characterization of oral lesions associated with inhibitors of mammalian target of rapamycin in cancer patients. *Cancer* 116, 210–215. doi: 10.1002/cncr.24696

Sonis, S. T. (1998). Mucositis as a biological process: a new hypothesis for the development of chemotherapy-induced stomatotoxicity. *Oral Oncol.* 34, 39–43. doi: 10.1016/S1368-8375(97)00053-5

Sonis, S. T. (2002). The biologic role for nuclear factor-kappaB in disease and its potential involvement in mucosal injury associated with anti-neoplastic therapy. *Crit. Rev. Oral Biol. Med.* 13, 380–389. doi: 10.1177/154411130201300502

Sonis, S. T. (2004). The pathobiology of mucositis. *Nat. Rev. Cancer* 4, 277–284. doi: 10.1038/nrc1318

Sonis, S. T. (2007). Pathobiology of oral mucositis: novel insights and opportunities. *J. Support Oncol.* 9 (Suppl 4), 3–11.

Sonis, S. T. (2010). Regimen-related gastrointestinal toxicities in cancer patients. *Curr. Opin. Support. Palliat. Care* 4, 26–30. doi: 10.1097/SPC.0b013e328335fb76

Sonis, S. T. (2011). *Oral Mucositis. Pocket Book for Cancer Supportive Care*. London: Springer Healthcare.

Sonis, S. T. (2013). Oral mucositis in head and neck cancer: risk, biology, and management. *Am. Soc. Clin. Oncol. Educ. Book* doi: 10.1200/EdBook_AM.2013.33.e236

Sonis, S. T., Eilers, J. P., Epstein, J. B., LeVeque, F. G., Liggett, W. H., Mulagha, M. T., et al. (1999). Validation of a new scoring system for the assessment of clinical trial research of oral mucositis induced by radiation or chemotherapy. Mucositis Study Group. *Cancer* 85, 2103–2113. doi: 10.1002/(sici)1097-0142(19990515)85:10<2103::aid-cncr2>3.0.co;2-0

Sonis, S. T., Elting, L. S., Keefe, D., Peterson, D. E., Schubert, M., Hauer-Jensen, M., et al. (2004). Perspectives on cancer therapy-induced mucosal injury: pathogenesis, measurement, epidemiology, and consequences for patients. *Cancer* 100, 1995–2025. doi: 10.1002/cncr.20162

Sonis, S. T., Hashemi, S., Epstein, J. B., Nair, R. G., and Raber-Durlacher, J. E. (2016). Could the biological robustness of low level laser therapy (Photobiomodulation) impact its use in the management of mucositis in head and neck cancer patients. *Oral Oncol.* 54, 7–14. doi: 10.1016/j.oraloncology.2016.01.005

Sonis, S. T., Tracey, C., Shklar, G., Jenson, J., and Florine, D. (1990). An animal model for mucositis induced by cancer chemotherapy. *Oral Surg. Oral Med. Oral Pathol.* 69, 437–443. doi: 10.1016/0030-4220(90)90376-4

Sorensen, J. B., Skovsgaard, T., Bork, E., Damstrup, L., and Ingeberg, S. (2008). Double-blind, placebo-controlled, randomized study of chlorhexidine prophylaxis for 5-fluorouracil-based chemotherapy-induced oral mucositis with nonblinded randomized comparison to oral cooling (cryotherapy) in gastrointestinal malignancies. *Cancer* 112, 1600–1606. doi: 10.1002/cncr.23328

Spielberger, R., Stiff, P., Bensinger, W., Gentile, T., Weisdorf, D., Kewalramani, T., et al. (2004). Palifermin for oral mucositis after intensive therapy for hematologic cancers. *N. Engl. J. Med.* 351, 2590–2598. doi: 10.1056/NEJMoa040125

Squier, C. A., and Kremer, M. J. (2001). Biology of oral mucosa and esophagus. *JNCI Monogr.* 2001, 7–15. doi: 10.1093/oxfordjournals.jncimonographs.a003443

Stein, A., Voigt, W., and Jordan, K. (2010). Chemotherapy-induced diarrhea: pathophysiology, frequency and guideline-based management. *Ther. Adv. Med. Oncol.* 2, 51–63. doi: 10.1177/1758834009355164

Stiff, P. J., Emmanouilides, C., Bensinger, W. I., Gentile, T., Blazar, B., Shea, T. C., et al. (2006a). Palifermin reduces patient-reported mouth and throat soreness and improves patient functioning in the hematopoietic stem-cell transplantation setting. *J. Clin. Oncol.* 24, 5186–5193. doi: 10.1200/JCO.2005.02.8340

Stiff, P. J., Erder, H., Bensinger, W. I., Emmanouilides, C., Gentile, T., Isitt, J., et al. (2006b). Reliability and validity of a patient self-administered daily questionnaire to assess impact of oral mucositis (OM) on pain and daily functioning in patients undergoing autologous hematopoietic stem cell transplantation (HSCT). *Bone Marrow Transplant.* 37, 393–401. doi: 10.1038/sj.bmt.1705250

Stringer, A. M., Al-Dasooqi, N., Bowen, J. M., Tan, T. H., Radzuan, M., Logan, R. M., et al. (2013). Biomarkers of chemotherapy-induced diarrhoea: a clinical study of intestinal microbiome alterations, inflammation and circulating matrix metalloproteinases. *Support. Care Cancer* 21, 1843–1852. doi: 10.1007/s00520-013-1741-7

Stringer, A. M., and Logan, R. M. (2015). The role of oral flora in the development of chemotherapy-induced oral mucositis. *J. Oral Pathol. Med.* 44, 81–87. doi: 10.1111/jop.12152

Svanberg, A., Öhrn, K., and Birgegård, G. (2015). Caphosol(®) mouthwash gives no additional protection against oral mucositis compared to cryotherapy alone in stem cell transplantation. A pilot study. *Eur. J. Oncol. Nurs.* 19, 50–53. doi: 10.1016/j.ejon.2014.07.011

Theis, V. S., Sripadam, R., Ramani, V., and Lal, S. (2010). Chronic radiation enteritis. *Clin. Oncol.* 22, 70–83. doi: 10.1016/j.clon.2009.10.003

Treister, N., Nieder, M., Baggott, C., Olson, E., Chen, L., Dang, H., et al. (2017). Caphosol for prevention of oral mucositis in pediatric myeloablative haematopoietic cell transplantation. *Br. J. Cancer* 116, 21–27. doi: 10.1038/bjc.2016.380

Trotti, A., Bellm, L. A., Epstein, J. B., Frame, D., Fuchs, H. J., Gwede, C. K., et al. (2003). Mucositis incidence, severity and associated outcomes in patients with head and neck cancer receiving radiotherapy with or without chemotherapy: a systematic literature review. *Radiother. Oncol.* 66, 253–262. doi: 10.1016/S0167-8140(02)00404-8

Tsujimoto, T., Yamamoto, Y., Wasa, M., Takenaka, Y., Nakahara, S., Takagi, T., et al. (2015). L-glutamine decreases the severity of mucositis induced by chemoradiotherapy in patients with locally advanced head and neck cancer: a double-blind, randomized, placebo-controlled trial. *Oncol. Rep.* 33, 33–39. doi: 10.3892/or.2014.3564

United States Department of Health and Human Services (2010). *Common Terminology Criteria for Adverse Events (CTCAE) - CTCAE_4.03.* Available at: https://evs.nci.nih.gov/ftp1/CTCAE/CTCAE_4.03_2010-06-14_QuickReference_8.5x11.pdf [accessed December 9, 2016].

Uçüncü, H., Ertekin, M. V., Yörük, O., Sezen, O., Ozkan, A., Erdoğan, F., et al. (2006). Vitamin E and L-carnitine, separately or in combination, in the prevention of radiation-induced oral mucositis and myelosuppression: a controlled study in a rat model. *J. Radiat. Res.* 47, 91–102. doi: 10.1269/jrr.47.91

Van Cutsem, E., Köhne, C.-H., Hitre, E., Zaluski, J., Chang Chien, C.-R., Makhson, A., et al. (2009). Cetuximab and chemotherapy as initial treatment for metastatic colorectal cancer. *N. Engl. J. Med.* 360, 1408–1417. doi: 10.1056/NEJMoa0805019

Van Cutsem, E., Köhne, C.-H., Láng, I., Folprecht, G., Nowacki, M. P., Cascinu, S., et al. (2011). Cetuximab plus irinotecan, fluorouracil, and leucovorin as first-line treatment for metastatic colorectal cancer: updated analysis of overall survival according to tumor KRAS and BRAF mutation status. *J. Clin. Oncol.* 29, 2011–2019. doi: 10.1200/JCO.2010.33.5091

Van Sebille, Y. Z. A., Stansborough, R., Wardill, H. R., Bateman, E., Gibson, R. J., and Keefe, D. M. (2015). Management of mucositis during chemotherapy: from pathophysiology to pragmatic therapeutics. *Curr. Oncol. Rep.* 17:50. doi: 10.1007/s11912-015-0474-9

Vasconcelos, R. M., Sanfilippo, N., Paster, B. J., Kerr, A. R., Li, Y., Ramalho, L., et al. (2016). Host-microbiome cross-talk in oral mucositis. *J. Dent. Res.* 95, 725–733. doi: 10.1177/0022034516641890

Venook, A. P., Niedzwiecki, D., Lenz, H.-J., Innocenti, F., Mahoney, M. R., O'Neil, B. H., et al. (2014). CALGB/SWOG 80405: phase III trial of irinotecan/5-FU/leucovorin (FOLFIRI) or oxaliplatin/5-FU/leucovorin (mFOLFOX6) with bevacizumab (BV) or cetuximab (CET) for patients (pts) with KRAS wild-type (wt) untreated metastatic adenocarcinoma of the colon or rectum (MCRC). *J. Clin. Oncol.* 32, 5s. doi: 10.1200/jco.2014.32.18_suppl.lba3

Viet, C. T., Corby, P. M., Akinwande, A., and Schmidt, B. L. (2014). Review of preclinical studies on treatment of mucositis and associated pain. *J. Dent. Res.* 93, 868–875. doi: 10.1177/0022034514540174

Villa, A., and Sonis, S. T. (2015). Mucositis: pathobiology and management. *Curr. Opin. Oncol.* 27, 159–164. doi: 10.1097/CCO.0000000000000180

Villa, A., and Sonis, S. T. (2016). Pharmacotherapy for the management of cancer regimen-related oral mucositis. *Expert Opin. Pharmacother.* 17, 1801–1807. doi: 10.1080/14656566.2016.1217993

Wardill, H. R., Bowen, J. M., Al-Dasooqi, N., Sultani, M., Bateman, E., Stansborough, R., et al. (2014). Irinotecan disrupts tight junction proteins within the gut : implications for chemotherapy-induced gut toxicity. *Cancer Biol. Ther.* 15, 236–244. doi: 10.4161/cbt.27222

Webb, G. J., Brooke, R., and De Silva, A. N. (2013). Chronic radiation enteritis and malnutrition. *J. Dig. Dis.* 14, 350–357. doi: 10.1111/1751-2980.12061

Wong, K. H., Kuciejewska, A., Sharabiani, M. T. A., Ng-Cheng-Hin, B., Hoy, S., Hurley, T., et al. (2016). A randomised controlled trial of Caphosol mouthwash in management of radiation-induced mucositis in head and neck cancer. *Radiother. Oncol.* 122, 207–211. doi: 10.1016/j.radonc.2016.06.015

Worthington, H. V., Clarkson, J. E., Bryan, G., Furness, S., Glenny, A.-M., Littlewood, A., et al. (2011). Interventions for preventing oral mucositis for patients with cancer receiving treatment. *Cochrane Database Syst. Rev.* 4:CD000978. doi: 10.1002/14651858.CD000978.pub5

Yamamoto, H., Ishihara, K., Takeda, Y., Koizumi, W., and Ichikawa, T. (2013). Changes in the mucus barrier during cisplatin-induced intestinal mucositis in rats. *BioMed Res. Int.* 2013:276186. doi: 10.1155/2013/276186

Yuan, A., and Sonis, S. (2014). Emerging therapies for the prevention and treatment of oral mucositis. *Expert Opin. Emerg. Drugs* 19, 343–351. doi: 10.1517/14728214.2014.946403

Zecha, J. A. E. M., Raber-Durlacher, J. E., Nair, R. G., Epstein, J. B., Sonis, S. T., Elad, S., et al. (2016). Low level laser therapy/photobiomodulation in the management of side effects of chemoradiation therapy in head and neck cancer: part 1: mechanisms of action, dosimetric, and safety considerations. *Support. Care Cancer* 24, 2781–2792. doi: 10.1007/s00520-016-3152-z

Conflict of Interest Statement: The authors declare that the research was conducted in the absence of any commercial or financial relationships that could be construed as a potential conflict of interest.

7

Dual Functional Capability of Dendritic Cells – Cytokine-Induced Killer Cells in Improving Side Effects of Colorectal Cancer Therapy

Paula Mosińska[1], Agata Gabryelska[1], Malwina Zasada[1,2] and Jakub Fichna[1]*

[1] Department of Biochemistry, Faculty of Medicine, Medical University of Łódź, Łódź, Poland, [2] Department of Cosmetic Raw Materials Chemistry, Faculty of Pharmacy, Medical University of Łódź, Łódź, Poland

The aim of cancer therapy is to eradicate cancer without affecting healthy tissues. Current options available for treating colorectal cancer (CRC), including surgery, chemotherapy or radiotherapy, usually elicit multiple adverse effects and frequently fail to completely remove the tumor cells. Thus, there is a constant need for seeking cancer cell-specific therapeutics to improve the course of cancer therapy and reduce the risk of relapse. In this review we elaborate on the mechanisms underlying the immunotherapy with dendritic cells (DCs) and cytokine-induced killer (CIK) cells, and summarize their effectiveness and tolerability available clinical studies. Finally, we discuss the up-to-date combinatorial adoptive anti-cancer immunotherapy with CIK cells co-cultured with DCs that recently showed encouraging efficacy and usefulness in treating malignant disease, including CRC.

Keywords: dendritic cells, cytokine-induced killer cells, colorectal cancer, immunotherapy, colorectal cancer treatment

Edited by:
Kulmira Nurgali,
Victoria University, Australia

Reviewed by:
Patrick Anthony Hughes,
University of Adelaide, Australia
Vasso Apostolopoulos,
Victoria University, Australia
Antonio Macciò,
A. Businco Hospital, Italy

****Correspondence:***
Paula Mosińska
paula.mosinska@gmail.com

INTRODUCTION

Colorectal cancer is the second in woman and the third in men most commonly diagnosed cancer worldwide (Siegel et al., 2015), accounted for approximately 1.2 million new cases and over 600.000 deaths annually (Torre et al., 2015). Surgical resection is the first choice procedure for patients suffering from CRC, and is frequently followed by radio- or chemotherapy. For early staged CRC patients, the combined course of treatment results in 5-year survival rate of up to 80% (Zhu et al., 2014). Nevertheless, surgical resection with adjuvant radio- or chemotherapy is often poorly tolerated by patients due to many severe side effects directly related to complications after surgery, including infections and bleedings, and indirectly to psychological trauma, nausea, vomiting, and fever. Therefore, new, more patient friendly and especially effective treatment is necessary to avoid tumor recurrence, and enhance the response rate to therapy.

Abbreviations: ADCC, antibody-dependent cell-mediated cytotoxicity; APCs, antigen presenting cells; CIK, cytokine-induced killer cells; CRC, colorectal cancer; CTT, cytotoxic T lymphocytes; DCs, dendritic cells; DTH, Delayed Type Hypersensitivity; ER, endoplasmic reticulum; i-DCs, induced DCs; IDO, indoleamine 2,3-dioxygenase; IFN-γ, interferon gamma; IFNs-I, interferons type I; IL-1, interleukin-1; IL-2, interleukin-2; IL-6, interleukin-6; IL-12, interleukin-12; LAKs, lymphokine-activated killers; mDCs, myeloid dendritic cells; MHC, major histocompatibility complex; MST, medium survival time; NOD, nucleotide oligomerization domain; OS, overall survival; PBMS, peripheral blood mononuclear cells; pDCs, plasmacytoid dendritic cells; PFS, progression-free survival; TAAs, tumor associated antigens; TAP, transporters for antigen presentation; Th cell, T helper cell.

Colorectal cancer is a heterogenous disease in terms of its molecular characteristics, clinical manifestations, and sensitivity to treatments. Along with accumulation of genetic alterations (e.g., genomic and chromosomal instabilities) and epigenetic changes that constitute the main forces for tumor development, immune pattern of the tumor microenvironment seems to be the major predictor of patient's survival in a variety of primary tumors (Maby et al., 2015). High density of T cells and $CD8^{+}$ T cells cytotoxic orientation or mature DCs are considered as a target in the treatment of large group of cancers such as colorectal, lung, breast, pancreatic and melanoma cancers (Al-Shibli et al., 2008; Pagès et al., 2009; Mahmoud et al., 2011; Remark et al., 2013). Adaptive and innate immune system can protect the host from tumor development through mechanisms of immunosurveillance (Mlecnik et al., 2010; Stoll et al., 2015). Cancer immunotherapy involves the use of therapeutic modalities, which stimulate the host's anti-tumor response by altering the effector cell number and secretion of soluble mediators, and decreases the host's suppressor mechanisms by modulating immune checkpoints. The immunotherapy represents the most promising new cancer treatment approach, also among CRC patients. Patients suffering from CRC are in an immunosuppressed state when they undergo radiotherapy, surgery, or chemotherapy and often exhibit compromised immune responses; therefore, it is recommended to target dysfunctional cells to achieve most promising therapeutic results and simultaneously recover anti-cancer immunity to support immune response to tumor cells. DCs, responsible for the activation of T-cells, and CIK cells, which induce the secretion of a diverse array of cytokines, are rapidly evolving immunotherapeutic targets in eradicating residual cancer cells (Yang et al., 2011). The therapy has already been used in the treatment of chronic myeloid leukemia and other types of cancer such as liver, kidney, breast, and prostate (Wang et al., 2009).

Understanding of the molecular interactions between immune system and tumor cells has significantly improved in the last decade, leading to the development of DC-CIK adoptive immunotherapy, which encompasses the introduction of DCs in combination with the CIK cells. The immunotherapy with DC-CIK reduces the severity of adverse effects, namely grade III and IV leukopenia, thrombocytopenia and anemia, which commonly occurs as a consequence of conventional cancer therapy, improves overall quality of life and prolongs the survival of CRC patients (Lin et al., 2016).

MECHANISM OF ACTION OF DCS

Dendritic cells are well-characterized APCs (Steinman, 1991), which reside in peripheral tissues. The role of DCs is to capture, process and present phagocytosed antigens, including TAAs, express lymphocyte costimulatory molecules and secrete cytokines, such as IL-12, IL-15 and type I interferons (IFNs I) to initiate primary immune response in resting naive T cells (Pulendran et al., 2008; Legitimo et al., 2014).

Dendritic cells comprise multiple subsets with different morphologic, phenotypic, and functional properties. There are two main classes of DCs, similar for both mice and humans: mDCs, also called classical DCs, and pDCs, which originate from CD34+ bone marrow precursors (**Figure 1**). Under certain conditions, both types can be also propagated from monocytes (Shortman and Naik, 2007; Pulendran et al., 2008). The two DC subsets possess distinct features: mDCs express CD11c marker and are considered as principal producers of IFNs I, whereas pDCs express mainly CD123 and IDO, an enzyme participating in the generation of regulatory T cells (Koido et al., 2013). A detailed discussion of DC subtypes can be found elsewhere (Dudek et al., 2013; Ma et al., 2013; Legitimo et al., 2014). In healthy conditions, DCs occur in an immature or semi-mature state and are usually localized in various non-lymphoid organs and tissues. Immature DCs are responsible for the uptake and process of peptides. They are able to respond to various inflammatory signals, e.g., toll-like receptors (TLR), NOD-like receptors, scavenger receptors, and inflammatory mediators, chemokines and cytokines (Niu et al., 2014). Upon activation, immature DCs migrate to lymphoid tissues and interact with T cells. Active DCs produce and secrete IL-12, which induces cell differentiation of lymphocytes T CD4 + into antigen-specific effector Th cells e.g., Th1, Th2, Th17, and increases production of interferon-gamma (IFN-γ) and cytotoxic activity of CTL, essential for antitumor immune activity (Koido et al., 2013). The distinction between mature and immature DCs relates to their phenotypic and functional properties. Maturation of DCs occurs when the cell can upregulate MHC class II molecules and several surface ligands, including CD80, CD83 and CD86 (Märten et al., 2001). Moreover, fully matured DCs can control the balance between inflammatory, e.g., IL-6, immunostimulatory, e.g., IL-12 cytokines and immunosuppressive cytokines (Xie et al., 2006). However, existing evidence suggests that DCs may occur in states, since they exhibit high functional plasticity, i.e., DCs are able to express immunostimulating and/or immunesuppresive factors depending on microenvironmental conditions that affect their differentiation, maturation, polarization and activation; however, even in multiple environmental milieus morphologically different DC subsets are able to stimulate T cell proliferation and modulate their response (Manicassamy and Pulendran, 2011).

Various endogenous and exogenous stimuli affect maturation of DCs by changing the processing and presentation of the antigen, e.g., activated natural killer (NK) cells acquire the ability to defeat DCs that have failed to undergo complete maturation. Moreover, DC–NK interaction induces generation of various cytokines by both cell types, and besides enhancing DC maturation, also promotes the proliferation of NK cells. Endogenous antigens are degraded into peptides by proteasomes in the cytosol and together with TAP are transferred to ER, where they create complexes with MHC class I molecules. The peptide-MHC I complexes is subsequently presented to CD8+ T cells. This form of antigen presentation is available not only for DCs but also for other nucleated cells (Ma et al., 2013). Exogenous antigens in turn are processed in endosomes, loaded onto MHC class II molecules, and activate CD4+ T cells and cause their further polarization to Th cells. This process is restricted only to APCs (Ma et al., 2013).

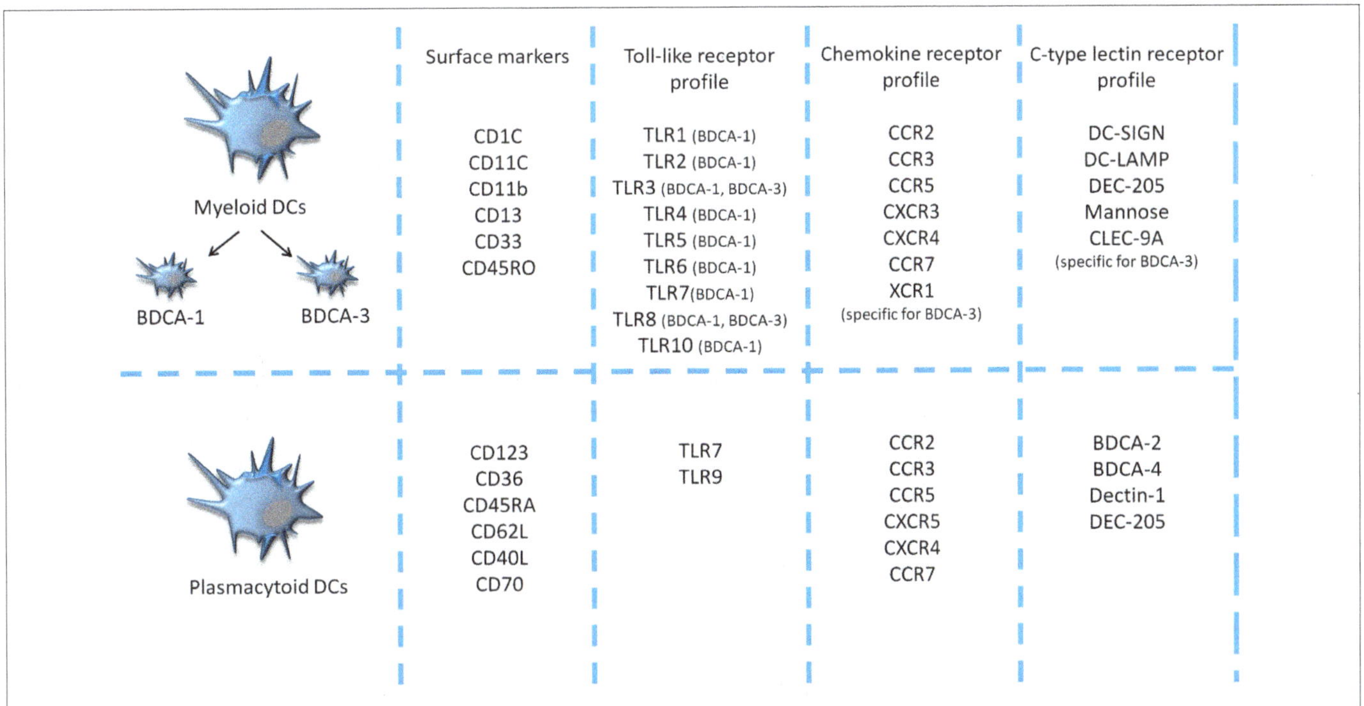

FIGURE 1 | Comparison of surface markers, toll-like receptor (TLR), chemokine receptors (CCR) and C-type lectin receptors (CLRs) profiles between two major populations of naturally circulating DCs- human blood myeloid and plasmacytoid DCs- in the peripheral blood of humans (Mckenna et al., 2005; Bamboat et al., 2009; Reizis et al., 2011).

Metastasis and tumor stage are related to higher infiltrations of DCs in the tumor tissue (Gordon et al., 2014). DCs modulate innate and adoptive immunity, affect oncogenesis, especially tumor progression, and therefore influence response to cancer therapy (Bloy et al., 2014). However, the presence of tumor cells may also drive DCs into state of tolerance and immunosuppression, resulting in their decreased or completely inhibited activity of initiating the immune response. Functional impairments of DCs have been reported in various types of cancer, such as chronic myeloid leukemia, liver cancer as well as CRC (Miller et al., 2004).

Dendritic cell-based interventions aim at (re)activating the endogenous cancer-specific immune response, which *de facto* constitutes an anti-cancer vaccine. Exploiting naturally circulating DCs can be performed either by isolating pDCs or mDCs and stimulating them *ex vivo* (with adjuvants and antigens), *in vivo* (by means of nanoparticles coated with antibodies against DCs-specific cell surface receptors), and DC-derived exosomes (Bol et al., 2013; Bloy et al., 2014).

GENERAL MECHANISM OF CIK CELLS

Cytokine-induced killer cells are *ex vivo* expanded heterogeneous population of lymphocytes T CD8+ with additional NK cells phenotype. They are generated by an *in vitro* extraction of PBMC and its further exposition to IFN-γ, anti CD-3 antibody, and prolong propagation in presence of high-dose IL-1 and IL-2 (Wang et al., 2011; Schlimper et al., 2012). After maturation, when the majority of cells exhibit granular lymphocyte morphology and express NK and T-cell markers, CIK cells are transferred to the recipient in autologous or allogeneic settings (Zhao et al., 2015).

The lytic activity of CIK cells is driven mainly by $CD3^{+}CD56^{+}$ cells that can coexpress both the T-cell marker CD3 and the NK cell marker CD56 (Pievani et al., 2011). They were first described in 1991 by Schmidt-Wolf et al. (1991), who concluded CIK cells to have higher proliferation and strengthened cytotoxic properties against tumor cells compared to their progenitors LAKs. CIK cells display non-MHC-restricted NK-like anti-tumor activity against allogenic and syngeneic hematological malignancies (Sangiolo et al., 2008). They secrete proinflammatory cytokines, predominantly IFN-γ and IL-4. Due to their CLT phenotype, CIK cells are also capable of eliminating cells presenting MHC molecules (Wang et al., 2009). Mechanisms used by CIK cells to terminate cancer cell include release of granules, such as granzymes and perforin. Along with NK cells, macrophages, monocytes, and neutrophils, CIK cells can mediate cytotoxicity through ADCC (Kohrt et al., 2012). It is therefore possible that besides recognizing cancer cells without prior antigen sensitization in a non-MHC restricted manner, CIK cells anti-tumor activity might be enhanced by adding specific monoclonal antibodies targeting ADCC (Wang et al., 2014). Since CIK cells can be produced by a simple approach and exert anti-tumor activity *in vitro*, they seem to be suitable tools for the treatment of solid and hematopoietic tumors (Li et al., 2012). Autologous and allogenic CIK cells have been already evaluated in the treatment of different tumor types (NCT0076910, NCT01186809, NCT02886897, NCT00394381, NCT00815321, NCT01871480, and NCT01232062).

DC–CIK INTERACTION

Based on available data the adoptive immunotherapy with DC-CIK encompass either the infusion of DCs (the amount of infused cells ranges from 1 to 5 $\times$ 10^7) following the administration of CIK cells (the amount of cells range from 2 to 15 $\times$ 10^9) or autologous tumor lysate pulsed DC-CIK cells infused intravenously (NCT02202928) (Zhu et al., 2014).

According to different clinical trials, DCs can be injected subcutaneously, intravenously or intradermally, in turn CIK cells are usually administered intravenously or intradermally (NCT01956630, NCT02491697, and NCT02202928).

Any dysfunction of either DC or CIK cells may cause inefficient immune response, which consequently enables cancer cells to spread. Interactions between molecules on the surface of mature DCs and CIK cells cause an increased activation of each of these populations; however, the exact mechanism of action is still not fully understood. The stage of DCs maturation determines DC–CIK interaction and its function (Lin et al., 2016). Mature DCs provide necessary signals for proliferation of CIK cells by increasing their cytotoxic and cytolytic capabilities; immature DCs are unable to trigger this reaction and are consequently killed by CIK cells (Qu et al., 2014). DC–CIK interaction also causes a significant increase in the number of costimulatory and antigen-presenting molecules on DCs surface, which provides the cell with greater tumor-fighting capabilities (**Figure 2**). Combination of DC-CIK in cancer therapy, compared to each therapy alone, results in an enhanced immune response in treated patients (n = 100) and greater therapeutic effects (Zhu et al., 2014). Numerous studies provide evidence that DC-CIK were effective in the treatment of multiple solid tumors, e.g., breast cancer, non-small-cell lung cancer, without causing any serious adverse reactions.

The fact that distinct subsets of DCs precursors can be activated and mobilized by various cytokines, e.g., in humans pDCs can be regulated *in vivo* with Flt4 ligand or G-CSF, whereas other blood DC subsets only by Flt3L, it additionally provides an individual approach for manipulating of immune responses in humans (Arpinati et al., 2000; Pulendran et al., 2000). This approach may constitute another way of improving the effect of therapy with DC-CIK.

However, it has to be mentioned that multiple parameters can modulate the quality of immune responses through DC targeting (Ueno et al., 2011). Thus, some major issues need consideration during DC vaccine development:

-biological function of the DC subsets that is anticipated to deliver antigens,

-the type of activation signaling and immune response that the DC can induce,

-the selection of antigens and their formulation that will induce the antigen-specific response

-the receptors expressed by the particular subset of DCs.

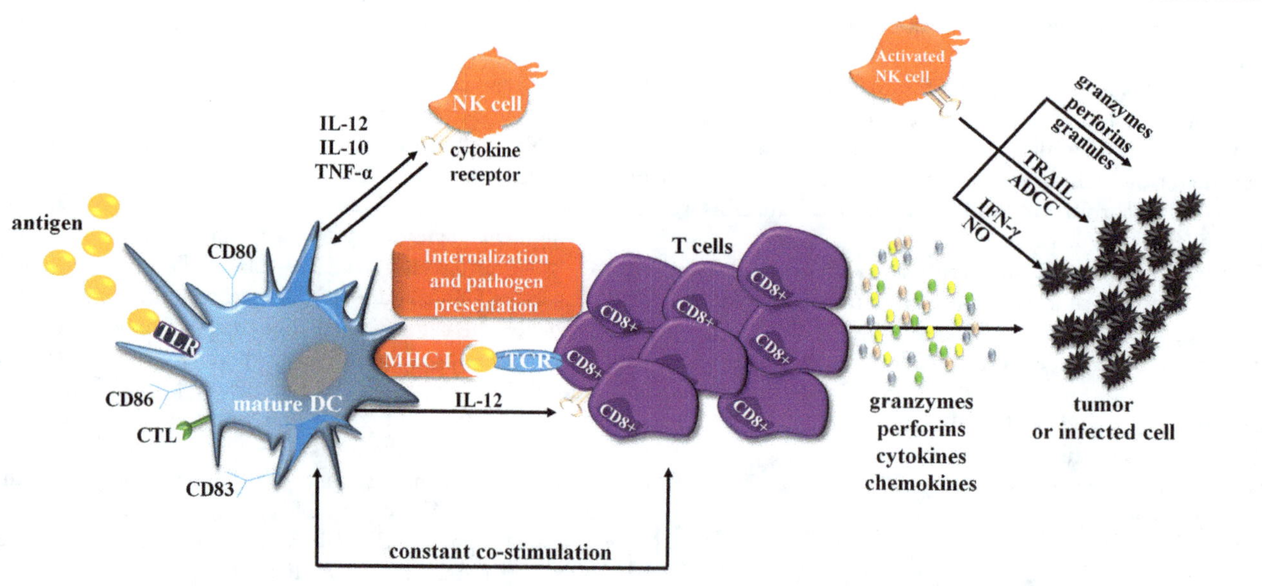

FIGURE 2 | Simplified scheme showing interactions between DCs and CIK cells. mDCs are also able to crosstalk with NK cells, prototypical effector cells of innate immunity. Both mDC and NK cells reciprocally stimulate and regulate their functions. For example upon activation, NK cells acquire the ability to defeat immature DCs. On the other hand, activated IFN-α-generating DCs can also stimulate NK cells and initiate antigen-specific T- and B-cell responses. The crosstalk appears via cell-to-cell interaction and largely involves the activation of NK cells via transmembrane TNF-α. Activated NK cells can also directly kill target tumor cells through several mechanisms involving TRAIL, ADCC, IFN-γ, NO or by the release of granzymes, perforins, granules. ADCC, antibody-dependent cellular cytotoxicity; CTL, C-type lectins; IFN-γ, interferon γ; MHC II, major histocompatibility complex II; NK cell, natural killer cell; NO, nitric oxide; TCR, toll-like receptors; TRAIL, tumor necrosis factor-related apoptosis-inducing ligand.

BENEFICIAL EFFECTS OF DC-CIK THERAPY

One of great advantages of immunotherapy is an easy evaluation and monitoring of patients' response to therapy based on DTH reaction. According to Zhu et al. (2014; Lin et al., 2016), among 100 patients with CRC, more than 60% developed positive cell-mediated cytotoxicity response to the treatment with DC-CIK, assessed in DTH skin test. Adverse events occurred in less than 30% of recruited patients and included fever, insomnia, sore joints and skin rush (Niu et al., 2014; Zhang et al., 2016). However, validity and efficacy of DTH can be affected by the tumor environment and therefore the obtained results should be treated with caution.

Dendritic cell-cytokine-induced killer cell-based immunotherapy combined with chemotherapy prolongs PFS in patients with CRC, and increases OS rate to almost 4 months, when compared to chemotherapy alone (Lin et al., 2016). Similar outcomes were reported in the study by Niu et al. (2014) in which 44 out of 70 patients with CRC developed positive immune response after DC-CIK-based immunotherapy, which prolonged their MST. No severe adverse events were observed; however, similarly to the study by Zhu et al. (2014) patients experienced mild inconveniences, e.g., insomnia, fever, anorexia, skin rush or joint soreness. The respective increase in PFS and OS were almost 9 and 15 months, respectively, for patients treated with DC-CIK therapy additionally to chemotherapy. The incorporation of the adjuvant immunotherapy for patients undergoing primary chemotherapy resulted in general improvement in quality of life, including physical strength, appetite, better sleep and increase in body weight (Zhan et al., 2012). Finally, DC-CIK therapy proved to decrease the recurrence and metastasis rate in CRC patients (Lin et al., 2016).

Dendritic cell-cytokine-induced killer therapy targets tumor cells without attacking other cells of the organism, which it is not associated with toxicity, and thus make it a viable treatment option for patients in poor health (Hui et al., 2009). As opposed to chemotherapy, DC-CIK therapy induces fewer and less severe adverse effects, and also limits the side effects caused by chemotherapy itself. Adjuvant DC-CIK therapy to primary chemotherapy lowers the frequency of severe treatment induced complications - hematological toxicities such as leukopenia, anemia and thrombocytopenia as well as nausea, vomiting and abdominal liver function (Lin et al., 2016).

Worth mentioning, tumors that develop radiation or chemotherapy resistance, still remain a suitable target for immunotherapy (Dasgupta et al., 2011). A combined approach to use conventional anti-cancer therapy to kill the bulk of cancer cells and immunotherapy (e.g., DCs as adjuvants) to improve immunization against tumor cells, can be even more effective in treating cancer.

Currently, there are few clinical trials, both ongoing and still recruiting, assessing the effect of the autologous tumor lysate pulsed DC-CIK treatment in CRC patients (NCT02202928, NCT01839539, and NCT02415699).

LIMITATIONS OF ANTI-CRC THERAPY

Chemotherapy has many imperfections: not only its sensitivity declines over time, but often causes numerous adverse effects, for example nausea and vomiting. This line of treatment is also associated with severe toxicity, which deteriorates general health of patients and leads to discontinuation of treatment (Dasgupta et al., 2011).

In contrast to chemotherapy, the side effects of immunotherapy include insomnia, fever, anorexia, diarrhea, joint soreness and general fatigue (Wood et al., 2000). They are minor, occur rarely and are mostly self-resolving; usually no special treatments and hospitalizations are necessary. In some cases, the anti-inflammatory drugs are used to resolve side effects such as fever. The treatment with DC-CIK does not prompt autoimmune reactions (Niu et al., 2014). In some singular cases limited toxicity may appear; however, lowering the dose of the treatment resolves the side effects and allows the patients to continue the treatment (Zhan et al., 2012). Nonetheless, because the positive cell-mediated cytotoxicity response to DC vaccine and CIK cell therapy is developed in around 60% of CRC patients, the therapy is not effective for all (Niu et al., 2014).

Currently, peripheral blood is the main source of DC-CIK. As the therapy should be personalized for each patient, the repeated collection of blood can be difficult and may imply a considerable costs, which narrow the number of recipients. In some cases, e.g., elderly patients or patients in poor health, obtaining the number of cytotoxic cells necessary for the therapy may pose a significant challenge and limit the utility of the therapy.

There is still insufficient number of clinical trials that evaluate the effectiveness of DC-CIK therapy in patients with CRC, and which determine the probability of the occurrence of adverse effects. Randomized controlled trials with larger sample sizes or meta-analysis are warranted to provide evidence for further application of this therapy.

CONCLUSION

Immunotherapy has fewer side effects than standard treatment with chemo- or radiotherapy and is generally more potent in preventing their onset. Recent studies present new treatment options for patients suffering from CRC, focusing predominantly on DC-CIK therapy, which stimulate the immune system of a patient against cancer. Being in the spotlight of cancer prevention, the therapy with DC-CIK shows a great potential in alleviating symptoms of CRC, improving the quality of life of patients and simultaneously prolonging their lifespan. Several studies recommend to include the DC-CIK therapy as adjuvant for currently applied anti-cancer therapy; however, the conclusions were drawn based on a small number clinical trials having possibly high heterogeneity and publication bias. Moreover, due to variability of studies (e.g., tumor stage, cell phenotype, cell purity) and parameters assessed throughout, the outcomes could not be unified. Despite promising outcomes obtained so far, there is no strong evidence that the DC-CIK therapy shows a clear advantage over currently used treatment options. Undoubtedly, combined immunotherapy and chemotherapy may have a synergistic effect on OS compared with chemotherapy alone. However, the definite efficacy of DC-CIK therapy is still not explicit and warrants evaluation.

AUTHOR CONTRIBUTIONS

PM and JF provided the overall concept and framework of the manuscript. AG, PM, and MZ researched and identified appropriate articles. PM and AG participated in writing the manuscript. PM, JF, and MZ revised the manuscript. All authors approved the final version of the manuscript.

ACKNOWLEDGMENTS

Supported by grants from the Medical University of Łódź (#503/1-156-04/503-01 to JF and 502-03/1-156-04/502-14-299 to PM) and grants from National Science Centre (#UMO-2013/11/B/NZ7/01301 and #UMO-2014/13/B/NZ4/01179 to JF, and 2016/21/N/NZ5/01932 to PM).

REFERENCES

Al-Shibli, K. I., Donnem, T., Al-Saad, S., Persson, M., Bremnes, R. M., and Busund, L.-T. (2008). Prognostic effect of epithelial and stromal lymphocyte infiltration in non-small cell lung cancer. *Clin. Cancer Res.* 14, 5220–5227. doi: 10.1158/1078-0432.CCR-08-0133

Arpinati, M., Green, C. L., Heimfeld, S., Heuser, J. E., and Anasetti, C. (2000). Granulocyte-colony stimulating factor mobilizes T helper 2-inducing dendritic cells. *Blood* 95, 2484–2490.

Bamboat, Z. M., Stableford, J. A., Plitas, G., Burt, B. M., Nguyen, H. M., Welles, A. P., et al. (2009). Human liver dendritic cells promote T cell hyporesponsiveness. *J. Immunol.* 182, 1901–1911. doi: 10.4049/jimmunol.0803404

Bloy, N., Pol, J., Aranda, F., Eggermont, A., Cremer, I., Herv Fridman, W., et al. (2014). Trial watch: dendritic cell-based anticancer therapy. *Oncoimmunology* 3:e963424. doi: 10.4161/21624011.2014.963424

Bol, K. F., Tel, J., Jolanda, I., De Vries, M., and Figdor, C. G. (2013). Naturally circulating dendritic cells to vaccinate cancer patients. *Oncoimmunology* 2:e23431. doi: 10.4161/onci.23431

Dasgupta, A., Shields, J. E., and Spencer, H. T. (2011). Treatment of a solid tumor using engineered drug-resistant immunocompetent cells and cytotoxic chemotherapy. *Hum. Gene Ther.* 23, 711–721. doi: 10.1089/hum.2011.172

Dudek, A. M., Martin, S., Garg, A. D., and Agostinis, P. (2013). Immature, semi-mature, and fully mature dendritic cells: toward a DC-cancer cells interface that augments anticancer immunity. *Front. Immunol.* 4:438. doi: 10.3389/fimmu.2013.00438

Gordon, J. R., Ma, Y., Churchman, L., Gordon, S. A., Dawicki, W., Butterfield, L. H., et al. (2014). Regulatory dendritic cells for immunotherapy in immunologic diseases. *Front. Immunol.* 31:7. doi: 10.3389/fimmu.2014.00007

Hui, D., Qiang, L., Jian, W., Ti, Z., and Da-Lu, K. (2009). A randomized, controlled trial of postoperative adjuvant cytokine-induced killer cells immunotherapy after radical resection of hepatocellular carcinoma. *Dig. Liver Dis.* 41, 36–41. doi: 10.1016/j.dld.2008.04.007

Kohrt, H. E., Houot, R., Marabelle, A., Cho, H. J., Osman, K., Goldstein, M., et al. (2012). Combination strategies to enhance antitumor ADCC. *Immunotherapy* 4, 511–527. doi: 10.2217/imt.12.38

Koido, S., Ohkusa, T., Homma, S., Namiki, Y., Takakura, K., Saito, K., et al. (2013). Immunotherapy for colorectal cancer. *World J. Gastroenterol.* 19, 8531–8542. doi: 10.3748/wjg.v19.i46.8531

Legitimo, A., Consolini, R., Failli, A., Orsini, G., and Spisni, R. (2014). Dendritic cell defects in the colorectal cancer. *Hum. Vaccines Immunother.* 10, 3224–3235. doi: 10.4161/hv.29857

Li, X.-D., Xu, B., Wu, J., Ji, M., Xu, B.-H., Jiang, J.-T., et al. (2012). Review of Chinese clinical trials on CIK cell treatment for malignancies. *Clin. Transl. Oncol.* 14, 102–108. doi: 10.1007/s12094-012-0768-4

Lin, T., Song, C., Chuo, D.-Y., Zhang, H., and Zhao, J. (2016). Clinical effects of autologous dendritic cells combined with cytokine-induced killer cells followed by chemotherapy in treating patients with advanced colorectal cancer: a prospective study. *Tumour Biol.* 37, 4367–4372. doi: 10.1007/s13277-015-3957-2

Ma, Y., Shurin, G. V., Peiyuan, Z., and Shurin, M. R. (2013). Dendritic cells in the cancer microenvironment. *J. Cancer* 4, 36–44. doi: 10.7150/jca.5046

Maby, P., Tougeron, D., Hamieh, M., Mlecnik, B., Kora, H., Bindea, G., et al. (2015). Correlation between density of CD8+ T-cell infiltrate in microsatellite unstable colorectal cancers and frameshift mutations: a rationale for personalized immunotherapy. *Cancer Res.* 75, 3446–3455. doi: 10.1158/0008-5472.CAN-14-3051

Mahmoud, S. M. A., Paish, E. C., Powe, D. G., Macmillan, R. D., Grainge, M. J., Lee, A. H. S., et al. (2011). Tumor-infiltrating CD8+ lymphocytes predict clinical outcome in breast cancer. *J. Clin. Oncol.* 29, 1949–1955. doi: 10.1200/JCO.2010.30.5037

Manicassamy, S., and Pulendran, B. (2011). Dendritic cell control of tolerogenic responses. *Immunol. Rev.* 241, 206–227. doi: 10.1111/j.1600-065X.2011.01015.x

Märten, A., Ziske, C., Schöttker, B., Renoth, S., Weineck, S., and Buttgereit, P. (2001). Interactions between dendritic cells and cytokine-induced killer cells lead to an activation of both populations. *J. Immunother.* 24, 502–510. doi: 10.1097/00002371-200111000-00007

Mckenna, K., Beignon, A.-S., and Bhardwaj, N. (2005). Plasmacytoid dendritic cells: linking innate and adaptive immunity. *J. Virol.* 79, 17–27. doi: 10.1128/JVI.79.1.17-27.2005

Miller, M. J., Hejazi, A. S., Wei, S. H., Cahalan, M. D., and Parker, I. (2004). T cell repertoire scanning is promoted by dynamic dendritic cell behavior and random T cell motility in the lymph node. *Proc. Natl. Acad. Sci. U.S.A.* 101, 998–1003. doi: 10.1073/pnas.0306407101

Mlecnik, B., Tosolini, M., Charoentong, P., Kirilovsky, A., Bindea, G., Berger, A., et al. (2010). Biomolecular network reconstruction identifies T-cell homing factors associated with survival in colorectal cancer. *Gastroenterology* 138, 1429–1440. doi: 10.1053/j.gastro.2009.10.057

Niu, J., Ren, Y., Zhang, T., Yang, X., Zhu, W., Zhu, H., et al. (2014). Retrospective comparative study of the effects of dendritic cell vaccine and cytokine-induced killer cell immunotherapy with that of chemotherapy alone and in combination for colorectal cancer. *Biomed. Res. Int.* 2014, 214727. doi: 10.1155/2014/214727

Pagès, F., Kirilovsky, A., Mlecnik, B., Asslaber, M., Tosolini, M., Bindea, G., et al. (2009). In situ cytotoxic and memory T cells predict outcome in patients with early-stage colorectal cancer. *J. Clin. Oncol.* 27, 5944–5951. doi: 10.1200/JCO.2008.19.6147

Pievani, A., Borleri, G., Pende, D., Moretta, L., Rambaldi, A., Golay, J., et al. (2011). Dual-functional capability of CD3 +CD56 + CIK cells, a T-cell subset that acquires NK function and retains TCR-mediated specific cytotoxicity. *Blood* 118, 3301–3310. doi: 10.1182/blood-2011-02-336321

Pulendran, B., Banchereau, J., Burkeholder, S., Kraus, E., Guinet, E., Chalouni, C., et al. (2000). Flt3-ligand and granulocyte colony-stimulating factor mobilize distinct human dendritic cell subsets in vivo. *J. Immunol.* 165, 566–572. doi: 10.4049/JIMMUNOL.165.1.566

Pulendran, B., Tang, H., and Denning, T. (2008). Division of labor, plasticity, and crosstalk between dendritic cell subsets. *Curr. Opin. Immunol.* 20, 61–67. doi: 10.1016/j.coi.2007.10.009

Qu, H.-Q., Zhou, X.-S., Zhou, X.-L., and Wang, J. (2014). Effect of DC-CIK cell on the proliferation, apoptosis and differentiation of leukemia cells. *Asian Pac. J. Trop. Med.* 7, 659–662. doi: 10.1016/S1995-7645(14)60111-5

Reizis, B., Bunin, A., Ghosh, H. S., Lewis, K. L., and Sisirak, V. (2011). Plasmacytoid dendritic cells: recent progress and open questions. *Annu. Rev. Immunol.* 29, 163–183. doi: 10.1146/annurev-immunol-031210-101345

Remark, R., Alifano, M., Cremer, I., Lupo, A., Dieu-Nosjean, M. C., Riquet, M., et al. (2013). Characteristics and clinical impacts of the immune environments in colorectal and renal cell carcinoma lung metastases: influence of tumor origin. *Clin. Cancer Res.* 19, 4079–4091. doi: 10.1158/1078-0432.CCR-12-3847

Sangiolo, D., Martinuzzi, E., Todorovic, M., Vitaggio, K., Vallario, A., Jordaney, N., et al. (2008). Alloreactivity and anti-tumor activity segregate within two distinct subsets of cytokine-induced killer (CIK) cells: implications for their infusion across major HLA barriers. *Int. Immunol.* 20, 841–848. doi: 10.1093/intimm/dxn042

Schlimper, C., Hombach, A. A., Abken, H., and Schmidt-Wolf, I. G. H. (2012). Improved activation toward primary colorectal cancer cells by antigen-specific targeting autologous cytokine-induced killer cells. *Clin. Dev. Immunol.* 2012, 1–8. doi: 10.1155/2012/238924

Schmidt-Wolf, I. G., Negrin, R. S., Kiem, H. P., Blume, K. G., and Weissman, I. L. (1991). Use of a SCID mouse/human lymphoma model to evaluate cytokine-induced killer cells with potent antitumor cell activity. *J. Exp. Med.* 174, 139–149. doi: 10.1084/jem.174.1.139

Shortman, K., and Naik, S. H. (2007). Steady-state and inflammatory dendritic-cell development. *Nat. Rev. Immunol.* 7, 19–30. doi: 10.1038/nri1996

Siegel, R., Miller, K., and Jemal, A. (2015). Cancer statistics, 2015. *CA Cancer J. Clin.* 65, 5–29. doi: 10.3322/caac.21254

Steinman, L. (1991). Prospects for immunotherapy directed to the T cell receptor in human autoimmune disease. *Ann. N. Y. Acad. Sci.* 636, 147–153. doi: 10.1111/j.1749-6632.1991.tb33445.x

Stoll, G., Bindea, G., Mlecnik, B., Galon, J., Zitvogel, L., and Kroemer, G. (2015). Meta-analysis of organ-specific differences in the structure of the immune infiltrate in major malignancies. *Oncotarget* 6, 11894–11909. doi: 10.18632/oncotarget.4180

Torre, L. A., Bray, F., Siegel, R. L., Ferlay, J., Lortet-tieulent, J., and Jemal, A. (2015). Global Cancer Statistics, 2012. *CA Cancer J. Clin.* 65, 87–108. doi: 10.3322/caac.21262

Ueno, H., Klechevsky, E., Schmitt, N., Ni, L., Flamar, A.-L., Zurawski, S., et al. (2011). Targeting human dendritic cell subsets for improved vaccines. *Semin. Immunol.* 23, 21–27. doi: 10.1016/j.smim.2011.01.004

Wang, K., Gao, X., Pang, J., Liu, X., Cai, Y., Zhang, Y., et al. (2009). Dendritic cells transduced with a PSMA-encoding adenovirus and cocultured with autologous cytokine-induced lymphocytes induce a specific and strong immune response against prostate cancer cells. *Urol. Oncol.* 27, 26–32. doi: 10.1016/j.urolonc.2007.09.003

Wang, X., Yu, W., Li, H., Yu, J., Zhang, X., Ren, X., et al. (2014). Can the dual-functional capability of CIK cells be used to improve antitumor effects? *Cell. Immunol.* 287, 18–22. doi: 10.1016/j.cellimm.2013.11.009

Wang, Y., Dai, H., Li, H., Lv, H., Wang, T., Fu, X., et al. (2011). Growth of human colorectal cancer SW1116 cells is inhibited by cytokine-induced killer cells. *Clin. Dev. Immunol.* 2011:621414. doi: 10.1155/2011/621414

Wood, G. W., Holladay, F. P., Turner, T., Wang, Y. Y., and Chiga, M. (2000). A pilot study of autologous cancer cell vaccination and cellular immunotherapy using anti-CD3 stimulated lymphocytes in patients with recurrent grade III/IV astrocytoma. *J. Neurooncol.* 48, 113–120. doi: 10.1023/A:1006456421177

Xie, Z.-J., Jia, L.-M., He, Y.-C., and Gao, J.-T. (2006). Morphological observation of tumor infiltrating immunocytes in human rectal cancer. *World J. Gastroenterol.* 21, 1757–1760. doi: 10.3748/wjg.v12.i11.1757

Yang, T., Xiang, Y., Li, Y., Shao, J., Li, Q., and Yu, H. (2011). Clinical study of co-treatment with DC-CIK cells for advanced solid carcinomas. *Chin. German J. Clin. Oncol.* 10, 354–359. doi: 10.1007/s10330-011-0785-8

Zhan, H.-L., Gao, X., Pu, X.-Y., Li, W., Li, Z.-J., Zhou, X.-F., et al. (2012). A randomized controlled trial of postoperative tumor lysate-pulsed dendritic cells and cytokine-induced killer cells immunotherapy in patients with localized and locally advanced renal cell carcinoma. *Chin. Med. J.* 125, 3771–3777.

Zhang, L., Yang, X., Sun, Z., Li, J., Zhu, H., Li, J., et al. (2016). Dendritic cell vaccine and cytokine-induced killer cell therapy for the treatment of advanced non-small cell lung cancer. *Oncol. Lett.* 11, 2605–2610. doi: 10.3892/ol.2016.4273

Zhao, Y.-J., Jiang, N., Song, Q.-K., Wu, J.-P., Song, Y.-G., Zhang, H.-M., et al. (2015). Continuous DC-CIK infusions restore CD8+ cellular immunity, physical activity and improve clinical efficacy in advanced cancer patients unresponsive to conventional treatments. *Asian Pac. J. Cancer Prev.* 16, 2419–2423. doi: 10.7314/APJCP.2015.16.6.2419

Zhu, H., Yang, X., Li, J., Ren, Y., Zhang, T., Zhang, C., et al. (2014). Immune response, safety, and survival and quality of life outcomes for advanced colorectal cancer patients treated with dendritic cell vaccine and cytokine-induced killer cell therapy. *Biomed. Res. Int.* 2014, 5–9. doi: 10.1155/2014/603871

Conflict of Interest Statement: The authors declare that the research was conducted in the absence of any commercial or financial relationships that could be construed as a potential conflict of interest.

The reviewer VA and handling Editor declared their shared affiliation, and the handling Editor states that the process nevertheless met the standards of a fair and objective review.

8

Biomarkers Associated with Cognitive Impairment in Treated Cancer Patients: Potential Predisposition and Risk Factors

Hélène Castel[1,2,3], Angeline Denouel[4], Marie Lange[4,5], Marie-Christine Tonon[1,2,3], Martine Dubois[1,2,3] and Florence Joly[3,4,5,6]*

[1] Laboratory of Neuronal and Neuroendocrine Differentiation and Communication, Institut National de la Santé et de la Recherche Médicale, DC2N, Normandie University, Rouen, France, [2] Institute for Research and Innovation in Biomedicine, Rouen, France, [3] Cancer and Cognition Platform, Ligue Nationale Contre le Cancer, Caen, France, [4] Institut National de la Santé et de la Recherche Médicale, U1086, Caen, France, [5] Medical Oncology Department, Centre François Baclesse, Caen, France, [6] Medical Oncology, University Hospital Center, Caen, France

Edited by:
R. Thomas Jagoe, McGill University, Canada

Reviewed by:
Charlotte K. Callaghan, Trinity College Dublin, Ireland
Loredana Bergandi, University of Turin, Italy

***Correspondence:**
Hélène Castel
helene.castel@univ-rouen.fr

Purpose: Cognitive impairment in cancer patients induced, at least in part, by treatment are frequently observed and likely have negative impacts on patient quality of life. Such cognitive dysfunctions can affect attention, executive functions, and memory and processing speed, can persist after treatment, and their exact causes remain unclear. The aim of this review was to create an inventory and analysis of clinical studies evaluating biological markers and risk factors for cognitive decline in cancer patients before, during, or after therapy. The ultimate objectives were to identify robust markers and to determine what further research is required to develop original biological markers to enable prevention or adapted treatment management of patients at risk.

Method: This review was guided by the PRISMA statement and included a search strategy focused on three components: "cognition disorders," "predictive factors"/"biological markers," and "neoplasms," searched in PubMed since 2005, with exclusion criteria concerning brain tumors, brain therapy, and imaging or animal studies.

Results: Twenty-three studies meeting the criteria were analyzed. Potential associations/correlations were identified between cognitive impairments and specific circulating factors, cerebral spinal fluid constituents, and genetic polymorphisms at baseline, during, and at the end of treatment in cancer populations. The most significant results were associations between cognitive dysfunctions and genetic polymorphisms, including APOE-4 and COMT-Val; increased plasma levels of the pro-inflammatory cytokine, IL-6; anemia; and hemoglobin levels during chemotherapy. Plasma levels of specific hormones of the hypothalamo-pituitary-adrenal axis are also modified by treatment.

Discussion: It is recognized in the field of cancer cognition that cancer and comorbidities, as well as chemotherapy and hormone therapy, can cause persistent cognitive dysfunction. A number of biological circulating factors and genetic polymorphisms, can predispose to the development of cognitive disorders. However, many predictive factors remain unproven and discordant findings are frequently reported, warranting additional clinical and preclinical longitudinal cohort studies, with goals of better characterization of potential biomarkers and identification of patient populations at risk and/or particularly deleterious treatments. Research should focus on prevention and personalized cancer management, to improve the daily lives, autonomy, and return to work of patients.

Keywords: cognitive disorders, biological markers, predictive factors, cancer, chemotherapy

INTRODUCTION

There have been improvements in the efficacy of cancer treatments, and also in the management of side effects and patient care over the last decade. However, cancer treatments, most often chemotherapy, may induce side effects on the bone marrow, heart, cardiac, or digestive system and often cause nausea, alopecia, or even cognitive impairments Ahles (2012). Chemotherapy can cross the blood brain barrier (BBB) and cause brain damage (Cheung et al., 2015; Wang et al., 2015), which could explain cognitive impairments, including of concentration, memory, executive functions, and processing speed, symptoms often referred to as "chemofog" or "chemobrain" (Vardy et al., 2008; Joly et al., 2015). These cognitive disorders can have major consequences on patient quality of life, return to work, or autonomy, and thus represent a major public health issue which requires investigation.

To identify and characterize subgroups of patients at risk of cognitive impairment induced by cancer and its treatment, and to adapt patient treatment, it is essential to discover biological factors mediating cognitive problems and/or risk factors, such as genetic polymorphisms, inflammatory indicators, or blood biomarkers (Kesler et al., 2013; Wang et al., 2015). Some biomarkers, that are either predictive of risk or produced in response to treatment or the cancer itself, can be relatively easily measured by blood sampling before, during, and after management of the cancer. Such biological predictive factors may also correlate with cerebral imaging, to provide information about brain structure and volume changes involved in cognitive impairment (Wang et al., 2015).

The objective of this review was to establish a summary of original articles published since 2005, including all biological predictive factors of cognitive changes in cancer patients, particularly after cancer treatment. Moreover, we discuss the limitations of these studies, concerning their different types, methods, results, and interpretation.

METHODS USED FOR INFORMATION STRATIFICATION

Articles were retrieved from PubMed using the following key words:

- MeSH terms: "cognition disorders," "neurotoxicity syndromes," "biological markers," "prognosis," "biological factors"
- PubMed terms: "predictive factors," "cancer," "chemobrain," "chemofog," "cognitive dysfunction," "cognitive impairments"

This review was guided by the PRISMA statement and used a search strategy focused on three components: "cognition disorders," "predictive factors"/"biological markers," and "neoplasms," searched in PubMed (with MeSH and PubMed terms). Original studies since 2005 were included, regardless of type (i.e., cross-sectional and longitudinal, randomized, and non-randomized, single center and multicenter). Selection was not based on cancer type; mainly acute lymphoblastic leukemia (ALL), acute myeloid leukemia (AML), myelodysplastic syndrome (MDS), breast, lung, prostate, and differentiated thyroid carcinoma were included; however, brain tumors and cancers involving brain metastasis were excluded, because of their mass effects and potential consequences of surgery/resection on the brain, which are likely to directly impact cognitive function (**Table 1**). Moreover, all types of cancer treatments were included, except encephalic radiotherapy, which can have direct effects on brain function, edema, and cognition (**Table 1**). Studies for which predictive factors were cerebral and/or imaging parameters (magnetic resonance imaging/hippocampal volume or metabolic activity) or that did not address one or more of the three components, cancer, cognition, or biological mechanisms, were also excluded, along with clinical, physiopathological, and psychological parameters. Only human studies were included, thus preclinical animal studies were not taken into account.

The first exclusion criterion, evaluated by reading abstracts, was the absence of at least one of the three domains, i.e., "cognition disorders," "predictive factors,"/"biological markers," and "neoplasms." Between 2005 and 2015, 65 studies at least partly covered the topic under investigation. Other exclusion criteria, determined by reading entire papers, concerned studies of brain tumors or cranial radiotherapy, or the absence of

---

Abbreviations: AC/CAF, Cyclophosphamide/cyclophosphamide plus fluorouracil; ALL, Acute lymphoblastic leukemia; APOE, Apolipoprotein E; Aβ40 and Aβ42, amyloid-β peptides 40 and 42; CMF, Cyclophosphamide, methotrexate, and fluorouracil; COMT, Catechol-O-methyltransferase; CRP, C-reactive protein; CSF, Cerebrospinal fluid; CT, Chemotherapy; DNA, Deoxyribonucleic acid; Dox, Doxorubicin; ELISA, Enzyme-linked immunosorbent assay; EPO, Erythropoietin; GnRH, Gonadotropin-releasing hormone; Hb, Hemoglobin; IL, Interleukin; INFγ, Interferon γ; LPC, Lysophosphatidylcholine; MCP-1, Monocyte chemoattractant protein 1; MMSE, Mini-mental State Examination; MTHFR, 5,10-methylenetetrahydrofolate; mRCC, Metastatic renal cell cancer; pNF-H, Phosphorylated neurofilament subunit H; SM, Sphingomyelin; TNFα, Tumor necrosis factor-alpha; TNF-RII, Tumor necrosis factor-receptor type II; VEGF, Vascular endothelial growth factor; VEGFR TKI, Tyrosine kinase VEGF receptor; RT, Radiotherapy.

TABLE 1 | Main antitumor treatments and their mechanisms of action reported within the 23 selected publications that can be linked to modified biological factors and cognitive dysfunctions.

Cancer type	Treatment	Mechanisms of action
Breast	Leuprolide	GnRH agonist: reduce estrogen levels by continuous (and not pulsate) infusion of a GnRH action mimic
	Tamoxifen	Adjuvant hormonal treatment: blockage of estrogenic receptors (ER) in early and advanced ER-positive breast cancers
	Exemestane	orally active aromatase[a] inhibitor: irreversible blockade of estrogen production
	Anti-aromatases	Competition with aromatase which blocks estrogen synthesis (not indicated in cited publications)
	Doxorubicin	Antibiotic intercalating DNA agent, inhibitor of Topoisomerase II, and oxygen free radical producer leading to toxicity
	Cyclophosphamide	Bifunctional inhibitor of DNA transcription and replication leading to mitotic cell apoptosis
	Docetaxel	Cytotoxic properties *via* inhibition of the microtubule dynamic during mitosis
	5-FU	Inhibition of thymidylate synthase (inhibition of DNA synthesis)
	Vincristine	Stop tubulin polymerization and block cell during metaphase
	Methotrexate	Inhibition of folic acid (cytotoxic effect) through inhibition of mitochondrial metabolism
ALL[b]	Methotrexate	Inhibition of folic acid (cytotoxic effect) through inhibition of mitochondrial metabolism
	Cytarabine	Block DNA synthesis during cell division
mRCC[c] or GIST[d]	Sunitinib	Inhibition of tyrosine kinase receptors involved in tumor growth
	Sorafenib	Kinase inhibitor which leads decrease of tumor cell proliferation
	VEGFR inhibitors	Angiogenesis inhibitor (stop tumor growth)
	Radiotherapy	Tumor cell apoptosis by DNA deterioration

[a]*Aromatase, enzyme responsible of the biosynthesis of estrogen.*
[b]*ALL, Acute lymphoblastic leukemia.*
[c]*mRCC, metastatic renal cancer carcinoma.*
[d]*GIST, Gastrointestinal solid tumor.*

clear data on cognition and/or biomarker levels. Of the initially selected 65 studies, 23 were finally included in the analysis (**Figure 1**). These studies aimed to evaluate and characterize changes in several biological factors predictive for cognitive alteration in cancer patients, often in association with treatment. Different domains of cognition were assessed by batteries of neuropsychological tests and self-reports of cognitive function. The biological factors covered in this review are summarized in **Tables 2–6**. Most often, blood and serum samples were analyzed as simple and rapid tests with potential to provide information about the risk of cancer patients developing cognitive issues, and to facilitate identification of optimal treatment regimens for specific patient populations.

BIOLOGICAL MARKERS AND COGNITIVE IMPAIRMENTS IN TREATED CANCER PATIENTS

Plasma Biomarkers

Plasma Inflammatory Responses

The main cytokines analyzed in the reviewed studies were the pro-inflammatory triad, interleukin-6 (IL-6), tumor necrosis factor-alpha (TNF-α), and interleukin 1β (IL-1β). As IL-6 is an early mediator of inflammation and a key component of the acute phase response, it can also moderate inflammation by dampening TNF-α and IL-1β responses. Currently, the exact mechanisms involved in the inflammatory response during cancer therapy are not fully understood. Nevertheless, in cancer patients, circulating levels of cytokines were often increased and could be significant determinants of the alteration of particular cognitive functions after chemotherapy (Meyers et al., 2005; Ishikawa et al., 2012; Cheung et al., 2015). Based on the study by Ishikawa et al. (2012), it was difficult to conclusively link the observed cognitive issues with chemotherapy treatment since (i) cytokines, including IL-6, were measured in patient populations suffering from various types of advanced and inoperable or recurrent cancers and (ii) the delay between the end of the treatment and the time of the plasma assay was not stated. The study conducted by Meyers demonstrated that at baseline, higher IL-6 levels were associated with poorer executive functions, confirming that cancers are associated with high levels of circulating cytokines, connected with cognitive dysfunction, before chemotherapy. A longitudinal study by Cheung et al. (2015) established that higher concentrations of IL-1β and IL-6 were associated with more severe cognitive disturbance, and that increased IL-1β specifically was associated with poorer response speed performance during or just after the end of a chemotherapy treatment episode (Cheung et al., 2015; **Table 2**). In contrast, elevated IL-4 levels were linked to better response speed and fewer cognitive complaints in patients with breast cancer (**Table 2**), suggesting that maintenance of IL-4 levels during cancer care is likely to be neuroprotective (Cheung et al., 2015). Interestingly, breast cancer patients treated with chemotherapy had significantly elevated IL-6 and TNF-α levels after approximately 5 years off-therapy, compared with healthy controls, with an interaction between these two cytokines (Kesler et al., 2013). This study was particularly informative, since it correlated increased cytokine levels with diminished hippocampal volume, which is associated with verbal memory function. In agreement, an independent

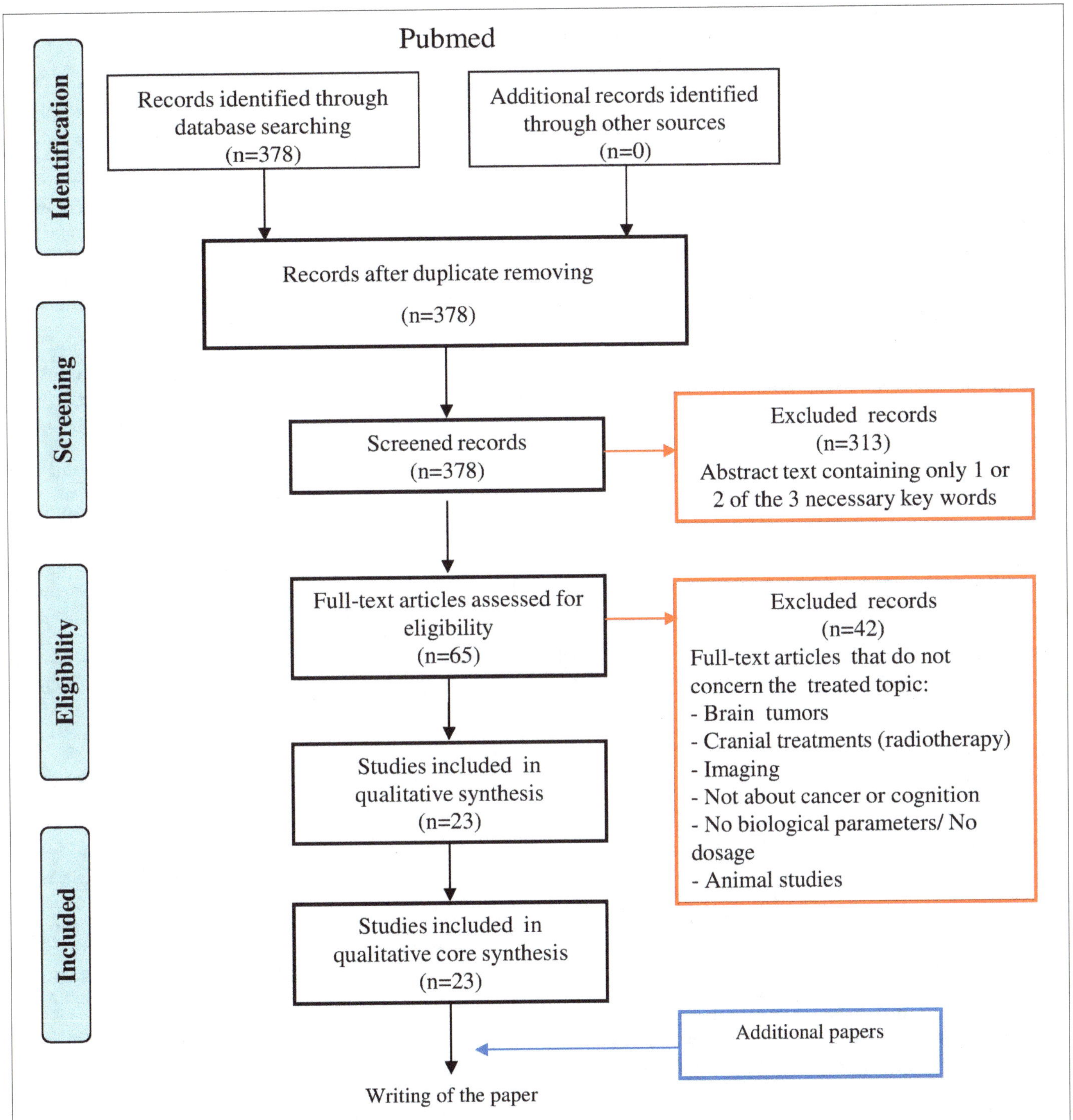

FIGURE 1 | PRISMA statement diagram illustrating the process of report identification, information selection and final inclusion for the present overview. The first exclusion criterion form the reading of the abstract, concerns the absence of the 3 combined domain, i.e., "cognition disorders," "predictive Factor"/"biological markers" and "neoplasms." The second exclusion criterion after reading of the entire papers, concerns brain tumors, cranial radiotherapy or the absence of clear data on cognition and/or biological marker dosage.

correlation between higher plasma IL-6 levels and deteriorated memory performance was described in breast cancer patients exposed to adjuvant local radiotherapy (**Table 2**; Shibayama et al., 2014). Together, these data suggest that cancer leads to increased plasma levels of selected pro-inflammatory cytokines, and that increased plasma IL-6 levels, likely resulting from chemotherapy or radiotherapy, may be a key systemic factor involved in, and/or predictive of, cognitive dysfunction (**Table 2**).

Besides IL-6, which was described as marker of both cancer-associated and cancer treatment-induced inflammation, studies of other cytokines were less frequently reported. A longitudinal cross-sectional study, including baseline measurements, demonstrated changes in a number of pro-inflammatory cytokines; however, only levels of TNF receptor type-II (TNF-RII) were significantly higher in plasma from chemotherapy-treated patients compared with those who did not receive chemotherapy, with no differences observed in IL-1ra, IL-6, or C-reactive protein (CRP; Ganz et al., 2013). In detail, significant correlations between plasma TNF-RII and self-reported memory complaints, but not cognitive dysfunction evaluated by neuropsychological tests, was demonstrated at baseline (associated with relatively diminished brain metabolism). The study also demonstrated increased TNF-RII over time in patients who had received radiotherapy (first end point), different chemotherapy regimens (second end point), and then endocrine therapy (third endpoint; **Table 2**), leading them to hypothesize that fatigue and cognitive complaints may be caused by disturbances in TNF pathways (Ganz et al., 2013).

In addition to cancer-related increases in circulating cytokine levels, data reported by Janelsins et al. (2012) support the idea that some cytokines may be specifically up-regulated in response to chemotherapy, and contribute to the development of cognitive difficulties. The study compared cytokine levels of IL-6, IL-8, and monocyte chemoattractant protein-1 (MCP-1) in patients receiving doxorubicin (Dox)-based cyclophosphamide/cyclophosphamide plus fluorouracil (AC/CAF) or Dox-based cyclophosphamide, methotrexate and fluorouracil (CMF) chemotherapy. The results demonstrated augmentation and diminution of cytokine levels in the AC/CAF and CMF groups, respectively, over time from baseline (prior to chemotherapy) and after two consecutive chemotherapy cycles, with a significant difference in levels of IL-6 between the two groups, suggesting that chemotherapy can induce specific cytokine changes. However, the study was under-powered and the time-points for blood sampling (before chemotherapy cycle) and cognitive evaluation (after chemotherapy cycle) did not match, hence it is difficult to conclusively evaluate the link between cytokine/chemokine changes and cognition, other than the reported negative correlation between MCP-1 and forgetfulness, difficulty with concentration, and thinking (subjective complaints, **Table 2**; Janelsins et al., 2012).

Circulating cytokines associated with cognitive impairment in cancer patients during the course of treatment, or in survivors after the end of treatment, represented the most measurable and measured factors, and studies converged to suggest that chemotherapy could dysregulate cytokine levels, which may interfere with brain functioning, leading to cognitive impairment (Ahles and Saykin, 2007). Indeed, some cytokines, including IL-6, IL-1β, and TNF-α, could have causal roles by crossing the BBB via active transporters (Cheung et al., 2015) and can interact with synapses (Wang et al., 2015), thereby leading to systemic communication between peripheral cytokines and the brain, rather than central cytokine production. This hypothesis is supported by a recent study by Hayslip et al. (2015), which proposed direct intravascular oxidative modification of plasma proteins by chemotherapy, leading to monocyte release of TNF-α which, by diffusing through the BBB, could then activate cascades of events potentially causing cognitive impairment (Hayslip et al., 2015). They demonstrated that the exogenous anti-oxidant, sodium-2-mercaptoethane sulfonate (mesna), present only in blood and urine, reduced plasma protein oxidation and TNF-α levels in patients receiving Dox-containing chemotherapy (Hayslip et al., 2015). Also, the observation that changes in plasma TNF-α levels were linked to reduced left hippocampal volume in cancer patients receiving chemotherapy (Kesler et al., 2013), suggests that cerebral apoptosis, or other cell death mechanisms, are likely responsible for altered verbal memory performance. Such cell death mechanisms could be counteracted by neutralization of circulating cytokines.

Although this hypothesis raises interesting therapeutic options, other studies did not show any significant correlation between plasma cytokine levels and cognitive impairment with or without chemotherapy (Pomykala et al., 2013). In fact, co-variations between metabolism in selected brain regions and cytokines were detected by comparing values at baseline and 1 year after treatment completion in a group of patients who received chemotherapy (Pomykala et al., 2013). Overall, there is a clear difficulty in postulating a direct link between any particular cytokine that may be specifically up-regulated by a specific chemotherapy and responsible for a selected type of cognitive dysfunction. The observed discrepancies between studies may be due to differences in chemotherapy regimens, time periods between measurement of cytokine plasma levels and the end of chemotherapy, measurements of cytokine levels in serum or plasma, or the variable sensitivities of the methods used for measurement. Principal tests applied were the enzyme-linked immunosorbent assay (ELISA), including different variants such as the high sensitivity multiplex immunoassay (Ganz et al., 2013; Kesler et al., 2013; Pomykala et al., 2013; Cheung et al., 2015), or regular and high sensitivity kits (Ganz et al., 2013). Currently, the detailed mechanisms underlying cognitive changes remain unclear and future studies are required to obtain more data about the direct or indirect links between inflammatory responses and brain disorders associated with cancer therapy. It will be important to further consider the role of cytokines as predictive biomarkers for cognitive impairment in cancer and cancer-treated patients and to propose new cytokine inhibitors or antagonists as therapeutic options.

Non-inflammatory Biomarkers in Blood and Serum Samples

Since tumors can expand through development of angiogenic features and via release of angiogenetic factors, including vascular endothelial growth factor (VEGF), recently introduced targeted therapies include inhibitors of tyrosine kinase VEGF receptor (VEGFR TKI) and drugs targeting VEGF itself. As VEGF is also involved in neurogenesis and brain vascularization, it might be supposed that levels of VEGF could be linked to cognitive impairments (**Table 3**, Ishikawa et al., 2012). Accordingly, its levels were determined in a cross-sectional study of metastatic renal cancer (mRCC) patients treated with VEGFR TKI (8 week treatment period). The patients exhibited elevated erythrocyte

TABLE 2 | Summary of methods and results from selected studies concerning inflammatory response.

Authors	Type of study	Age Mean ± (*SD* or range)	Cancer location (*n*)	Treatment type	Studied factors	Measurements			Results	
						Biological tests	Assessed cognitive domains	Time of assessment	Observed cognitive impairments	Association with studied predictive factors
INFLAMMATORY RESPONSE										
Cheung et al., 2015	Multi-center prospective cohort	50.5 ± 8.4	Breast ($n = 99$)	Chemotherapy (anthracycline)	IL-1β, IL-2, IL-4, IL-6, IL-8, IL-10, GM-CSF, IFN-γ, TNF-α	Sensitive multiplex immunoassay (Venipuncture)	- Processing speed - Response speed - Memory - Attention (battery of tests) - + Self-report functioning	➢ T1: Before chemotherapy ➢ T2: 6 weeks ➢ T3: 12 weeks after initiation of chemotherapy	- Response speed performance (2.2% of patients) - Memory (13.2%) - Attention (7.3%) - Processing speed (2.2%) - Response speed (4.2%) + Self-perceived cognitive disturbances (29.3%)	↗ IL-1β: Poorer response speed performance ↗ IL-4: better response speed and less cognitive complaints ↗ IL-6: more severe cognitive complaints
Ganz et al., 2013	Prospective, cross-sectional at basal line, longitudinal and observational cohort	51.3 ± 7.8	Breast (patient-received CT[a]: $n = 49$; No CT patients: $n = 44$)	Radiotherapy Chemotherapy (FEC[c] or AC-T[b])	IL-6, IL-1, TNF-α RII, CRP	Sensitivity ELISA tests (Venipuncture)	- Psychomotor - Executive functions - Verbal learning and memory - Visual learning and memory - Visuo-spatial and motor speed (battery of tests) - Cognitive complaints	➢ T1: before therapy ➢ T2: 6 months later ➢ T3: 12 months later	Memory complaints	↗ TNF-RII: memory complaints

(Continued)

TABLE 2 | Continued

Authors	Type of study	Age Mean ± (*SD* or range)	Cancer location (*n*)	Treatment type	Studied factors	Measurements			Results	
						Biological tests	Assessed cognitive domains	Time of assessment	Observed cognitive impairments	Association with studied predictive factors
Ishikawa et al., 2012	Cross-sectional, case-control	63 (23–83)	Solid malignancies (various types: advanced, inoperable or recurrent) (Patients: $n = 50$ Healthy controls: $n = 33$)	Chemotherapy	IL-1β, IL-1Ra, IL-2, IL-4, IL-5, IL-6, IL-7, IL-8, IL-9, IL-10, IL-12, IL-13, IL-15, IL-17, basic FGF, eotaxin, G-CSF, GM-CSF, IFN-γ, IP10, MCP-1, MIP-1α, MIP-1β, PDGF-BB, RANTES, TNF-α, VEGF	Multiplex cytokine array system (Venipuncture)	Cognitive complaints (2 items of the EORTC QLQ-C30)	➢ After chemotherapy	Not specified	IL-6 and VEGF: negative correlation with subjective cognitive functioning
Janelsins et al., 2012	Stratified, randomized, double-blinded, and longitudinal	52.2 ± 10.2	Breast (AC/CAF[d]: $n = 27$ CMF[e]: $n = 27$)	Chemotherapy (AC/CAF or CMF)	IL-6, IL-8, MCP-1	Colorimetric ELISA kits (Venipuncture)	- Heavy-headed - Thoughts muddled - Difficulty thinking - Concentration and forgetful - Self-report functioning	➢ Prior to on-study chemotherapy cycle 2 ➢ After 2 consecutive chemotherapy cycles	All subjective domains (12-44% of patients)	- AC/CAF: No significant correlation between IL-6 or IL-8 and cognitive complaints. Significant correlation between MCP-1 and forgetfulness, difficulties with concentration and thinking. - CMF: No significant correlation

(Continued)

TABLE 2 | Continued

Authors	Type of study	Age Mean ± (*SD* or range)	Cancer location (*n*)	Treatment type	Studied factors	Measurements			Results	
						Biological tests	Assessed cognitive domains	Time of assessment	Observed cognitive impairments	Association with studied predictive factors
Kesler et al., 2013	Cross-sectional, case-control	54.6 ± 6.5	Breast (Case: *n* = 42 Healthy Control: *n* = 35)	Chemotherapy Number of regimens	IL-6, TNF-αs	Sandwich immunoassay (ELISA) (Venipuncture)	- Verbal memory - Learning - Global intelligence (battery of tests) - + Cognitive complaints	➢ Mean 4.8 ± 3.4 years off-therapy	Verbal memory (objective and subjective)	-↗ IL-6, ↗ TNF-α levels: ↗ Memory difficulties. In the breast cancer group, ↘ left hippocampal volume associated with ↗ TNF-α and ↘ IL-6, with a significant interaction between these two cytokines
Meyers et al., 2005	Longitudinal	60.2 (21–84)	Acute Myelogenous Leukemia (AML) or Myelodysplastic syndrome (MDS) (*n* = 54)	Chemotherapy: lipodaunocin plus Cytoxan or topotecan, plus or minus thalidomide	IL-1, IL-1RA, IL-6, IL-8, TNF-α, (+ Hb)	Standard enzyme-linked immunoabsorbant assays	- Attention, - Graphomotor speed - Verbal fluency - Visual-motor scanning speed - Executive functions - Fine motor dexterity - Memory (battery of tests)	➢ Before treatment ➢ and after 1 month of therapy	- Memory - Verbal fluency - Cognitive processing speed - Executive function and fine motor dexterity	↗ IL-6 level: ↘ executive function ↗ IL-8 level: ↗ memory performance

(Continued)

TABLE 2 | Continued

Authors	Type of study	Age Mean ± (*SD* or range)	Cancer location (*n*)	Treatment type	Studied factors	Measurements			Results	
						Biological tests	Assessed cognitive domains	Time of assessment	Observed cognitive impairments	Association with studied predictive factors
Mulder et al., 2014	Cross-sectional, case-control	60 (38-81) (+ TKI)	Metastatic renal cell cancer (mRCC) or Gastrointestinal stromal tumor (GIST) (VEGFR TKI group: *n* = 30, patient controls: *n* = 20, healthy controls: *n* = 30)	VEGFR TKI[f] (Sunitinib or Sorafenib)	Testosterone, sex hormone binding globuline, estradiol, albumin, vitamin B12, thyroid function, CRP, ESR[g], LDH[h] Serum IL-1β, IL-2, IL-4, IL-5, IL-6, IL-8, IL-10, IL-12, TNF-α, TNF-β, IFN-γ	Specific ELISA (Venipuncture)	- Learning and memory - Attention and concentration - Executive functions (battery of tests) - + Self-report functioning	➢ Sunitinib or sorafenib for at least 8 weeks	- Learning and memory, and executive functions:Both patient groups significantly worse than healthy - Cognitive complaints > VEGFR TKI patients vs. healthy	- ↗ levels of ESR: ↘ scores learning, memory, attention, concentration and executive function - CRP and neutrophils: ↘ scores learning and memory (VEGFR TKI group). - Correlation between markers of systemic inflammation and worse cognitive performances - No correlation between serum IL-8 and cognitive functioning, or between free testosterone or estradiol and neuropsychological tests
Shibayama et al., 2014	Cross-sectional	47 ± 52 (+RT) 46.6 ± 6.2 (-RT)	Breast (Exposition to adjuvant RT with 25 CT: *n* = 51, Unexposed with 26 CT: *n* = 54)	Adjuvant regional RT	Plasma IL-6	Chemiluminescent enzyme immunoassay (Venipuncture)	- Attention/ concentration - Immediate verbal and visual memory - Delayed recall (battery of tests)	➢ 1 year after the initial therapy	- Delayed recall and immediate verbal memory in radiotherapy group	↘ delayed recall mediated by ↗ plasma IL-6 level

[a]*CT, Chemotherapy.*
[b]*AC-T, Cyclophosphamide, doxycycline plus taxane.*
[c]*FEC, Fluorouracil, cyclophosphamide plus taxane.*
[d]*AC/CAF: cyclophosphamide, or cyclophosphamide plus fluorouracil.*
[e]*CMF, cyclophosphamide, methotrexate and fluorouracil.*
[f]*VEGFR TKI, Vascular endothelial growth factor receptor tyrosine kinase inhibitors.*
[g]*ESR, Erythrocyte sedimentation rate.*
[h]*LDH, Lactate dehydrogenase.*

TABLE 3 | Summary of methods and results from selected studies concerning other factors in blood and serum samples.

Authors	Type of study	Age mean ± (*SD* or range)	Cancer location (*n*)	Treatment type	Studied factors	Measurements			Results	
						Biological tests	Assessed cognitive domains	Time of assessment	Observed cognitive impairments	Association with studied predictive factors
BLOOD AND SERUM SAMPLES										
Fan et al., 2009	Non-randomized sub-study	53 to 50	Breast (Patients received hEPO: $n = 45$, Patients with standard care: $n = 42$)	Chemotherapy as adjuvant or neoadjuvant treatment	Hb	Blood tests	- Global efficiency (MMSE) - Verbal memory - + Self-report functioning	➢ After chemotherapy	No significant difference between groups	- No association between Hb and cognitive functioning. - Protective effect of hEPO against delayed cognitive dysfunction not shown
Iconomou et al., 2008	Prospective, single-center, non-randomized	58.9 ± 9.9	Solid malignancy ($n = 50$) Breast, colorectal, lung, genitourinary	Chemotherapy	Anemia, Hb hEPO	Hb levels (Venipuncture)	- Global efficiency: - Orientation - Recording - Attention - Calculation - Recall - Language - Copying (MMSE)	➢ T1 = baseline ➢ Study completion-T2 = week 12	No clinically significant alterations during hEPO treatment	Change of Hb not related with change of objective or subjective cognitive performance
Mancuso et al., 2006	Prospective, observational	76.6 ± 4.8	Lung ($n = 42$)	Chemotherapy	Anemia, Hb	Haemoglobin level	- Global efficiency - Orientation - Recording - Attention - Calculation - Recall - Language and copying (MMSE)	➢ Before chemotherapy (baseline) ➢ after each CT cycle	Not specified	↗ Hb: positive correlation with MMSE value
Massa et al., 2006	Longitudinal	71.4 (68–75)	Solid malignancy: Lung, oral cavity, ovary, breast, endometrial colon, stomach (Cancer patients with anemia related to cancer chemotherapy: $n = 10$)	Chemotherapy + rHuEPO	Hb level	Blood tests	- Global efficiency	➢ Prior to start chemotherapy ➢ After 4, 8 and 12 weeks of treatment	Better cognitive functions	↗ Hb levels: ↗ cognitive functioning assessed by MMSE after 4, 8 and 12 weeks of rHuEPO treatment

(Continued)

TABLE 3 | Continued

Authors	Type of study	Age mean ± (*SD* or range)	Cancer location (*n*)	Treatment type	Studied factors	Measurements			Results	
						Biological tests	Assessed cognitive domains	Time of assessment	Observed cognitive impairments	Association with studied predictive factors
Natori et al., 2015	Cross-sectional	45.5 to 50	Breast (pNF-H positive: $n = 18$ pNF-H negative: $n = 58$)	Chemotherapy Many regimens	pNF-H level	ELISA (Venipuncture)	- Nonverbal - Intellectual capacity - Premorbid intellectual quotient (battery of tests) - + Self-report functioning	➢ Naïve ➢ Different cycles of chemotherapy 1, 3 or 7 cycles, ➢ Completed chemotherapy for at least 24 months	No difference among the patient groups	- ↗ serum pNF-H level but no association with cognitive deficits
Tan et al., 2013	Longitudinal	71 (59–89)	Prostate ($n = 50$)	Leuprolide	Plasma Aβ40 and Aβ42[a]	ELISA	- Global efficiency - ± verbal episodic memory	➢ Before the first leuprolide injection (baseline), ➢ At 2, 4 and 12 months	Better memory performance (practice effect)	No association between Plasma Aβ40 and Aβ42 levels and cognitive efficiency or memory functions

[a] *Aβ40 and Aβ42 : amyloid-β peptides 40 and 42.*

TABLE 4 | Summary of methods and results from selected studies concerning hormonal factors.

Authors	Type of study	Age mean ± (*SD* or range)	Cancer location (*n*)	Treatment type	Studied factors	Measurements			Results	
						Biological tests	Assessed cognitive domains	Time of assessment	Observed cognitive impairments	Association with studied predictive factors
HORMONAL FACTORS										
Andreano et al., 2012	Longitudinal, Case-control	41.9 (27–49)	Breast (Case: $n=$ 20 Natural cycling women Control: $n=20$)	Lupron (Leuprolide)	Cortisol, estradiol, progesterone, glucocorticoids	Salivary ELISA for cortisol, estradiol and progesterone + physiological stressor	- Working memory - Verbal paired associate memory - Narrative recall (level of emotional arousal was considered) (battery of tests)	➢ After treatment for cases ➢ during the mid-luteal phase of menstrual cycles for controls	Narrative recall: delayed recall for emotional material	-↘ ovarian hormone levels - No difference of salivary cortisol level after stress -↘ glucocorticoid responsiveness: absence of enhancement of memory consolidation for emotional material in cases
Jenkins et al., 2005	Prospective, longitudinal, case-control	67.5 ± 4.7	Prostate (Case: n = 32 Control: $n=18$)	Leuprolide	Free and bound testosterone, β-estradiol, sex hormone-binding globulin	Serum, Not specified	- Auditory/verbal memory - Visual memory, - Working memory and attention, - Processing speed - Vigilance - Intelligence	➢ Before drug treatment (Baseline T1) ➢ at 3 months before radiotherapy (T2) ➢ 9 months later (T3)	- Verbal - Visual spatial - Processing speed	↘ bioavailable testosterone, but no correlation with cognitive performance
Moon et al., 2014	, Cross-sectional, case-control	70.9 ± 5.0	Differentiated Thyroid Carcinoma (Case: $n=50$ Control: $n=90$)	TSH-suppressive therapy	Free T_4 and TSH levels	RIA (Venipuncture)	- Verbal fluency - language - global cognitive function - memory - visuospatial function - attention - executive function	➢ After at least 5 years of TSH-suppressive treatment	° No difference between patient and control groups	↗ T_4 level: ↗ global cognitive and visuospatial functions

TABLE 5 | Summary of methods and results from selected studies concerning genetic predictive factors.

Authors	Type of study	Age mean ± (*SD* or range)	Cancer location (*n*)	Treatment type	Studied factors	Measurements			Results	
						Biological tests	Assessed cognitive domains	Time of assessment	Observed cognitive impairments	Association with studied predictive factors
GENETIC PREDICTORS										
Kamdar et al., 2011	Prospective cohort	4.4 ± 3.9 –12.1 ± 11.3	ALL ($n = 62$)	Methotrexate chemotherapy	6 Genotype polymorphisms (folate pathway: MTHFR[a] 677C>T MTHFR 1298A>C SHMT[b] 1420C>T MS[c] 2759 A>G MTRR[d] 66A>G TSER[e]2R/3R TSER3R/3R	Genotyping essay by PCR (Venipuncture)	- Attention - Processing speed - Verbal fluency - Visuo-spatial motor speed (battery of tests)	Years after end of therapy: 5.3± 4.4	Global cognitive functioning: 44.3% of patients	Combined effect of multiple folate pathway polymorphisms (MS and MTHFR): ↗cognitive disturbance probability (attention and processing speed)
Krull et al., 2013a	Cohort	7.0 ± 3.11	ALL ($n = 243$)	Chemotherapy (without prophylactic cranial irradiation)	Many genetic polymorphisms	Genotyping by PCR (Venipuncture)	- General intelligence - Processing speed - Working memory - Sustained attention - + cognitive complaints (assessed by parents)	2 years completion of consolidation therapy	Sustained attention and attention difficulties reported by parents	MS (/ MAOA[f]/ APOE[g]) polymorphisms: ↗ Cognitive disturbance probability (attentiveness and response speed)
Small et al., 2011	Cross-sectional, Case-control	56.93 ± 9.01 (RT) 51.22 ± 8.63 (CT)	Breast (RT: $n = 58$ CT: $n = 72$ Healthy Controls: $n = 204$)	Chemotherapy and radiotherapy	COMT[h] Genotype COMT-Val COMT-Met	DNA collection by saliva and genotyping	- Overall cognition - Episodic memory - Attention - Complex cognition - Verbal fluency - Motor speed (battery of tests)	6 months after end of treatments	° COMT-Val+ carriers performed worse than COMT-Met homozygote carriers: Attention, verbal fluency and motor speed	COMT-Val homozygote: ↗ Cognitive disturbances probability

[a]*MTHFR: 5,10-methylenetetrahydrofolate reductase.*
[b]*SHMT: serine hydroxylmethyltransferase.*
[c]*MS: methionine synthase.*
[d]*MTRR: methionine synthase reductase.*
[e]*TSER: thymidylate synthase enhancer region.*
[f]*MAOA : Monoamine oxidase A.*
[g]*APOE: Apolipoprotein E.*
[h]*COMT: Catechol-O-Methyltransferase.*

TABLE 6 | Summary of methods and results from selected studies concerning cerebrospinal fluid.

Authors	Type of study	Age mean ± (*SD* or range)	Cancer location (*n*)	Treatment type	Studied factors	Measurements			Results	
						Biological tests	Assessed cognitive domains	Time of assessment	Observed cognitive impairments	Association with studied predictive factors
CEREBROSPINAL FLUID										
Krull et al., 2013b	Longitudinal	7.0 ± 3.11	ALL ($n = 76$)	Chemotherapy Methotrexate	CSF phospholipids (PE[a], PI[b], PC[c], SM[d], LPC[e])	Extraction and separation by chromatography (lumbar punctures)	- General cognitive abilities - Processing speed - Working memory - Visual-motor integration - Academic functions (battery of tests)	➢ After completion of induction therapy (initial assessment) ➢ Consolidation period:- one year after the initial assessment, - 2 years after - 3 years after	- Motor speed - Verbal and visual working memory - Motor speed	- Association between early variations in SM and motor speed and in LPC and verbal working memory; - Association between later elevation in SM with decline in visual working memory
Moore et al., 2008	Longitudinal	7.83 ± 2.87	ALL ($n = 26$ with 7 with low-risk, 13 with standard-risk and 6 with high-risk ALL)	Chemotherapy Methotrexate	CSF monounsaturated and saturated fatty acids: (palmitic, stearic, palmitoleic and oleic acids)	Gas chromatography	- General intelligence - Visual-motor skills - Academic abilities (battery of tests)	➢ At diagnosis, prior treatments (fatty acids) ➢ achieved remission (baseline) ➢ 1 year later (cognitive abilities)	- Global intelligence - Academic math abilities - Visual motor skills declines	-↗ ratio stearic/oleic acids: negative correlation with global intelligence and academic math abilities -↗ ratio palmitic/palmitoleic acids: negative correlation with global intelligence
Protas et al., 2009	Longitudinal	7.59 (range 2–16)	ALL ($n = 38$)	Chemotherapy Number of regimens	CSF Tau protein	ELISA	- Intelligence quotient (verbal performance) (battery of tests)	➢ At diagnosis ➢ after induction treatment ➢ during consolidation ➢ before maintenance therapy	Not specified	Tau protein level (at the initiation of maintenance therapy) negatively correlated with verbal abilities

[a]*PE, Phosphatidylethanolamine.*
[b]*PI, Phosphatidylinositol.*
[c]*PC, Phosphatidylcholine.*
[d]*SM, Sphingomyelin.*
[e]*LPC, Lysophosphatidylcholine.*

sedimentation rates (ERS), CRP levels, and neutrophil counts, that were negatively correlated with learning, memory, attention, concentration, and executive functions (Mulder et al., 2014); however, no correlations were found with cytokine, hemoglobin (Hb), or electrolyte levels, leucocyte counts, or VEGF levels in blood samples. In a more recent longitudinal study, 30% of mRCC patients treated with anti-angiogenics were found to develop fatigue and cognitive disorders, while VEGF plasma levels measured at baseline, and 3 and 6 months from baseline, were associated with fatigue, but not with cognitive dysfunction (Joly et al., 2016). The impact of TKI, and of cancer itself, should be investigated further to clarify the exact effects of TKI on inflammatory responses and other circulating plasma markers, such as Hb, detrimental to cognitive performance.

Several studies investigating the contribution of chemotherapy-induced anemia to cognitive impairment in cancer patients suggested that changes in Hb were linked to the development of cognitive impairment during chemotherapy. This was stressed in the elderly cancer population studied by Mancuso et al. (2006), were Hb levels were associated with quality of life, functional capacity, mental decline, and depression, suggesting that maintenance of normal Hb levels is essential to prevent cognitive decline during chemotherapy. Low powered studies on treatments with specific therapies, such as recombinant human erythropoietin (rHuEPO), led to show improved Hb levels which were correlated with better cognitive function (**Table 3**; Mancuso et al., 2006; Massa et al., 2006). When rHuEPO is administered several times each week, it can compensate for cancer and chemotherapy-induced anemia after approximately 3 weeks of chemotherapy. In a larger cohort study, Iconomou et al. (2008) observed no significant changes in cognitive function in responders, exhibiting increased Hb levels after 12 weeks of rHuEPO treatment, despite improvement of physical function and diminished fatigue (Iconomou et al., 2008). In contrast, other studies using the same types of cognitive tests failed to detect evidence for a protective effect of erythropoietin (EPO) against delayed cognitive dysfunction (24 months from the end of the treatment) in groups of patients with breast cancer receiving chemotherapy (Fan et al., 2009; **Table 3**).

Other systemic biological markers were also highlighted. A relationship between androgen receptors and amyloid precursors has been described (Takayama et al., 2009). Increased levels of amyloid-β40 (Aβ40), a marker associated with the Alzheimer disease, did not appear to be associated with cognitive mini-mental state examination (MMSE) scores after leuprolide treatment in prostate cancer patients (Tan et al., 2013). However, this study had some limitations, including a lack of evaluation of the ratio Aβ40/Aβ42 in plasma, indicating that the interesting hypothesis of a possible impact of cancer treatment on Aβ plasma levels and cognition deserves further investigation (**Table 3**).

Another candidate plasma marker for cognitive dysfunction following therapy-induced brain damage is axonal phosphorylated neurofilament subunit H (pNF-H), levels of which are increased in the blood of patients who have had acute brain ischemic stroke compared with controls, and are associated with the severity of the stroke (Singh et al., 2011; Andreano et al., 2012). Thus, Natori et al. (2015) considered that pNF-H would constitute an interesting systemic biomarker of neuronal lesions and measured its levels in the serum of breast cancer patients at baseline, after one to seven cycles of different chemotherapy regimens, and 1 month–1 year after the end of therapy. They established that pNF-H levels increased with the number of chemotherapy doses administered, but did not find any correlation with neuropsychological scores (Natori et al., 2015; **Table 4**). This suggests that measurement of serum pNF-H in chemotherapy-treated cancer patients, alongside the application of more sensitive batteries of cognitive tests, may be worthwhile to further evaluate pNF-H as a biomarker of neural axonal damage and cognitive impairment.

Hormonal Factors

Endocrine function, specifically gonadal and stress hormones, may also contribute to cognitive difficulties during cancer treatment. To date, the results of research into hormonal factors remain inconclusive, and studies are often related to patients receiving hormonal therapy. For example, significant reductions in free testosterone and β-estradiol levels were detected in prostate cancer patients after 3 months exposure to leuprolide, and some changes in spatial memory also were observed during treatment; however, there was no association between the changes in hormonal factors and those in cognition (Jenkins et al., 2005; **Table 5**). When therapy to suppress thyroid-stimulating hormone (TSH) was administered to patients with differentiated thyroid carcinoma, a positive correlation between free serum T_4 levels and cognitive processing speed was detected (Moon et al., 2014), suggesting that exogenous T_4 supplementation can improve cognitive function in this group of patients. In addition, given that gonadal hormonal levels can influence the hypothalamic-pituitary-adrenal axis (HPA), the cognitive and endocrine effects of the cortisol activating stressor, cold pressor stress (CPS), were tested in breast cancer patients previously treated with chemotherapy, and then receiving Lupron (Andreano et al., 2012). The glucocorticoid (cortisol) response to CPS was absent in the cancer patient group compared with controls, and delayed recall performance was also impaired in the individuals with cancer (Andreano et al., 2012). Thus, stress-induced cortisol favoring memory consolidation can be selectively altered in cancer patients. Other than this interesting study relating regulation of the HPA axis to cognitive impairment in cancer patients, there is little evidence to link the role of chemotherapy, stress, and/or cancer on circulating hormone levels and cognition.

Genetic Factors

There is relative heterogeneity among cancer patients regarding (i) the various domains of cognition that can be affected, including working memory, executive functions, verbal memory, and processing speed; and (ii) the proportion of patients exhibiting long-term cognitive deficits, independent of fatigue or emotional disturbances. This has prompted medical researchers to investigate potential predisposing factors for the development of cognitive impairment during cancer and its treatment. Indeed, immune status, cancer diagnosis in the elderly, and/or a number of key genetic polymorphisms can predispose to cognitive changes (Ahles and Saykin, 2007; Mandelblatt et al., 2013; Janelsins et al., 2014). Should studies clearly demonstrate genetic predisposition, this could enable adaption of treatment to specific patient populations. Accordingly, recent studies have shown that genetic factors may be linked to cognitive impairments in cancer patients after therapy; for example, the gene encoding apolipoprotein E (APOE), located in chromosome 19, which functions in lipid transport and regulation of inflammation. APOE has three allelic variants (E2, E3, and E4), which include various combinations of two single nucleotide polymorphisms, rs7412 and rs429358. Chemotherapy-treated breast cancer patients carrying APOE-4 allele E4, a well-known risk factor for Alzheimer's disease (Ahles, 2012), have a higher risk of cognitive dysfunction during the course of cancer treatment (Mandelblatt et al., 2013). Consistent with these findings, Krull et al. analyzed various polymorphisms among childhood ALL survivors, and identified three that were associated with neurocognitive disorders, such as attentiveness, response speed, or parent-reported attention problems. In particular, an association between APOE-4 and attention deficit was described in survivors (**Table 5**). This study also identified associations between a single nucleotide polymorphism in the genes encoding methionine synthase (MS), which is responsible for the conversion of homocysteine to methionine, and monoamine oxidase A (MAOA), which catalyzes the deamination of amines such as dopamine, serotonin, or norepinephrine, and attention difficulties (Krull et al., 2013a).

The key role of neurotransmitters as potential predisposing markers, is stressed by the other polymorphism commonly reported as linked to cognitive impairments, the Val158 Met encoding single-nucleotide polymorphism in catechol-O-methyltransferase (COMT), which catalyzes the metabolic breakdown of catecholamines through the methylation of dopamine and noradrenaline (Ahles and Saykin, 2007). In detail, codon 158 of COMT on chromosome 22q11, can encode for either a valine or a methionine residue (Small et al., 2011). The valine-containing variant protein exhibits elevated activity, leading to enhanced neurotransmitter degradation and consequent diminished neurotransmission (**Table 5**). This polymorphism predisposed a subgroup of patients with breast cancer to a higher risk of diminished cognitive performance, including attention, verbal fluency, and motor speed, evaluated 6 months after the end of chemotherapy (Small et al., 2011).

Other genetic polymorphisms also appear to be implicated in cognitive changes, such as those regulating folate pathways. Kamdar et al. (2011) investigated six different polymorphisms in genes involved in the folate pathway in childhood ALL survivors (Kamdar et al., 2011; **Table 5**), and described two genotypes in genes encoding 10-methylenetetrahydrofolate reductase and sphingomyelin (SM) as significantly correlated with general neurocognitive impairment (Kamdar et al., 2011).

Biological Factors in Cerebrospinal Fluid

When attempting to identify direct biological factors associated with cognitive alterations in cancer patients, variations in levels detected in cerebrospinal fluid (CSF) would be expected to provide better information about causal links with, or consequences of, treatment. Relationships between alterations in phospholipids, SM, and lysophosphatidylcholine (LPC) concentrations, as markers of white matter integrity, and some domains of cognitive function, were identified in children with ALL before and during long periods of chemotherapy (methotrexate administration over a period of years; Krull et al., 2013b). SM and LPC were shown to increase in CSF following chemotherapy induction and were associated with motor speed or visual working memory, and verbal working memory, respectively (**Table 6**; Krull et al., 2013b). These data indicate the occurrence of early cerebral neurochemical and neurocognitive alterations during chemotherapy, suggesting that, in addition to the effects of cancer itself, there is a direct and rapid impact of chemotherapy on the brain (white matter), and that brain imaging of the white matter may be beneficial during methotrexate administration. Methotrexate alters mitochondrial oxidative metabolism by inhibiting recycling of nicotinamide adenine dinucleotide, leading to accumulation of monounsaturated fatty acids. Thus, Moore et al. (2008) evaluated fatty acid levels (ratio between monounsaturated/saturated) in the CSF of patients with childhood ALL treated with methotrexate for more than 3 years (Moore et al., 2008). The number of intrathecal methotrexate doses received during the first year was significantly correlated with an increase in the stearic/oleic acid ratio, which was negatively correlated with decreased global intelligence and academic mathematics ability, while the palmitic/palmitoleic acid ratio was negatively correlated with global intelligence alone (**Table 6**; Moore et al., 2008). Hence, these two studies strongly support a specific deleterious impact of chemotherapy on beta-oxidation and fatty acid metabolism in the brain, suggesting that membrane and myelin defects may accompany cognitive dysfunction in some populations of cancer patients.

CSF analysis can also provide inform about the microtubule-associated protein tau, whose CSF levels have already been associated with neurotoxicity and neurodegenerative pathologies. There is a significant increase in tau protein after induction and during consolidation, compared with at the time of diagnosis, in ALL patients. The level of tau measured before maintenance therapy was negatively correlated with verbal abilities (Protas et al., 2009), suggesting probable neural cell injury.

Overall, studies of patients with ALL receiving methotrexate-containing chemotherapy regimens for long periods demonstrate robust links between cognitive domains, such as working memory or verbal abilities, and modified CSF components, such as fatty acids, phospholipids, and even tau protein, which plays an important role in Alzheimer's disease (**Table 6**). Although the sampling method to obtain CSF by lumbar puncture is more invasive than blood tests, it appears to provide promising predictive biological information relating to cognitive function in cancer patients, which could be highly useful in various settings.

Co-Morbidities and Limitations

It is important to consider clinical, physiopathological, and psychological factors in addition to biological markers, in relation to cognitive impairment of patients with cancer. In particular, to evaluate the contribution of co-morbidities and associated treatments, is essential to understand patient history and knowledge of these factors can help to predict cognitive impairments and determine the significance of changes in circulating factors in cancer patients during treatment. In support of this idea, in a study aiming to identify predictors of cognitive performance in breast cancer patients, treatment for hypertension was identified as having a significant negative impact on verbal fluency and working memory performance, and treatment for diabetes mellitus, was found to detrimentally affect executive functioning and reaction speed (Schilder et al., 2010). The same study also demonstrated that a higher number of "reproductive years" (as an indicator of lifetime estrogen exposure) appears to predict worse executive functioning. A longitudinal cohort study by Bender et al. (2013) demonstrated that before adjuvant chemotherapy, post-menopausal breast cancer patients exhibit poorer cognitive function than matched healthy controls; however, factors related to oral contraception were better predictors of verbal memory and attention in both controls and cancer patients (Bender et al., 2013), likely due to the positive biological impact of estrogen on brain function. The roles of various other factors, such as surgery, sleep disorders, anxiety, and cancer itself, on cognitive impairments specifically observed in cancer patients before chemotherapy, remain unknown. More generally, a study by Mandelblatt et al. (2014) revealed that elderly breast cancer patients with more advanced cancer or high levels of co-morbidity (including diabetes and cardiovascular disease) had higher rates of cognitive impairment than those with low co-morbidity levels, unlike matched control groups (Mandelblatt et al., 2014). These results highlight that some cancer patient populations are at risk of developing cognitive deficits as a result of cancer management, including chemotherapy.

Several limitations should be noted in the studies analyzed in this report. There is an absence of meta-analyses, and the majority of available studies were prospective cross-sectional trials, mostly composed of small samples, and consequently had relatively low statistical power. Also, the studies included are not strictly comparable, because of the different methods used. Biological measurement methods are the main limit, and thus the variability in assessed cognitive domains and tests analyzed should also be considered in evaluation of this review. Indeed, some studies use global efficiency analyses, such as MMSE, whereas others applied batteries of tests, which are more sensitive for objective measurement of cognitive impairments. It should also be noted that practice effects can modify test results, particularly in longitudinal studies repeatedly using the same tests on patients after short periods of time. Finally, the large diversity of chemotherapy regimens used, inconsistent sampling points, and various cognitive assessment methods remain the major obstacles to identification of clear correlations between circulating biological factors levels and performance in specific domains of cognition. In addition, brain imaging could be an interesting approach to correlation of brain activity and biological markers in patients exhibiting no obvious cognitive impairment (Ferguson et al., 2007).

CONCLUSION

A number of potential predictive markers have been identified that require validation in large series. Indeed, initial studies of factors, such as selected cytokines, stress hormones, CSF proteins, lipids, or Hb levels, have provided interesting information about changes in biomarkers that evolve during the course of the treatment of cancer patients, and also about genetic polymorphisms predisposing to cognitive deficits. Additional longitudinal studies, and investigation of other factors, previously identified in different pathological situations as associated with fatigue or aging, should facilitate better characterization of risk of cognitive impairment in cancer.

The question addressed in this study is among the priorities in cancer patient care and the ability to use biological risk factors to predict, better understand, and help to prevent cognitive issues, or adjust treatments for specific populations of patients identified as at risk, would be of major benefit. Such markers would also likely facilitate identification of biological mechanisms underlying neurotoxicity, and could open new avenues for testing and evaluation of therapeutic strategies designed to prevent cognitive dysfunction during cancer treatment, leading to improved quality of life, autonomy, and return to work rates of cancer survivors.

AUTHOR CONTRIBUTIONS

HC and AD selected, read and analyzed articles. ML, MT, and MD built tables and analyzed cognitive domains evaluated in each study. HC and FJ supervised, organized and wrote the manuscript.

FUNDING

Academic French governemental organization: Inserm and Normandie University, Anti-cancer center: Baclesse center, Caen, France

ACKNOWLEDGMENTS

We thank Inserm, the Baclesse Center, the Normandie Rouen and Caen Université, and the Cancéropôle Nord-Ouest that aided the efforts of the authors.

REFERENCES

Ahles, T. A. (2012). Brain vulnerability to chemotherapy toxicities. *Psychooncology* 21, 1141–1148. doi: 10.1002/pon.3196

Ahles, T. A., and Saykin, A. J. (2007). Candidate mechanisms for chemotherapy-induced cognitive changes. *Nat. Rev. Cancer* 7, 192–201. doi: 10.1038/nrc2073

Andreano, J. M., Waisman, J., Donley, L., and Cahill, L. (2012). Effects of breast cancer treatment on the hormonal and cognitive consequences of acute stress. *Psychooncology* 21, 1091–1098. doi: 10.1002/pon.2006

Bender, C. M., Sereika, S. M., Ryan, C. M., Brufsky, A. M., Puhalla, S., and Berga, S. L. (2013). Does lifetime exposure to hormones predict pretreatment cognitive function in women before adjuvant therapy for breast cancer? *Menopause* 20, 922–929. doi: 10.1097/GME.0b013e3182843eff

Cheung, Y. T., Ng, T., Shwe, M., Ho, H. K., Foo, K. M., Cham, M. T., et al. (2015). Association of proinflammatory cytokines and chemotherapy-associated cognitive impairment in breast cancer patients: a multi-centered, prospective, cohort study. *Ann. Oncol.* 26, 1446–1451. doi: 10.1093/annonc/mdv206

Fan, H. G. M., Park, A., Xu, W., Yi, Q.-L., Braganza, S., Chang, J., et al. (2009). The influence of erythropoietin on cognitive function in women following chemotherapy for breast cancer. *Psychooncology* 18, 156–161. doi: 10.1002/pon.1372

Ferguson, R. J., McDonald, B. C., Saykin, A. J., and Ahles, T. A. (2007). Brain structure and function differences in monozygotic twins: possible effects of breast cancer chemotherapy. *J. Clin. Oncol.* 25, 3866–3870. doi: 10.1200/JCO.2007.10.8639

Ganz, P. A., Bower, J. E., Kwan, L., Castellon, S. A., Silverman, D. H. S., Geist, C., et al. (2013). Does tumor necrosis factor-alpha (TNF-α) play a role in post-chemotherapy cerebral dysfunction? *Brain. Behav. Immun.* 30(Suppl.), S99–S108. doi: 10.1016/j.bbi.2012.07.015

Hayslip, J., Dressler, E. V., Weiss, H., Taylor, T. J., Chambers, M., Noel, T., et al. (2015). Plasma TNF-α and soluble TNF receptor levels after doxorubicin with or without Co-Administration of Mesna-A randomized, cross-over clinical study. *PLoS ONE* 10:e0124988. doi: 10.1371/journal.pone.0124988

Iconomou, G., Koutras, A., Karaivazoglou, K., Kalliolias, G. D., Assimakopoulos, K., Argyriou, A. A., et al. (2008). Effect of epoetin alpha therapy on cognitive function in anaemic patients with solid tumours undergoing chemotherapy. *Eur. J. Cancer Care (Engl)* 17, 535–541. doi: 10.1111/j.1365-2354.2007.00857.x

Ishikawa, T., Kokura, S., Sakamoto, N., Okajima, M., Matsuyama, T., Sakai, H., et al. (2012). Relationship between circulating cytokine levels and physical or psychological functioning in patients with advanced cancer. *Clin. Biochem.* 45, 207–211. doi: 10.1016/j.clinbiochem.2011.09.007

Janelsins, M. C., Kesler, S. R., Ahles, T. A., and Morrow, G. R. (2014). Prevalence, mechanisms, and management of cancer-related cognitive impairment. *Int. Rev. Psychiatry* 26, 102–113. doi: 10.3109/09540261.2013.864260

Janelsins, M. C., Mustian, K. M., Palesh, O. G., Mohile, S. G., Peppone, L. J., Sprod, L. K., et al. (2012). Differential expression of cytokines in breast cancer patients receiving different chemotherapies: implications for cognitive impairment research. *Support. Care Cancer* 20, 831–839. doi: 10.1007/s00520-011-1158-0

Jenkins, V. A., Bloomfield, D. J., Shilling, V. M., and Edginton, T. L. (2005). Does neoadjuvant hormone therapy for early prostate cancer affect cognition? Results from a pilot study. *BJU Int.* 96, 48–53. doi: 10.1111/j.1464-410X.2005.05565.x

Joly, F., Giffard, B., Rigal, O., De Ruiter, M. B., Small, B. J., Dubois, M., et al. (2015). Impact of cancer and its treatments on cognitive function: advances in research from the Paris International Cognition and Cancer Task Force Symposium and update since 2012. *J. Pain Symptom Manag.* 50, 830–841. doi: 10.1016/j.jpainsymman.2015.06.019

Joly, F., Heutte, N., Duclos, B., Noal, S., Léger, I., Dauchy, S., et al. (2016). Prospective evaluation of the impact of antiangiogenic treatment on fatigue and cognitive functions in metastatic renal cancer. *Eur. Urol. Focus.* doi: 10.1016/j.euf.2016.04.009

Kamdar, K. Y., Krull, K. R., El-Zein, R. A., Brouwers, P., Potter, B. S., Harris, L. L., et al. (2011). Folate pathway polymorphisms predict deficits in attention and processing speed after childhood leukemia therapy. *Pediatr. Blood Cancer* 57, 454–460. doi: 10.1002/pbc.23162

Kesler, S., Janelsins, M., Koovakkattu, D., Palesh, O., Mustian, K., Morrow, G., et al. (2013). Reduced hippocampal volume and verbal memory performance associated with interleukin-6 and tumor necrosis factor-alpha levels in chemotherapy-treated breast cancer survivors. *Brain. Behav. Immun.* 30(Suppl.), S109–S116. doi: 10.1016/j.bbi.2012.05.017

Krull, K. R., Bhojwani, D., Conklin, H. M., Pei, D., Cheng, C., Reddick, W. E., et al. (2013a). Genetic mediators of neurocognitive outcomes in survivors of childhood acute lymphoblastic leukemia. *J. Clin. Oncol.* 31, 2182–2188. doi: 10.1200/JCO.2012.46.7944

Krull, K. R., Hockenberry, M. J., Miketova, P., Carey, M., and Moore, I. M. (2013b). Chemotherapy-related changes in central nervous system phospholipids and neurocognitive function in childhood acute lymphoblastic leukemia. *Leuk. Lymphoma* 54, 535–540. doi: 10.3109/10428194.2012.717080

Mancuso, A., Migliorino, M., De Santis, S., Saponiero, A., and De Marinis, F. (2006). Correlation between anemia and functional/cognitive capacity in elderly lung cancer patients treated with chemotherapy. *Ann. Oncol.* 17, 146–150. doi: 10.1093/annonc/mdj038

Mandelblatt, J. S., Hurria, A., McDonald, B. C., Saykin, A. J., Stern, R. A., VanMeter, J. W., et al. (2013). Cognitive effects of cancer and its treatments at the intersection of aging: what do we know; what do we need to know? *Semin. Oncol.* 40, 709–725. doi: 10.1053/j.seminoncol.2013.09.006

Mandelblatt, J. S., Stern, R. A., Luta, G., McGuckin, M., Clapp, J. D., Hurria, A., et al. (2014). Cognitive impairment in older patients with breast cancer before systemic therapy: is there an interaction between cancer and comorbidity? *J. Clin. Oncol.* 32, 1909–1918. doi: 10.1200/JCO.2013.54.2050

Massa, E., Madeddu, C., Lusso, M. R., Gramignano, G., and Mantovani, G. (2006). Evaluation of the effectiveness of treatment with erythropoietin on anemia, cognitive functioning and functions studied by comprehensive geriatric assessment in elderly cancer patients with anemia related to cancer chemotherapy. *Crit. Rev. Oncol. Hematol.* 57, 175–182. doi: 10.1016/j.critrevonc.2005.06.001

Meyers, C. A., Albitar, M., and Estey, E. (2005). Cognitive impairment, fatigue, and cytokine levels in patients with acute myelogenous leukemia or myelodysplastic syndrome. *Cancer* 104, 788–793. doi: 10.1002/cncr.21234

Moon, J. H., Ahn, S., Seo, J., Han, J. W., Kim, K. M., Choi, S. H., et al. (2014). The effect of long-term thyroid-stimulating hormone suppressive therapy on the cognitive function of elderly patients with differentiated thyroid carcinoma. *J. Clin. Endocrinol. Metab.* 99, 3782–3789. doi: 10.1210/jc.2013-4454

Moore, I. M. K., Miketova, P., Hockenberry, M., Krull, K., Pasvogel, A., Carey, M., et al. (2008). Methotrexate-induced alterations in beta-oxidation correlate with cognitive abilities in children with acute lymphoblastic leukemia. *Biol. Res. Nurs.* 9, 311–319. doi: 10.1177/1099800407313268

Mulder, S. F., Bertens, D., Desar, I. M. E., Vissers, K. C. P., Mulders, P. F. A., Punt, C. J. A., et al. (2014). Impairment of cognitive functioning during Sunitinib or Sorafenib treatment in cancer patients: a cross sectional study. *BMC Cancer* 14:219. doi: 10.1186/1471-2407-14-219

Natori, A., Ogata, T., Sumitani, M., Kogure, T., Yamauchi, T., and Yamauchi, H. (2015). Potential role of pNF-H, a biomarker of axonal damage in the central nervous system, as a predictive marker of chemotherapy-induced cognitive impairment. *Clin. Cancer Res.* 21, 1348–1352. doi: 10.1158/1078-0432.CCR-14-2775

Pomykala, K. L., Ganz, P. A., Bower, J. E., Kwan, L., Castellon, S. A., Mallam, S., et al. (2013). The association between pro-inflammatory cytokines, regional cerebral metabolism, and cognitive complaints following adjuvant chemotherapy for breast cancer. *Brain Imaging Behav.* 7, 511–523. doi: 10.1007/s11682-013-9243-2

Protas, P. T., Muszynska-Roslan, K., Holownia, A., Grabowska, A., Wielgat, P., Krawczuk-Rybak, M., et al. (2009). Negative correlation between cerebrospinal fluid tau protein and cognitive functioning in children with acute lymphoblastic leukemia. *Pediatr. Blood Cancer* 53, 105–108. doi: 10.1002/pbc.900022029

Schilder, C. M. T., Seynaeve, C., Linn, S. C., Boogerd, W., Beex, L. V., Gundy, C. M., et al. (2010). Cognitive functioning of postmenopausal breast cancer patients before adjuvant systemic therapy, and its association with medical and psychological factors. *Crit. Rev. Oncol. Hematol.* 76, 133–141. doi: 10.1016/j.critrevonc.2009.11.001

Shibayama, O., Yoshiuchi, K., Inagaki, M., Matsuoka, Y., Yoshikawa, E., Sugawara, Y., et al. (2014). Association between adjuvant regional radiotherapy and cognitive function in breast cancer patients treated with conservation therapy. *Cancer Med.* 3, 702–709. doi: 10.1002/cam4.174

Singh, P., Yan, J., Hull, R., Read, S., O'Sullivan, J., Henderson, R. D., et al. (2011). Levels of phosphorylated axonal neurofilament subunit H (pNfH) are increased in acute ischemic stroke. *J. Neurol. Sci.* 304, 117–121. doi: 10.1016/j.jns.2011.01.025

Small, B. J., Rawson, K. S., Walsh, E., Jim, H. S. L., Hughes, T. F., Iser, L., et al. (2011). Catechol-O-methyltransferase genotype modulates cancer treatment-related cognitive deficits in breast cancer survivors. *Cancer* 117, 1369–1376. doi: 10.1002/cncr.25685

Takayama, K., Tsutsumi, S., Suzuki, T., Horie-Inoue, K., Ikeda, K., Kaneshiro, K., et al. (2009). Amyloid precursor protein is a primary androgen target gene that promotes prostate cancer growth. *Cancer Res.* 69, 137–142. doi: 10.1158/0008-5472.CAN-08-3633

Tan, W. W., Heckman, M. G., Vishnu, P., Crook, J. E., Younkin, L. H., Covil, E. G., et al. (2013). Effect of leuprolide on serum amyloid-β peptide levels and memory in patients with prostate cancer with biochemical recurrence. *Urology* 81, 150–154. doi: 10.1016/j.urology.2012.08.066

Vardy, J., Wefel, J. S., Ahles, T., Tannock, I. F., and Schagen, S. B. (2008). Cancer and cancer-therapy related cognitive dysfunction: an international perspective from the Venice cognitive workshop. *Ann. Oncol.* 19, 623–629. doi: 10.1093/annonc/mdm500

Wang, X.-M., Walitt, B., Saligan, L., Tiwari, A. F. Y., Cheung, C. W., and Zhang, Z.-J. (2015). Chemobrain: a critical review and causal hypothesis of link between cytokines and epigenetic reprogramming associated with chemotherapy. *Cytokine* 72, 86–96. doi: 10.1016/j.cyto.2014.12.006

Conflict of Interest Statement: The authors declare that the research was conducted in the absence of any commercial or financial relationships that could be construed as a potential conflict of interest.

9

New Insights toward Colorectal Cancer Chemotherapy using Natural Bioactive Compounds

*Saúl Redondo-Blanco, Javier Fernández, Ignacio Gutiérrez-del-Río, Claudio J. Villar and Felipe Lombó **

Departamento de Biología Funcional, Área de Microbiología, Facultad de Medicina, Instituto Universitario de Oncología del Principado de Asturias (IUOPA), Universidad de Oviedo, Oviedo, Spain

Combination therapy consists in the simultaneous administration of a conventional chemotherapy drug (or sometimes, a radiotherapy protocol) together with one or more natural bioactives (usually from plant or fungal origin) of small molecular weight. This combination of anticancer drugs may be applied to cell cultures of tumor cells, or to an animal model for a cancer type (or its xenograft), or to a clinical trial in patients. In this review, we summarize current knowledge describing diverse synergistic effects on colorectal cancer cell cultures, animal models, and clinical trials of various natural bioactives (stilbenes, flavonoids, terpenes, curcumin, and other structural families), which may be important with respect to diminish final doses of the chemotherapy drug, although maintaining its biological effect. This is important as these approaches may help reduce side effects in patients under conventional chemotherapy. Also, these molecules may exerts their synergistic effects via different cell cycle pathways, including different ones to those responsible of resistance phenotypes: transcription factors, membrane receptors, adhesion and structural molecules, cell cycle regulatory components, and apoptosis pathways.

Keywords: CRC, nutraceutical, chemotherapy, radiotherapy, combination therapy, apoptosis

Edited by:
Kulmira Nurgali,
Victoria University, Australia

Reviewed by:
Amit K. Tyagi,
University of Texas MD Anderson Cancer Center, USA
Stefania Nobili,
University of Florence, Italy

****Correspondence:***
Felipe Lombó
lombofelipe@uniovi.es

INTRODUCTION

CRC is the third most common cancer in men (after lung and prostate cancers) and the second in women (after breast cancer) worldwide, with a prevalence of 10.0 and 9.2%, respectively (Merrill and Anderson, 2011; Bray et al., 2013; Ferlay et al., 2015). CRC is also one of the leading death causes and, despite the improvement in our knowledge in this disease achieved in recent years, current treatments are not enough to control metastatic forms of CRC (Santandreu et al., 2011). Surgery is the main procedure in patients with potentially curable CRC, but neoadjuvant chemotherapy and/or radiotherapy is sometimes given before or after surgery depending on disease stage. However, these treatment regimens are not enough to control CRC, since 30% of patients with stage I–III and up to 65% of patients with stage IV will develop recurrent disease (van der Stok et al., 2016), highlighting the urgency of finding new and more effective treatment schemes.

The potential of nutraceutical natural compounds such as flavonoids, anthocyanidins, carotenoids, or terpenoids for cancer prevention has been widely investigated, and there are many evidences supporting that moderate consumption of fruits and vegetables is correlated with decreased risk of CRC (Fernández et al., 2016). Some members of these families of compounds have the ability to modulate signaling pathways as well as to regulate the expression of genes involved in cell cycle regulation, differentiation, and apoptosis (Pan et al., 2011). Besides being useful in prevention, some of these molecules could be also helpful for the treatment of CRC, especially in combination with other drugs.

Combination therapy allows targeting simultaneously different pathways involved in cancer, taking advantage of different mechanisms of action in order to reduce the development of tumor drug resistance (Housman et al., 2014). In the case of CRC, diverse cell cycle alterations are involved in its establishment and development, as in the case of chromosomal instability versions (CIN; around two-thirds of cases), the DNA mismatch repair phenotype (around 15% of CRC cases) and other less frequent CRC versions as abnormal DNA methylation, colon inflammation status, and microRNA triggering effects (Colussi et al., 2013). In CIN CRC phenotypes, for example, diverse signaling pathways become affected, as those involving APC, β-catenin, Tcf, and WNT proteins (Morin et al., 1997; Sparks et al., 1998). Several studies published in recent years have shown that cancer treatment through combinatorial approach is much more effective than the use of drugs individually (Singh et al., 2013). Also, chemosensitization by means of phytochemicals, based on the use of a natural compound to increase the activity of a drug through modulation of its resistance pathways, is one of the strategies proposed to overcome chemoresistance, one of the main challenges in CRC treatment (Amiri et al., 2013).

Combinations of two drugs onto a biological system may produce improved (synergistic), reduced (antagonistic), or identical (additive) effects compared to their effects when acting separately. Since combinatorial approach to cancer treatment with natural compounds is a promising way to avoid resistances (by affecting more than one target) and to enhance the potency of chemotherapy (through chemosensitization; Majumdar et al., 2009; Gupta et al., 2011), it is necessary for researchers to mathematically assess the nature of these interactions between molecules. This is often made by using the Chou-Talay combination index (CI), based on the median-effect equation: $CI = a/A + b/B$ (Chou and Talalay, 1984). A and B are, respectively, the doses of drug A (alone) and B (alone) needed to produce a specified effect while a and b is the dose in combination that produces the same effect. CI shows an additive interaction between two drugs when it is equal to 1, synergism when CI < 1, and antagonism when CI > 1 (Tallarida, 2002).

STILBENES

Resveratrol (**Figure 1A**) is a stilbene found in more than 70 plant species, including edible plants such as grapes, raspberries, blueberries, or peanuts, and the Japanese knotweed (*Polygonum cuspidatum*), which contains the highest naturally occurring levels of this molecule (Burns et al., 2002). Resveratrol is a phytoalexin, a natural inhibitor of cell proliferation, synthesized by plants in response to environmental stress and pathogenic invasion (Singh et al., 2013).

Since the publication in 1997 of the chemopreventive activity of topically applied resveratrol in a mouse model of skin cancer (Jang et al., 1997), this natural compound has been extensively studied for the prevention and also treatment of many diseases, including CRC. The promising *in vitro* results of these studies have made resveratrol one of the natural compounds that have attracted more attention in recent times, even among mainstream media. For example, resveratrol can interfere with some hallmarks of cancer, protecting against both tumor initiation and cancer progression by interfering with cytochrome P_{450} isoenzymes, inhibiting cyclooxygenase (COX) enzymes and decreasing DNA binding activity of NF-kB, which is usually upregulated in cancer. Resveratrol can also mimic the effects of caloric restriction and protect against metabolic disease, through activation of the SIRT1 histone deacetylase and AMPK (Gescher et al., 2013; Carter et al., 2014).

Beyond its potential usefulness in cancer chemoprevention or even treatment, recent studies have shown that resveratrol can exert synergistic activities used in combination with other chemotherapeutic agents (**Table 1**). This would allow to establish a new and more effective treatment with fewer side effects (Singh et al., 2013). An overview of the studies published to date analyzing combinations of resveratrol with antitumor drugs is reviewed below.

Combinations of resveratrol and quercetin have been shown to synergistically induce apoptosis in the MOLT-4 leukemia cell line (Mertens-Talcott and Percival, 2005). Based on this study, the effects of different concentrations of a 1:1 combination of quercetin and resveratrol on the HT-29 CCR cell line were analyzed, focusing on its effect on Sp transcription factors, usually overexpressed in tumors. The combination of both compounds induced apoptosis in the HT-29 line, decreasing RNA and protein levels of survivin, Sp1, Sp3, and Sp4, in a pathway in which the microRNA-27a appears to be involved. It should be noted that in this study no synergistic effect can be detected between the two compounds since all the tests were carried out with combinations of both compounds and their effects alone were not analyzed (Del Follo-Martinez et al., 2013).

Using an azoxymethane-induced mouse model of colon carcinogenesis, recent studies showed that a combination of resveratrol and grape seed extract reduced the incidence of tumors as much as the nonsteroidal anti-inflammatory drug sulindac, without occurrence of toxicity. In addition, *in vitro* assays performed with isolated human colon cancer stem cells (CSCs) showed that this combination of compounds suppressed proliferation, sphere formation and nuclear translocation of β-catenin through the downregulation of c-Myc and cyclin D, downstream proteins of Wnt/β-catenin pathway (Reddivari et al., 2016).

In 2004, it was discovered that resveratrol sensitizes HCT116 CRC cells to 5-Fluorouracil (5-FU; Fulda and Debatin, 2004). The first experiments were conducted in SHEP neuroblastoma cells, finding that resveratrol induces apoptosis in cooperation with several antitumor drugs (VP16, doxorubicin, cytarabine, actinomycin D, taxol, or methotrexate).

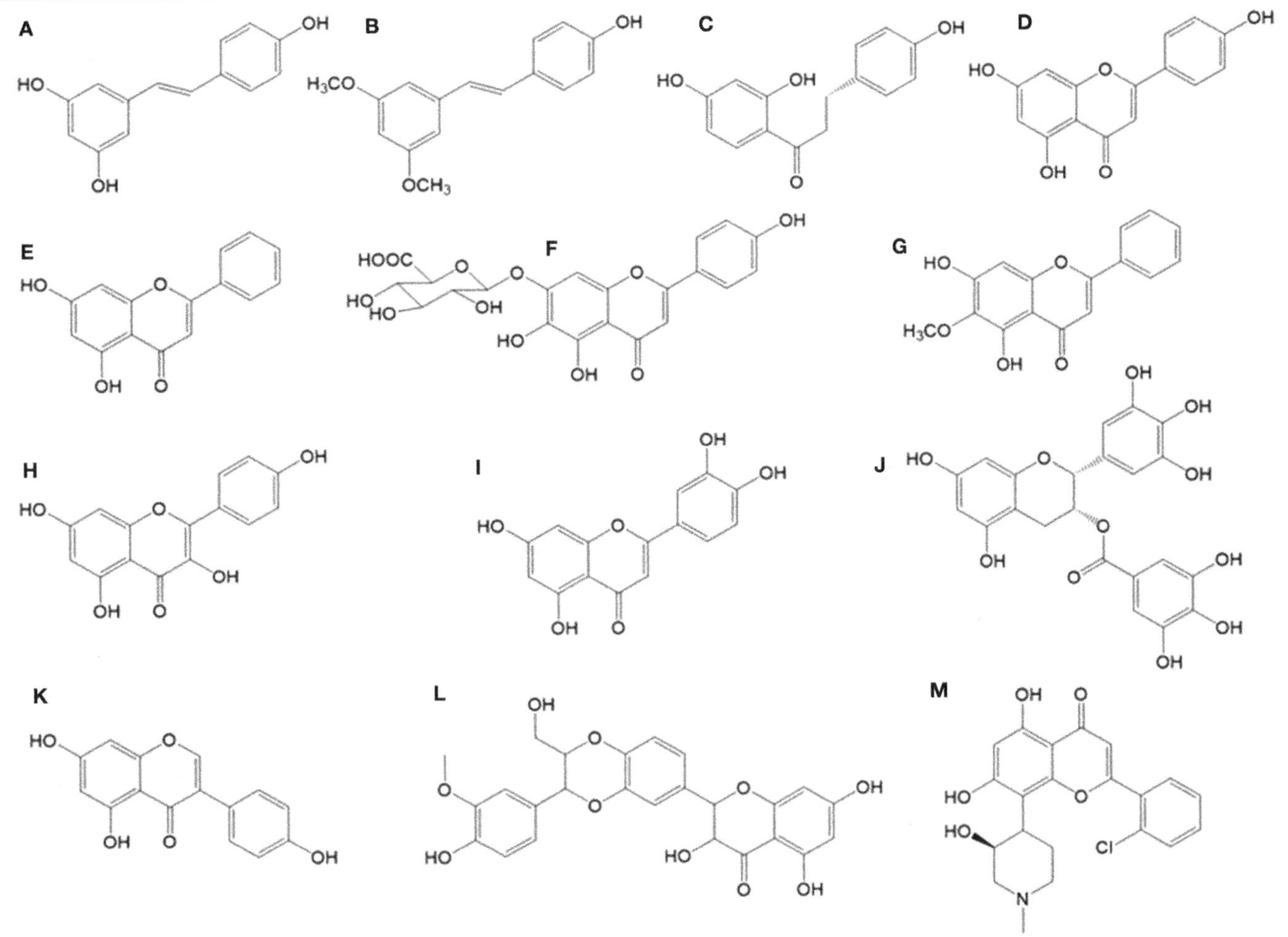

FIGURE 1 | Chemical structures of bioactive stilbenes and flavonoids described in the text. (A) Resveratrol, **(B)** pterostilbene, **(C)** isoliquiritigenin, **(D)** apigenin, **(E)** chrysin, **(F)** quercetin, **(G)** oroxylin, **(H)** kaempferol, **(I)** genistein, **(J)** flavopiridol, **(K)** silibinin, **(L)** scutellarin, **(M)** EGCG.

Interestingly, pretreatment with resveratrol prior to exposure of these antitumor drug was more effective than concurrent or subsequent treatment. In order to test the role of p53 in the chemosensitizing effect of resveratrol, additional experiments were performed with wild-type p53 and p53-deficient HCT116 CRC cells. Pretreatment with 30 μM resveratrol for 24 h increased apoptosis induced by 5-FU (at 10, 30, and 100 μM during the next 24 h) on both cell lines. These results suggest that resveratrol can induce cell cycle arrest and apoptosis independently of p53 status (Fulda and Debatin, 2004). Nevertheless, other researchers have reported that p53 upregulation could play an important role on the synergistic effect between resveratrol and etoposide, a topoisomerase II inhibitor used as an antineoplastic drug (Amiri et al., 2013).

Resveratrol also sensitizes HT-29 and SW620 CRC cell lines to cytotoxic oxidative stress induced by 5-FU, by inhibiting their endogenous antioxidant capacity (Santandreu et al., 2011). Moderate resveratrol concentration (15 μM) in combination with very low 5-FU (0.5 μM) concentration causes a significant inhibition of cell proliferation, migration, and cell cycle arrest at S phase, leading to apoptosis in HCT-116 cells. The same study provides evidence suggesting that its mechanism of action may be related with the activation of the MAPK pathway through upregulation of p-JNK and p-p38, with no p-ERK changes (Mohapatra et al., 2011). Similar results were found in a study with etoposide resistant HT-29 cells, where resveratrol was able to chemosensitize HT-29 cells promoting cell cycle inhibition, reactive oxygen species (ROS) generation, AMPK activation, and apoptosis induction (Hwang et al., 2007a).

Inter-cellular junctions could play an important role in the synergism observed between resveratrol and 5-FU, a drug which can induce an increase of mesenchymal features and loss of epithelial ones in CRC cells; those related to cancer proliferation, motility, drug resistance and metastasis. Resveratrol chemosensitizes CRC cells to 5-FU through inhibition of EMT (epithelial–mesenchymal transition) factors (vimentin and SNAI2 proteins), up-regulation of intercellular junctions (desmosomes, gap and tight junctions, and adhesion molecules such as E-cadherin) and by down-regulation of NF-kB pathway (**Table 1**; Buhrmann et al., 2015).

TABLE 1 | Summary of main *in vitro* and *in vivo* synergistic effects of combinations of stilbenes and chemotherapeutic compounds against CRC.

References	Tested molecule	In combination with	Experimental model	Main result	Proposed mechanism
Ali and Braun, 2014	Resveratrol	Mitomycin C	CRC cell culture (primary cell lines from resected colorectal tumors)	Synergistic suppression of cell proliferation by resveratrol and Mitomycin C	Up-regulation of $p21^{WAF1/CIP1}$
Amiri et al., 2013	Resveratrol	Etoposide	CRC cell culture (HCT-116)	Synergistic effect of resveratrol on etoposide	Up-regulation of *TP53* expression
Buhrmann et al., 2015	Resveratrol	5-Flourouracil	CRC cell culture (HCT-116, SW480) in a 3D-alginate microenviroment	Synergistic activity between resveratrol and 5-Fu decreasing viability and inducing apoptosis	Up-regulation of desmosomes, gap and tight junction adhesion molecules. Inhibition of EMT factors. Down-regulation of NF-kB activation
Kaminski et al., 2014	Resveratrol	Oxaliplatin	CRC cell culture (Caco-2)	Positive: CRC cells chemosensitization by resveratrol. Synergistic activity of resveratrol and oxaliplatin inhibiting CRC cell growth	Induction of cell death
Kumazaki et al., 2013	Resveratrol	5-Fluorouracil	CRC cell culture (DLD-1, SW480, COLO201)	Synergistic enhancement of growth inhibition and apoptosis	Up-regulation of miR-34a expression causing a down-regulation of *E2F3*
Majumdar et al., 2009	Resveratrol	Curcumin	CRC cell culture (HCT-116) and mouse xenograft CRC models	Synergism between curcumin and resveratrol inhibiting growth of CRC cells *in vitro* and *in vivo*	Attenuation of NF-κB activity. Inhibition of constitutive activation of EGFR
Mohapatra et al., 2011	Resveratrol	5-Fluorouracil	CRC cell culture (HCT-116)	Synergistic induction of apoptosis	Cell cycle arrest in S phase, enhanced DNA damage
Santandreu et al., 2011	Resveratrol	5-Fluorouracil	CRC cell culture (HT-29, SW620)	Positive: Resveratrol sensitize CCR cells to 5-Fluorouracil	Increase in oxidative stress, inactivation or down-regulation of redox-sensitive proteins
Yang S. et al., 2015	Resveratrol	Oxaliplatin	CRC cell culture (HCT-116, HT-29) and mouse xenograft CRC model	Synergistic effect of resveratrol and oxaliplatin in a *miR-34c* dependent manner	Up-regulation of *miR-34c*
Fulda and Debatin, 2004	Resveratrol	5-Fluorouracil	CRC cell culture (HCT-116) and other human cancer cell lines	Positive: Resveratrol sensitizes CRC cells for subsequent treatment with 5-Fu	Cell cycle arrest and apoptosis by downregulation of surviving, irrespective of p53 status
Hwang et al., 2007a	Resveratrol	Etoposide	CRC cell culture (HT-29)	Positive: Resveratrol chemosensitizes CRC cells for subsequent treatment with etoposide	inhibition of cell growth, increase of ROS generation, activation of AMPK, induction of apoptosis
Tolba and Abdel-Rahman, 2015	Pterostilbene	5-Fluorouracil	CRC cell culture (HCT-116, Caco-2)	Synergistic effect of pterostilbene on cytotoxic effects of 5-FU	Supression of Akt and ERK phosphorylation. Increase of FOXO-1 and p27kip1 levels

A new mechanism based on miR-34a has been also described which may partially explain the synergistic inhibition of HCT116 growth induced by resveratrol and 5-FU. Here, resveratrol promoted suppression of PI3K/Akt and MAPK Erk1/2 signaling pathways and upregulation of miR-34a expression, which downregulates *E2F3* gene expression and its downstream target *Sirt1* gene (Kumazaki et al., 2013).

Other recent study shows that resveratrol chemosensitizes HT-29 and HCT-116 CRC cells to oxaliplatin through up-regulation of miR-34c, which in turn knocked down its target KITLG. This result was confirmed in xenograft mice, where the combination treatment with oxaliplatin and resveratrol was more effective inhibiting tumor growth than individual treatments (Yang S. et al., 2015). Also, resveratrol and oxaliplatin combinations synergistically inhibit cell growth of Caco-2 CRC cells via apoptosis and necrosis induction (Kaminski et al., 2014).

Mitomycin C is another drug that can be potentially enhanced by resveratrol. Unlike mitomycin C, resveratrol can induce $p21^{WAF1/CIP1}$ overexpression regardless of p53 status, and a combined treatment of these two compounds has inhibited synergistically the proliferation of mitomycin C-resistant CRC cells (Ali and Braun, 2014).

Pterostilbene (**Figure 1B**), a structural analog to resveratrol, characterized by the presence of two methoxy groups instead of resveratrol hydroxyl groups, is able to enhance 5-FU treatment in CRC cells. This synergistic effect is stronger in Caco-2 cells, which express higher levels of ER-β (estrogen receptor beta) compared with HCT116 cells (Tolba and Abdel-Rahman, 2015).

Despite all these promising features of resveratrol as chemopreventive, chemotherapeutic and chemosensitizer agent, clinical trials and other *in vivo* evidences suggest that there may be limitations in clinical application, mainly due to its low systemic availability. Between 70 and 80% of orally consumed resveratrol is quickly absorbed via passive diffusion in the enterocytes. After that, conjugated resveratrol derivatives (glucuronides and sulfates) are rapidly formed, and only 2% of unmodified trans-resveratrol is found in the blood, reaching its maximum concentration between 30 and 60 min after ingestion (Carter et al., 2014). For example, a single 25 mg dose of resveratrol results in a 2 mM (490 ng/mL) serum peak for resveratrol and all of its metabolites, with only trace amounts of unmodified resveratrol (<5 ng/mL; Walle et al., 2004). Furthermore, it has been observed that resveratrol absorption and pharmacokinetics are strongly influenced by food matrix (Rotches-Ribalta et al., 2012) and by its metabolism by gastrointestinal microbiota (Bode et al., 2013). Also, resveratrol dosage in patients and volunteers over 1 g per day has shown gastrointestinal adverse effects such as diarrhea, flatulence, nausea, and abdominal pain (Brown et al., 2010). Anyway, resveratrol and its metabolites have been identified in normal and tumor colorectal human tissue samples, in higher concentrations than those found in blood samples after intake doses of 0.5–1 g/day. Thus, colorectum is a suitable target tissue for chemoprevention and combination therapy by oral resveratrol, as observed concentrations in this tissue are able to produce pharmacological effects (Patel et al., 2010).

FLAVONOIDS

Flavonoids are one of the most numerous and widely distributed family of bioactive compounds in plants. These polyphenolic secondary metabolites are essential for plants morphology and physiology. Flavonoids are involved in flowers, seeds, stems, and leaves pigmentation, as well as in its growth and reproduction (to attract pollinators), while at the same time they protect plants against microbial infections and ultraviolet radiation (Harborne and Williams, 2000). Chemically, flavonoids are characterized by showing a 15-C skeleton (structured as C6-C3-C6) with two phenyl aromatic rings (A and B) plus one heterocycle aromatic ring (ring C), all of them tailored with one or more hydroxyl groups (Manach et al., 2004). Flavonoids are further subdivided into several subgroups depending on the degree of substitution: chalcones (as isoliquiritigenin); flavanones (as naringenin), flavones (as apigenin and luteolin), flavonols (as quercetin and kaempferol), flavanols (as epigallocatechin), isoflavones (as genistein), and anthocyanins. Flavonoids are the largest group of diet polyphenols, with more than 4,000 representatives (Manach et al., 2004; Kumar and Pandey, 2007).

Although, flavonoids are not necessary nutrients for well-being in the short-term, there are several evidences that claim that a moderate intake has beneficial long-term health effects. These compounds, the same as stilbenes, are powerful antioxidants that prevent the appearance of tumors, cardiovascular diseases and osteoporosis, improve cognitive functions and diabetes; or have phytoestrogenic, anti-inflammatory, antibacterial, or antiviral actions, having therefore a strong impact on human health (Kumar and Pandey, 2013).

Isoliquiritigenin

Isoliquiritigenin (**Figure 1C**), a chalcone originated from dried roots of several *Glycyrrhiza* species (licorice plants), exhibits antioxidant, estrogenic, and anti-tumor activities (Guo et al., 2008). It has shown synergistic effect in combination with cisplatin in a xenograft mice model for CRC using CT-26 mouse CRC cells. In this mice model, an oral dose of 1 mg/kg of this chalcone, plus an intraperitoneal cisplatin injection of 5 mg/kg were able to reduce 79% the tumor growth. Also, addition of isoliquiritigenin to this cisplatin treatment was able to reduce liver and kidney damage, as transaminases (AST, ALT), creatinine and blood urea nitrogen levels were kept at normal concentrations, in contrast with control cisplatin treatment. With respect to oxidative damage, this combination therapy with isoliquiritigenin reduced nitric oxide serum levels, lipid peroxidation and GSH levels, in contrast to cisplatin treatment alone (**Table 2**; Lee et al., 2008). This point is very interesting, as major hepatic damages caused by cisplatin are bound to increased oxidative damage due to depletion in GSH levels and an increase in malonaldehyde and membrane peroxidation. Cisplatin treatment is also associated to increased serum levels of transaminases and bilirubin, two important markers for hepatic damage, following histopathological changes as necrosis and hepatocytes degeneration with infiltration of inflammatory cells around portal vein (Caro and Cederbaum, 2004; Dasari and Tchounwou, 2014). Increased liver damage due to cisplatin has been observed in patients with higher expression levels of cytochrome P450-2E1 (Caro and Cederbaum, 2004). The reduction achieved in cisplatin doses, if transferred to *in vivo* experiments, would contribute to a potential reduction in side effects caused by this drug, which usually are associated to ototoxicity, gastrotoxicity, myelosuppression, hepatotoxicity (due to ROS causing a reduction in GSH levels and an increase in malonaldehyde), cardiotoxicity (due to depletion in cardiac myocytes of lactate dehydrogenase and creatine kinase, following membrane peroxidation in these cells), and nephrotoxicity (due to inhibition of carnitine synthesis and its reabsorption by the proximal tube; Dasari and Tchounwou, 2014)(**Figure 3**).

Apigenin

Apigenin (**Figure 1D**) is one of the most widely distributed flavones in fruits and vegetables, such as parsley, Chinese cabbage, bell pepper, garlic, celery, and guava (Manach et al., 2004). It is a chemopreventive agent that has been shown to present strong cytostatic and anti-angiogenic effects *in vitro* (Hirano et al., 1989; Engelmann et al., 2002). *In vitro,* apigenin induces growth inhibition, cell cycle arrest, and apoptosis in CRC cells (Zhong et al., 2010; Lee Y. et al., 2014; Yang L. et al., 2015). Moreover, apigenin is a strong inhibitor of ABC transporters (ATP-Binding Cassette), which are responsible for the increase in the efflux of chemotherapeutic drugs in the lumen (apical) face of colonocytes, thereby significantly reducing its bioavailability and leading to its active detoxification (Katayama et al., 2007). Finally,

TABLE 2 | Summary of main *in vitro* and *in vivo* synergistic effects of combinations of flavonoids and chemotherapeutic compounds against CRC.

References	Tested molecule	In combination with	Experimental model	Main result	Proposed mechanism
Horinaka et al., 2006	Apigenin	TRAIL	CRC cell culture (DLD-1)	Synergistic potentiation of TRAIL-induced apoptosis	Up-regulation of DR5
Shao et al., 2013	Apigenin	ABT-263 (Navitoclax)	CRC cell culture (HTC-116) and SCID mice bearing HTC-116 xenografts	Synergistic induction of apoptosis, antagonism effect on ABT-263-induced Mcl-1 up-regulation and greater tumour growth inhibition	Down-regulation of Mcl-1, inhibition of PI3K/AKT pathway and ERK phosphorylation
Yoshida et al., 2008	Kaempferol	TRAIL	CRC cell culture (SW480 and DLD-1)	Positive: Increase in apoptotic induction in a kaempferol-dose dependent manner	Up-regulation of DR5
Li et al., 2010	Chrysin	TNFα	CRC cell culture (HCT-116)	Positive: Increase in cell death	Inhibition of TNFα-induced NF-κβ activation
Khan et al., 2012	Chrysin	Cisplatin	Wistar rats	Positive: Prophylactic effect against colon toxicity	Reducing oxidative stress
Ding et al., 2012	Chrysin	TRAIL	CRC cell culture (HT-29)	Positive: Enhanced TRAIL-induced cell death	Suppression of c-FLIP and up-regulation of DR5
León et al., 2015	Chrysin	Vanadyl cation	CRC cell culture (HT-29)	Positive: Cell cycle arrest in G2/M phase	Decrease in GSH levels
Hwang et al., 2005	Genistein	5-FU	CRC cell culture (HT-29)	Synergistic effect on cell growth blocking	Over-expression of pro-apoptotic p53 and p21, down-regulation of Glut-1 and down-regulation of COX-2
Hu et al., 2014	Genistein	Cisplatin	CRC cell culture (HT-29)	Positive: Inhibited cell growth and induced apoptosis in an additive manner	Inhibition of TK
Park et al., 2001	Genistein	Dexamethasone	CRC cell culture (Colo320 HSR)	Synergistic effect on blocking cell cycle	Increase in p21 levels
Son et al., 2013	Genistein	Radiotherapy	BALB/c mice bearing CT26 xenografts	Positive: Less non-tumorigenic apoptotic cells and improved morphological changes in healthy intestinal tissue	Activation of antioxidant systems
Gruca et al., 2014	Genistein	Radiotherapy	CRC cell culture (HCT-116)	Synergistic effect on clonogenic survival	Enhanced EGFR inhibition and prolonged inhibition of AKT and ERK
Kumazaki et al., 2013; Wubetu et al., 2015	EGCG	5-FU	CRC cell culture (DLD-1, SW480 and COLO201)	Synergistic growth suppression	Regulation of ABC transporter-related genes
Saldanha et al., 2014	EGCG	Sodium butyrate	CRC cell culture (HT-29)	Synergistic induction of apoptosis	Down-regulation of survivin
Ohishi et al., 2002	EGCG	Sulindac	Azoxymethane colon cancer induction in rats	Synergistic induction of apoptosis	Enhanced inhibition of COX-2
Ambrosini et al., 2008	Flavopiridol	SN-38	HCT116 cell line	Synergistic effect on the apoptotic effects of SN-38	Down-regulation of Rad51 by p53 and Cdk9 inhibition.
Darpolor et al., 2011	Flavopiridol	Irinotecan	Mice xenograft (HCT116)	Improves tumor response	Reduces cytokine activity
Fornier et al., 2007	Flavopiridol	Docetaxel	Phase I trial	Partial responses and a complete response in one patient	Unknown
Guo et al., 2006	Flavopiridol	Docetaxel and 5-FU	Mice xenograft (HCT116)	Significant decrease in a tumor volume	Unknown
Motwani et al., 2001	Flavopiridol	SN-38	Mouse xenograft model	Flavopiridol enhances a reduction in tumors	The effect is produced by p21
Colombo et al., 2011	Silymarin	Doxorubicin and paclitaxel	LoVo cell line	Synergistic effect in LoVo cells and additive in LoVo/DX	Low expression of p-gp pump
León et al., 2015	Silymarin	Vanadium compounds	HT29 cell line	Improves cytotoxic effect	Inhibits topoisomerase IB activity and NF-κB
Tsai et al., 2015	Silibinin	Metformin	COLO205 cell line	Reduction cell viability more than 60%	Increase caspase 3 activation and AIF expression

(Continued)

TABLE 2 | Continued

References	Tested molecule	In combination with	Experimental model	Main result	Proposed mechanism
Psahoulia et al., 2007	Quercetin	TRAIL	Caco-2, SW620 and HT29 cell lines	Sensitizes the cells to the treatment	Distribution of death factors in raft domains that are the initiators of apoptosis
Xavier et al., 2011	Quercetin	5-FU	Co115 and HCT15 cell lines	Enhances apoptosis more than 100 times	The effect is mediated by p53
Osman et al., 2015	Luteolin	Aspirin	Colorectal cancer in rats	Highly significant reduction in polyps number and size	Enhance inhibition the inflammatory response
Chan et al., 2009	Scutellarin	5-FU	HCT116 cell line	A significant increase in apoptosis levels	p53-regulated caspase-6 activation mechanism
Lee et al., 2008	Isoliquiritigenin	Cisplatin	Mice xenograft (CT26)	Reduce 79% tumor growth and reduces adverse effects	Mechanism in combination is unknown
Ha et al., 2012	Oroxylin	5-FU	HT29 cell line and mice xenografts (HT29)	Reduce 66% tumor growth and shows synergistic effects in HT29 cell line	Inhibition of COX-2 gene expression
Cheah et al., 2014	Procyanidins	5-FU	Caco-2 cell line	Increase cytotoxicity	Unknown

apigenin is also responsible for NAG-1 [Nonsteroidal Anti-inflammatory Drug (NSAID) Activated Gene-1] overexpression in CRC cells, a member of the TGF-B (Transforming Growth Factor-B) superfamily which shows pro-apoptotic and antitumor activities (Yang et al., 2014). In fact, apigenin increases in a dose-dependent way in CRC cells, both *in vivo* and *in vitro*, NAG-1 and p53 expression, reducing intestinal tumor load and number (Zhong et al., 2010). Therefore, apigenin has a promising application as a safe antitumor agent. However, it has a modest antitumor activity against cancer cells when used alone, so new strategies are needed in order to enhance its effectiveness, as those based on combination therapy of this flavonoid with CRC drugs.

CD26 is a multifunctional cell-surface protein that is involved in the suppression of pathways responsible for tumor growth and metastasis. In fact, CD26 is down-regulated in several types of tumors including colon cancer and this protein is normally expressed in the epithelial cells of the human colon. Therefore, compounds which enhance CD26 levels are expected to have antitumor potential.

It has been shown that apigenin alone is able to cause an increase of 56.3% in the cell surface abundance and activity of CD26 in different CRC cell lines (HT-29 and HRT-18), so some authors have studied whether this flavone is able to enhance the up-regulation in CD26 cell surface expression of irinotecan, 5-FU and oxaliplatin, that are three chemotherapeutic agents used for the treatment of colorectal cancer. In the case of 5-FU and oxaliplatin, no specific interaction was reported with the action of apigenin; however, the ability of apigenin to potentiate CD26 was much more robust when was combined with increasing concentrations of irinotecan, generating a 4.2-fold increase in the potency of this drug (with a reduction of EC_{50} for irinotecan from 4.68 to 1.26 μg/mL). An interaction was also observed when the experimental design was reversed, adding a fixed dose of irinotecan to a series of apigenin concentrations, increasing by 30 times the capacity of apigenin to enhance CD26 expression, lowering its EC_{50} from 32.8 to 1.10 μM. Therefore, it was observed that in the case of irinotecan (a topoisomerase I inhibitor), but not of 5-FU or oxaliplatin, there is a specific interaction with the action of apigenin due to a cross-talk in the mechanism of action of apigenin with irinotecan, as apigenin is able to inhibit toposimorease I-DNA complex which overlaps with the primary mechanism of action of irinotecan (Lefort and Blay, 2011). This presupposes that part of the mechanism of action of apigenin is intimately related to topoisomerases.

TRAIL (tumor necrosis factor-related apoptosis-inducing protein), a member of the TNF superfamily, is able to induce apoptosis through interaction with the death receptor 5 (DR5), whose expression is regulated by the tumor suppressor p53. TRAIL is not toxic in normal cells because non-neoplastic cells express high levels of decoy receptors (DcR) for TRAIL, which could interfere with TRAIL signaling; it shows acquired resistance in cancer cells (Almasan and Ashkenazi, 2003; Du et al., 2016).

Apigenin induces the expression of DR5 in a dose-dependent manner preventing the degradation of this protein by acting as a proteasome inhibitor and increasing its expression in the membrane, so this up-regulation of DR5 acts in a synergic form sensitizing to the treatment with exogenous soluble recombinant human tumor necrosis factor-related apoptosis-inducing ligand (TRAIL) in CRC DLD-1 cells, showing a greater apoptotic effect than the treatment with TRAIL alone. As said before, TRAIL is an attractive candidate for cancer therapy because it selectively induces apoptosis in cancer cells, and it has been shown that combination of TRAIL with apigenin did not induce expression of DR5 protein and enhanced TRAIL-induced apoptosis in normal human PBMCs cells (Horinaka et al., 2006). Therefore, the combined treatment of apigenin and TRAIL is a promising anticancer therapy.

Diverse anti-apoptotic proteins as Bcl-XL, Bcl-2, Bcl-w, and Mcl-1 can prevent cell death in tumor cells. ABT-263 (Navitoclax) is a novel oral inhibitor for Bcl-2 family proteins, acting as a Bcl-2 homology 3 (BH3) mimetic, and leading to apoptosis, except in tumor cells with Mcl-1 overexpression (Tolcher et al., 2015). As apigenin induces apoptosis in tumor cells by modulating different kinds of signaling pathways, including downregulation of Mcl-1 mRNA (Shi et al., 2015), this apigenin Mcl-1 downregulation may enhance the ABT-263 antitumor activity (Shao et al., 2013; Erdogan et al., 2016). Furthermore, the inhibitory effect of apigenin on ERK phosphorylation levels is significant when CRC HCT116 cells are cotreated with ABT-263 (Shao et al., 2013). All these findings were verified *in vivo* in a SCID mice model bearing HCT116 xenografts, in which treatment with ABT-263 or apigenin alone resulted in a 30% inhibition of tumor growth compared with untreated control, but this percentage was increased to 70% by combination therapy, with decreased Mcl-1 levels as well as phosphorylated prosurvival mediators ERK or AKT (**Table 2**; Shao et al., 2013).

Summing up, both apigenin and ABT-263 alone induced low apoptosis rates in HCT116, DLS1, SW48, HT29, and HCT-8 tumor cells, but in combination therapy, an increase of 80% in apoptosis was recorded via a caspase dependent mechanism. The combination index of these combinations was below 1.0, indicating a synergistic effect (Shao et al., 2013).

Chrysin

Chrysin (**Figure 1E**) is another flavone found in honey, propolis, and various plant extracts such as chamomile and blue passion flower (*Passiflora caerulea*; Renuka et al., 2016). Chrysin has multiple biological activities, including antitumor effects in diverse cancer cell lines and tumor animal models (Kasala et al., 2015).

Several studies in SW480 CRC cells have shown that this flavone is able to induce cell cycle arrest at G2/M transition in a dose-dependent manner. Combination of chrysin plus apigenin doubled the proportion of SW480 cells in G2/M arrest; indicating that both flavones cooperate in slowing down tumor progression (Wang et al., 2004). *In vitro* studies on DLD1 CRC cells have demonstrated a chemoprotective effect of chrysin due to induction of AhR activity (Aryl Hydrocarbon Receptor) accompanied by p21 overexpression, a cell cycle important inhibitor (Ronnekleiv-Kelly et al., 2012). At early tumorigenesis stages, chrysin shows a chemopreventive activity by modulating normal cryptal cells proliferation and by activating apoptosis in aberrant cryptal cells (as those generated in an azoxymethane animal model for CRC). These activities are carried out by downregulating PCNA (Proliferating Cell Nuclear Antigen) and growth factors such as IGF-1 (Miyamoto et al., 2006, 2010; Kasala et al., 2015).

Tumor necrosis factor-alpha (TNF-α) is a pro-inflammatory cytokine with a wide range of biological activities also including both cell progression and death. These TNFα conflicting activities rely on TNF receptor 1 (TNFR1) activation of two different pathways: a caspase cascade for induction of apoptotic events, and nuclear transcription factor kappa-β (NF-kβ), which is a cell survival mechanism. Generally, most tumor cells are refractory to TNFα-induced apoptosis if they keep a working NF-kβ pathway (Chen and Goeddel, 2002; Karin et al., 2004). But chrysin sensitizes HCT116 CRC cells (highly resistant to TNFα apoptosis induction) toward TNFα-induced apoptosis due to its blocking of NF-kβ/caspase 8 pathway, by downregulating its trigger, c-FLIP-I (Li et al., 2010). Combination therapy with chrysin and TNFα together showed a 40% increase in cell death compared to monotherapy, due to caspase 8 activation (**Table 2**; Chen et al., 2004; Romier et al., 2008; Li et al., 2010).

TRAIL binding to death receptors as DR5 results in adaptor protein FADD (Fas-associated protein with death domain) and procaspase 8 or 10 recruitment, which then activate this death pathway. The main negative regulator of this pathway is the cellular caspase-8 (FLICE) inhibitory protein (c-FLIP). Its overexpression causes resistance to this apoptotic process, thereby limiting the therapeutic use of TRAIL. In order to overcome these resistances, a combination with TRAIL pathway sensitizers targeting c-FLIP expression may be a promising approach. In this sense, chrysin is able to suppress c-FLIP expression and to enhance DR5 expression in HT-29 cells, enhancing TRAIL-induced cell death in CRC cells (Ding et al., 2012).

Flavonoids antioxidant activity can also reduce chemotherapy side effects. Cisplatin generates a wide variety of ROS that interact with DNA, lipids, and proteins in CRC cells, including Pt-DNA adducts that hinder cell division and DNA synthesis/repair, leading to apoptotic events (Dasari and Tchounwou, 2014). In this sense, the prophylactic effect of chrysin against colon toxicity due to cisplatin was tested in Wistar rats, confirming a protective effect by reducing oxidative stress (Khan et al., 2012). Although, cisplatin is not used in CRC patients' treatment, these experiments in rats show interesting effects of chrysin with respect to ROS inducing agents.

With a similar action to cisplatin, vanadium compounds are considered a new class of non-platinum metal compounds with eventual low toxicity, although they are not used in clinical praxis. *In vitro,* these compounds inhibit cell cycle even at low doses, by generating ROS, which leads to DNA cleavage and apoptosis. Chrysin complexation with vanadyl cation increased antitumor activity in HT-29 cells (cell cycle arrest in G2/M transition) compared to the monotherapy treatment. Chrysin vanadate complex reduced to 56% the HT-29 cell survival vs. 88% in the case of cisplatin. This chrysin potentiating effect may be due to a reduction in GSH levels, one of the most important antioxidant defenses in mammals (León et al., 2015). In order to avoid gastrointestinal damage in preclinical trials, different vanadium complexes have been generated with flavonoids (Evangelou, 2002).

Scutellarin

Scutellarin is a glycoside of the flavone scutellarein (**Figure 1F**), isolated from the traditional Chinese medicine plant *Scutellaria barbata* (Xing et al., 2011). It has been used in HCT116 cells as chemosensitizing agent (at 100 μM) combined with resveratrol (at 200 μM) and 5-FU (at 500 μM). These experiments showed an increase in apoptosis, due co caspase 6 activation, which was absent in p53 (−/−) versions of this cell line (Chan et al., 2009).

Oroxylin

Oroxylin A is a O-methylated flavone (**Figure 1G**) extracted from the herb *Scutellariae radix*. Oroxylin A inhibits iNOS and COX-2 gene expression by blocking NF-κB. Also, this flavone inhibits LPS-induced NF-kB activation by blocking IκB degradation, the protein which usually binds NF-kB in the cytosol, keeping it in its inactive form (Chen et al., 2000).

Combination of oroxylin A with 5-FU (1:5) both *in vivo* and *ex vivo* in a CRC model using HT-29 cells showed a synergistic action, with COX-2 inhibition and increased ROS generation, which led to HT-20 sensitization to 5-FU. 5-FU IC_{50} in HT-29 is 4.63 mmol/L, but when combined with oroxylin A, this value diminishes to 764 μmol/L. To corroborate this synergistic effect, in a nude mice xenograft model for HT-29, 100 mg/kg oroxylin A plus 20 mg/kg 5-FU showed a 66% tumor size decrease, in comparison with 36 and 42% reduction in the monotherapies, respectively (**Table 2**; Ha et al., 2012). Therefore, oroxylin combination therapy could be a valuable tool in order to reduce 5-FU doses and subsequent *in vivo* side effects.

Kaempferol

Kaempferol (**Figure 1H**) is a flavonol present in black tea, broccoli, propolis, grapefruit, and other plant sources. This compound has a marked antitumor potential on different types of cancer cells (Gutiérrez-del-Río et al., 2016). In CRC cells, it induces p53-dependent growth inhibition and, at the same time, apoptosis by inducing cytochrome c mitochondrial release and caspase-3 cleavage activation (Li W. et al., 2009; Lee H. S. et al., 2014b). In HT-29 cells, this flavonol induces apoptosis and inhibits IGF-IR and ErbB3 signaling (Lee H. S. et al., 2014a). Kaempferol is also able to induce G1 and G2/M cell cycle arrest by inhibiting the activity of CDK2, CDK4, and Cdc2 (Cho et al., 2013).

Monotherapy with kaempferol or TRAIL alone showed a slight effect on apoptosis induction in SW480 and DLD-1 CRC cells, while the combination therapy induced a dramatic apoptosis increase in a kaempferol dose-dependent manner. This means that kaempferol is able to sensitize these CRC cells to TRAIL-induced apoptosis. Interestingly, this combination of drugs showed very low cytotoxicity in PBMC normal cells (Yoshida et al., 2008).

Quercetin

Quercetin (**Figure 1I**) is an ubiquitous flavonol in nature, where it is found in onion, apples, and many other vegetables and fruits. Quercetin inhibits RASA1 expression in CRC cell lines, avoiding RAS activation and therefore its proliferative effects (Ranelletti et al., 2000). Quercetin was combined with TRAIL for treatment of three CRC cell lines, Caco-2 (adenoma), SW-620, and HT-29 (adenocarcinomas); demonstrating that this flavonol is a potent sensitizer to TRAIL-induced apoptosis in a synergistic manner (SW-620 and HT-29), whereas this combination resulted in an additive effect in the case of adenoma cells (Caco-2). These pro-apoptotic effects seem to be associated with a membrane distribution of quercetin in lipid rafts domains, regions which are rich in cholesterol, sphingolipids, and TRAIL death receptors. This membrane distribution could be the initiator for signal cascades causing TRAIL-mediated apoptosis (Psahoulia et al., 2007).

Quercetin has been also used in combination with 5-FU *in vitro*, treating CO115 (p53 positive) and HCT15 (p53 negative) CRC cell lines. This combination of drugs showed higher apoptosis levels in CO115 cell line, in a synergistic manner, but an additive effect in HCT15 cells. This enhanced apoptosis was even higher than with 100 times higher 5-FU concentration in monotherapy. p53 may elicit this synergistic pro-apoptotic effects by enhancing caspase 3 activation and diminishing Bcl-2 (anti-apoptotic) levels. This involvement of p53 is reinforced when a siRNA is used to silence p53 expression in CO115 cells, losing the synergistic effect of this combination of drugs (**Table 2**; Xavier et al., 2011).

Epigallocatechin

(-)-Epigallocatechin-3-gallate (EGCG, **Figure 1J**) is the major polyphenolic constituent of green tea, representing 200–300 mg/brewed cup (Singh et al., 2011). The antitumor effects of this and other flavanols are widely supported by epidemiological, *in vitro*, animal and clinical studies (Singh et al., 2011). For example, different concentrations of grape seed extracts [rich in (-)-epicatechin] were tested in combination with 5-FU 100 μM in Caco-2 cells, showing a slightly synergistic effect on cell apoptosis (Cheah et al., 2014).

EGCG and related compounds are able to inhibit several critical signal transduction pathways in cancer cells. For example, EGCG inhibits multiple RTKs (Receptor Tyrosine Kinase) as the IGF/IGF1R system, EGFR, and HER2 receptors, which play key roles in CRC cell proliferation (Shimizu et al., 2005; Adachi et al., 2008, 2009). EGCG also blocks cell proliferation and cell migration in CRC cells, by inhibiting the signaling pathway TF (Tissue Factor)/VIIa/PAR2 (Protease-Activated Receptor 2) that usually mediates ERK1/2 phosphorylation and final activation of the pro-inflammatory NF-kβ. This lower activity of the transcription factor NF-kB induces an up-regulation of caspase-7 and a down-regulation of MMP-9 matrix metalloprotease expression, affecting proliferation and migration of tumor cells (**Table 2**; Zhou et al., 2012).

Furthermore, EGCG is an epigenetic regulator, which contributes to degradation of DNMT3A (DNA Methyltransferase 3A) and HDACs (Histone Deacetylases) through a process of ubiquitination in CRC cells sensitive to methylation. These effects, together with histones deacetylation, are very important epigenetic mechanisms in tumorigenesis, as they are responsible for silencing various tumor suppressor genes and other ones involved in cell cycle regulation and apoptosis (Moseley et al., 2013). Therefore, EGCG is able to restore the expression of genes involved in tumor suppression such as RXRalpha (Retinoid X Receptor alpha) that are silenced by epigenetic processes in tumor cells (Morris et al., 2016).

Also, it is remarkable the effect exerted by EGCG at the level of CSCs, downregulating *Notch* signaling, a membrane receptor, which is directly involved in the differentiation and proliferation of CRC stem cells (Jin et al., 2013).

Based on these anti-proliferative, anti-metastatic and epigenetic activities for EGCG, its effectiveness in combination with anticancer drugs has been tested. The combination of 5-FU with EGCG resulted in a synergistic growth inhibition in several human CRC cell lines (DLD-1, SW480, and COLO201) (Kumazaki et al., 2013). The same combination on HT-29 and HTC-116 CRC cells reduced cell viability significantly compared with the monotherapies. The EGCG potentiating effect on the 5-FU is supposed to be due to a downregulation in the expression of ABC transporters, which causes higher intracellular 5-FU concentrations (Hwang et al., 2007b; Wubetu et al., 2015).

Sodium butyrate is a non-toxic compound naturally produced in the colon after microbial fermentation of dietary fiber, which shows strong antitumor effects only on transformed colonocytes. Combination of EGCG and sodium butyrate on HT-29 tumor cells caused a synergistic reduction in survivin protein and mRNA levels, an anti-apoptotic protein highly expressed in CRC (Saldanha et al., 2014).

Another compound inducing apoptosis in tumor colonocytes, sulindac, is a NSAID inhibiting COX-1 (expressed constitutively in all tissues) and COX-2 (highly expressed in CRC and induced by cytokines). Although, sulindac has side effects due to this broad cyclooxygenases inhibition, its combination with EGCG reduces them due to an enhanced inhibition of COX-2 (Suganuma et al., 1999). This synergistic effect has been also observed in rats developing CRC by induction with the chemical inducer azoxymethane (Ohishi et al., 2002).

Genistein

Genistein (**Figure 1K**) is an isoflavone which can be found in high concentrations in soybeans, lentils, beans, and chickpeas. Numerous epidemiological studies have reported a negative correlation between the incidence of CRC and diets rich in soybean (Spector et al., 2003; Rossi et al., 2006). This isoflavone has a growing interest as a pro-apoptotic agent because of its specific and almost exclusively activity against tumor cells (as CRC) rather than normal ones (Marín et al., 2015). Genistein acts by increasing the expression of pro-apoptotic proteins as Bax or p21 (Yu et al., 2004), by inhibiting NF-kβ (Luo et al., 2014) and topoisomerase II (Mizushina et al., 2013), by regulating ERB expression (Pampaloni et al., 2014), by suppressing the carcinogen induction of WNT/β-catenin signaling pathway (Zhang et al., 2013), by increasing the expression of antioxidant enzymes such as glutathione peroxidase (Ganai and Farooqi, 2015), and by preventing human CRC metastases due to MMP2 metalloproteases inhibition (Xiao et al., 2015). All these activities can be exploited by combinatory approaches in order to prevent or to treat CRC.

As it has been mentioned above, 5-FU is widely used in the treatment of solid tumors such as CRC, but its main clinical limitation is the development of resistant phenotypes by the over-expression of anti-apoptotic proteins or cell proliferation factors. In order to overcome this resistance problems, a combinated treatment with genistein on HT-29 cells resistant to 5-FU showed a significant reduction in cell viability compared to the monotherapy. These experiments demonstrated a synergistic effect on cell growth inhibition by over-expression of pro-apoptotic *p53* and *p21* genes and downregulation of survival genes such as *Glut-1*. However, the main mechanism involved in this combination was due to COX-2 expression inhibition (Hwang et al., 2005). In a similar way, combination of genistein with cisplatin also inhibited cell growth and induced apoptosis in a synergistic manner in HT-29 CRC cells, by inhibiting tyrosine kinases (Hu et al., 2014). Finally, combination with dexamethasone also shows synergistic effects by increasing p21 levels in Colo320 HSR cells, inhibiting their growth (Park et al., 2001).

Together with chemotherapy, radiotherapy also plays a crucial role in the treatment of rectal cancer, however, in more than 70% of patients, it causes side effects on the gastrointestinal system, as mucositis due to the generation of free radicals by ionizing radiation, which causes oxidative damage to normal colonocytes. A solution to this problem would be to combine radiotherapy with natural radioprotective agents (Jagetia, 2007). In this sense, the remarkable antioxidant activity of genistein, combined with its ability to activate antioxidant pathways, makes it a perfect candidate to protect against radiation cellular damage. Following this hypothesis, CT26 CRC cells were injected into BALB/c mice, and animals were treated with radiotherapy in the abdominal area. After a combination with genistein, this isoflavone reduced the apoptosis in normal cells and improved morphological changes in healthy intestinal mucosa. Also, tumors size was lower in mice subjected to combination therapy (**Table 2**; Son et al., 2013).

The epidermal growth factor receptor (EGFR) plays a very important role in tumor progression because binding of its ligands initiates a cascade of intracellular phosphorylations that ultimately triggers genes associated with cell proliferation, survival, or invasion. This receptor is over-expressed in tumor cells and diverse drugs inhibit this tyrosine kinase, although resistance phenotypes usually appear after irradiation (Singh et al., 2016). Interestingly, pretreatment with genistein during 24 h before irradiation was able to perform a synergistic effect on irradiated HTC116 cells survival (CI < 0.7), due to an enhanced EGFR inhibition (Gruca et al., 2014).

Silymarin

Silymarin is a flavolignan extract from milk thistle (*Sylibum marianum*). This flavolignans mixture contains silibinin (silybin A and B, the most active compounds, **Figure 1L**), isosilybin (A, B), silydianin, and silychrystin (Lee et al., 2006). Silybins induce cell cycle arrest and apoptosis by acting on cyclin dependent kinases (CDKs).

Silymarin has been tested in combination with doxorubicin and paclitaxel against CRC cells, in a cell line sensitive to doxorubicin (LoVo) and its multidrug resistant isogenic version (LoVo/DX). Twenty-four hour prior to treatment with both drugs, silymarin was used in these cells, showing a synergistic effect in LoVo cell line, but not in LoVo/DX cells, where an additive effect was observed. This additive effect may be valuable when dealing with *in vivo* experiments, as any contribution to reduce doxorubicin doses would also reduce its side effects, mainly associated to cardiotoxicity (**Figure 3**). This cardiotoxicity is due to formation of iron-related free radicals, as well as damages to mitochondrial NAD(P)H oxidase complex

(Thorn et al., 2011). Silymarin causes higher intracellular drug concentrations in LoVo cells due to a repression of P-gp pump (P-glycoprotein, MDR1). However, in LoVo/DX cells, the strong P-gp overexpression prevents this sensitizing effect (Colombo et al., 2011).

Silibinin also enhances metformin antiproliferative effects. Combination of this antidiabetic agent at 10 mmol/L plus 100 μmol/L of silibinin in COLO205 CRC cell line showed a synergistic inhibition of 60% in cell survival, which did not affect normal HCoEpiC cells. Monotherapy at these concentrations had no effects. This combination of drugs increased caspase 3 activation and AIF expression, resulting in apoptosis activation by extrinsic and mitochondrial ways. A role for the PTEN/Akt pathway in this apoptosis induction in cancer cells was also observed, with increased PTEN levels and decreased phosphorylated protein kinase B (p-Akt) (**Table 2**; Tsai et al., 2015).

Vanadium (IV) complexes have been tested in combination with silibinin and chrysin against HT-29 cell line, showing increased cytotoxic effects at 100 μM vanadyl ion in comparison with monotherapies (280 μM vanadyl). In this combination, chrysin induces cell cycle arrest in G_2/M transition, while silibinin induces apoptosis due to caspases activation and NF-κB inhibition (León et al., 2015).

Flavopiridol

Flavopiridol (Alvocidib, **Figure 1M**) is a semi-synthetic flavonoid-like derivative, generated from rohitukine, an alkaloid from the bark of *Dysoxylum binectariferum*, a tree from India (Kelland, 2000). Flavopiridol inhibits cyclin-dependent kinases (CDKs), targeting the ATP-binding pocket of their catalytic subunit, as Cdk1, Cdk2, Cdk4, Cdk6, Cdk7, and Cdk9. Also, it inhibits other kinases like PKA, PKC, Erk-1, EGFR, and other receptor associated protein kinases. Flavopiridol blocks cell cycle in G_1/S and G_2/M transitions by lowering expression levels of cyclin D1, $p27^{Kip1}$, and $p21^{Waf1/Cip1}$. Low cyclin D1 levels cause a reduction in Cdk4 concentration, leading to an accumulation of hypophosphorylated retinoblastoma protein (Rb), which causes cell cycle arrest. Low $p27^{Kip1}$ or $p21^{Waf1/Cip1}$ levels also cause a reduction in Cdk2 concentration, inducing cell cycle arrest in G_1phase and inhibiting EEF1B2 elongation factor, which blocks RNApol II transcription of Newcomb (2004).

Flavopiridol is a potent apoptosis inducer in tumor cells, via the mitochondrial pathway (release of cytochrome c or caspases activation), but also via AIF (apoptosis-inducing factor) pathway (Achenbach et al., 2000). This pro-apoptotic effect is enhanced as flavopiridol also inhibits Akt activation, leading to NF-κB inactivation and therefore to an inhibition of proliferation processes (Takada and Aggarwal, 2004). Therefore, this flavonoid derivative triggers apoptosis and at the same time inhibits proliferation.

Irinotecan, a semisynthetic analog of the natural alkaloid camptothecin, and SN-38, the irinotecan bioactive metabolite, prevents DNA from unwinding by inhibiting topoisomerase 1. Combination of SN-38 treatment followed by flavopiridol in HCT116 cell line and its null isogenic p53 (−/−) equivalent showed apoptosis induction only in the p53 wild type cell line. Here, p53 produced Rad51 mRNA downregulation, a gene coding for a DNA-repair protein (Ambrosini et al., 2008).

In a mouse xenograft model with HCT116 cell line, irinotecan treatment followed by flavopiridol showed a significant decrease in tumor growth compared to monotherapies. This study suggests changes in the choline kinase activity and decreased phosphocholine (Motwani et al., 2001; Darpolor et al., 2011). Since diarrhea is one of the most common side effect associated to irinotecan treatment, this synergistic effect among flavopiridol and irinotecan may be a valuable combination for preventing or reducing this gastrointestinal toxicity associated to this camptothecin derivative (Fuchs et al., 2003) (**Figure 3**).

Sequential treatment with docetaxel, flavopiridol, and 5-FU in HCT116 cell line showed an 8-fold increase in caspase activity, with much lower increase if the three compounds were added simultaneously, in pairs or separately. Using this triple combination in mice xenografts with HCT116 caused a decrease in tumor volume by 95% (50% reduction for single drug treatment, 70% reduction for two drugs combination; **Table 2**; Guo et al., 2006).

A phase I trial of weekly, sequential docetaxel followed by flavopiridol (after 4 h first treatment) in patients with advanced solid tumors showed that this combination of drugs was well tolerated, with one dose-limiting toxicity occurring at 70 mg/m^2 flavopiridol. Docetaxel common toxicity effects are mostly associated to neutropenia (Ho and Mackey, 2014). Also, one complete response was observed in a patient with pancreatic carcinoma, as well as four partial responses in pancreatic (1), breast (2), and ovarian (1) tumors. Stable disease was observed in ten patients (27 patients in total; Fornier et al., 2007).

TERPENES

Another large and diverse class of organic compounds where some of them have shown a promising role against CRC in combination with other drugs are the terpenes. Terpenes are the structurally most diverse class of all plant and fungal bioactive metabolites, with more than 50,000 molecules. All terpenes derive from the condensation of dimethylallyl diphosphate (DMAPP) and isopentenyl diphosphate (IPP) precursors, which may be linked together "head to tail" to form linear chains or may be arranged to form rings (Klein-Marcuschamer et al., 2007). Terpenes are classified, according to the number of biosynthetic isoprene units, in monoterpenes (10 carbon atoms, C10), sesquiterpenes (C15), diterpenes (C20), triterpenes (C30), and tetraterpenes (C40) (Misawa, 2011). In addition, terpenes that have undergone oxidation steps are called terpenoids. Some examples are essential oils such as limonene (C10, flavoring agent), vitA (C20), β-carotene (C40), and steroids (C30, cholesterol, testosterone).

Artesunate

Artesunate (**Figure 2C**) is the hemisuccinate ester of artemisin, a sesquiterpene found in *Artemisa annua* (a traditional Chinese herb), widely used for malaria treatment as ROS inducer in the *Plasmodium* parasite (Meshnick, 2002). Artesunate is

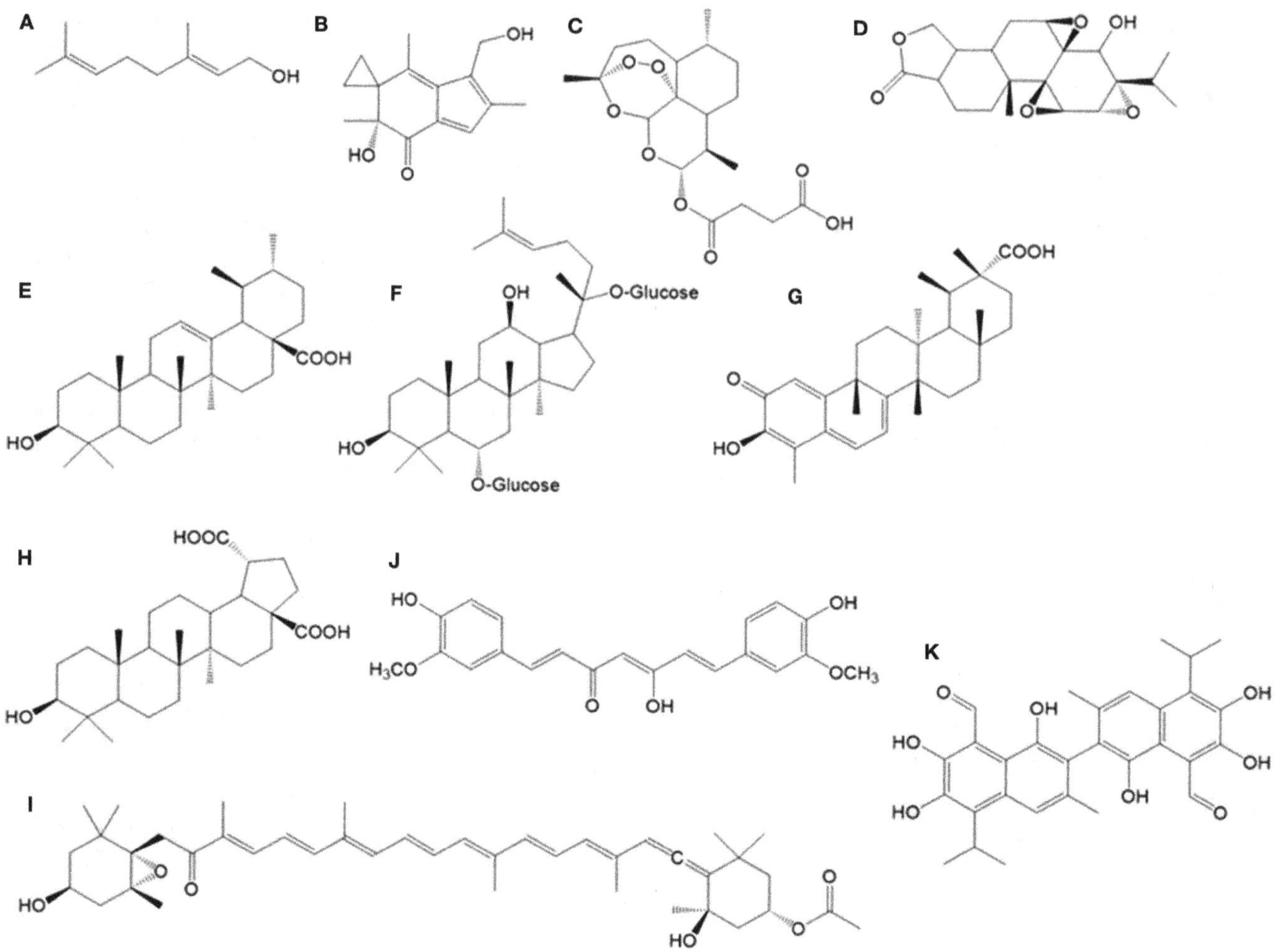

FIGURE 2 | Chemical structures of bioactive terpenoids and other compounds described in the text. (A) geraniol, **(B)** irofulven, **(C)** artesunate, **(D)** triptolide, **(E)** ursolic acid, **(F)** ginsenoside, **(G)** celastrol, **(H)** betulinic acid, **(I)** fucoxanthin, **(J)** curcumin, **(K)** gossypol.

cytotoxic in HCT116 cells, inducing a cell cycle arrest at G_1, due to cyclin D1 downregulation and p21 overexpression. The treatment of these CRC cells with artesunate (1.9 μM) or oxaliplatin (another agent also causing ROS stress in cells, together with other alkylating activities on DNA; 4 μM) causes 50% cell killing. However, the same effect can be obtained with a combination of just 0.65 μM artesunate plus 1.6 μM oxaliplatin, which reinforces the used of artesunate as a possible adjuvant chemotherapy molecule (Liu et al., 2011).

Geraniol

The monoterpene geraniol (**Figure 2A**) is a main component in commercially important essential oils (rose, lemon, etc.), with wide use in perfumes. *In vitro* combination of geraniol (150 μM, IC_{30}) plus 5-FU (0.25 μM, IC_{30}) on Caco-2 cells increased the cell death in comparison with monotherapy, causing over 20% reductions cell survival. In a tumor xenograft model for TC118 CRC cell line, combination of geraniol (150 mg/kg) plus 5-FU (40 mg/kg) showed a clear 83% reduction in tumors size, whereas monotherapies with these concentrations caused only 26 and 30% tumor reductions, respectively (Carnesecchi et al., 2004).

In a CRC animal model using the mutagen dimethylhydrazine, oral geraniol (25 mg/100 g) was administered in order to test its effects in CRC prevention at early stages (aberrant crypt foci reduction in colon mucosa, ACF). After 9 weeks, a significant 37% reduction in colon ACF was observed with respect to control animals, together with enhanced apoptosis parameters. This protection was also accompanied by a 30% reduction in the cellular levels of Bcl-2 in geraniol treated animals, an anti-apoptotic protein, whose low levels may explain the geraniol antitumor effect in colon mucosa (**Table 3**). These results may open the path to the study of other non-cyclic monoterpenes as antitumor agents (Vieira et al., 2011).

Irofulven

Irofulven (**Figure 2B**) is a semi-synthetic derivative of illudin S, a sesquiterpene isolated from the mushroom *Omphalotus illudens*.

TABLE 3 | Summary of main *in vitro* and *in vivo* synergistic effects of terpenoids and other compounds in combination with chemotherapeutic compounds against CRC.

References	Tested molecule	In combination with	Experimental model	Main result	Proposed mechanism
Carnesecchi et al., 2004; Vieira et al., 2011	Geraniol	5-FU	Caco-2 cell line	Synergistic: 20% reduction in cell survival	Down-regulation of Bcl-2
Carnesecchi et al., 2004	Geraniol	5-FU	Mice xenograft (TC118)	Synergistic: 80% reduction in tumor size	Unknown
Serova et al., 2006	Irofulven	Oxaliplatin	HT-29 cell line	Synergistic: reduced cell survival	Unknown
Britten et al., 1999	Irofulven	Irinotecan	Mice xenograft (HT-29)	Synergistic: tumor size reduction	Unknown
Liu et al., 2011	Artesunate	Oxaliplatin	HCT116 cell line	Synergistic: 50% cell killing	ROS induction
Liu et al., 2014	Triptolide	Oxaliplatin	SW480 cell line	Synergistic: 62% cell killing	Apoptosis induction, blocking of β-catenin translocation to nucleus
Liu et al., 2014	Triptolide	Oxaliplatin	Mice xenograft (SW480)	Synergistic: 60% tumor growth reduction	Unknown
Koh et al., 2012; Prasad et al., 2012	Ursolic acid	Radiotherapy	CT26 and HCT116 cell lines	Synergistic: 55% cell killing	Apoptosis induction, caspase 3 activation, ROS increase, GSH, NF-kB and Bcl-2 reductions
Wang et al., 2015	Ginsenolides	5-FU	Mice xenograft (HCT116)	Synergistic: reduced tumor size	G_1 arrest
Kim et al., 2009	Ginsenolides	Docetaxel	HCT116 cell line	Synergistic: increased cell death	NF-kB inhibiton, Bcl-2 repression
Zhu et al., 2010	Calastrol	TRAIL	SW620 cell line	Synergistic: increased cell killing	Apoptosis induction
Jung et al., 2007	Betulinic acid	5-FU, oxaliplatin, irinotecan	SNU-C5 cell line	Synergistic: increased cell killing, reduction in chemoresistance	Apoptosis induction (caspase 3)
Li et al., 2007	Curcumin	Oxaliplatin	Lo-Vo cell line	Synergistic: growth inhibition	Unknown
Anitha et al., 2014	Curcumin	5-FU	HT-29	Synergistic: increased cells killing	Apoptosis induction
Murakami et al., 2013	Curcumin	Turmerones	CRC mouse model (dimethyl-hydrazine)	Synergistic: tumor size reduction	Apoptosis induction
Yue et al., 2016b	Curcumin	Bevacizumab	Mice xenograft (HT-29)	Synergistic: tumor size reduction	Apoptosis induction
Zhang et al., 2003; Lan et al., 2015	Gossypol	5-FU	Mice xenograft (HT-29)	Synergistic: tumor size reduction	Apoptosis induction, chemical sensitization

It shows potent growth inhibition on a wide variety of human solid tumor cell lines and primary tumor cell types. *In vivo* testing has demonstrated excellent dose-related antitumor activity in several human tumor mice xenograft models.

Combination of irofulven with radiation or chemotherapeutic agents such as paclitaxel, irinotecan, 5-FU, mitomycin C, thiotepa, topotecan, and cisplatin have produced additive and/or synergistic inhibition of cellular proliferation in a variety of tumor types. With respect to CRC, simultaneous exposure to irofulven and cisplatin is at least additive for HCT116 cells, whereas simultaneous exposure to irofulven and 5-FU is additive for HT-29 cells and synergistic for the irofulven-resistant HCT116 cell line (Poindessous et al., 2003). Combination of irofulven with oxaliplatin also led to synergistic activity in HT-29 cell line (Serova et al., 2006). In a mice xenograft model for HT-29 cells, combination of irofulven and irinotecan, significant reduction in tumor weights occurred with partial responses in nearly all of the animals and some animals achieving complete responses (**Table 3**; Britten et al., 1999).

Triptolide

Triptolide (**Figure 2D**) is a diterpene from *Tripterygium wilfordii* tree, used as anti-inflammatory and antitumor in traditional Chinese medicine. Individual treatments with triptolide or oxaliplatin during 48 h in SW480 cell line showed IC_{50} values of 16.7 ng/mL and 20.8 μg/mL, respectively. However, in combination with 10 μg/mL oxaliplatin, 8 ng/mL of this diterpene was able to induce 62% apoptosis. This synergistic effect was due to an inhibition of nuclear translocation of the transcription factor β-catenin under combinatory conditions, causing that this cell progression factor remains accumulated in the cytoplasm. Also, in a mice xenograft model for this cell line, combination of triptolide (0.1 mg/kg) with oxaliplatin (5 mg/kg) also showed this synergistic effect, reducing tumors growth by 60% (**Table 3**). This positive effect was not accompanied by a significant increase in ALT and AST transaminases (biomarkers for hepatic damage) nor in blood urea nitrogen (biomarker for renal damage; Liu et al., 2014). In a similar way, combination of triptolide (0.15 mg/kg) plus 5-FU (12 mg/kg) in another xenograft model with HT-29 cell line caused a reduction of 96% tumor growth for 3 weeks treatment, with no side effects observed (Tang et al., 2007). These results open the way for the use of triptolide in the treatment of solid tumors in preclinical trials (Jiang et al., 2001; Fidler et al., 2003).

Ursolic Acid

The triterpene ursolic acid (**Figure 2E**) is found in diverse herb species as basil and rosemary. This antioxidant compound is able

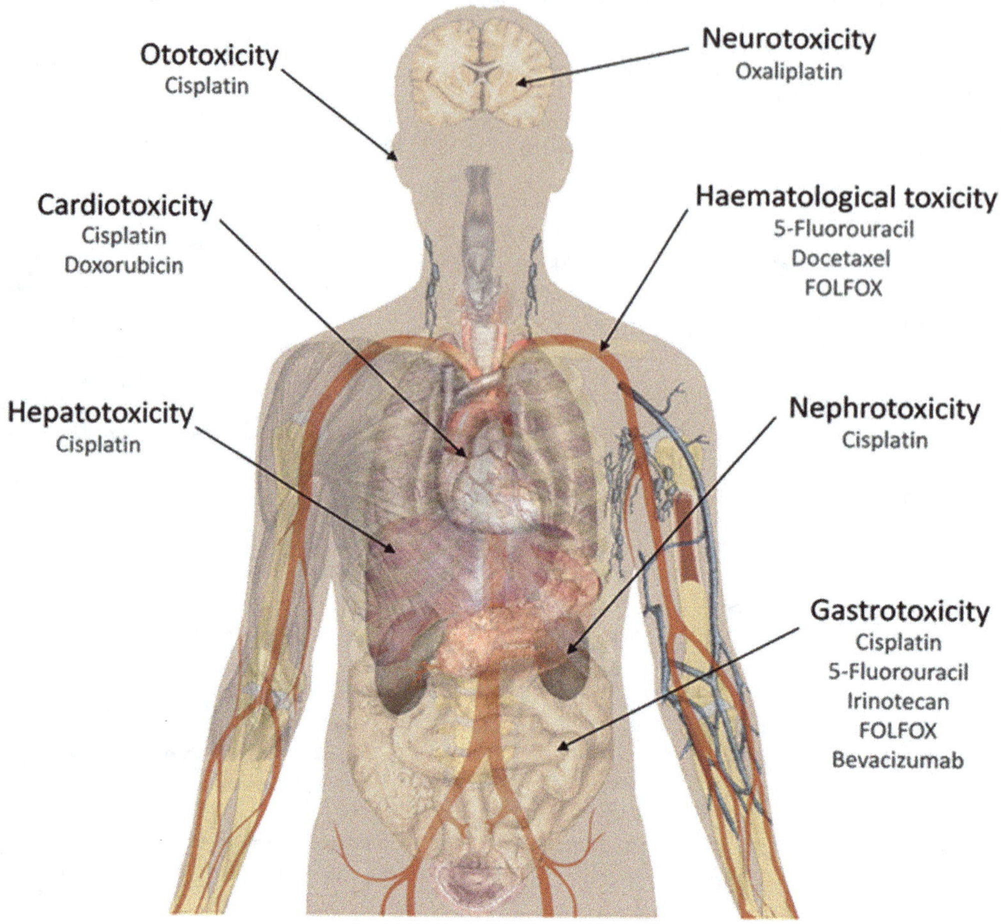

FIGURE 3 | Chemotherapy compounds that have been mentioned in this work and their main side effects.

to modulate cellular redox status in normal cells, but in tumor cells it exerts pro-oxidative action. This is an important fact when dealing with tumor cells and radiotherapy, as ionizing radiation works by increasing cell oxidative damage in transformed cells, leading to apoptosis. In this sense, radio-resistance status can be avoided or reverted by using drugs able to increase ROS and its mitochondrial, DNA and membranes damages.

Using *in vitro* experiments with CT26 mouse CRC cells, a synergistic effect has been described for a combination of ursolic acid plus radiotherapy, where apoptosis was enhanced 55%, via caspase 3 activation. In these co-treated tumor cells, it was observed higher peroxides formation, lower GSH levels and extended mitochondrial damage (Koh et al., 2012). These pro-apoptotic effects of ursolic acid have been reproduced in other CRC cell lines as HCT116, where this compound was able to reduce the pro-inflammatory NF-kB cytokine, the pro-metastatic MMP-9 matrix metalloprotease, and the survival effectors Bcl-2 and survivin. All these changes in expression of key cancer modulators were reinforced when conducting these *in vitro* experiments with ursolic acid and capecitabine together (**Table 3**; Prasad et al., 2012).

In a mouse xenograft model with HCT116 cells, combination of ursolic acid with capecitabine caused a 68% reduction in tumor volume, also diminishing distant metastasis to lung around 60% (Prasad et al., 2012).

Ginsenosides

Panaxadiol is a ginsenosides (**Figure 2F**) triterpene found both in ginseng (*Panax ginseng*) and in notoginseng (*Panax pseudoginseng*). Previous studies have shown the antitumor activities of these compound on several cell lines and their targeting on multiple cancer signaling pathways (Park et al., 1999; Jin et al., 2003; Gao et al., 2013). Notoginseng extract, which contains high amounts of ginsenosides, enhances 5-FU induced apoptosis in human CRC cells (Wang et al., 2007a,b). Looking for specific bioactive components in these extracts, panaxadiol was found to be the component which caused enhanced apoptosis in HCT116 cell line (Li X. L. et al., 2009). Similar results were obtained with protopanaxadiol, another ginseng metabolite that significantly enhanced 5-FU effects on HCT116 cells by inducing arrest in G_1 phase and apoptosis. These *in vitro* data were confirmed by using an *in vivo* mice xenograft model, showing that protopanaxadiol and 5-FU co-administration very significantly reduced the tumor size in a dose-related manner (**Table 3**; Wang et al., 2015).

Another member of this family, ginsenoside Rg3, is able to repress NF-kB expression in HCT116 cell line, leading to apoptosis, with a IC_{50} value of 100 μM. NF-kB is usually activated in these and other tumor cells. Twenty-four hour combination of 50 μM ginsenoside R3 plus 5 μM docetaxel in this cell line resulted in a synergistic NF-kB inhibition, absent in the monotherapy experiments at these concentrations. This pro-apoptosis effect was due to Bcl-2 repression and expression of the pro-apoptotic proteins caspase 3 and Bax, which demonstrated the chemosensitization of these tumor cells to docetaxel in the presence of ginsenosides R3 (Kim et al., 2009).

Celastrol

Celastrol (**Figure 2G**) is a triterpene from the bark of the *T. wilfordii* tree. This compound inhibits the heat shock protein HSP90, blocking its interaction with Cdc37. TRAIL addition to cultures of SW620 CRC cells shows an IC_{50} value of 423.5 ng/mL, whereas this parameter is reduced to only 121.1 ng/mL in the presence of 2 μM celastrol during 72 h, due to apoptosis induction via caspase 3; therefore, celastrol shows a synergistic effect in combination with TRAIL (Zhu et al., 2010).

Betulinic Acid

Betulinic acid (**Figure 2H**) is an anti-inflammatory and antimalarial triterpene isolated from diverse plants, as *Betula pubescens* tree (birch) and many others. This compound exerts apoptosis through caspase 3 induction in SNU-C5 CRC cell line with IC_{50} value of 1 μg/mL. Three resistance variants were originated from this cell line, showing increased resistance to 5-FU (total resistance, instead IC_{50} of 6 μg/mL in parental cell line), irinotecan (5.55-fold IC_{50} instead of IC_{50} of 18 μg/mL in parental cell line), and oxaliplatin (total resistance, instead IC_{50} of 100 μg/mL in parental cell line). These three resistant variants were more sensitive to betulinic acid alone than the parental cell line, but more interestingly, combination of betulinic acid plus 5-FU reverted apoptosis induction in the 5-FU resistant cells. A similar reversion effect was observed with a combination of betulinic acid plus oxaliplatin in oxaliplatin-resistant cells. These results clearly demonstrate that in some cases it is possible to circumvent acquired chemoresistance by combination therapy of anticancer drugs with chemosensitizers as betulinic acid (Jung et al., 2007).

Fucoxanthin

Fucoxanthin (**Figure 2I**) is a tetraterpenoid carotenoid found in the edible macroalga *Undaria pinnatifida*, which has been associated to prevention of CRC (Kim et al., 1998). *In vitro* studies with Caco-2 cell line have shown that this carotenoid is able to induce apoptosis after 72 h exposure at 22.6 μM. This apoptosis induction was due to an 80% reduction in Bcl-2 protein levels, a survival factor (Hosokawa et al., 2004).

CURCUMIN

Curcumin (**Figure 2J**) is a diarylheptanoid found in turmeric (*Curcuma longa*) that is frequently described as a chemopreventive agent for CRC (Chauhan, 2002; Goel et al., 2008; Prasad et al., 2014). Curcumin protects against chemically induced intestinal tumorigenesis in mice and rats (Huang et al., 1992, 1994; Rao et al., 1993; Kim et al., 1998; Kawamori et al., 1999) and prevents adenoma development in the gastrointestinal tract of *apc*(±) mice, a model of human familial adenomatous polyposis (Perkins et al., 2002).

A combination of liposomal curcumin with oxaliplatin *in vitro* at equimolar concentrations resulted in no significant enhanced growth inhibition compared with monotherapies results. However, 4:1 molar ration combinations in LoVo cells resulted in a synergistic effect. However, there was no synergistic effect for both drugs *in vivo* using Colo205 and LoVo mice xenografts (Li et al., 2007).

Dasatinib is a potent Src and Abl kinases inhibitor. Curcumin showed synergistic effect with this inhibitor in HCT116 and HT-29 cells under FOLFOX treatment (5-FU, leucovorin plus oxaliplatin) resistant phenotype. This combination of drugs is preferred to single agent regimens, as oxaliplatin alone, which has limited activity. FOLFOX inhibited cellular growth, invasion and colonosphere formation and also reduced CSCs populations as evidenced by the decreased expression of their specific markers (CD133, CD44, CD166, and ALDH; Nautiyal et al., 2011).

Different studies have also reported the potential enhancement of 5-FU antitumor efficacy in combination with curcumin/hexahydrocurcumin, both *in vitro* (Du et al., 2006; Srimuangwong et al., 2012a) and *in vivo* (Srimuangwong et al., 2012b). Curcumin can potentiate as well the pro-apoptotic and anti-metastatic effects of capecitabine, a prodrug that is enzymatically converted to 5-FU in the body (Kunnumakkara et al., 2009). In a recent phase I clinical trial using a combination of curcumin with FOLFOX, this combination of drugs enhanced anti-proliferative effects in patient-derived explants, indicating that curcumin can reduce CRC cells survival (Patel et al., 2008; James et al., 2015). Oxaliplatin treatment causes neurosensory toxicity and paresthesia, but combination therapy with FOLFOX regimen leads to common neutropenia, neurotoxicity, and diarrhea (Braun and Seymour, 2011) (**Figure 3**).

Curcumin is relatively safe for normal cells, but it can induce tumor apoptosis by different pathways (Hanif et al., 1997; Ravindran et al., 2009; Kantara et al., 2014), as it has demonstrated in several clinical trials (Bar-Sela et al., 2010; Gupta et al., 2013). However, its poor bioavailability is still regarded as a major problem for its therapeutic use (Anand et al., 2007). One approach to enhance curcumin absorption by colonocytes, to increase *in vitro* bioactivity and *in vivo* bioavailability is nanoencapsulation. This promising process reduces the non-selective exposure of this nutraceutical and improves the plasma half-life of the drug (Tsai et al., 2011; Yallapu et al., 2012). For example, 5-FU and curcumin were individually entrapped in chemically modified chitosan nanoparticles that were characterized for its *in vitro* hemocompatibility, drug release profile, cellular internalization, *in vitro* combinatorial antitumor effects in HT-29 cells and plasma concentration time profile by pharmacokinetics (in Swiss Albino mouse model). These experiments demonstrated that nanoparticles were blood-compatible, the release profile over a period of 4 days was sustained, the antitumor effects on CRC cells were enhanced and the plasma concentrations of both components in the mouse model were improved and prolonged up to 72 h, longer than bare drugs (Anitha et al., 2014).

A synergistic combination of curcumin and resveratrol has been also described. Both agents, acting together, inhibited the constitutive activation of EGFRs and IGF-1R in HCT-116 CRC cells. A test with a mice xenograft mouse model of CRC showed that the combination of resveratrol and curcumin (at doses of 50 and 500 mg/kg, respectively, administered by gavage for 3 weeks) is highly effective in inhibiting tumor growth and stimulating apoptosis of CRC cells *in vivo*, through attenuation of NF-κB activity (**Table 1**; Majumdar et al., 2009).

Turmerones are several structurally related non-polar sesquiterpenes found in turmeric ethanol extracts, which could increase curcumin accumulation inside colonocytes, but this curcumin-free fraction also exhibits biological activities. Pharmacokinetic results showed that plasma curcumin levels in mice fed with turmeric extract were the highest ones (Aggarwal et al., 2013; Yue et al., 2016b). Interestingly, the combination of curcumin and turmerones abolishes tumor formation when fed to a dimethyl-hydrazine-initiated and DSS-promoted mouse model of CRC (Murakami et al., 2013). Also, in a HT-29 tumor xenograft mice model, feeding with turmeric ethanol extract caused a greater tumor size reduction than feeding with curcumin (Yue et al., 2016a,b). The presence of turmerones increases curcumin accumulation inside colonocytes and could enhance curcumin antitumor activity in mice models. Bevacizumab is a monoclonal antibody targeting vascular endothelial growth factor. It has been used in combination with turmeric ethanol extract (including curcumin) for treatment of mice harboring HT-29 xenografts. Also, a combination therapy of turmeric extract plus bevacizumab treatment significantly inhibited tumor growth. These inhibitory effects were comparable with those of FOLFOX plus bevacizumab, with no observable side-effect induced by turmeric extract treatment while significant side effects were found in FOLFOX-treated mice (**Table 3**; Yue et al., 2016b). Potential synergistic effects of turmerones, curcumin, and bevacizumab could eventually allow a future reduction in this antibody dosage to patients, if applied in clinic. This would lead to reduction/prevention of some rare side effects associated to bevacizumab therapy, as thrombosis, arterial hypertension, proteinuria, perforation of the gastrointestinal tract, or nasal septum, wound healing abnormalities (which may lead to postoperative bleeding in CRC surgery), irreversible leuco-encephalopathy syndrome, allergic skin rash, and hypersensitivity reactions (including flashing, pruritus, arterial hypertension, rigors, broncho-constriction, chest pain, and sweats). These side effects also include rare spontaneous delayed (sometimes even several months after surgery) leakage from colon or rectal anastomosis after treatment with bevacizumab (Pavlidis and Pavlidis, 2013).

GOSSYPOL

Gossypol (**Figure 2K**) is a natural phenolic aldehyde derived from the cotton plant (*Gossypium*). Its antitumor properties have been studied in a variety of tumors since the 1980s, being currently evaluated in phase I and II clinical trials for its use as a single agent or in combination with other antitumor agents in a variety of hematologic, lymphoid, and solid tumors. Gossypol inhibits cell proliferation and induces apoptosis and autophagy in a variety of CRC cell lines. Also, it inhibits CRC growth in a mouse xenograft model after oral administration (Zhang et al., 2003; Lan et al., 2015). Gossypol sensitizes the antitumor activity of 5-FU, causing a synergistic cytotoxic effect in HT-29, HCT116, and RKO cells, compared with monotherapies (**Table 3**; Yang D. et al., 2015).

CONCLUSIONS

As a general rule, designing of combinations involving a traditional chemotherapy drug (or radiotherapy protocol) plus one or more natural bioactive compounds (including in some cases well-known nutraceuticals), could be a promising approach in order to potentially achieve improvements in the partial or complete remission of CRC tumors; and at the same time this could minimize side effects which could be associated with this drug treatment or radiotherapy (neutropenia, diarrhea, cardiotoxicity, nephrotoxicity, hepatotoxicity, etc.) (**Figure 3**). Most synergistic effects of these combinations have been reported in *in vitro* and using animal tumor models and are due to antioxidant bioactivity, apoptosis induction (via the mitochondrial or extrinsic pathways) and/or cell cycle arrest (at any checkpoint).

These beneficial effects due to the addition of a natural bioactive to the canonical drug treatment, are enhanced by the fact that these natural compounds and nutraceuticals can reinforce the drug effective concentration, which is needed in order to achieve the same therapeutic result. Also, interestingly, in some cases, addition of the bioactive compound may allow to overcome the intrinsic or acquired chemo- or radio-resistance occurring in some tumor cells, as these plant or fungal compounds may modulate simultaneously diverse target pathways in the neoplastic cell, overcoming those altered cell regulatory routes which may be responsible for a particular resistance mechanism.

Finally, in many cases, these bioactives are small molecular weight compounds present in medicinal plants and foods, which would allow their potential easy oral administration, independently of painful or stressful administration methods (peritoneal, catheters, etc.). In the specific case of CRC therapy, this is a fact of enormous importance, as these molecules can easily reach the transformed colon mucosa cells.

AUTHOR CONTRIBUTIONS

Introduction and resveratrol section were written by SR, flavonoids section was written by JF and IG, terpenoids section was written by CV and FL. Final revision was made by FL.

FUNDING

Authors wish to thank to MINECO (Spanish Ministry or Economy and Competitiveness) for grant AGL-2010-20622.

REFERENCES

Achenbach, T. V., Muller, R., and Slater, E. P. (2000). Bcl-2 independence of flavopiridol-induced apoptosis. Mitochondrial depolarization in the absence of cytochrome c release. *J. Biol. Chem.* 275, 32089–32097. doi: 10.1074/jbc.M005267200

Adachi, S., Nagao, T., To, S., Joe, A. K., Shimizu, M., Matsushima-Nishiwaki, R., et al. (2008). (-)-Epigallocatechin gallate causes internalization of the epidermal growth factor receptor in human colon cancer cells. *Carcinogenesis* 29, 1986–1993. doi: 10.1093/carcin/bgn128

Adachi, S., Shimizu, M., Shirakami, Y., Yamauchi, J., Natsume, H., Matsushima-Nishiwaki, R., et al. (2009). (-)-Epigallocatechin gallate downregulates EGF receptor via phosphorylation at Ser1046/1047 by p38 MAPK in colon cancer cells. *Carcinogenesis* 30, 1544–1552. doi: 10.1093/carcin/bgp166

Aggarwal, B. B., Yuan, W., Li, S., and Gupta, S. C. (2013). Curcumin-free turmeric exhibits anti-inflammatory and anticancer activities: identification of novel components of turmeric. *Mol. Nutr. Food Res.* 57, 1529–1542. doi: 10.1002/mnfr.201200838

Ali, I., and Braun, D. P. (2014). Resveratrol enhances mitomycin C-mediated suppression of human colorectal cancer cell proliferation by up-regulation of p21WAF1/CIP1. *Anticancer Res.* 34, 5439–5446.

Almasan, A., and Ashkenazi, A. (2003). Apo2L/TRAIL: apoptosis signaling, biology, and potential for cancer therapy. *Cytokine Growth Factor Rev.* 14, 337–348. doi: 10.1016/S1359-6101(03)00029-7

Ambrosini, G., Seelman, S. L., Qin, L.-X., and Schwartz, G. K. (2008). The cyclin-dependent kinase inhibitor flavopiridol potentiates the effects of topoisomerase I poisons by suppressing Rad51 expression in a p53-dependent manner. *Cancer Res.* 68, 2312–2320. doi: 10.1158/0008-5472.CAN-07-2395

Amiri, F., Zarnani, A.-H., Zand, H., Koohdani, F., Jeddi-Tehrani, M., and Vafa, M. (2013). Synergistic anti-proliferative effect of resveratrol and etoposide on human hepatocellular and colon cancer cell lines. *Eur. J. Pharmacol.* 718, 34–40. doi: 10.1016/j.ejphar.2013.09.020

Anand, P., Kunnumakkara, A. B., Newman, R. A., and Aggarwal, B. B. (2007). Bioavailability of curcumin: problems and promises. *Mol. Pharm.* 4, 807–818. doi: 10.1021/mp700113r

Anitha, A., Sreeranganathan, M., Chennazhi, K. P., Lakshmanan, V. K., and Jayakumar, R. (2014). *In vitro* combinatorial anticancer effects of 5-fluorouracil and curcumin loaded *N,O*-carboxymethyl chitosan nanoparticles toward colon cancer and *in vivo* pharmacokinetic studies. *Eur. J. Pharm. Biopharm.* 88, 238–251. doi: 10.1016/j.ejpb.2014.04.017

Bar-Sela, G., Epelbaum, R., and Schaffer, M. (2010). Curcumin as an anti-cancer agent: review of the gap between basic and clinical applications. *Curr. Med. Chem.* 17, 190–197. doi: 10.2174/092986710790149738

Bode, L. M., Bunzel, D., Huch, M., Cho, G., Ruhland, D., Bunzel, M., et al. (2013). *In vivo* and *in vitro* metabolism of trans-resveratrol by human gut microbiota. *Am. J. Clin. Nutr.* 97, 295–309. doi: 10.3945/ajcn.112.049379

Braun, M. S., and Seymour, M. T. (2011). Balancing the efficacy and toxicity of chemotherapy in colorectal cancer. *Ther. Adv. Med. Oncol.* 3, 43–52. doi: 10.1177/1758834010388342

Bray, F., Ren, J.-S., Masuyer, E., and Ferlay, J. (2013). Global estimates of cancer prevalence for 27 sites in the adult population in 2008. *Int. J. Cancer* 132, 1133–1145. doi: 10.1002/ijc.27711

Britten, C. D., Hilsenbeck, S. G., Eckhardt, S. G., Marty, J., Mangold, G., MacDonald, J. R., et al. (1999). Enhanced antitumor activity of 6-hydroxymethylacylfulvene in combination with irinotecan and 5-fluorouracil in the HT29 human colon tumor xenograft model. *Cancer Res.* 59, 1049–1053.

Brown, V. A., Patel, K. R., Viskaduraki, M., Crowell, J. A., Perloff, M., Booth, T. D., et al. (2010). Repeat dose study of the cancer chemopreventive agent resveratrol in healthy volunteers: safety, pharmacokinetics, and effect on the insulin-like growth factor axis. *Cancer Res.* 70, 9003–9011. doi: 10.1158/0008-5472.CAN-10-2364

Buhrmann, C., Shayan, P., Kraehe, P., Popper, B., Goel, A., and Shakibaei, M. (2015). Resveratrol induces chemosensitization to 5-fluorouracil through up-regulation of intercellular junctions, Epithelial-to-mesenchymal transition and apoptosis in colorectal cancer. *Biochem. Pharmacol.* 98, 51–68. doi: 10.1016/j.bcp.2015.08.105

Burns, J., Yokota, T., Ashihara, H., Lean, M. E. J., and Crozier, A. (2002). Plant foods and herbal sources of resveratrol. *J. Agric. Food Chem.* 50, 3337–3340. doi: 10.1021/jf0112973

Carnesecchi, S., Bras-Gonçalves, R., Bradaia, A., Zeisel, M., Gossé, F., Poupon, M. F., et al. (2004). Geraniol, a component of plant essential oils, modulates DNA synthesis and potentiates 5-fluorouracil efficacy on human colon tumor xenografts. *Cancer Lett.* 215, 53–59. doi: 10.1016/j.canlet.2004.06.019

Caro, A. A., and Cederbaum, A. I. (2004). Oxidative stress, toxicology, and pharmacology of CYP2E1. *Annu. Rev. Pharmacol. Toxicol.* 44, 27–42. doi: 10.1146/annurev.pharmtox.44.101802.121704

Carter, L. G., D'Orazio, J. A., and Pearson, K. J. (2014). Resveratrol and cancer: focus on *in vivo* evidence. *Endocr. Relat. Cancer* 21, R209–R225. doi: 10.1530/ERC-13-0171

Chan, J. Y., Tan, B. K. H., and Lee, S. C. (2009). Scutellarin sensitizes drug-evoked colon cancer cell apoptosis through enhanced caspase-6 activation. *Anticancer Res.* 29, 3043–3047.

Chauhan, D. P. (2002). Chemotherapeutic potential of curcumin for colorectal cancer. *Curr. Pharm. Des.* 8, 1695–1706. doi: 10.2174/1381612023394016

Cheah, K. Y., Howarth, G. S., Bindon, K. A., Kennedy, J. A., and Bastian, S. E. P. (2014). Low molecular weight procyanidins from grape seeds enhance the impact of 5-Fluorouracil chemotherapy on Caco-2 human colon cancer cells. *PLoS ONE* 9:e98921. doi: 10.1371/journal.pone.0098921

Chen, C.-C., Chow, M.-P., Huang, W.-C., Lin, Y.-C., and Chang, Y.-J. (2004). Flavonoids inhibit tumor necrosis factor-alpha-induced up-regulation of intercellular adhesion molecule-1 (ICAM-1) in respiratory epithelial cells through activator protein-1 and nuclear factor-kappaB: structure-activity relationships. *Mol. Pharmacol.* 66, 683–693. doi: 10.1124/mol.66.3

Chen, G., and Goeddel, D., V (2002). TNF-R1 signaling: a beautiful pathway. *Science* 296, 1634–1635. doi: 10.1126/science.1071924

Chen, Y. C., Yang, L. L., and Lee, T. J. F. (2000). Oroxylin A inhibition of lipopolysaccharide-induced iNOS and COX-2 gene expression via suppression of nuclear factor- kappaB activation. *Biochem. Pharmacol.* 59, 1445–1457. doi: 10.1016/S0006-2952(00)00255-0

Cho, H. J., Han, J., and Park, Y. (2013). Kaempferol induces cell cycle arrest in HT-29 human colon cancer cells. *J. Cancer Prev.* 18, 1–7. doi: 10.15430/JCP.2013.18.3.257

Chou, T. C., and Talalay, P. (1984). Quantitative analysis of dose-effect relationships: the combined effects of multiple drugs or enzyme inhibitors. *Adv. Enzyme Regul.* 22, 27–55. doi: 10.1016/0065-2571(84)90007-4

Colombo, V., Lupi, M., Falcetta, F., Forestieri, D., D'Incalci, M., and Ubezio, P. (2011). Chemotherapeutic activity of silymarin combined with doxorubicin or paclitaxel in sensitive and multidrug-resistant colon cancer cells. *Cancer Chemother. Pharmacol.* 67, 369–379. doi: 10.1007/s00280-010-1335-8

Colussi, D., Brandi, G., Bazzoli, F., and Ricciardiello, L. (2013). Molecular pathways involved in colorectal cancer: implications for disease behavior and prevention. *Int. J. Mol. Sci.* 14, 16365–16385. doi: 10.3390/ijms140816365

Darpolor, M. M., Kennealey, P. T., Le, H. C., Zakian, K. L., Ackerstaff, E., Rizwan, A., et al. (2011). Preclinical study of treatment response in HCT-116 cells and xenografts with ^{1}H-decoupled ^{31}P MRS. *NMR Biomed.* 24, 1159–1168. doi: 10.1002/nbm.1674

Dasari, S., and Tchounwou, P. B. (2014). Cisplatin in cancer therapy: molecular mechanisms of action. *Eur. J. Pharmacol.* 740, 364–378. doi: 10.1016/j.ejphar.2014.07.025

Del Follo-Martinez, A., Banerjee, N., Li, X., Safe, S., and Mertens-Talcott, S. (2013). Resveratrol and quercetin in combination have anticancer activity in colon cancer cells and repress oncogenic microRNA-27a. *Nutr. Cancer* 65, 494–504. doi: 10.1080/01635581.2012.725194

Ding, J., Polier, G., Kohler, R., Giaisi, M., Krammer, P. H., and Li-Weber, M. (2012). Wogonin and related natural flavones overcome tumor necrosis factor-related apoptosis-inducing ligand (TRAIL) protein resistance of tumors by down-regulation of c-FLIP protein and up-regulation of TRAIL receptor 2 expression. *J. Biol. Chem.* 287, 641–649. doi: 10.1074/jbc.M111.286526

Du, B., Jiang, L., Xia, Q., and Zhong, L. (2006). Synergistic inhibitory effects of curcumin and 5-fluorouracil on the growth of the human colon cancer cell line HT-29. *Chemotherapy* 52, 23–28. doi: 10.1159/000090238

Du, J., Wang, Y., Chen, D., Ji, G., Ma, Q., Liao, S., et al. (2016). BAY61-3606 potentiates the anti-tumor effects of TRAIL against colon cancer through up-regulating DR4 and down-regulating NF-κB. *Cancer Lett.* 383, 145–153. doi: 10.1016/j.canlet.2016.10.002

Engelmann, C., Blot, E., Panis, Y., Bauer, S., Trochon, V., Nagy, H. J., et al. (2002). Apigenin – strong cytostatic and anti-angiogenic action *in vitro* contrasted by lack of efficacy *in vivo*. *Phytomedicine* 9, 489–495. doi: 10.1078/09447110260573100

Erdogan, S., Doganlar, O., Doganlar, Z. B., Serttas, R., Turkekul, K., Dibirdik, I., et al. (2016). The flavonoid apigenin reduces prostate cancer CD44(+) stem cell survival and migration through PI3K/Akt/NF-κB signaling. *Life Sci.* 162, 77–86. doi: 10.1016/j.lfs.2016.08.019

Evangelou, A. M. (2002). Vanadium in cancer treatment. *Crit. Rev. Oncol. Hematol.* 42, 249–265. doi: 10.1016/S1040-8428(01)00221-9

Ferlay, J., Soerjomataram, I., Dikshit, R., Eser, S., Mathers, C., Rebelo, M., et al. (2015). Cancer incidence and mortality worldwide: sources, methods and major patterns in GLOBOCAN 2012. *Int. J. Cancer* 136, E359–E386. doi: 10.1002/ijc.29210

Fernández, J., Redondo-Blanco, S., Gutiérrez-del-Río, I., Miguélez, E. M., Villar, C. J., and Lombó, F. (2016). Colon microbiota fermentation of dietary prebiotics towards short-chain fatty acids and their roles as anti-inflammatory and antitumour agents: a review. *J. Funct. Foods* 25, 511–522. doi: 10.1016/j.jff.2016.06.032

Fidler, J. M., Li, K., Chung, C., Wei, K., Ross, J. A., Gao, M., et al. (2003). PG490-88, a derivative of triptolide, causes tumor regression and sensitizes tumors to chemotherapy. *Mol. Cancer Ther.* 2, 855–862.

Fornier, M. N., Rathkopf, D., Shah, M., Patil, S., O'Reilly, E., Tse, A. N., et al. (2007). Phase I dose-finding study of weekly docetaxel followed by flavopiridol for patients with advanced solid tumors. *Clin. Cancer Res.* 13, 5841–5846. doi: 10.1158/1078-0432.CCR-07-1218

Fuchs, C. S., Moore, M. R., Harker, G., Villa, L., Rinaldi, D., and Hecht, J. R. (2003). Phase III comparison of two irinotecan dosing regimens in second-line therapy of metastatic colorectal cancer. *J. Clin. Oncol.* 21, 807–814. doi: 10.1200/JCO.2003.08.058

Fulda, S., and Debatin, K.-M. (2004). Sensitization for anticancer drug-induced apoptosis by the chemopreventive agent resveratrol. *Oncogene* 23, 6702–6711. doi: 10.1038/sj.onc.1207630

Ganai, A. A., and Farooqi, H. (2015). Bioactivity of genistein: a review of *in vitro* and *in vivo* studies. *Biomed. Pharmacother.* 76, 30–38. doi: 10.1016/j.biopha.2015.10.026

Gao, J. L., Lv, G. Y., He, B. C., Zhang, B. Q., Zhang, H., Wang, N., et al. (2013). Ginseng saponin metabolite 20(S)-protopanaxadiol inhibits tumor growth by targeting multiple cancer signaling pathways. *Oncol. Rep.* 30, 292–298. doi: 10.3892/or.2013.2438

Gescher, A., Steward, W. P., and Brown, K. (2013). Resveratrol in the management of human cancer: how strong is the clinical evidence? *Ann. N.Y. Acad. Sci.* 1290, 12–20. doi: 10.1111/nyas.12205

Goel, A., Kunnumakkara, A. B., and Aggarwal, B. B. (2008). Curcumin as "Curecumin": from kitchen to clinic. *Biochem. Pharmacol.* 75, 787–809. doi: 10.1016/j.bcp.2007.08.016

Gruca, A., Krawczyk, Z., Szeja, W., Grynkiewicz, G., and Rusin, A. (2014). Synthetic genistein glycosides inhibiting egfr phosphorylation enhance the effect of radiation in HCT 116 colon cancer cells. *Molecules* 19, 18558–18573. doi: 10.3390/molecules191118558

Guo, J., Liu, A., Cao, H., Luo, Y., Pezzuto, J. M., and van Breemen, R. B. (2008). Biotransformation of the chemopreventive agent 2′,4′,4-trihydroxychalcone (isoliquiritigenin) by UDP-glucuronosyltransferases. *Drug Metab. Dispos.* 36, 2104–2112. doi: 10.1124/dmd.108.021857

Guo, J., Zhou, A., Fu, Y., Verma, U. N., Tripathy, D., Frenkel, E. P., et al. (2006). Efficacy of sequential treatment of HCT116 colon cancer monolayers and xenografts with docetaxel, flavopiridol, and 5-fluorouracil. *Acta Pharmacol. Sin.* 27, 1375–1381. doi: 10.1111/j.1745-7254.2006.00421.x

Gupta, S. C., Kannappan, R., Reuter, S., Kim, J. H., and Aggarwal, B. B. (2011). Chemosensitization of tumors by resveratrol. *Ann. N.Y. Acad. Sci.* 1215, 150–160. doi: 10.1111/j.1749-6632.2010.05852.x

Gupta, S. C., Patchva, S., and Aggarwal, B. B. (2013). Therapeutic roles of curcumin: lessons learned from clinical trials. *AAPS J.* 15, 195–218. doi: 10.1208/s12248-012-9432-8

Gutiérrez-del-Río, I., Villar, C. J., and Lombó, F. (2016). "Chapter 3. Therapeutic uses of kaempferol: anticancer and anti-inflammatory activity," in *Kaempferol: Biosynthesis, Food Sources and Therapeutic Uses*, eds T. Garde-Cerdán and A. Gonzalo-Diago (New York, NY: Nova Science Publishers), 71–100.

Ha, J., Zhao, L., Zhao, Q., Yao, J., Zhu, B.-B., Lu, N., et al. (2012). Oroxylin A improves the sensitivity of HT-29 human colon cancer cells to 5-FU through modulation of the COX-2 signaling pathway. *Biochem. Cell Biol.* 90, 521–531. doi: 10.1139/o2012-005

Hanif, R., Qiao, L., Shiff, S. J., and Rigas, B. (1997). Curcumin, a natural plant phenolic food additive, inhibits cell proliferation and induces cell cycle changes in colon adenocarcinoma cell lines by a prostaglandin-independent pathway. *J. Lab. Clin. Med.* 130, 576–584. doi: 10.1016/S0022-2143(97)90107-4

Harborne, J. B., and Williams, C. A. (2000). Advances in flavonoid research since 1992. *Phytochemistry* 55, 481–504. doi: 10.1016/S0031-9422(00)00235-1

Hirano, T., Oka, K., and Akiba, M. (1989). Antiproliferative effects of synthetic and naturally occurring flavonoids on tumor cells of the human breast carcinoma cell line, ZR-75-1. *Res. Commun. Chem. Pathol. Pharmacol.* 64, 69–78.

Ho, M. Y., and Mackey, J. R. (2014). Presentation and management of docetaxel-related adverse effects in patients with breast cancer. *Cancer Manag. Res.* 6, 253–259. doi: 10.2147/CMAR.S40601

Horinaka, M., Yoshida, T., Shiraishi, T., Nakata, S., Wakada, M., and Sakai, T. (2006). The dietary flavonoid apigenin sensitizes malignant tumor cells to tumor necrosis factor-related apoptosis-inducing ligand. *Mol. Cancer Ther.* 5, 945–951. doi: 10.1158/1535-7163.MCT-05-0431

Hosokawa, M., Kudo, M., Maeda, H., Kohno, H., Tanaka, T., and Miyashita, K. (2004). Fucoxanthin induces apoptosis and enhances the antiproliferative effect of the PPARgamma ligand, troglitazone, on colon cancer cells. *Biochim. Biophys. Acta* 1675, 113–119. doi: 10.1016/j.bbagen.2004.08.012

Housman, G., Byler, S., Heerboth, S., Lapinska, K., Longacre, M., Snyder, N., et al. (2014). Drug resistance in cancer: an overview. *Cancers (Basel).* 6, 1769–1792. doi: 10.3390/cancers6031769

Hu, X. J., Xie, M. Y., Kluxen, F. M., and Diel, P. (2014). Genistein modulates the anti-tumor activity of cisplatin in MCF-7 breast and HT-29 colon cancer cells. *Arch. Toxicol.* 88, 625–635. doi: 10.1007/s00204-013-1184-4

Huang, M. T., Lou, Y. R., Ma, W., Newmark, H. L., Reuhl, K. R., and Conney, A. H. (1994). Inhibitory effects of dietary curcumin on forestomach, duodenal, and colon carcinogenesis in mice. *Cancer Res.* 54, 5841–5847.

Huang, M.-T., Wang, Z. Y., Georgiadis, C. A., Laskin, J. D., and Conney, A. H. (1992). Inhibitory effects of curcumin on tumor initiation by benzo[a]pyrene and 7,12-dimethylbenz[a]anthracene. *Carcinogenesis* 13, 2183–2186. doi: 10.1093/carcin/13.11.2183

Hwang, J. T., Ha, J., and Ock, J. P. (2005). Combination of 5-fluorouracil and genistein induces apoptosis synergistically in chemo-resistant cancer cells through the modulation of AMPK and COX-2 signaling pathways. *Biochem. Biophys. Res. Commun.* 332, 433–440. doi: 10.1016/j.bbrc.2005.04.143

Hwang, J. T., Ha, J., Park, I. J., Lee, S. K., Baik, H. W., Kim, Y. M., et al. (2007b). Apoptotic effect of EGCG in HT-29 colon cancer cells via AMPK signal pathway. *Cancer Lett.* 247, 115–121. doi: 10.1016/j.canlet.2006.03.030

Hwang, J. T., Kwak, D. W., Lin, S. K., Kim, H. M., Kim, Y. M., and Park, O. J. (2007a). Resveratrol induces apoptosis in chemoresistant cancer cells via modulation of AMPK signaling pathway. *Ann. N.Y. Acad. Sci.* 1095, 441–448. doi: 10.1196/annals.1397.047

Jagetia, G. C. (2007). Recent advances in indian herbal drug research guest editor: thomas paul asir devasagayam radioprotective potential of plants and herbs against the effects of ionizing radiation. *J. Clin. Biochem. Nutr.* 40, 74–81. doi: 10.3164/jcbn.40.74

James, M. I., Iwuji, C., Irving, G., Karmokar, A., Higgins, J. A., Griffin-Teal, N., et al. (2015). Curcumin inhibits cancer stem cell phenotypes in *ex vivo* models of colorectal liver metastases, and is clinically safe and tolerable in combination with FOLFOX chemotherapy. *Cancer Lett.* 364, 135–141. doi: 10.1016/j.canlet.2015.05.005

Jang, M., Cai, L., Udeani, G. O., Slowing, K. V., Thomas, C. F., Beecher, C. W., et al. (1997). Cancer chemopreventive activity of resveratrol, a natural product derived from grapes. *Science* 275, 218–220. doi: 10.1126/science.275.5297.218

Jiang, X. H., Wong, B. C., Lin, M. C., Zhu, G. H., Kung, H. F., Jiang, S. H., et al. (2001). Functional p53 is required for triptolide-induced apoptosis and AP-1 and nuclear factor-kappaB activation in gastric cancer cells. *Oncogene* 20, 8009–8018. doi: 10.1038/sj.onc.1204981

Jin, H., Gong, W., Zhang, C., and Wang, S. (2013). Epigallocatechin gallate inhibits the proliferation of colorectal cancer cells by regulating Notch signaling. *Onco Targets Ther.* 6, 145–153. doi: 10.2147/OTT.S40914

Jin, Y. H., Choi, J. S., Shin, S., Lee, K. Y., Park, J. H., and Lee, S. K. (2003). Panaxadiol selectively inhibits cyclin A-associated Cdk2 activity by elevating p21WAF1/CIP1 protein levels in mammalian cells. *Carcinogenesis* 24, 1767–1772. doi: 10.1093/carcin/bgg097

Jung, G. R., Kim, K. J., Choi, C. H., Lee, T. B., Han, S. I., Han, H. K., et al. (2007). Effect of betulinic acid on anticancer drug-resistant colon cancer cells. *Basic Clin. Pharmacol. Toxicol.* 101, 277–285. doi: 10.1111/j.1742-7843.2007.00115.x

Kaminski, B. M., Weigert, A., Scherzberg, M.-C., Ley, S., Gilbert, B., Brecht, K., et al. (2014). Resveratrol-induced potentiation of the antitumor effects of oxaliplatin is accompanied by an altered cytokine profile of human monocyte-derived macrophages. *Apoptosis* 19, 1136–1147. doi: 10.1007/s10495-014-0988-x

Kantara, C., O'Connell, M., Sarkar, S., Moya, S., Ullrich, R., and Singh, P. (2014). Curcumin promotes autophagic survival of a subset of colon cancer stem cells, which are ablated by DCLK1-siRNA. *Cancer Res.* 74, 2487–2498. doi: 10.1158/0008-5472.CAN-13-3536

Karin, M., Yamamoto, Y., and Wang, Q. M. (2004). The IKK NF-kappa B system: a treasure trove for drug development. *Nat. Rev. Drug Discov.* 3, 17–26. doi: 10.1038/nrd1279

Kasala, E. R., Bodduluru, L. N., Madana, R. M., V, A. K., Gogoi, R., and Barua, C. C. (2015). Chemopreventive and therapeutic potential of chrysin in cancer: mechanistic perspectives. *Toxicol. Lett.* 233, 214–225. doi: 10.1016/j.toxlet.2015.01.008

Katayama, K., Masuyama, K., Yoshioka, S., Hasegawa, H., Mitsuhashi, J., and Sugimoto, Y. (2007). Flavonoids inhibit breast cancer resistance protein-mediated drug resistance: transporter specificity and structure-activity relationship. *Cancer Chemother. Pharmacol.* 60, 789–797. doi: 10.1007/s00280-007-0426-7

Kawamori, T., Lubet, R., Steele, V. E., Kelloff, G. J., Kaskey, R. B., Rao, C. V., et al. (1999). Chemopreventive effect of curcumin, a naturally occurring anti-inflammatory agent, during the promotion/progression stages of colon cancer. *Cancer Res.* 59, 597–601.

Kelland, L. R. (2000). Flavopiridol, the first cyclin-dependent kinase inhibitor to enter the clinic: current status. *Expert Opin. Investig. Drugs* 9, 2903–2911. doi: 10.1517/13543784.9.12.2903

Khan, R., Khan, A. Q., Qamar, W., Lateef, A., Tahir, M., Rehman, M. U., et al. (2012). Chrysin protects against cisplatin-induced colon. toxicity via amelioration of oxidative stress and apoptosis: probable role of p38MAPK and p53. *Toxicol. Appl. Pharmacol.* 258, 315–329. doi: 10.1016/j.taap.2011.11.013

Kim, J. M., Araki, S., Kim, D. J., Park, C. B., Takasuka, N., Baba-Toriyama, H., et al. (1998). Chemopreventive effects of carotenoids and curcumins on mouse colon carcinogenesis after 1,2-dimethylhydrazine initiation. *Carcinogenesis* 19, 81–85. doi: 10.1093/carcin/19.1.81

Kim, S. M., Lee, S. Y., Yuk, D. Y., Moon, D. C., Choi, S. S., Kim, Y., et al. (2009). Inhibition of NF-kB by ginsenoside Rg3 enhances the susceptibility of colon cancer cells to docetaxel. *Arch. Pharm. Res.* 32, 755–765. doi: 10.1007/s12272-009-1515-4

Klein-Marcuschamer, D., Ajikumar, P. K., and Stephanopoulos, G. (2007). Engineering microbial cell factories for biosynthesis of isoprenoid molecules: beyond lycopene. *Trends Biotechnol.* 25, 417–424. doi: 10.1016/j.tibtech.2007.07.006

Koh, S. J., Tak, J. K., Kim, S. T., Nam, W. S., Kim, S. Y., Park, K. M., et al. (2012). Sensitization of ionizing radiation-induced apoptosis by ursolic acid. *Free Radic. Res.* 46, 339–345. doi: 10.3109/10715762.2012.656101

Kumar, S., and Pandey, A. K. (2007). Chemistry and biological activities of flavonoids: an overview. *Sci. World J.* 73, 637–670. doi: 10.1155/2013/162750

Kumar, S., and Pandey, A. K. (2013). Chemistry and biological activities of flavonoids: an overview. *Sci. World J.* 2013:162750. doi: 10.1155/2013/162750

Kumazaki, M., Noguchi, S., Yasui, Y., Iwasaki, J., Shinohara, H., Yamada, N., et al. (2013). Anti-cancer effects of naturally occurring compounds through modulation of signal transduction and miRNA expression in human colon cancer cells. *J. Nutr. Biochem.* 24, 1849–1858. doi: 10.1016/j.jnutbio.2013.04.006

Kunnumakkara, A. B., Diagaradjane, P., Anand, P., Kuzhuvelil, H. B., Deorukhkar, A., Gelovani, J., et al. (2009). Curcumin sensitizes human colorectal cancer to capecitabine by modulation of cyclin D1, COX-2, MMP-9, VEGF and CXCR4 expression in an orthotopic mouse model. *Int. J. Cancer* 125, 2187–2197. doi: 10.1002/ijc.24593

Lan, L., Appelman, C., Smith, A. R., Yu, J., Larsen, S., Marquez, R. T., et al. (2015). Natural product (-)-gossypol inhibits colon cancer cell growth by targeting RNA-binding protein Musashi-1. *Mol. Oncol.* 9, 1406–1420. doi: 10.1016/j.molonc.2015.03.014

Lee, C. K., Son, S. H., Park, K. K., Park, J. H. Y., Lim, S. S., and Chung, W. Y. (2008). Isoliquiritigenin inhibits tumor growth and protects the kidney and liver against chemotherapy-induced toxicity in a mouse xenograft model of colon carcinoma. *J. Pharmacol. Sci.* 106, 444–451. doi: 10.1254/jphs.FP0071498

Lee, H. S., Cho, H. J., Kwon, G. T., Han, J., and Park, Y. (2014a). Kaempferol Downregulates Insulin-like growth factor-I receptor and ErbB3 signaling in HT-29 human colon cancer cells. *J. Cancer Prev.* 19, 161–169. doi: 10.15430/JCP.2014.19.3.161

Lee, H. S., Cho, H. J., Yu, R., Lee, K. W., Chun, H. S., and Park, J. H. Y. (2014b). Mechanisms underlying apoptosis-inducing effects of kaempferol in HT-29 human colon cancer cells. *Int. J. Mol. Sci.* 15, 2722–2737. doi: 10.3390/ijms15022722

Lee, J. I., Hsu, B. H., Wu, D., and Barrett, J. S. (2006). Separation and characterization of silybin, isosilybin, silydianin and silychristin in milk thistle extract by liquid chromatography-electrospray tandem mass spectrometry. *J. Chromatogr. A* 1116, 57–68. doi: 10.1016/j.chroma.2006.03.053

Lee, Y., Sung, B., Kang, Y. J., Kim, D. H., Jang, J. Y., Hwang, S. Y., et al. (2014). Apigenin-induced apoptosis is enhanced by inhibition of autophagy formation in HCT116 human colon cancer cells. *Int. J. Oncol.* 44, 1599–1606. doi: 10.3892/ijo.2014.2339

Lefort, É. C., and Blay, J. (2011). The dietary flavonoid apigenin enhances the activities of the anti-metastatic protein CD26 on human colon carcinoma cells. *Clin. Exp. Metastasis* 28, 337–349. doi: 10.1007/s10585-010-9364-6

León, I. E., Cadavid-Vargas, J. F., Tiscornia, I., Porro, V., Castelli, S., Katkar, P., et al. (2015). Oxidovanadium(IV) complexes with chrysin and silibinin: anticancer activity and mechanisms of action in a human colon adenocarcinoma model. *J. Biol. Inorg. Chem.* 20, 1175–1191. doi: 10.1007/s00775-015-1298-7

Li, L., Ahmed, B., Mehta, K., and Kurzrock, R. (2007). Liposomal curcumin with and without oxaliplatin: effects on cell growth, apoptosis, and angiogenesis in colorectal cancer. *Mol. Cancer Ther.* 6, 1276–1282. doi: 10.1158/1535-7163.MCT-06-0556

Li, W., Du, B., Wang, T., Wang, S., and Zhang, J. (2009). Kaempferol induces apoptosis in human HCT116 colon cancer cells via the Ataxia-Telangiectasia mutated-p53 pathway with the involvement of p53 upregulated modulator of apoptosis. *Chem. Biol. Interact.* 177, 121–127. doi: 10.1016/j.cbi.2008.10.048

Li, X., Huang, Q., Ong, C.-N., Yang, X.-F., and Shen, H.-M. (2010). Chrysin sensitizes tumor necrosis factor-α-induced apoptosis in human tumor cells via suppression of nuclear factor-kappaB. *Cancer Lett.* 293, 109–116. doi: 10.1016/j.canlet.2010.01.002

Li, X. L., Wang, C. Z., Mehendale, S. R., Sun, S., Wang, Q., and Yuan, C. S. (2009). Panaxadiol, a purified ginseng component, enhances the anti-cancer effects of 5-fluorouracil in human colorectal cancer cells. *Cancer Chemother. Pharmacol.* 64, 1097–1104. doi: 10.1007/s00280-009-0966-0

Liu, W. M., Gravett, A. M., and Dalgleish, A. G. (2011). The antimalarial agent artesunate possesses anticancer properties that can be enhanced by combination strategies. *Int. J. Cancer* 128, 1471–1480. doi: 10.1002/ijc.25707

Liu, Y., Xiao, E., Yuan, L., and Li, G. (2014). Triptolide synergistically enhances antitumor activity of oxaliplatin in colon carcinoma *in vitro* and *in vivo*. *DNA Cell Biol.* 33, 418–425. doi: 10.1089/dna.2014.2356

Luo, Y., Wang, S.-X., Zhou, Z.-Q., Wang, Z., Zhang, Y.-G., Zhang, Y., et al. (2014). Apoptotic effect of genistein on human colon cancer cells via inhibiting the nuclear factor-kappa B (NF-B) pathway. *Tumour Biol.* 35, 11483–11488. doi: 10.1007/s13277-014-2487-7

Majumdar, A. P. N., Banerjee, S., Nautiyal, J., Patel, B. B., Patel, V., Du, J., et al. (2009). Curcumin synergizes with resveratrol to inhibit colon cancer. *Nutr. Cancer* 61, 544–553. doi: 10.1080/01635580902752262

Manach, C., Scalbert, A., Morand, C., Rémésy, C., and Jiménez, L. (2004). Polyphenols: food sources and bioavailability. *Am. J. Clin. Nutr.* 79, 727–747.

Marín, L., Miguélez, E. M., Villar, C. J., and Lombó, F. (2015). Bioavailability of dietary polyphenols and gut microbiota metabolism: antimicrobial properties. *Biomed Res. Int.* 2015:905215. doi: 10.1155/2015/905215

Merrill, R. M., and Anderson, A. E. (2011). Risk-adjusted colon and rectal cancer incidence rates in the United States. *Dis. Colon Rectum* 54, 1301–1306. doi: 10.1097/DCR.0b013e3182242bd3

Mertens-Talcott, S. U., and Percival, S. S. (2005). Ellagic acid and quercetin interact synergistically with resveratrol in the induction of apoptosis and cause transient cell cycle arrest in human leukemia cells. *Cancer Lett.* 218, 141–151. doi: 10.1016/j.canlet.2004.06.007

Meshnick, S. R. (2002). Artemisinin: mechanisms of action, resistance and toxicity. *Int. J. Parasitol.* 32, 1655–1660. doi: 10.1016/S0020-7519(02)00194-7

Misawa, N. (2011). Pathway engineering for functional isoprenoids. *Curr. Opin. Biotechnol.* 22, 627–633. doi: 10.1016/j.copbio.2011.01.002

Miyamoto, S., Kohno, H., Suzuki, R., Sugie, S., Murakami, A., Ohigashi, H., et al. (2006). Preventive effects of chrysin on the development of azoxymethane-induced colonic aberrant crypt foci in rats. *Oncol. Rep.* 15, 1169–1173. doi: 10.3892/or.15.5.1169

Miyamoto, S., Yasui, Y., Ohigashi, H., Tanaka, T., and Murakami, A. (2010). Dietary flavonoids suppress azoxymethane-induced colonic preneoplastic lesions in male C57BL/KsJ-db/db mice. *Chem. Biol. Interact.* 183, 276–283. doi: 10.1016/j.cbi.2009.11.002

Mizushina, Y., Shiomi, K., Kuriyama, I., Takahashi, Y., and Yoshida, H. (2013). Inhibitory effects of a major soy isoflavone, genistein, on human DNA topoisomerase II activity and cancer cell proliferation. *Int. J. Oncol.* 43, 1117–1124. doi: 10.3892/ijo.2013.2032

Mohapatra, P., Preet, R., Choudhuri, M., Choudhuri, T., and Kundu, C. N. (2011). 5-fluorouracil increases the chemopreventive potentials of resveratrol through DNA damage and MAPK signaling pathway in human colorectal cancer cells. *Oncol. Res.* 19, 311–321. doi: 10.3727/096504011X13079697132844

Morin, P. J., Sparks, A. B., Korinek, V., Barker, N., Clevers, H., Vogelstein, B., et al. (1997). Activation of beta-catenin-Tcf signaling in colon cancer by mutations in beta-catenin or APC. *Science* 275, 1787–1790. doi: 10.1126/science.275.5307.1787

Morris, J., Moseley, V. R., Cabang, A. B., Coleman, K., Wei, W., Garrett-Mayer, E., et al. (2016). Reduction in promotor methylation utilizing EGCG (Epigallocatechin-3-gallate) restores RXRalpha expression in human colon cancer cells. *Oncotarget* 7, 11–17. doi: 10.18632/oncotarget.9204

Moseley, V. R., Morris, J., Knackstedt, R. W., and Wargovich, M. J. (2013). Green tea polyphenol epigallocatechin 3-gallate, contributes to the degradation of DNMT3A and HDAC3 in HCT 116 human colon cancer cells. *Anticancer Res.* 33, 5325–5334.

Motwani, M., Jung, C., Sirotnak, F. M., She, Y., Shah, M. A., Gonen, M., et al. (2001). Augmentation of apoptosis and tumor regression by flavopiridol in the presence of CPT-11 in Hct116 colon cancer monolayers and xenografts. *Clin. Cancer Res.* 7, 4209–4219.

Murakami, A., Furukawa, I., Miyamoto, S., Tanaka, T., and Ohigashi, H. (2013). Curcumin combined with turmerones, essential oil components of turmeric, abolishes inflammation-associated mouse colon carcinogenesis. *Biofactors* 39, 221–232. doi: 10.1002/biof.1054

Nautiyal, J., Kanwar, S. S., Yu, Y., and Majumdar, A. P. (2011). Combination of dasatinib and curcumin eliminates chemo-resistant colon cancer cells. *J. Mol. Signal.* 6:7. doi: 10.1186/1750-2187-6-7

Newcomb, E. W. (2004). Flavopiridol: pleiotropic biological effects enhance its anti-cancer activity. *Anticancer Drugs* 15, 411–419. doi: 10.1097/01.cad.0000127332.06439.47

Ohishi, T., Kishimot, Y., Hara, Y., Hasegawa, J., and Isemura, M. (2002). Synergistic effects of (-)-epigallocatechin gallate with sulindac against colon carcinogenesis of rats treated with azoxymethane. *Cancer Lett.* 177, 118–121. doi: 10.1016/S0304-3835(01)00767-4

Osman, N. H. A., Said, U. Z., El-Waseef, A. M., and Ahmed, E. S. A. (2015). Luteolin supplementation adjacent to aspirin treatment reduced dimethylhydrazine-induced experimental colon carcinogenesis in rats. *Tumour Biol.* 36, 1179–1190. doi: 10.1007/s13277-014-2678-2

Pampaloni, B., Palmini, G., Mavilia, C., Zonefrati, R., Tanini, A., and Brandi, M. L. (2014). *In vitro* effects of polyphenols on colorectal cancer cells. *World J. Gastrointest. Oncol.* 6, 289–300. doi: 10.4251/wjgo.v6.i8.289

Pan, M.-H., Lai, C.-S., Wu, J.-C., and Ho, C.-T. (2011). Molecular mechanisms for chemoprevention of colorectal cancer by natural dietary compounds. *Mol. Nutr. Food Res.* 55, 32–45. doi: 10.1002/mnfr.201000412

Park, J. H., Oh, E. J., Choi, Y. H., Kang, C. D., Kang, H. S., Kim, D. K., et al. (2001). Synergistic effects of dexamethasone and genistein on the expression of Cdk inhibitor p21WAF1/CIP1 in human hepatocellular and colorectal carcinoma cells. *Int. J. Oncol.* 18, 997–1002. doi: 10.3892/ijo.18.5.997

Park, M. T., Cha, H. J., Jeong, J. W., Kim, S. I., Chung, H. Y., Kim, N. D., et al. (1999). Glucocorticoid receptor-induced down-regulation of MMP-9 by ginseng components, PD and PT contributes to inhibition of the invasive capacity of HT1080 human fibrosarcoma cells. *Mol. Cells* 9, 476–483.

Patel, B. B., Sengupta, R., Qazi, S., Vachhani, H., Yu, Y., Rishi, A. K., et al. (2008). Curcumin enhances the effects of 5-fluorouracil and oxaliplatin in mediating growth inhibition of colon cancer cells by modulating EGFR and IGF-1R. *Int. J. Cancer* 122, 267–273. doi: 10.1002/ijc.23097

Patel, K. R., Brown, V. A., Jones, D. J. L., Britton, R. G., Hemingway, D., Miller, A. S., et al. (2010). Clinical pharmacology of resveratrol and its metabolites in colorectal cancer patients. *Cancer Res.* 70, 7392–7399. doi: 10.1158/0008-5472.CAN-10-2027

Pavlidis, E. T., and Pavlidis, T. E. (2013). Role of bevacizumab in colorectal cancer growth and its adverse effects: a review. *World J. Gastroenterol.* 19, 5051–5060. doi: 10.3748/wjg.v19.i31.5051

Perkins, S., Verschoyle, R. D., Hill, K., Parveen, I., Threadgill, M. D., Sharma, R. A., et al. (2002). Chemopreventive efficacy and pharmacokinetics of curcumin in the min/+ mouse, a model of familial adenomatous polyposis. *Cancer Epidemiol. Biomarkers Prev.* 11, 535–540.

Poindessous, V., Koeppel, F., Raymond, E., Cvitkovic, E., Waters, S. J., and Larsen, A. K. (2003). Enhanced antitumor activity of irofulven in combination with 5-fluorouracil and cisplatin in human colon and ovarian carcinoma cells. *Int. J. Oncol.* 23, 1347–1355. doi: 10.3892/ijo.23.5.1347

Prasad, S., Tyagi, A. K., and Aggarwal, B. B. (2014). Recent developments in delivery, bioavailability, absorption and metabolism of curcumin: the golden pigment from golden spice. *Cancer Res. Treat.* 46, 2–18. doi: 10.4143/crt.2014.46.1.2

Prasad, S., Yadav, V. R., Sung, B., Reuter, S., Kannappan, R., Deorukhkar, A., et al. (2012). Ursolic acid inhibits growth and metastasis of human, colorectal cancer in an orthotopic nude mouse model by targeting multiple cell signaling pathways: chemosensitization with capecitabine. *Clin. Cancer Res.* 18, 4942–4953. doi: 10.1158/1078-0432.CCR-11-2805

Psahoulia, F. H., Drosopoulos, K. G., Doubravska, L., Andera, L., and Pintzas, A. (2007). Quercetin enhances TRAIL-mediated apoptosis in colon cancer cells by inducing the accumulation of death receptors in lipid rafts. *Mol. Cancer Ther.* 6, 2591–2599. doi: 10.1158/1535-7163.MCT-07-0001

Ranelletti, F. O., Maggiano, N., Serra, F. G., Ricci, R., Larocca, L. M., Lanza, P., et al. (2000). Quercetin inhibits p21-RAS expression in human colon cancer cell lines and in primary colorectal tumors. *Int. J. Cancer* 85, 438–445. doi: 10.1002/(SICI)1097-0215(20000201)85:3<438::AID-IJC22>3.0.CO;2-F

Rao, C. V., Simi, B., and Reddy, B. S. (1993). Inhibition by dietary curcumin of azoxymethane-induced ornithine decarboxylase, tyrosine protein kinase, arachidonic acid metabolism and aberrant crypt foci formation in the rat colon. *Carcinogenesis* 14, 2219–2225. doi: 10.1093/carcin/14.11.2219

Ravindran, J., Prasad, S., and Aggarwal, B. B. (2009). Curcumin and cancer cells: how many ways can curry kill tumor cells selectively? *AAPS J.* 11, 495–510. doi: 10.1208/s12248-009-9128-x

Reddivari, L., Charepalli, V., Radhakrishnan, S., Vadde, R., Elias, R. J., Lambert, J. D., et al. (2016). Grape compounds suppress colon cancer stem cells *in vitro* and in a rodent model of colon carcinogenesis. *BMC Complement. Altern. Med.* 16:278. doi: 10.1186/s12906-016-1254-2

Renuka, M., Vijayakumar, N., and Ramakrishnan, A. (2016). Chrysin, a flavonoid attenuates histological changes of hyperammonemic rats: a dose dependent study. *Biomed. Pharmacother.* 82, 345–354. doi: 10.1016/j.biopha.2016.05.013

Romier, B., Van De Walle, J., During, A., Larondelle, Y., and Schneider, Y.-J. (2008). Modulation of signalling nuclear factor-kappaB activation pathway by polyphenols in human intestinal Caco-2 cells. *Br. J. Nutr.* 100, 542–551. doi: 10.1017/S0007114508966666

Ronnekleiv-Kelly, S. M., Geiger, P. G., and Kennedy, G. D. (2012). Chrysin activates the aryl hydrocarbon receptor and reduces colon cancer cell viability. *J. Surg. Res.* 172:305. doi: 10.1016/j.jss.2011.11.536

Rossi, M., Negri, E., Talamini, R., Bosetti, C., Parpinel, M., Gnagnarella, P., et al. (2006). Flavonoids and colorectal cancer in Italy. *Cancer Epidemiol. Biomarkers Prev.* 15, 1555–1558. doi: 10.1158/1055-9965.EPI-06-0017

Rotches-Ribalta, M., Andres-Lacueva, C., Estruch, R., Escribano, E., and Urpi-Sarda, M. (2012). Pharmacokinetics of resveratrol metabolic profile in healthy humans after moderate consumption of red wine and grape extract tablets. *Pharmacol. Res.* 66, 375–382. doi: 10.1016/j.phrs.2012.08.001

Saldanha, S. N., Kala, R., and Tollefsbol, T. O. (2014). Molecular mechanisms for inhibition of colon cancer cells by combined epigenetic-modulating epigallocatechin gallate and sodium butyrate. *Exp. Cell Res.* 324, 40–53. doi: 10.1016/j.yexcr.2014.01.024

Santandreu, F. M., Valle, A., Oliver, J., and Roca, P. (2011). Resveratrol potentiates the cytotoxic oxidative stress induced by chemotherapy in human colon cancer cells. *Cell. Physiol. Biochem.* 28, 219–228. doi: 10.1159/000331733

Serova, M., Calvo, F., Lokiec, F., Koeppel, F., Poindessous, V., Larsen, A. K., et al. (2006). Characterizations of irofulven cytotoxicity in combination with cisplatin and oxaliplatin in human colon, breast, and ovarian cancer cells. *Cancer Chemother. Pharmacol.* 57, 491–499. doi: 10.1007/s00280-005-0063-y

Shao, H., Jing, K., Mahmoud, E., Huang, H., Fang, X., and Yu, C. (2013). Apigenin sensitizes colon cancer cells to antitumor activity of ABT-263. *Mol. Cancer Ther.* 12, 2640–2650. doi: 10.1158/1535-7163.MCT-13-0066

Shi, M.-D., Shiao, C.-K., Lee, Y.-C., and Shih, Y.-W. (2015). Apigenin, a dietary flavonoid, inhibits proliferation of human bladder cancer T-24 cells via blocking cell cycle progression and inducing apoptosis. *Cancer Cell Int.* 15:33. doi: 10.1186/s12935-015-0186-0

Shimizu, M., Deguchi, A., Lim, J. E., Moriwaki, H., Kopelovich, L., and Weinstein, I. B. (2005). (-)-Epigallocatechin gallate and polyphenon e inhibit growth and activation of the epidermal growth factor receptor and human epidermal growth factor receptor-2 signaling pathways in human colon cancer cells. *Clin. Cancer Res.* 11, 2735–2746. doi: 10.1158/1078-0432.ccr-04-2014

Singh, B. N., Shankar, S., and Srivastava, R. K. (2011). Green tea catechin, epigallocatechin-3-gallate (EGCG): mechanisms, perspectives and clinical applications. *Biochem. Pharmacol.* 82, 1807–1821. doi: 10.1016/j.bcp.2011.07.093

Singh, C. K., George, J., and Ahmad, N. (2013). Resveratrol-based combinatorial strategies for cancer management. *Ann. N.Y. Acad. Sci.* 1290, 113–121. doi: 10.1111/nyas.12160

Singh, D., Attri, B. K., Gill, R. K., and Bariwal, J. (2016). Review on EGFR inhibitors: critical updates. *Mini Rev. Med. Chem.* 16, 1134–1166. doi: 10.2174/1389557516666160321114917

Son, T., Gong, E., Bae, M., Kim, S., Heo, K., Moon, C., et al. (2013). Protective effect of genistein on radiation-induced intestinal injury in tumor bearing mice. *BMC Complement. Altern. Med.* 13:103. doi: 10.1186/1472-6882-13-103

Sparks, A. B., Morin, P. J., Vogelstein, B., and Kinzler, K. W. (1998). Mutational analysis of the APC/beta-catenin/Tcf pathway in colorectal cancer. *Cancer Res.* 58, 1130–1134.

Spector, D., Anthony, M., Alexander, D., and Arab, L. (2003). Soy consumption and colorectal cancer. *Nutr. Cancer* 47, 1–12. doi: 10.1207/s15327914nc4701_1

Srimuangwong, K., Tocharus, C., Chintana, P. Y., Suksamrarn, A., and Tocharus, J. (2012a). Hexahydrocurcumin enhances inhibitory effect of 5-fluorouracil on HT-29 human colon cancer cells. *World J. Gastroenterol.* 18, 2383–2389. doi: 10.3748/wjg.v18.i19.2383

Srimuangwong, K., Tocharus, C., Tocharus, J., Suksamrarn, A., and Chintana, P. Y. (2012b). Effects of hexahydrocurcumin in combination with 5-fuorouracil on dimethylhydrazine-induced colon cancer in rats. *World J. Gastroenterol.* 18, 6951–6959. doi: 10.3748/wjg.v18.i47.6951

Suganuma, M., Okabe, S., Kai, Y., Sueoka, N., Sueoka, E., and Fujiki, H. (1999). Synergistic effects of (−)-epigallocatechin gallate with (−)-epicatechin, sulindac, or tamoxifen on cancer-preventive activity in the human lung cancer cell line PC-9. *Cancer Res.* 59, 44–47.

Takada, Y., and Aggarwal, B. B. (2004). Flavopiridol inhibits NF-kappaB activation induced by various carcinogens and inflammatory agents through inhibition of IkappaBalphakinase and p65 phosphorylation. Abrogation of cyclin D1, cyclooxygenase-2, and matrix metalloprotease-9. *J. Biol. Chem.* 279, 4750–4759. doi: 10.1074/jbc.M304546200

Tallarida, R. J. (2002). The interaction index: a measure of drug synergism. *Pain* 98, 163–168. doi: 10.1016/S0304-3959(02)00041-6

Tang, X., Zhu, Y., Tao, W., Wei, B., and Lin, X. (2007). Synergistic effect of triptolide combined with 5-fluorouracil on colon carcinoma. *Postgrad. Med. J.* 83, 338–343. doi: 10.1136/pgmj.2006.055426

Thorn, C. F., Oshiro, C., Marsh, S., Hernandez-Boussard, T., McLeod, H., Klein, T. E., et al. (2011). Doxorubicin pathways: pharmacodynamics and adverse effects. *Pharmacogenet. Genomics* 21, 440–446. doi: 10.1097/FPC.0b013e32833ffb56

Tolba, M. F., and Abdel-Rahman, S. Z. (2015). Pterostilbine, an active component of blueberries, sensitizes colon cancer cells to 5-fluorouracil cytotoxicity. *Sci. Rep.* 5:15239. doi: 10.1038/srep15239

Tolcher, A. W., LoRusso, P., Arzt, J., Busman, T. A., Lian, G., Rudersdorf, N. S., et al. (2015). Safety, efficacy, and pharmacokinetics of navitoclax (ABT-263) in combination with irinotecan: results of an open-label, phase 1 study. *Cancer Chemother. Pharmacol.* 76, 1041–1049. doi: 10.1007/s00280-015-2882-9

Tsai, C.-C., Chuang, T.-W., Chen, L.-J., Niu, H.-S., Chung, K.-M., Cheng, J.-T., et al. (2015). Increase in apoptosis by combination of metformin with silibinin in human colorectal cancer cells. *World J. Gastroenterol.* 21, 4169–4177. doi: 10.3748/wjg.v21.i14.4169

Tsai, Y. M., Chien, C. F., Lin, L. C., and Tsai, T. H. (2011). Curcumin and its nano-formulation: the kinetics of tissue distribution and blood-brain barrier penetration. *Int. J. Pharm.* 416, 331–338. doi: 10.1016/j.ijpharm.2011.06.030

van der Stok, E. P., Spaander, M. C. W., Grünhagen, D. J., Verhoef, C., and Kuipers, E. J. (2016). Surveillance after curative treatment for colorectal cancer. *Nat. Rev. Clin. Oncol.* doi: 10.1038/nrclinonc.2016.199. [Epub ahead of print].

Vieira, A., Heidor, R., Cardozo, M. T., Scolastici, C., Purgatto, E., Shiga, T. M., et al. (2011). Efficacy of geraniol but not of β-ionone or their combination for the chemoprevention of rat colon carcinogenesis. *Brazilian J. Med. Biol. Res.* 44, 538–545. doi: 10.1590/S0100-879X2011000600007

Walle, T., Hsieh, F., DeLegge, M. H., Oatis, J. E., and Walle, U. K. (2004). High absorption but very low bioavailability of oral resveratrol in humans. *Drug Metab. Dispos.* 32, 1377–1382. doi: 10.1124/dmd.104.000885

Wang, C. Z., Luo, X., Zhang, B., Song, W. X., Ni, M., Mehendale, S., et al. (2007a). Notoginseng enhances anti-cancer effect of 5-fluorouracil on human colorectal cancer cells. *Cancer Chemother. Pharmacol.* 60, 69–79. doi: 10.1007/s00280-006-0350-2

Wang, C. Z., Xie, J. T., Zhang, B., Ni, M., Fishbein, A., Aung, H. H., et al. (2007b). Chemopreventive effects of Panax notoginseng and its major constituents on SW480 human colorectal cancer cells. *Int. J. Oncol.* 31, 1149–1156.

Wang, C. Z., Zhang, Z., Wan, J. Y., Zhang, C. F., Anderson, S., He, X., et al. (2015). Protopanaxadiol, an active ginseng metabolite, significantly enhances the effects of fluorouracil on colon cancer. *Nutrients* 7, 799–814. doi: 10.3390/nu7020799

Wang, W., VanAlstyne, P. C., Irons, K. A., Chen, S., Stewart, J. W., and Birt, D. F. (2004). Individual and interactive effects of apigenin analogs on G2/M cell-cycle arrest in human colon carcinoma cell lines. *Nutr. Cancer* 48, 106–114. doi: 10.1207/s15327914nc4801_14

Wubetu, G. Y., Shimada, M., Morine, Y., Ikemoto, T., Ishikawa, D., Iwahashi, S., et al. (2015). Epigallocatechin gallate hinders human hepatoma and colon cancer sphere formation. *J. Gastroenterol. Hepatol.* 31, 256–264. doi: 10.1111/jgh.13069

Xavier, C. P. R., Lima, C. F., Rohde, M., and Pereira-Wilson, C. (2011). Quercetin enhances 5-fluorouracil-induced apoptosis in MSI colorectal cancer cells through p53 modulation. *Cancer Chemother. Pharmacol.* 68, 1449–1457. doi: 10.1007/s00280-011-1641-9

Xiao, X., Liu, Z., Wang, R., Wang, J., Zhang, S., Cai, X., et al. (2015). Genistein suppresses FLT4 and inhibits human colorectal cancer metastasis. *Oncotarget* 6, 3225–3239. doi: 10.18632/oncotarget.3064

Xing, J., You, H., Dong, Y., Lu, J., Chen, S., Zhu, H., et al. (2011). Metabolic and pharmacokinetic studies of scutellarin in rat plasma, urine, and feces. *Acta Pharmacol. Sin.* 32, 655–663. doi: 10.1038/aps.2011.11

Yallapu, M. M., Jaggi, M., and Chauhan, S. C. (2012). Curcumin nanoformulations: a future nanomedicine for cancer. *Drug Discov. Today* 17, 71–80. doi: 10.1016/j.drudis.2011.09.009

Yang, D., Qu, J., Qu, X., Cao, Y., Xu, L., Hou, K., et al. (2015). Gossypol sensitizes the antitumor activity of 5-FU through down-regulation of thymidylate synthase in human colon carcinoma cells. *Cancer Chemother. Pharmacol.* 76, 575–586. doi: 10.1007/s00280-015-2749-0

Yang, L., Allred, K. F., Dykes, L., Allred, C. D., and Awika, J. M. (2015). Enhanced action of apigenin and naringenin combination on estrogen receptor activation in non-malignant colonocytes: implications on sorghum-derived phytoestrogens. *Food Funct.* 6, 749–755. doi: 10.1039/C4FO00300D

Yang, M. H., Kim, J., Khan, I. A., Walker, L. A., and Khan, S. I. (2014). Nonsteroidal anti-inflammatory drug activated gene-1 (NAG-1) modulators from natural products as anti-cancer agents. *Life Sci.* 100, 75–84. doi: 10.1016/j.lfs.2014.01.075

Yang, S., Li, W., Sun, H., Wu, B., Ji, F., Sun, T., et al. (2015). Resveratrol elicits anti-colorectal cancer effect by activating miR-34c-KITLG *in vitro* and *in vivo*. *BMC Cancer* 15:969. doi: 10.1186/s12885-015-1958-6

Yoshida, T., Konishi, M., Horinaka, M., Yasuda, T., Goda, A. E., Taniguchi, H., et al. (2008). Kaempferol sensitizes colon cancer cells to TRAIL-induced apoptosis. *Biochem. Biophys. Res. Commun.* 375, 129–133. doi: 10.1016/j.bbrc.2008.07.131

Yu, Z., Li, W., and Liu, F. (2004). Inhibition of proliferation and induction of apoptosis by genistein in colon cancer HT-29 cells. *Cancer Lett.* 215, 159–166. doi: 10.1016/j.canlet.2004.06.010

Yue, G. G. L., Jiang, L., Kwok, H. F., Lee, J. K. M., Chan, K. M., Fung, K. P., et al. (2016b). Turmeric ethanolic extract possesses stronger inhibitory activities on colon tumour growth than curcumin - the importance of turmerones. *J. Funct. Foods* 22, 565–577. doi: 10.1016/j.jff.2016.02.011

Yue, G. G. L., Kwok, H.-F., Lee, J. K.-M., Jiang, L., Wong, E. C.-W., Gao, S., et al. (2016a). Combined therapy using bevacizumab and turmeric ethanolic extract (with absorbable curcumin) exhibited beneficial efficacy in colon cancer mice. *Pharmacol. Res.* 111, 43–57. doi: 10.1016/j.phrs.2016.05.025

Zhang, M., Liu, H., Guo, R., Ling, Y., Wu, X., Li, B., et al. (2003). Molecular mechanism of gossypol-induced cell growth inhibition and cell death of HT-29 human colon carcinoma cells. *Biochem. Pharmacol.* 66, 93–103. doi: 10.1016/S0006-2952(03)00248-X

Zhang, Y., Li, Q., Zhou, D., and Chen, H. (2013). Genistein, a soya isoflavone, prevents azoxymethane-induced up-regulation of WNT/β-catenin signalling and reduces colon pre-neoplasia in rats. *Br. J. Nutr.* 109, 33–42. doi: 10.1017/S0007114512000876

Zhong, Y., Krisanapun, C., Lee, S. H., Nualsanit, T., Sams, C., Peungvicha, P., et al. (2010). Molecular targets of apigenin in colorectal cancer cells: involvement of p21, NAG-1 and p53. *Eur. J. Cancer* 46, 3365–3374. doi: 10.1016/j.ejca.2010.07.007

Zhou, F., Zhou, H., Wang, T., Mu, Y., Wu, B., Guo, D., et al. (2012). Epigallocatechin-3-gallate inhibits proliferation and migration of human colon cancer SW620 cells *in vitro*. *Acta Pharmacol. Sin.* 33, 120–126. doi: 10.1038/aps.2011.139

Zhu, H., Ding, W.-J., Wu, R., Weng, Q.-J., Lou, J.-S., Jin, R.-J., et al. (2010). Synergistic anti-cancer activity by the combination of TRAIL/APO-2L and celastrol. *Cancer Invest.* 28, 23–32. doi: 10.3109/07357900903095664

Conflict of Interest Statement: The authors declare that the research was conducted in the absence of any commercial or financial relationships that could be construed as a potential conflict of interest.

10

Profile of Antiemetic Activity of Netupitant Alone or in Combination with Palonosetron and Dexamethasone in *Ferrets* and *Suncus murinus* (House Musk Shrew)

John A. Rudd[1,2], Man P. Ngan[1], Zengbing Lu[1], Guy A. Higgins[3], Claudio Giuliano[4], Emanuela Lovati[4] and Claudio Pietra[4]*

[1] *Emesis Research Group, School of Biomedical Sciences, Faculty of Medicine, The Chinese University of Hong Kong, Hong Kong, China,* [2] *Brain and Mind Institute, The Chinese University of Hong Kong, Hong Kong, China,* [3] *Intervivo Solutions Inc., Toronto, ON, Canada,* [4] *Research and Preclinical, Helsinn Healthcare SA., Lugano, Switzerland*

Edited by:
Raquel Abalo,
King Juan Carlos University, Spain

Reviewed by:
Rosane Vianna-Jorge,
Instituto Nacional do Câncer, Brazil
Lorand Bartho,
University of Pécs, Hungary
Joel C. Bornstein,
University of Melbourne, Australia

****Correspondence:***
John A. Rudd
jar@cuhk.edu.hk

Background and Aims: Chemotherapy-induced acute and delayed emesis involves the activation of multiple pathways, with 5-hydroxytryptamine (5-HT; serotonin) playing a major role in the initial response. Substance P tachykinin NK_1 receptor antagonists can reduce emesis induced by disparate emetic challenges and therefore have a clinical utility as broad inhibitory anti-emetic drugs. In the present studies, we investigate the broad inhibitory anti-emetic profile of a relatively new NK_1 receptor antagonist, netupitant, alone or in combination with the long acting $5\text{-}HT_3$ receptor antagonist, palonosetron, for a potential to reduce emesis in ferrets and shrews.

Materials and Methods: Ferrets were pretreated with netupitant and/or palonosetron, and then administered apomorphine (0.125 mg/kg, s.c.), morphine (0.5 mg/kg, s.c.), ipecacuanha (1.2 mg/kg, p.o.), copper sulfate (100 mg/kg, intragastric), or cisplatin (5–10 mg/kg, i.p.); in other studies netupitant was administered to *Suncus murinus* before motion (4 cm horizontal displacement, 2 Hz for 10 min).

Results: Netupitant (3 mg/kg, p.o.) abolished apomorphine-, morphine-, ipecacuanha- and copper sulfate-induced emesis. Lower doses of netupitant (0.03–0.3 mg/kg, p.o.) dose-dependently reduced cisplatin (10 mg/kg, i.p.)-induced emesis in an acute (8 h) model, and motion-induced emesis in *S. murinus*. In a ferret cisplatin (5 mg/kg, i.p.)-induced acute and delayed emesis model, netupitant administered once at 3 mg/kg, p.o., abolished the first 24 h response and reduced the 24–72 h response by 94.6%; the reduction was markedly superior to the effect of a three times per day administration of ondansetron (1 mg/kg, i.p.). A single administration of netupitant (1 mg/kg, p.o.) plus palonosetron (0.1 mg/kg, p.o.) combined with dexamethasone (1 mg/kg, i.p., once per day), also significantly antagonized cisplatin-induced acute and delayed emesis and was comparable with a once-daily regimen of ondansetron (1 mg/kg, p.o.) plus aprepitant (1 mg/kg, p.o.) in combination with dexamethasone (1 mg/kg, i.p.).

Conclusion: In conclusion, netupitant has potent and long lasting anti-emetic activity against a number of emetic challenges indicating broad inhibitory properties. The convenience of protection afforded by the single dosing of netupitant together with palonosetron was demonstrated and also is known to provide an advantage over other therapeutic strategies to control emesis in man.

Keywords: anti-emetic, nausea, vomiting, chemotherapy, 5-HT$_3$, NK$_1$, ferret

INTRODUCTION

The treatment of cancer with chemotherapeutic agents such as cisplatin is documented to be associated with a number of side effects including nausea and emesis, which can be reduced by agents blocking 5-HT$_3$ and substance P NK$_1$ receptors (Rudd and Andrews, 2004; Hesketh, 2008). It has been hypothesized that there is an initial release of 5-HT (serotonin) from enterochromaffin cells in the gastrointestinal tract to activate 5-HT$_3$ receptors located on vagal afferents (Naylor and Rudd, 1996; Minami et al., 2003). The mechanism of release is not entirely known but may involve free radical generation and/or cellular damage, which subsequently leads to the involvement of other neurotransmitter systems and/or mediators (Andrews and Rudd, 2015). The response occurring over the first 0–24 h has become known as the acute response, and 'first generation' 5-HT$_3$ receptor antagonists, such as ondansetron and granisetron, have been used widely to reduce nausea and emesis during this phase (Hesketh, 2008). However, 5-HT$_3$ receptor antagonists are less effective to control nausea and emesis occurring during the post 24 h period, which became known as the delayed phase of emesis (Rudd and Andrews, 2004).

To improve the overall control of acute and delayed emesis, 5-HT$_3$ receptor antagonists were initially combined with glucocorticoids such as dexamethasone (Hesketh et al., 1994; Ioannidis et al., 2000). Subsequently, preclinical studies identified that brain penetrating tachykinin NK$_1$ receptor antagonists had a broad inhibitory profile to inhibit emesis induced by disparate challenges (Bountra et al., 1993; Tattersall et al., 1993, 1994; Andrews and Rudd, 2004). It was also shown that NK$_1$ receptor antagonists had anti-emetic activity in a ferret model of acute and delayed emesis prompting clinical testing (Rudd et al., 1996; Singh et al., 1997; Tattersall et al., 2000; Tsuchiya et al., 2002). The standard regimen to control both phases of emesis in man quickly changed to a triple regimen of a 5-HT$_3$ receptor antagonist, in combination with the first licensed NK$_1$ receptor antagonist for chemotherapy-induced emesis, aprepitant, plus a glucocorticoid (Jordan et al., 2005; Roila et al., 2010; Bayo et al., 2012). Unfortunately, however, even with these advances, there still remains a proportion of patients not adequately protected from chemotherapy-induced nausea and emesis (Navari, 2004; Aranda Aguilar et al., 2005).

Palonosetron is a 'second generation' 5-HT$_3$ receptor antagonist that is an order of magnitude more potent than older compounds at blocking 5-HT$_3$ receptors and has excellent bioavailability following oral administration (F 99%); it also has a plasma half-life that is approximately three times longer, enabling a convenient once per day administration (Wong et al., 1995; Grunberg and Koeller, 2003; De Leon, 2006). In the clinical setting, palonosetron was shown to be superior to the first generation 5-HT$_3$ receptor antagonists, particularly in its ability to reduce delayed nausea and emesis (Rubenstein, 2004; Geling and Eichler, 2005; Tonini et al., 2005). It was speculated that the unique profile of palonosetron may relate to its additional ability to prevent 5-HT$_3$ receptor re-cycling and/or a potential to reduce substance P responses mediated via NK$_1$ receptors by preventing 5-HT$_3$ and NK$_1$ receptor cross-talk (Rojas et al., 2008, 2010b, 2014; Stathis et al., 2012).

Since the clinical introduction of aprepitant, there have also been advances in the design of more potent and longer acting tachykinin NK$_1$ receptor antagonists (Reddy et al., 2006; Rojas et al., 2014). Netupitant is a novel orally active compound that penetrates into the brain and has a long duration of action and an insurmountable blocking activity at NK$_1$ receptors (Rizzi et al., 2012). Studies using NG108-15 cells have shown that netupitant and palonosetron have synergistic effects to antagonize substance P-induced calcium mobilization; synergism was not seen when netupitant was combined with ondansetron or granisetron (Stathis et al., 2012). Clinically, netupitant plus dexamethasone was shown to be superior to palonosetron plus dexamethasone against moderately emetogenic chemotherapy (Aapro et al., 2014), but the combination of netupitant and palonosetron with dexamethasone provided an excellent control of highly emetogenic chemotherapy induced-acute and delayed emesis, showing improvements over ondansetron and aprepitant combinations, with efficacy being maintained over multiple cycles (Gralla et al., 2014; Hesketh et al., 2014; Navari, 2015).

In the present studies, we used the ferret, a species with proven translational value in anti-emetic research (Percie du Sert et al., 2011), to explore the potential of a single administration of netupitant alone or in combination with palonosetron to inhibit cisplatin-induced acute and delayed emesis following an oral administration, compared with the control of emesis afforded by the three times per day administration of ondansetron alone, or when ondansetron was used daily combined with aprepitant and dexamethasone (Tattersall et al., 2000). An attempt was also made to characterize the spectrum of anti-emetic activity of netupitant to reduce emesis induced by other challenges. Apomorphine and morphine were selected to induce emesis via the area postrema (Lau et al., 2005; Percie du Sert et al., 2009), and intragastric copper sulfate was chosen to induce emesis via peripheral vagal and splanchnic pathways from the gastrointestinal tract (Kan et al., 2006). Ipecacuanha was selected as an emetogen inducing emesis via mixed central and peripheral pathways (Ariumi et al., 2000; Hasegawa et al., 2002). We also utilized *Suncus murinus* (house musk shrew) to investigate the potential of netupitant to reduce provocative motion-induced emesis that involves central pathways via vestibular inputs (Ueno et al., 1988; Ito et al., 2003). The studies described represent a reference point for others to compare the anti-emetic activity of new chemical entities or therapeutic strategies for the treatment of emesis.

MATERIALS AND METHODS

Animals

Male castrated ferrets (0.8–1.8 kg) were obtained from the University of Leeds (England) or Southland Ferrets (Invercargill, New Zealand). Water and food (SDS Diet 'C,' Special Diet Services, Ltd., UK, or TriPro super premium chicken meal formula dog food, American Nutrition, USA) were given *ad libitum* unless otherwise stated. Male *S. murinus* (45–65 g) were obtained from the University of Bradford (Bradford, U.K.). Dry pelleted trout pellets (Aquatic 3, Special Diet Services, UK) and water were given *ad libitum* unless otherwise stated. Animals were housed in temperature-controlled rooms at 20–24 ± 1°C under artificial lighting, with lights on between 06:00 and 18:00 h. The relative humidity was maintained at 50 ± 5%. All experiments were conducted under license from the respective Governments of England, Switzerland and Hong Kong, and were approved by the relevant Animal Experimentation Ethics committees.

Determination of the Plasma Half-Life of Netupitant in Ferrets

Ferrets were anesthetized with halothane (3%) in oxygen and the left jugular vein was cannulated and exteriorized to the back of the neck using standard surgical techniques (Barnes et al., 1991). Animals were then allowed to recover for 2 weeks. On the day of the experiment, at $t = 0$, a 1.5 ml blood sample was withdrawn before administering netupitant (3 mg/kg, p.o.). Subsequently, further blood sampling (1.5 ml) was continued at 1, 3, 6, 12, 24, 36, 48, 60, 72, 84, and 96 h. Each sample was centrifuged at 10,000 *g* for 10 min and the plasma was stored at −80°C prior to analysis. The analytical method used to determine the plasma concentration of netupitant was essentially the same as described by Huskey et al. (2003).

Experiments in Ferrets Involving Apomorphine, Morphine, Ipecacuanha, and Cisplatin during Acute Observation Times

On the day of experiment, the animals were transferred to individual cages where they were allowed at least 30 min to adapt before being presented with approximately 100 g of food. Netupitant (0.03–3 mg/kg) or vehicle [0.3% (v/v) Tween 80 in saline; 2 ml/kg] was then administered orally 2 h before the subcutaneous administration of apomorphine (0.125 mg/kg, s.c.), morphine (0.5 mg/kg, s.c.), ipecacuanha (1.2 mg/kg, p.o.), copper sulfate (100 mg/kg, i.g.), or cisplatin (10 mg/kg, i.p.). Animal behavior was recorded for up to 8 h using a closed circuit video recording system.

Experiments Involving *Suncus murinus* and Provocative Motion

The protocol used for the provocative motion-induced emesis experiments have been described previously (Chan et al., 2007). Briefly, the animals were transferred to the behavioral laboratory and given 30 min to habituate before being administered netupitant (0.03–3 mg/kg) or vehicle [0.3% (v/v) Tween 80 in saline; 2 ml/kg] orally. After 105 min, they were transferred to individual chambers (21 cm × 14 cm × 13 cm) and given 15 min to adapt before starting the provocative motion stimulus (i.e., 120 min post netupitant/vehicle administration; 4 cm horizontal displacement, 2 Hz, using a Heidolph Promax 2020 desktop shaker, Labplant, England). Animal behavior was recorded for 10 min using a closed circuit video recording system (Chan et al., 2007).

Experiments to Assess Anti-Emetic Potency on Cisplatin-Induced Acute and Delayed Emesis

The ferret acute and delayed emesis model has been described previously (Rudd and Naylor, 1996). Animals were transferred to individual observation cages where they were allowed at least 48 h to adapt. A dry pellet diet (Laboratory Feline Diet 5003, PMI Nutrition Inc., St. Louis, MO, USA) and water was available *ad libitum*. Animals were presented with 100 g of commercially available cat food (Whiskas®, Effem Foods Pty. Ltd., Wodonga, Australia) 30 min prior to drug/vehicle administration. In an initial series of experiments, ferrets were administered with cisplatin (5 mg/kg) intraperitoneally followed immediately by the oral administration of vehicle [0.3% (v/v) Tween 80 in saline; 2 ml/kg], netupitant (1–3 mg/kg), or ondansetron (1 mg/kg); the administration of vehicle or ondansetron was repeated at 8 h intervals.

In other experiments, ferrets were allowed a 2-day habituation period. Some ferrets were administered ondansetron (1 mg/kg, p.o.), or netupitant (3 mg/kg, p.o.), 2 h prior to the administration of cisplatin (5 mg/kg, i.p.); the administration of ondansetron was repeated at 8 h intervals. In other experiments, ferrets were administered palonosetron (0.1 mg/kg, p.o.) and/or netupitant (1 mg/kg, p.o.), in combination with dexamethasone (1 mg/kg, i.p.), or respective vehicles (2 ml/kg) 15 min before cisplatin (5 mg/kg, i.p.); dexamethasone (1 mg/kg, i.p.) or vehicle (distilled water, 1 ml/kg) was administered 15 min before cisplatin (5 mg/kg, i.p.) and then repeated at 24 h intervals. Some animals were also randomized as positive controls and administered ondansetron (1 mg/kg, p.o.) plus aprepitant (1 mg/kg, p.o.) orally 15 min before cisplatin and dexamethasone (1 mg/kg, i.p.) 15 min before cisplatin; ondansetron, and dexamethasone administrations were repeated at 24 h intervals. Respective vehicle controls (distilled water, 2 ml/kg) were also utilized.

Measurement of Emesis

Emesis was characterized by rhythmic abdominal contractions that were either associated with the forceful oral expulsion of solid or liquid material from the gastrointestinal tract (i.e., vomiting), or not associated with the passage of material

TABLE 1 | Ability of netupitant to abolish retching and vomiting induced by apomorphine, morphine, ipecacuanha, and copper sulfate pentahydrate.

Treatment	Apomorphine (0.125 mg/kg, s.c.)	Morphine (0.5 mg/kg, s.c.)	Ipecacuanha (1.2 mg/kg, p.o.)	Copper Sulphate (100 mg/kg, intragastric)
Vehicle	26.2 ± 2.8	43.8 ± 3.7	37.5 ± 6.8	78.8 ± 6.5
Netupitant 3 mg/kg, p.o.	0.0 ± 0.0**	0.0 ± 0.0**	0.0 ± 0.0**	0.0 ± 0.0**

*Netupitant (3 mg/kg) or vehicle, was administered orally 2 h prior to challenge with emetic drugs. Data represents the mean ± SEM of the number of retches + vomits recorded during a 30–60 min observation period. Significant differences relative to the vehicle control treated animals are indicated as **P < 0.01 (Student's unpaired t-test; n = 6).*

(i.e., retching movements). For ferrets, consecutive episodes of retching and/or vomiting were considered separate when the animal changed its location in the observation cage, or when the interval between episodes exceeded 5 s (Rudd and Naylor, 1996). For *S. murinus*, episodes of emesis were also characterized as described above, except that the interval to demarcate two consecutive episodes of retching and/or vomiting was 2 s (Rudd et al., 1999). At the end of the observation period, animals were terminated by an intraperitoneal injection of pentobarbitone sodium (80 mg/kg).

Data Analysis

Data are expressed as the mean ± SEM, unless otherwise stated. Half-life values and ID_{50} values were calculated from data expressed as a percentage of the control response using linear and non-linear regression analysis, respectively. In all cases, differences between treatment groups were considered significant when $P < 0.05$ (Student's T-test, or one way ANOVA and Tukey's multiple comparison tests, as appropriate; GraphPad Prism version 5.0, Inc. Version, San Diego, CA, USA).

Drug Formulation

Ondansetron hydrochloride d-hydrate, dexamethasone 21-phosphate disodium salt, and D-mannitol were from Sigma–Aldrich, St. Louis, MO, USA. Cisplatin (1 mg/ml in 0.1% mannitol in saline) was from David Bull Laboratories, Mulgrave, VIC, Australia. Palonosetron hydrochloride, aprepitant and netupitant were from Helsinn Advanced Synthesis SA, Switzerland. Ondansetron, dexamethasone, and palonosetron were dissolved in distilled water. Netupitant was dissolved in 0.3% Tween 80 in Saline (0.9% w/v). Aprepitant was dissolved in a solution of ethanol:propylene glycol:distilled water in the ratio of 1:6:3. Doses are expressed as the free base and dosing volumes were 1 ml/kg.

RESULTS

Pharmacokinetic Profile of Netupitant in Ferrets

The plasma level of netupitant peaked 1–3 h following its oral administration; the T_{max} was 2.5 ± 0.5 h and the C_{max} was 397.3 ± 19.7 ng/ml ($n = 4$). The plasma level of netupitant was measurable up to 96 h and had a flat terminal profile with a terminal half-life of 78.5 ± 17.0 h ($n = 4$).

Anti-Emetic of Activity of Netupitant against Drug- and Motion-Induced Emesis in the Ferret

No retching or vomiting was observed during the habituation periods and there were no obvious differences in the behavior of the animals randomized to the treatment groups prior to drug/vehicle administration. Netupitant was not associated with emesis during the pre-treatment period. Apomorphine, morphine and copper sulfate subsequently induced emesis in the vehicle treated animals following a short latency of ~ 5 min (data not shown). The range of retches + vomits recorded during the 30 min observation periods were: apomorphine, 21–35; morphine, 33–55; and copper sulfate, 60–100. The oral administration of netupitant at 3 mg/kg completely prevented the retching and vomiting response to these challenges ($P < 0.01$; **Table 1**). A more detailed dose-ranging experiment against apomorphine (control retches + vomits range: 17–32) revealed that a significant 33.8% reduction of retching + vomiting could be observed at doses of netupitant as low as 0.03 mg/kg ($P < 0.05$); increasing the doses to 0.1 mg/kg reduced emesis by 75.6% ($P < 0.01$) and 0.3 mg/kg prevented emesis completely ($P < 0.01$; **Figure 1**). The ID_{50} to inhibit apomorphine-induced retching + vomiting was 0.08 mg/kg, p.o. In the experiments involving ipecacuanha, the vehicle treated control animals exhibited emesis following a latency period of approximately 20 min (data not shown) that comprised ~38 retches + vomits during the 60 min observation period. The emetic response induced by ipecacuanha was similarly prevented completely by netupitant at 3 mg/kg, p.o. ($P < 0.05$; **Table 1**). No dose-ranging experiments were done against ipecacuanha, copper sulfate or morphine, so ID_{50} values could not be calculated.

In the experiments involving the use of cisplatin at 10 mg/kg, i.p., the vehicle treated control animals exhibited emesis after 60–90 min that comprised ~145 retches + vomits (range: 103–173) during the 8 h observation period. Netupitant at 0.1 mg/kg antagonized significantly the retching + vomiting response by 27.1% ($P < 0.05$) and increasing the dose of netupitant to 0.3 mg/kg, p.o., antagonized the response by 95.2% (**Figure 2**; $P < 0.01$); the ID_{50} to inhibit emesis was approximately 0.1 mg/kg, p.o.

Anti-Emetic of Activity of Netupitant against Provocative Motion (4 cm Horizontal Displacement at 2 Hz for 10 min)-Induced Emesis

In the experiments involving provocative motion, five out of six vehicle treated control animals exhibited emesis after a short

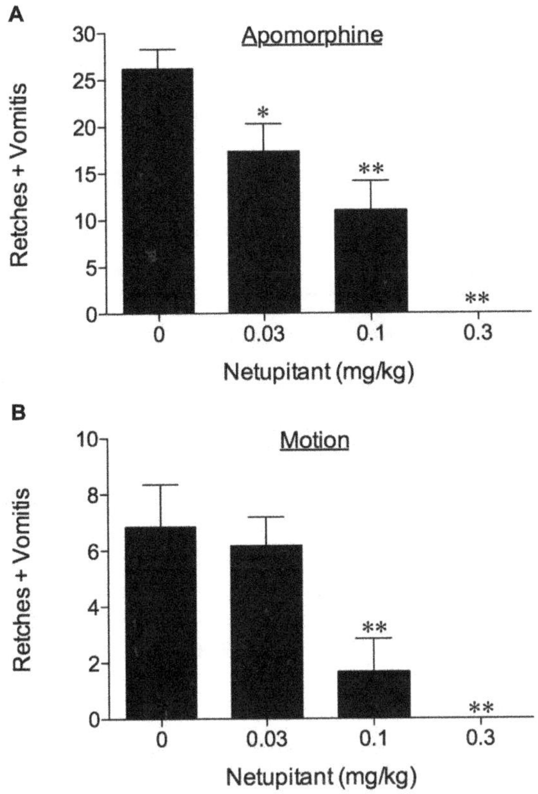

FIGURE 1 | The effect of netupitant on (A) apomorphine (0.125 mg/kg, s.c.)-induced emesis in ferrets and (B) motion-induced emesis in *Suncus murinus*. Netupitant (0.03–0.3 mg/kg) or vehicle was administered orally 2 h prior to apomorphine (0.125 mg/kg, s.c.) or motion (4 cm horizontal displacement, 2 Hz for 10 min). Significant differences relative to vehicle treated animals (0 mg/kg) are indicated as $^{*}P < 0.05$ or $^{**}P < 0.01$ (one way ANOVA followed by Tukey's multiple comparison testing).

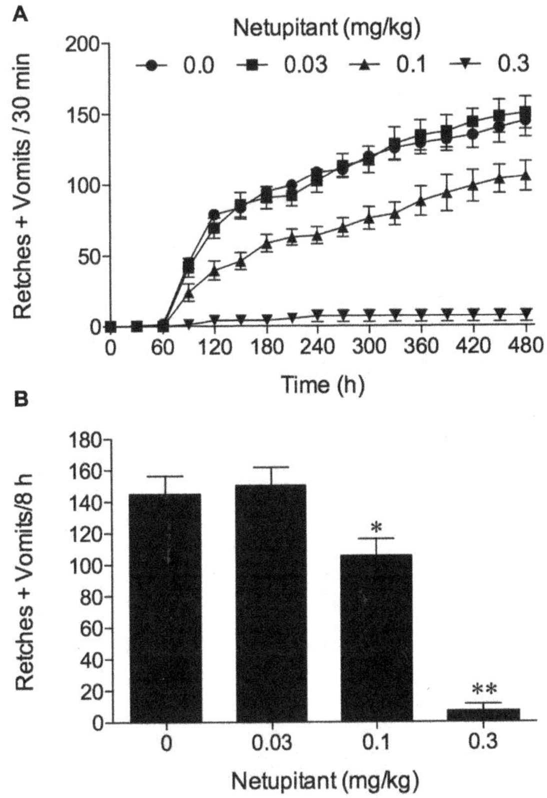

FIGURE 2 | The effect of netupitant on cisplatin (10 mg/kg, i.p.)-induced emesis in ferret. Netupitant (0.03–0.3 mg/kg) or vehicle was administered orally 2 h prior to cisplatin (10 mg/kg, i.p.; $t = 0$). Data represents the mean ± SEM of **(A)** cumulative numbers of retches + vomits per 30 min, or **(B)** the total numbers of retches + vomits occurring over 8 h ($n = 5$–6). Significant differences relative to vehicle treated animals (0 mg/kg) are indicated as $^{*}P < 0.05$, $^{**}P < 0.01$ (one way ANOVA followed by Tukey's multiple comparison testing).

latency (~2-4 min) that comprised ~8 retches + vomits (range: 7-11) during the 10 min observation period. Netupitant at 0.1 mg/kg, p.o. antagonized significantly the retching + vomiting response by 75.6% ($P < 0.01$), and increasing the dose of netupitant to 0.3 mg/kg, p.o., prevented the response completely (**Figure 1**; $P < 0.01$); the ID_{50} to inhibit emesis was 0.08 mg/kg, p.o.

Anti-Emetic Potential of Netupitant Compared with Ondansetron to Inhibit Cisplatin (5 mg/kg, i.p.)-Induced Acute and Delayed Emesis

In vehicle treated animals, cisplatin induced 148.7 ± 11.5 and 242.2 ± 24.0 retches + vomits during the acute (0–24 h) and delayed (24-3-72 h) periods, respectively (**Figure 3**). The three times per day administration of ondansetron, 1 mg/kg, p.o., reduced the acute response significantly by 67.8% ($P < 0.01$) and also reduced the delayed response by 48.3% ($P < 0.01$; **Figure 3**).

Netupitant at 3 mg/kg, p.o., administered 2 h prior to the injection of cisplatin, prevented completely the acute response ($P < 0.05$) and reduced the delayed response significantly by 94.6% ($P < 0.01$; **Figure 3**). In fact, the single administration of netupitant was almost twice as effective as the three times administration of ondansetron to prevent the acute and delayed retching and vomiting response ($P < 0.01$; **Figure 3**).

Comparison of the Anti-Emetic Activity of the Once Only Administration of Palonosetron and Netupitant with the Standard Regimen of Ondansetron and Aprepitant

In vehicle treated animals, cisplatin induced 205.6 ± 40.5 and 471.0 ± 98.3 retches + vomits during the acute (0–24 h) and delayed (24–72 h) periods, respectively (**Figure 4**). Both the standard regimen of ondansetron (1 mg/kg, p.o., every 24 h) plus aprepitant (1 mg/kg, p.o., administered once) and dexamethasone (1 mg/kg, i.p., every 24 h), and the single administration of netupitant (1 mg/kg, p.o.) plus palonosetron (0.1 mg/kg, p.o.) in combination with daily dexamethasone

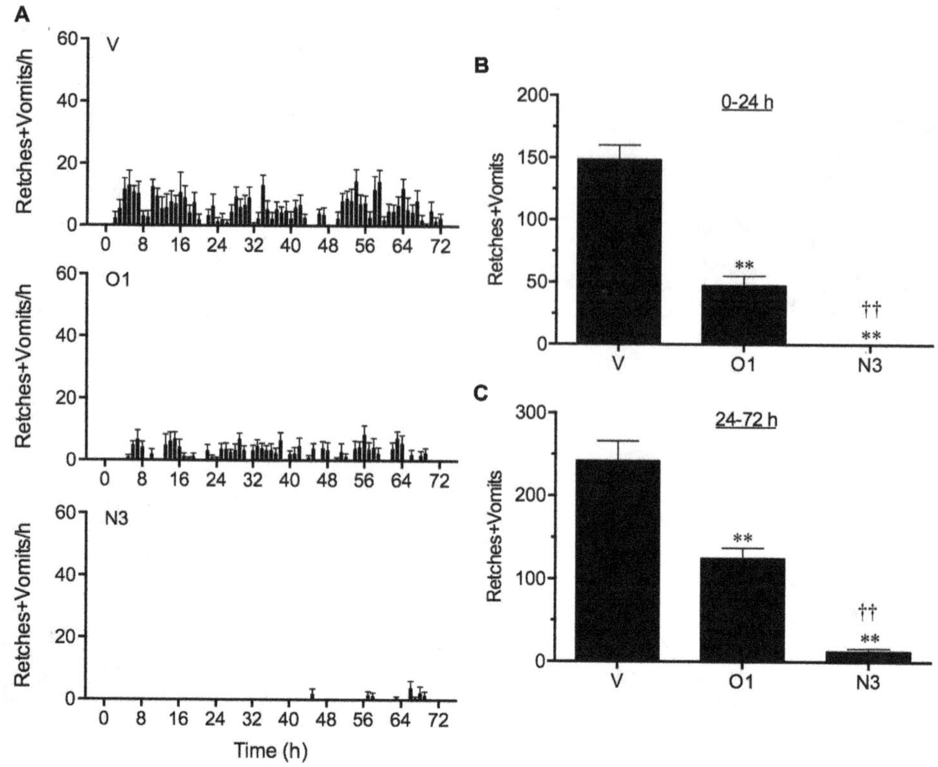

FIGURE 3 | The effect of ondansetron (O1) or netupitant (N3) on the profile of retching and/or vomiting induced by cisplatin in the ferret. Ondansetron, (1 mg/kg, p.o.), was administered 15 min before cisplatin (5 mg/kg, i.p.; $t = 0$) and then at regular 8 h intervals; netupitant (3 mg/kg, p.o.) was administered once, 2 h prior to cisplatin. Data represents the mean ± SEM of the total numbers of retches + vomits occurring in **(A)** 1, **(B)** 0–24, or **(C)** 24–72 h time intervals, as appropriate ($n = 5$–6). Significant differences relative to vehicle treated animals (V) are indicated as $^{**}P < 0.01$; significant differences relative to ondansetron treated animals are indicated as $^{\dagger\dagger}P < 0.01$ (one way ANOVA followed by Tukey's multiple comparison testing).

(1 mg/kg, i.p.) were highly effective to reduce the acute response significantly by 99.7 ($P < 0.01$) and 97.3% ($P < 0.01$), respectively (**Figure 4**). The standard regimen of ondansetron plus aprepitant and dexamethasone also reduced significantly the delayed emetic response by 86.3% ($P < 0.01$). The netupitant plus palonosetron and dexamethasone regimen reduced delayed emesis to a lesser extent by 60.2% ($P < 0.05$). However, there were no significant differences in the control of acute or delayed emesis by the two anti-emetic regimens ($P > 0.05$).

DISCUSSION

Netupitant was orally active to antagonize emesis induced by diverse emetogenic stimuli in ferrets and *S. murinus*. This profile is consistent with other NK_1 receptor antagonists that are presumed to be capable of penetrating the blood brain barrier to reach sites in the dorsal vagal complex and/or sites thought to be adjacent to the semi-compact part of the nucleus ambiguous (Tattersall et al., 1996; Fukuda et al., 1999; Andrews and Rudd, 2004). This is particularly relevant for centrally acting emetogens, such as apomorphine and morphine, or motion, but for other stimuli that may also cause a release of substance P in the periphery, the mechanism may in part also involve NK_1 receptors on the vagus or perhaps those located elsewhere in the periphery (Minami et al., 1998; Darmani et al., 2008; Ray et al., 2009).

The broad inhibitory anti-emetic profile in ferrets encompassed five challenges where acute emesis was induced: apomorphine [mechanism involving D_2 receptors at the level of the area postrema; (Lau et al., 2005)], morphine [emetic mechanism involving opioid receptors at the level of the area postrema; (Rudd and Naylor, 1995; Percie du Sert et al., 2009)], copper sulfate [mechanism predominantly involving gastric irritation and vagal and/or splanchnic nerves, but where the transmitter systems are not completely characterized; (Makale and King, 1992; Kan et al., 2006)], ipecacuanha [mechanism involving 5-HT_3 receptors and vagal and/or splanchnic nerves; (Ariumi et al., 2000; Hasegawa et al., 2002)] and cisplatin [high-dose model – mechanism involving a release of 5-HT from enterochromaffin cells, 5-HT_3 receptors and vagal and/or splanchnic nerves and activation of the area postrema; (Percie du Sert et al., 2009)]. Several doses of netupitant were utilized to compare potency to inhibit apomorphine- and cisplatin-induced emesis yielding ID_{50} values of ~0.1 mg/kg, p.o., which is five times below its reported potency in the gerbil foot tapping assay [$ID_{50} = 0.5$ mg/kg, p.o.; (Rizzi et al., 2012)]; at 0.3 mg/kg netupitant inhibited the emetic responses completely.

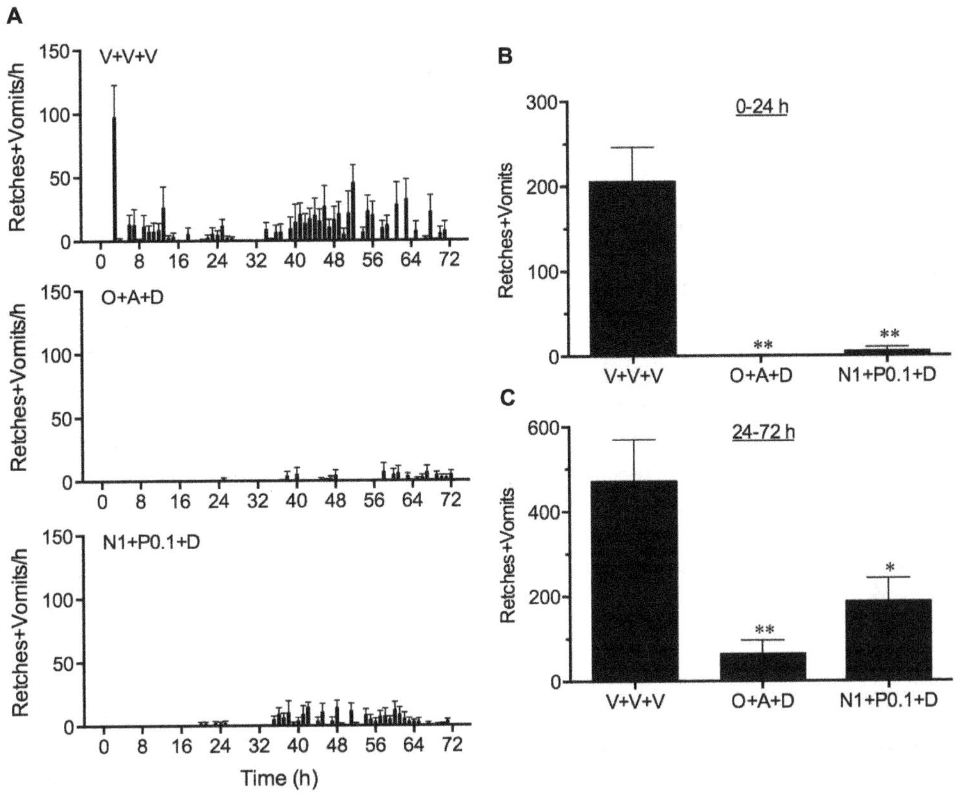

FIGURE 4 | A comparison of the effect of ondansetron plus aprepitant in combination with dexamethasone (O+A+D) with netupitant plus palonosetron in combination with dexamethasone (N1+P0.1+D) on cisplatin-induced retching and/or vomiting. Ondansetron, (1 mg/kg, p.o.), aprepitant (1 mg/kg, p.o.), palonosetron (0.1 mg/kg, p.o.), netupitant (1 mg/kg, p.o.), or dexamethasone (1 mg/kg, i.p.), or vehicle, were administered 15 min before cisplatin (5 mg/kg, i.p.; $t = 0$); the administration of ondansetron (1 mg/kg, p.o.) or dexamethasone (1 mg/kg, i.p.) or vehicle was repeated at 24 h intervals. Data represents the mean ± SEM of the total numbers of retches + vomits occurring in **(A)** 1, **(B)** 0–24, or **(C)** 24–72 h time intervals, as appropriate (n = 5–6). Significant differences relative to vehicle treated animals (V+V+V) are indicated as $^{*}P < 0.05$, or $^{**}P < 0.01$ (one way ANOVA followed by Tukey's multiple comparison testing).

A remarkably similar relative potency difference of other NK_1 receptor antagonists in the ferret cisplatin-induced emesis assay and the gerbil foot-tapping assay has been reported following intravenously administered brain penetrating NK_1 receptor antagonists, GR203040, CP-99,994, and L-742,694 (ID_{50} values in foot taping assay ~0.85 mg/kg; ID_{50} values in the cisplatin assay were ~0.18 mg/kg; Rupniak et al., 1997). The consistency of relative potency of the antagonists between studies may reflect netupitant's excellent bioavailability following oral administration (present investigations). It is also relevant that netupitant binds with high affinity to human NK_1 receptors (pKi = 9.0), with 1,000 fold selectivity over other tachykinin and G-protein coupled receptors (Rizzi et al., 2012). Predictably, in our studies, the use of netupitant at 3 mg/kg, p.o., abolished morphine- and ipecacuanha-induced emesis; a similar spectrum of effects has been reported for several other NK_1 receptor antagonists against these emetic stimuli [for a review, see (Andrews and Rudd, 2004)].

We also explored the anti-emetic potential of netupitant in the ferret cisplatin (low-dose 5 mg/kg)-induced acute and delayed emesis model (Rudd et al., 1994; Rudd and Naylor, 1997; Sam et al., 2001). In the present studies, the single oral administration of netupitant at 3 mg/kg was shown to be far superior to the three times per day administration of ondansetron (1 mg/kg, i.p.) at antagonizing both the acute (netupitant abolished acute emesis; ondansetron only reduced acute emesis by ~68%) and delayed response (netupitant reduced delayed emesis by ~95%; ondansetron reduced delayed emesis by ~49%) to cisplatin; the antagonism afforded by ondansetron is comparable to previously published data in this species (Rudd and Naylor, 1994, 1997; Rudd et al., 1996; Singh et al., 1997; Watanabe et al., 2008). These data demonstrate that netupitant has an exceptionally long duration of action which may relate to its exceptionally long plasma half-life of ~79 h (present studies), whereas the plasma half-life of ondansetron is reported to be ~2.3 h (Minami et al., 1991). If we place this in perspective, the first NK_1 receptor antagonist tested in the ferret acute and delayed emesis model, CP-99,994, [IC_{50} of 1.9 nM to displace [125I]-Bolton Hunter Substance P from ferret brain membranes (Watson et al., 1995)], had a short plasma half-life of ~1.4 h [data from cat, (Lucot et al., 1997)], and even when administered every 8 h at 10 mg/kg, only reduced cisplatin-induced acute emesis by 34% and reduced delayed emesis by ~87% (Rudd et al., 1996); this was the dose of CP-99,994 that was also shown to prevent apomorphine, morphine, ipecacuanha, cisplatin (high-dose)-induced emesis (Bountra et al., 1993; Tattersall et al., 1993; Zaman et al., 2000). Critically, aprepitant, which has an IC_{50} value of 0.7 nM at ferret NK_1 receptors (0.1 nM for human NK_1 receptors), and plasma half-life of 10 h [ferret; (Huskey et al., 2003); plasma half-life in humans, 10–29 h; (Bubalo et al., 2012)], only produces a similar level of inhibition of acute and delayed emesis when orally administered at 16 mg/kg (Tattersall et al., 2000).

Palonosetron (RS 25259-197) was first described as a high affinity 5-HT_3 receptor antagonist [pKi ~10; Wong et al., 1995)] and was subsequently shown to have a plasma half-life of ~40 h in humans (Siddiqui and Scott, 2004; Stoltz et al., 2004). It has been reported to inhibit cisplatin-induced emesis (10 mg/kg, i.v.; 5 h test) in ferrets and dogs with ID_{50} values of 0.003 and 0.008 mg/kg, respectively; the dose of 0.1 mg/kg, p.o., inhibited emesis by almost 100% in both species (Eglen et al., 1995). Indeed, palonosetron was revealed as being twice as potent as ondansetron to inhibit cisplatin-induced emesis in ferrets following oral administration (Eglen et al., 1995). Clinically, palonosetron is recognized as being superior to other 5-HT_3 receptor antagonists, particularly against chemotherapy-induced delayed emesis (Navari, 2009; Saito et al., 2009). In fact, the magnitude of difference, particularly in the control of delayed emesis, was unexpected; prompting speculation that palonosetron has properties distinct from other selective 5-HT_3 receptor antagonists. There is strong evidence that it may have a different mechanism of action to ondansetron at the 5-HT_3 receptor, including an ability to cause receptor internalization, with continued binding to the internalized receptor to prolong the inhibition of its function (not seen with ondansetron and granisetron) and, more recently, an indirect inhibition of substance P responses, *in vivo* (Rojas et al., 2008, 2010a,b).

In the cisplatin (5 mg/kg, i.p.) acute and delayed emesis model, we compared the anti-emetic potential of a regimen of netupitant and palonosetron (both administered before cisplatin) in combination with dexamethasone (administered before cisplatin and then every 24 h), with a regimen comprising ondansetron (administered before cisplatin and then every 24 h) and aprepitant (administered once before cisplatin) in combination with dexamethasone (administered before cisplatin and then every 24 h). Both treatment regimens were highly effective to antagonize acute emesis and were indistinguishable from each other. Indeed, the anti-emetic effect of the regimen of netupitant and palonosetron in combination with dexamethasone was still evident during the delayed phase of the response, and was not significantly different from the control of emesis seen following the more frequent dosing regimen of ondansetron and aprepitant in combination with dexamethasone. These data compare favorably with previous studies investigating aprepitant, ondansetron, and dexamethasone in ferrets (Tattersall et al., 2000).

Palonosetron has also been studied in the *Cryptotis parva* (least shrew). Across a subcutaneous dose range of 0.1–10 mg/kg, palonosetron dose-dependently antagonized the emesis induced by either the 5-HT_3 receptor agonist, 2 methyl-5-HT (5 mg/kg), i.p., or the L-type calcium channel opener, FLP 64176 (10 mg/kg, i.p.; Darmani et al., 2014). It is unknown why palonosetron could not completely inhibit 2-methyl-5-HT-induced emesis in this species, but the level of inhibition was similar to that reported for tropisetron against the same stimulus (Darmani, 1998).

Palonosetron administered as a single treatment, is not noted to have a U-shaped dose-response curve in ferrets or man against chemotherapy-induced emesis. However, in the least shrew, palonosetron appears to have a species-specific biphasic anti-emetic action against the initial 2 h of emesis induced by cisplatin (10 mg/kg, i.p.), with a significant reduction at 0.1 and 2.5 mg/kg, s.c; while at 0.5 and 5 mg/kg the protection was lost (Darmani et al., 2014). In a subsequent set of experiments, palonosetron was tested at 0.1 mg/kg, s.c., against the same dose of cisplatin but over an extended observation period of 40 h (Darmani et al., 2015). Palonosetron reduced the emesis occurring during the initial first 16 h of the experiment by 83% compared to vehicle pretreated cisplatin controls. An assessment of emesis during the 27–40 h period also recorded a non-significant reduction of 73% (Darmani et al., 2015). Comparatively, netupitant at a high dose of 5 mg/kg, s.c., non-significantly reduced the emesis occurring during the first 16 h by 70% and abolished emesis during the 27–40 h period (Darmani et al., 2015). When both palonosetron and netupitant were combined together, the emesis occurring during the first 16 h was reduced by approximately 94%, and the reduction of emesis in the 27–40 h period was still significantly reduced (Darmani et al., 2015). Thus, the combination of palonosetron and netupitant resulted in a greater level of protection against both acute and 'delayed' phases of cisplatin-induced emesis in the least shrew than either treatment administered alone.

Suncus murinus is a more commonly used shrew species to study mechanisms of emesis, but its tachykinin receptor has a distinct pharmacology compared to the human and rodent NK_1 receptor (Tattersall et al., 1995; Rudd et al., 1999). However, in the present studies, netupitant dose-dependently reduced motion-induced emesis, with a dose of 0.3 mg/kg, p.o., preventing the response completely. In comparison with data in the literature, netupitant appears more potent than other NK_1 receptor antagonists including CP-99,994, GR203040, GR205171, and RP67580 to antagonize motion-induced emesis in this species (Gardner et al., 1995, 1996; Rudd et al., 1999). It is known that patients with a history of motion sickness also have a higher incidence of chemotherapy-induced emesis (e.g., Morrow, 1984; Shih et al., 2009), post-operative nausea and vomiting, and pregnancy sickness (Bouganim et al., 2012; Warr, 2014). Therefore, it may be expected that netupitant would be useful to control emesis in such patients, where pathways involving motion sickness have been stimulated or perturbed.

CONCLUSION

The present studies revealed that netupitant has a broad inhibitory profile to inhibit emesis both in ferrets and *S. murinus*. In particular, a single dose of netupitant at 3 mg/kg given 3 h prior to the administration of cisplatin, provided almost complete protection from acute and delayed emesis; a lower dose of 1 mg/kg, in combination with a single oral dose of palonosetron at 0.1 mg/kg, in combination with daily administrations of dexamethasone (1 mg/kg, i.p.), was also highly effective to reduce acute and delayed emesis, being relatively comparable to a more frequent dosing regimen of ondansetron plus aprepitant in combination with dexamethasone. The convenience of oral dosing, efficacy, and long duration of action are consistent with clinical data. This has been realized by the successful formulation and use of palonosetron plus netupitant in a single pill (Akynzeo®) for the treatment of chemotherapy-induced acute and delayed nausea and emesis (Thompson, 2014; Lorusso et al., 2015; Navari, 2015).

AUTHOR CONTRIBUTIONS

JR, GH, CG, EL, and CP conceived and designed the experiments. JR, GH, MN, and ZL performed the experiments and data analysis. All authors contributed equally to writing the manuscript.

FUNDING

This work was supported in part by Helsinn SA grant. Other support was from the Emesis Research Group, the Chinese University of Hong Kong.

REFERENCES

Aapro, M., Rugo, H., Rossi, G., Rizzi, G., Borroni, M. E., Bondarenko, I., et al. (2014). A randomized phase III study evaluating the efficacy and safety of NEPA, a fixed-dose combination of netupitant and palonosetron, for prevention of chemotherapy-induced nausea and vomiting following moderately emetogenic chemotherapy. *Ann. Oncol.* 25, 1328–1333. doi: 10.1093/annonc/mdu101

Andrews, P. L. R., and Rudd, J. A. (2004). "The role of tachykinins and the tachykinin receptor in nausea and emesis," in *Handbook of Experimental Pharmacology*, ed. P. Holzer (Berlin: Springer-Verlag), 359–440.

Andrews, P. L. R., and Rudd, J. A. (2015). "The physiology and pharmacology of nausea and vomiting induced by anti-cancer chemotherapy in humans," in *Management of Chemotherapy-Induced Nausea and Vomiting: New Agents and New Uses of Current Agents*, ed. R. Navari (London: Springer Health Care Publishers).

Aranda Aguilar, E., Constenla Figueiras, M., Cortes-Funes, H., Diaz-Rubio Garcia, E., Gascon Vilaplana, P., Guillem, V., et al. (2005). Clinical practice guidelines on antiemetics in oncology. *Expert Rev. Anticancer Ther.* 5, 963–972. doi: 10.1586/14737140.5.6.963

Ariumi, H., Saito, R., Nago, S., Hyakusoku, M., Takano, Y., and Kamiya, H. (2000). The role of tachykinin NK-1 receptors in the area postrema of ferrets in emesis. *Neurosci. Lett.* 286, 123–126. doi: 10.1016/S0304-3940(00)01113-7

Barnes, N. M., Bunce, K. T., Naylor, R. J., and Rudd, J. A. (1991). The actions of fentanyl to inhibit drug-induced emesis. *Neuropharmacology* 30, 1073–1083. doi: 10.1016/0028-3908(91)90136-Y

Bayo, J., Fonseca, P. J., Hernando, S., Servitja, S., Calvo, A., Falagan, S., et al. (2012). Chemotherapy-induced nausea and vomiting: pathophysiology and therapeutic principles. *Clin. Transl. Oncol.* 14, 413–422. doi: 10.1007/s12094-012-0818-y

Bouganim, N., Dranitsaris, G., Hopkins, S., Vandermeer, L., Godbout, L., Dent, S., et al. (2012). Prospective validation of risk prediction indexes for acute and delayed chemotherapy-induced nausea and vomiting. *Curr. Oncol.* 19, e414–e421. doi: 10.3747/co.19.1074

Bountra, C., Bunce, K., Dale, T., Gardner, C., Jordan, C., Twissell, D., et al. (1993). Anti-emetic profile of a non-peptide neurokinin NK1 receptor. *Eur. J. Pharmacol.* 249, R3–R4. doi: 10.1016/0014-2999(93)90673-6

Bubalo, J. S., Cherala, G., McCune, J. S., Munar, M. Y., Tse, S., and Maziarz, R. (2012). Aprepitant pharmacokinetics and assessing the impact of aprepitant on cyclophosphamide metabolism in cancer patients undergoing hematopoietic stem cell transplantation. *J. Clin. Pharmacol.* 52, 586–594. doi: 10.1177/0091270011398243

Chan, S. W., Rudd, J. A., Lin, G., and Li, P. (2007). Action of anti-tussive drugs on the emetic reflex of *Suncus murinus* (house musk shrew). *Eur. J. Pharmacol.* 559, 196–201. doi: 10.1016/j.ejphar.2006.12.008

Darmani, N. A. (1998). Serotonin 5-HT3 receptor antagonists prevent cisplatin-induced emesis in *Cryptotis parva*: a new experimental model of emesis. *J. Neural Transm.* 105, 1143–1154. doi: 10.1007/s007020050118

Darmani, N. A., Wang, Y., Abad, J., Ray, A. P., Thrush, G. R., and Ramirez, J. (2008). Utilization of the least shrew as a rapid and selective screening model for the antiemetic potential and brain penetration of substance P and NK1 receptor antagonists. *Brain Res.* 1214, 58–72. doi: 10.1016/j.brainres.2008.03.077

Darmani, N. A., Zhong, W., Chebolu, S., and Mercadante, F. (2015). Differential and additive suppressive effects of 5-HT3 (palonosetron)- and NK1 (netupitant)-receptor antagonists on cisplatin-induced vomiting and ERK1/2, PKA and PKC activation. *Pharmacol. Biochem. Behav.* 131, 104–111. doi: 10.1016/j.pbb.2015.02.010

Darmani, N. A., Zhong, W., Chebolu, S., Vaezi, M., and Alkam, T. (2014). Broad-spectrum antiemetic potential of the L-type calcium channel antagonist nifedipine and evidence for its additive antiemetic interaction with the 5-HT(3) receptor antagonist palonosetron in the least shrew (*Cryptotis parva*). *Eur. J. Pharmacol.* 722, 2–12. doi: 10.1016/j.ejphar.2013.08.052

De Leon, A. (2006). Palonosetron (Aloxi): a second-generation 5-HT(3) receptor antagonist for chemotherapy-induced nausea and vomiting. *Proc. (Bayl. Univ. Med. Cent.)* 19, 413–416.

Eglen, R. M., Lee, C. H., Smith, W. L., Johnson, L. G., Clark, R., Whiting, R. L., et al. (1995). Pharmacological characterization of RS 25259-197, a novel and selective 5-HT3 receptor antagonist, in vivo. *Br. J. Pharmacol.* 114, 860–866. doi: 10.1111/j.1476-5381.1995.tb13283.x

Fukuda, H., Nakamura, E., Koga, T., Furukawa, N., and Shiroshita, Y. (1999). The site of the anti-emetic action of tachykinin NK1 receptor antagonists may exist in the medullary area adjacent to the semicompact part of the nucleus ambiguus. *Brain Res.* 818, 439–449. doi: 10.1016/S0006-8993(98)01324-9

Gardner, C. J., Armour, D. R., Beattie, D. T., Gale, J. D., Hawcock, A. B., Kilpatrick, G. J., et al. (1996). GR205171: a novel antagonist with high affinity for the tachykinin NK1 receptor, and potent broad-spectrum anti-emetic activity. *Regul. Pept.* 65, 45–53. doi: 10.1016/0167-0115(96)00071-7

Gardner, C. J., Twissell, D. J., Dale, T. J., Gale, J. D., Jordan, C. C., Kilpatrick, G. J., et al. (1995). The broad-spectrum anti-emetic activity of the novel non-peptide tachykinin NK1 receptor antagonist GR203040. *Br. J. Pharmacol.* 116, 3158–3163. doi: 10.1111/j.1476-5381.1995.tb15118.x

Geling, O., and Eichler, H. G. (2005). Should 5-hydroxytryptamine-3 receptor antagonists be administered beyond 24 hours after chemotherapy to prevent delayed emesis? Systematic re-evaluation of clinical evidence and drug cost implications. *J. Clin. Oncol.* 23, 1289–1294. doi: 10.1200/JCO.2005.04.022

Gralla, R. J., Bosnjak, S. M., Hontsa, A., Balser, C., Rizzi, G., Rossi, G., et al. (2014). A phase III study evaluating the safety and efficacy of NEPA, a fixed-dose combination of netupitant and palonosetron, for prevention of chemotherapy-induced nausea and vomiting over repeated cycles of chemotherapy. *Ann. Oncol.* 25, 1333–1339. doi: 10.1093/annonc/mdu096

Grunberg, S. M., and Koeller, J. M. (2003). Palonosetron: a unique 5-HT3-receptor antagonist for the prevention of chemotherapy-induced emesis. *Expert Opin. Pharmacother.* 4, 2297–2303. doi: 10.1517/14656566.4.12.2297

Hasegawa, M., Sasaki, T., Sadakane, K., Tabuchi, M., Takeda, Y., Kimura, M., et al. (2002). Studies for the emetic mechanisms of ipecac syrup (TJN-119) and its active components in ferrets: involvement of 5-hydroxytryptamine receptors. *Jpn. J. Pharmacol.* 89, 113–119. doi: 10.1254/jjp.89.113

Hesketh, P. J. (2008). Chemotherapy-induced nausea and vomiting. *N. Engl. J. Med.* 358, 2482–2494. doi: 10.1056/NEJMra0706547

Hesketh, P. J., Harvey, W. H., Harker, W. G., Beck, T. M., Ryan, T., Bricker, L. J., et al. (1994). A randomized, double-blind comparison of intravenous ondansetron alone and in combination with intravenous dexamethasone in the prevention of high-dose cisplatin-induced emesis. *J. Clin. Oncol.* 12, 596–600.

Hesketh, P. J., Rossi, G., Rizzi, G., Palmas, M., Alyasova, A., Bondarenko, I., et al. (2014). Efficacy and safety of NEPA, an oral combination of netupitant and palonosetron, for prevention of chemotherapy-induced nausea and vomiting following highly emetogenic chemotherapy: a randomized dose-ranging pivotal study. *Ann. Oncol.* 25, 1340–1346. doi: 10.1093/annonc/mdu110

Huskey, S. E., Dean, B. J., Bakhtiar, R., Sanchez, R. I., Tattersall, F. D., Rycroft, W., et al. (2003). Brain penetration of aprepitant, a substance P receptor antagonist, in ferrets. *Drug Metab. Dispos.* 31, 785–791. doi: 10.1124/dmd.31.6.785

Ioannidis, J. P., Hesketh, P. J., and Lau, J. (2000). Contribution of dexamethasone to control of chemotherapy-induced nausea and vomiting: a meta-analysis of randomized evidence. *J. Clin. Oncol.* 18, 3409–3422.

Ito, H., Nishibayashi, M., Kawabata, K., Maeda, S., Seki, M., and Ebukuro, S. (2003). Induction of Fos protein in neurons in the medulla oblongata after motion- and X-irradiation-induced emesis in musk shrews (*Suncus murinus*). *Auton. Neurosci.* 107, 1–8. doi: 10.1016/S1566-0702(03)00026-2

Jordan, K., Kasper, C., and Schmoll, H. J. (2005). Chemotherapy-induced nausea and vomiting: current and new standards in the antiemetic prophylaxis and treatment. *Eur. J. Cancer* 41, 199–205. doi: 10.1016/j.ejca.2004.09.026

Kan, K. K., Rudd, J. A., and Wai, M. K. (2006). Differential action of anti-emetic drugs on defecation and emesis induced by prostaglandin E2 in the ferret. *Eur. J. Pharmacol.* 544, 153–159. doi: 10.1016/j.ejphar.2006.06.034

Lau, A. H., Ngan, M. P., Rudd, J. A., and Yew, D. T. (2005). Differential action of domperidone to modify emesis and behaviour induced by apomorphine in the ferret. *Eur. J. Pharmacol.* 516, 247–252. doi: 10.1016/j.ejphar.2005.05.028

Lorusso, V., Karthaus, M., and Aapro, M. (2015). Review of oral fixed-dose combination netupitant and palonosetron (NEPA) for the treatment of chemotherapy-induced nausea and vomiting. *Future Oncol.* 11, 565–577. doi: 10.2217/fon.14.260

Lucot, J. B., Obach, R. S., McLean, S., and Watson, J. W. (1997). The effect of CP-99994 on the responses to provocative motion in the cat. *Br. J. Pharmacol.* 120, 116–120. doi: 10.1038/sj.bjp.0700888

Makale, M. T., and King, G. L. (1992). Surgical and pharmacological dissociation of cardiovascular and emetic responses to intragastric $CuSO_4$. *Am. J. Physiol.* 263, R284–R291.

Minami, M., Endo, T., Hirafuji, M., Hamaue, N., Liu, Y., Hiroshige, T., et al. (2003). Pharmacological aspects of anticancer drug-induced emesis with emphasis on serotonin release and vagal nerve activity. *Pharmacol. Ther.* 99, 149–165. doi: 10.1016/S0163-7258(03)00057-3

Minami, M., Endo, T., Kikuchi, K., Ihira, E., Hirafuji, M., Hamaue, N., et al. (1998). Antiemetic effects of sendide, a peptide tachykinin NK1 receptor antagonist, in the ferret. *Eur. J. Pharmacol.* 363, 49–55. doi: 10.1016/S0014-2999(98)00784-5

Minami, M., Endo, T., Monma, Y., and Shiroshita, Y. (1991). Phamracology of emesis induced by ant-cancer drugs. *J. Toxicol. Sci.* 16, 35–39. doi: 10.2131/jts.16.SupplementII_35

Morrow, G. R. (1984). Susceptibility to motion sickness and chemotherapy-induced side-effects. *Lancet* 1, 390–391. doi: 10.1016/S0140-6736(84)90436-7

Navari, R. M. (2004). Role of neurokinin-1 receptor antagonists in chemotherapy-induced emesis: summary of clinical trials. *Cancer Invest.* 22, 569–576. doi: 10.1081/CNV-200027137

Navari, R. M. (2009). Pharmacological management of chemotherapy-induced nausea and vomiting: focus on recent developments. *Drugs* 69, 515–533. doi: 10.2165/00003495-200969050-00002

Navari, R. M. (2015). Profile of netupitant/palonosetron (NEPA) fixed dose combination and its potential in the treatment of chemotherapy-induced nausea and vomiting (CINV). *Drug Des. Devel. Ther.* 9, 155–161. doi: 10.2147/DDDT.S76158

Naylor, R. J., and Rudd, J. A. (1996). Mechanisms of chemotherapy/radiotherapy-induced emesis in animal models. *Oncology* 53(Suppl. 1), 8–17. doi: 10.1159/000227634

Percie du Sert, N., Rudd, J. A., Apfel, C. C., and Andrews, P. L. (2011). Cisplatin-induced emesis: systematic review and meta-analysis of the ferret model and the effects of 5-HT(3) receptor antagonists. *Cancer Chemother. Pharmacol.* 67, 667–686. doi: 10.1007/s00280-010-1339-4

Percie du Sert, N., Rudd, J. A., Moss, R., and Andrews, P. L. (2009). The delayed phase of cisplatin-induced emesis is mediated by the area postrema and not the abdominal visceral innervation in the ferret. *Neurosci. Lett.* 465, 16–20. doi: 10.1016/j.neulet.2009.08.075

Ray, A. P., Chebolu, S., Ramirez, J., and Darmani, N. A. (2009). Ablation of least shrew central neurokinin NK1 receptors reduces GR73632-induced vomiting. *Behav. Neurosci.* 123, 701–706. doi: 10.1037/a0015733

Reddy, G. K., Gralla, R. J., and Hesketh, P. J. (2006). Novel neurokinin-1 antagonists as antiemetics for the treatment of chemotherapy-induced emesis. *Support. Cancer Ther.* 3, 140–142. doi: 10.3816/SCT.2006.n.011

Rizzi, A., Campi, B., Camarda, V., Molinari, S., Cantoreggi, S., Regoli, D., et al. (2012). In vitro and in vivo pharmacological characterization of the novel NK(1) receptor selective antagonist Netupitant. *Peptides* 37, 86–97. doi: 10.1016/j.peptides.2012.06.010

Roila, F., Herrstedt, J., Aapro, M., Gralla, R. J., Einhorn, L. H., Ballatori, E., et al. (2010). Guideline update for MASCC and ESMO in the prevention of chemotherapy- and radiotherapy-induced nausea and vomiting: results of the Perugia consensus conference. *Ann. Oncol.* 21(Suppl. 5), v232–v243. doi: 10.1093/annonc/mdq194

Rojas, C., Li, Y., Zhang, J., Stathis, M., Alt, J., Thomas, A. G., et al. (2010a). The antiemetic 5-HT3 receptor antagonist Palonosetron inhibits substance P-mediated responses in vitro and in vivo. *J. Pharmacol. Exp. Ther.* 335, 362–368. doi: 10.1124/jpet.110.166181

Rojas, C., Thomas, A. G., Alt, J., Stathis, M., Zhang, J., Rubenstein, E. B., et al. (2010b). Palonosetron triggers 5-HT(3) receptor internalization and causes prolonged inhibition of receptor function. *Eur. J. Pharmacol.* 626, 193–199. doi: 10.1016/j.ejphar.2009.10.002

Rojas, C., Raje, M., Tsukamoto, T., and Slusher, B. S. (2014). Molecular mechanisms of 5-HT(3) and NK(1) receptor antagonists in prevention of emesis. *Eur. J. Pharmacol.* 722, 26–37. doi: 10.1016/j.ejphar.2013.08.049

Rojas, C., Stathis, M., Thomas, A. G., Massuda, E. B., Alt, J., Zhang, J., et al. (2008). Palonosetron exhibits unique molecular interactions with the 5-HT3 receptor. *Anesth. Analg.* 107, 469–478. doi: 10.1213/ane.0b013e318172fa74

Rubenstein, E. B. (2004). Palonosetron: a unique 5-HT(3) receptor antagonist indicated for the prevention of acute and delayed chemotherapy-induced nausea and vomiting. *Clin. Adv. Hematol. Oncol.* 2, 284–288.

Rudd, J. A., and Andrews, P. L. R. (2004). "Mechanisms of acute, delayed and anticipatory vomiting in cancer and cancer treatment," in *Management of Nausea and Vomiting in Cancer and Cancer Treatment*, ed. P. Hesketh (New York, NY: Jones and Barlett Publishers Inc.), 15–66.

Rudd, J. A., Jordan, C. C., and Naylor, R. J. (1994). Profiles of emetic action of cisplatin in the ferret: a potential model of acute and delayed emesis. *Eur. J. Pharmacol.* 262, R1–R2. doi: 10.1016/0014-2999(94)90048-5

Rudd, J. A., Jordan, C. C., and Naylor, R. J. (1996). The action of the NK1 tachykinin receptor antagonist, CP 99,994, in antagonizing the acute and delayed emesis induced by cisplatin in the ferret. *Br. J. Pharmacol.* 119, 931–936. doi: 10.1111/j.1476-5381.1996.tb15761.x

Rudd, J. A., and Naylor, R. J. (1994). Effects of 5-HT3 receptor antagonists on models of acute and delayed emesis induced by cisplatin in the ferret. *Neuropharmacology* 33, 1607–1608. doi: 10.1016/0028-3908(94)90136-8

Rudd, J. A., and Naylor, R. J. (1995). "Opioid receptor involvement in emesis and anti-emesis," in *Serotonin and the Scientific Basis of Anti-Emetic Therapy*, eds P. L. R. Andrew, D. J. M. Reynolds, and C. J. Davis (London: Oxford Clincal Communications), 208–219.

Rudd, J. A., and Naylor, R. J. (1996). An interaction of ondansetron and dexamethasone antagonizing cisplatin-induced acute and delayed emesis in the ferret. *Br. J. Pharmacol.* 118, 209–214. doi: 10.1111/j.1476-5381.1996.tb15388.x

Rudd, J. A., and Naylor, R. J. (1997). The actions of ondansetron and dexamethasone to antagonise cisplatin-induced emesis in the ferret. *Eur. J. Pharmacol.* 322, 79–82. doi: 10.1016/S0014-2999(97)00073-3

Rudd, J. A., Ngan, M. P., and Wai, M. K. (1999). Inhibition of emesis by tachykinin NK1 receptor antagonists in *Suncus murinus* (house musk shrew). *Eur. J. Pharmacol.* 366, 243–252. doi: 10.1016/S0014-2999(98)00920-0

Rupniak, N. M., Tattersall, F. D., Williams, A. R., Rycroft, W., Carlson, E. J., Cascieri, M. A., et al. (1997). In vitro and in vivo predictors of the anti-emetic activity of tachykinin NK1 receptor antagonists. *Eur. J. Pharmacol.* 326, 201–209. doi: 10.1016/S0014-2999(97)85415-5

Saito, M., Aogi, K., Sekine, I., Yoshizawa, H., Yanagita, Y., Sakai, H., et al. (2009). Palonosetron plus dexamethasone versus granisetron plus dexamethasone for prevention of nausea and vomiting during chemotherapy: a double-blind, double-dummy, randomised, comparative phase III trial. *Lancet Oncol.* 10, 115–124. doi: 10.1016/S1470-2045(08)70313-9

Sam, T. S., Chan, S. W., Rudd, J. A., and Yeung, J. H. (2001). Action of glucocorticoids to antagonise cisplatin-induced acute and delayed emesis in the ferret. *Eur. J. Pharmacol.* 417, 231–237. doi: 10.1016/S0014-2999(01)00915-3

Shih, V., Wan, H. S., and Chan, A. (2009). Clinical predictors of chemotherapy-induced nausea and vomiting in breast cancer patients receiving adjuvant doxorubicin and cyclophosphamide. *Ann. Pharmacother.* 43, 444–452. doi: 10.1345/aph.1L437

Siddiqui, M. A., and Scott, L. J. (2004). Palonosetron. *Drugs* 64, 1125–1132; discussion1133–1124. doi: 10.2165/00003495-200464100-00006

Singh, L., Field, M. J., Hughes, J., Kuo, B. S., Suman-Chauhan, N., Tuladhar, B. R., et al. (1997). The tachykinin NK1 receptor antagonist PD 154075 blocks cisplatin-induced delayed emesis in the ferret. *Eur. J. Pharmacol.* 321, 209–216. doi: 10.1016/S0014-2999(96)00950-8

Stathis, M., Pietra, C., Rojas, C., and Slusher, B. S. (2012). Inhibition of substance P-mediated responses in NG108-15 cells by netupitant and palonosetron exhibit synergistic effects. *Eur. J. Pharmacol.* 689, 25–30. doi: 10.1016/j.ejphar.2012.05.037

Stoltz, R., Cyong, J. C., Shah, A., and Parisi, S. (2004). Pharmacokinetic and safety evaluation of palonosetron, a 5-hydroxytryptamine-3 receptor antagonist, in U.S. and Japanese healthy subjects. *J. Clin. Pharmacol.* 44, 520–531. doi: 10.1177/0091270004264641

Tattersall, F. D., Rycroft, W., Cumberbatch, M., Mason, G., Tye, S., Williamson, D. J., et al. (2000). The novel NK1 receptor antagonist MK-0869 (L-754,030) and its water soluble phosphoryl prodrug, L-758,298, inhibit acute and delayed cisplatin-induced emesis in ferrets. *Neuropharmacology* 39, 652–663. doi: 10.1016/S0028-3908(99)00172-0

Tattersall, F. D., Rycroft, W., Francis, B., Pearce, D., Merchant, K., MacLeod, A. M., et al. (1996). Tachykinin NK1 receptor antagonists act centrally to inhibit emesis induced by the chemotherapeutic agent cisplatin in ferrets. *Neuropharmacology* 35, 1121–1129. doi: 10.1016/S0028-3908(96)00020-2

Tattersall, F. D., Rycroft, W., Hargreaves, R. J., and Hill, R. G. (1993). The tachykinin NK1 receptor antagonist CP-99,994 attenuates cisplatin induced emesis in the ferret. *Eur. J. Pharmacol.* 250, R5–R6. doi: 10.1016/0014-2999(93)90649-3

Tattersall, F. D., Rycroft, W., Hill, R. G., and Hargreaves, R. J. (1994). Enantioselective inhibition of apomorphine-induced emesis in the ferret by the neurokinin1 receptor antagonist CP-99,994. *Neuropharmacology* 33, 259–260. doi: 10.1016/0028-3908(94)90018-3

Tattersall, F. D., Rycroft, W., Marmont, N., Cascieri, M., Hill, R. G., and Hargreaves, R. J. (1995). Enantiospecific inhibition of emesis induced by nicotine in the house musk shrew (*Suncus murinus*) by the neurokinin1 (NK1) receptor antagonist CP-99,994. *Neuropharmacology* 34, 1697–1699. doi: 10.1016/0028-3908(95)00164-6

Thompson, C. A. (2014). Netupitant-palonosetron combination approved by FDA. *Am. J. Health Syst. Pharm.* 71, 2000. doi: 10.2146/news140079

Tonini, G., Vincenzi, B., and Santini, D. (2005). New drugs for chemotherapy-induced nausea and vomiting: focus on palonosetron. *Expert Opin. Drug Metab. Toxicol.* 1, 143–149. doi: 10.1517/17425255.1.1.143

Tsuchiya, M., Fujiwara, Y., Kanai, Y., Mizutani, M., Shimada, K., Suga, O., et al. (2002). Anti-emetic activity of the novel nonpeptide tachykinin NK1 receptor antagonist ezlopitant (CJ-11,974) against acute and delayed cisplatin-induced emesis in the ferret. *Pharmacology* 66, 144–152. doi: 10.1159/0000 63796

Ueno, S., Matsuki, N., and Saito, H. (1988). *Suncus murinus* as a new experimental model for motion sickness. *Life Sci.* 43, 413–420. doi: 10.1016/0024-3205(88)90520-6

Warr, D. (2014). Prognostic factors for chemotherapy induced nausea and vomiting. *Eur. J. Pharmacol.* 722, 192–196. doi: 10.1016/j.ejphar.2013.10.015

Watanabe, Y., Okamoto, M., Ishii, T., Takatsuka, S., Taniguchi, H., Nagasaki, M., et al. (2008). Long-Lasting Anti-emetic Effect of T-2328, a Novel NK(1) Antagonist. *J. Pharmacol. Sci.* 107, 151–158. doi: 10.1254/jphs.08027FP

Watson, J. W., Gonsalves, S. F., Fossa, A. A., McLean, S., Seeger, T., Obach, S., et al. (1995). The anti-emetic effects of CP-99,994 in the ferret and the dog: role of the NK1 receptor. *Br. J. Pharmacol.* 115, 84–94. doi: 10.1111/j.1476-5381.1995.tb16324.x

Wong, E. H., Clark, R., Leung, E., Loury, D., Bonhaus, D. W., Jakeman, L., et al. (1995). The interaction of RS 25259-197, a potent and selective antagonist, with 5-HT3 receptors, in vitro. *Br. J. Pharmacol.* 114, 851–859. doi: 10.1111/j.1476-5381.1995.tb13282.x

Zaman, S., Woods, A. J., Watson, J. W., Reynolds, D. J., and Andrews, P. L. (2000). The effect of the NK1 receptor antagonist CP-99,994 on emesis and c-fos protein induction by loperamide in the ferret. *Neuropharmacology* 39, 316–323. doi: 10.1016/S0028-3908(99)00113-6

Conflict of Interest Statement: The authors declare that the research was conducted in the absence of any commercial or financial relationships that could be construed as a potential conflict of interest.

11

Tempol Ameliorates and Prevents Mechanical Hyperalgesia in a Rat Model of Chemotherapy-Induced Neuropathic Pain

Hee Kee Kim*, Seon-Hee Hwang and Salahadin Abdi*

Department of Pain Medicine, Division of Anesthesiology and Critical Care, The University of Texas MD Anderson Cancer Center, Houston, TX, USA

Chemotherapy-induced neuropathic pain is difficult to treat and prevent. Tempol decreases cellular superoxide radical levels and oxidative stress. The aims of our study were to investigate the analgesic and preventive effects of tempol on paclitaxel-induced neuropathic pain in rats and to identify the associated mechanisms of action. Neuropathic pain was induced with intraperitoneally injected paclitaxel on four alternate days in male Sprague–Dawley rats. Tempol was administered systemically as a single injection and a continuous infusion before or after the injection of paclitaxel. The mechanical threshold for allodynia, protein levels, and free radical levels were measured using von Frey filaments, Western blotting, and live cell imaging, respectively. After the rats developed neuropathic pain behavior, a single intraperitoneal injection and continuous infusion of tempol ameliorated paclitaxel-induced mechanical allodynia. Systemic infusion of tempol in the early phase of the development of pain behavior prevented the development of paclitaxel-induced pain behavior. Paclitaxel increased the levels of phosphorylated protein kinase C, phosphorylated nuclear factor κB, phosphodiesterase 4D (PDE4D), IL-1β, and monocyte chemoattractant protein-1 in the lumbar dorsal root ganglia; however, tempol decreased these levels. Paclitaxel also increased superoxide levels in a culture of primary dorsal root ganglion cells and tempol decreased these levels. In conclusion, tempol alleviates and prevents chemotherapy-induced neuropathic pain in rats by reducing the levels of inflammatory cytokines and free radicals in dorsal root ganglia.

Keywords: chemotherapy, neuropathic pain, free radical, inflammatory cytokines, paclitaxel, tempol

Edited by:
Raquel Abalo,
Universidad Rey Juan Carlos, Spain

Reviewed by:
David Balayssac,
Institut National de la Santé et de la Recherche Médicale (INSERM), France
David Pascual,
Universidad Rey Juan Carlos, Spain

****Correspondence:***
Hee Kee Kim
hkim9@mdanderson.org
Salahadin Abdi
sabdi@mdanderson.org

INTRODUCTION

Chemotherapeutic agents, including taxanes (e.g., paclitaxel, docetaxel), vinca alkaloids (e.g., vincristine, vinblastine), platinum agents (e.g., cisplatin, carboplatin, oxaliplatin), and others (e.g., thalidomide, bortezomib, lenalidomide), produce peripheral pain in the distal extremities in a symmetrical glove and stocking distribution (Yazdani and Abdi, 2014). Chemotherapy-induced neuropathic pain is a dose-limiting adverse effect that can take place at any time during the course of the treatment or even after its termination (Windebank and Grisold, 2008). This neuropathy can significantly decrease the overall quality of life in cancer patients (Mols et al., 2014; Rivera and Cianfrocca, 2015).

To date, analgesic drugs such as opioids, non-steroidal anti-inflammatory agents, anticonvulsants, antidepressants, and sodium channel blockers show little or no analgesic effects in paclitaxel-induced neuropathic pain (PINP) models (Xiao et al., 2008). It has also been reported that glutamine, glutathione, *N*-acetylcysteine, oxcarbazepine, and xaliproden did not prevent chemotherapy-induced neuropathy (Wolf et al., 2008). On the other hand, there have been several preclinical reports indicating cannabinoids might have some effects in reducing chemotherapy-induced peripheral neuropathy (Deng et al., 2012, 2015; Khasabova et al., 2012; Guindon et al., 2013; Vera et al., 2013; Harris et al., 2016), but their clinical efficacy has not been proved yet. Therefore, currently, no effective medications are available to treat or prevent neuropathic pain (Lee and Swain, 2006; Wolf et al., 2008; Hershman et al., 2014) and new alternatives need to be explored.

Several pain models have shown that systemic or spinal administration of free radical scavengers, including phenyl *N*-tert-butylnitrone and vitamin E, reduce pain behavior (Kim et al., 2004, 2006). In addition, tempol, a membrane-permeable superoxide dismutase mimetic, was reported to attenuate zymosan-induced visceral pain behavior and peroxynitrite-enhanced carrageenan-induced hyperalgesia (Khattab, 2006; Ji et al., 2015). Tempol is a member of nitroxide compounds and reacts with superoxide anion to form hydrogen peroxide. In addition, the sensitivity of tempol was greatest for hydroxyl radical, intermediate for hydrogen peroxide, and least for superoxide radical (Soule et al., 2007; Wilcox and Pearlman, 2008). The toxic doses of tempol are about 172.25–344.5 mg/kg when animals were intraperitoneally injected (Hahn et al., 1998). Tempol reduced oxidative damage in cerebral synaptosomes from gerbils and reduced exacerbated hypoxic brain damage (Howard et al., 1996; MacGregor et al., 2003). Tempol blocked the enhanced *N*-methyl-D-aspartate-induced neurotoxicity in cultured cortical brain cells (Hewett et al., 1994; Teichner et al., 2003). In addition, several studies have reported that tempol reduced tumor growth and incidence of cancer. Tempol decreased glioma formation in rats and delayed the development of tumors, and prolonged the lifespan of cancer-prone mice (Gariboldi et al., 2003; Erker et al., 2005; Zhang et al., 2008). However, the analgesic and preventive effects of tempol on chemotherapy-induced neuropathic pain have not been studied. The aims of this study were to investigate (1) the analgesic effects of tempol on PINP in rats, (2) the preventive effects of tempol on the development of PINP in rats, and (3) the mechanisms of action of tempol in the dorsal root ganglia (DRGs).

MATERIALS AND METHODS

Experimental Animals

Male adult Sprague–Dawley rats (200–350 g; Harlan Sprague–Dawley Company, Houston, TX, USA) were used for the experiment. They had free access to food and water and were housed in a room with a normal light-dark cycle (light cycle: 7:00 a.m. to 7:00 p.m.). All animals were habituated for 1 week before the experiments. The experimental protocol was approved by the institutional animal care and use committees of The University of Texas MD Anderson Cancer Center.

Paclitaxel-Induced Neuropathic Pain

Paclitaxel (Sigma, St. Louis, MO, USA) was dissolved in a vehicle solution (4% dimethyl sulfoxide and 4% Tween 80 in sterile saline) and was injected intraperitoneally at a dose of 2 mg/kg on days 0, 2, 4, and 6 (Polomano et al., 2001; Kim et al., 2010). Control rats were injected with the same volume of vehicle without paclitaxel.

Measurement of Mechanical Allodynia

To measure mechanical allodynia, we used a behavior test that has been described previously (Chaplan et al., 1994). Briefly, rats were placed in a plastic chamber on top of a mesh screen, and the mechanical threshold of the left hind paw was determined by the up-down method (Dixon, 1980) using monofilaments (0.45–14.45 g). A filament was applied to the most sensitive parts of the paw's plantar surface – the center of the paw or the base of the third or fourth toes – for 3–4 s. A sudden withdrawal of the foot during stimulation or immediately after removal of the filament was considered to be a positive response. A 50% mechanical threshold value was calculated. The investigator who conducted the behavioral tests was blinded to the control or treatment status of the rats.

Western Blot Analysis

The rats were anesthetized deeply with 4% isoflurane for induction for 5 min and then 3% for the maintenance. During anesthesia, rats were removed hair, opened chest cavity, and then perfused with cold saline. The L1-6 DRGs were removed, frozen in liquid nitrogen, and then stored in deep freezer (−80°C). They were homogenized in 150 μl of RIPA cell lysis buffer with a protease inhibitor on ice by homogenizer four times for 20 s (interval time: 2 min) and centrifuged at 17,000 × *g* at 4°C for 10 min. And then supernatants were loaded in 10% sodium dodecyl sulfate-polyacrylamide gels and transferred to polyvinylidene fluoride membranes. Blots were incubated with primary antibody against IL-1β (1:1000; Santa Cruz Biotechnology, Dallas, TX, USA), MCP-1 (1:500; Santa Cruz Biotechnology, Dallas, TX, USA), PDE4D (1:5000; Abcam, Cambridge, MA, USA), phosphorylated nuclear factor κB (p-NF-κB, 1:1000; Cell Signaling Technology, Danvers, MA, USA), phosphorylated protein kinase C (p-PKC, 1:1000; Cell Signaling Technology, Danvers, MA, USA), and GAPDH (1:5000; Santa Cruz Biotechnology, Dallas, TX, USA) overnight at 4°C. The blots were then incubated with anti-rabbit horseradish peroxidase-conjugated secondary antibody (1:5000; GenDepot, Katy, TX, USA) or anti-goat horseradish peroxidase-conjugated secondary antibody (1:5000; GenDepot, Katy, TX, USA). The immunoblots were analyzed with a chemiluminescence detection system and normalized to GAPDH. For equalizing protein loading, GAPDH expression was used as a control.

Behavioral Testing for Sedation

Behavioral testing for sedation was based on five-point scales of posture (0 = normal, 4 = flaccid atonia) and righting reflexes

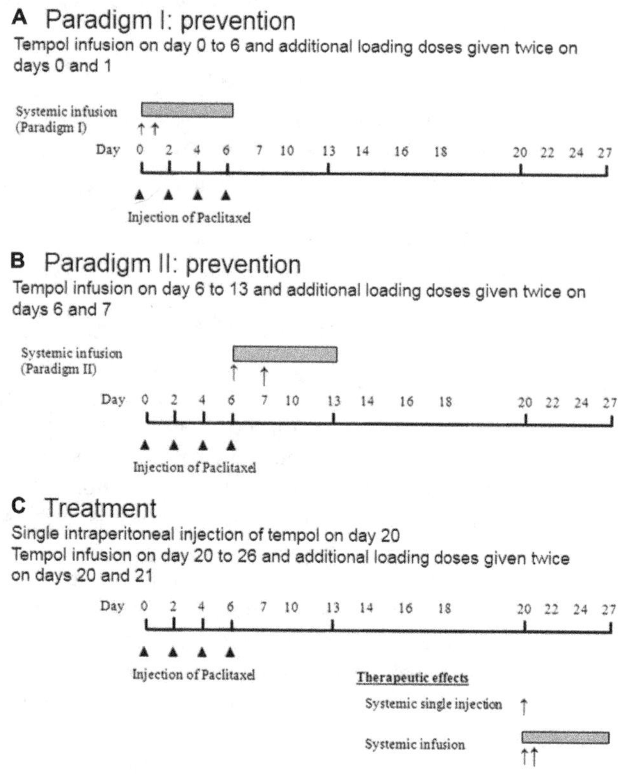

FIGURE 1 | Schematic overview of the experimental design. Note, ▲ represented single intraperitoneal injection of paclitaxel, ↑ represented single intraperitoneal injection of tempol, and ▭ represented intraperitoneal infusion of tempol.

(0 = struggles, 4 = no movement; Devor and Zalkind, 2001; Kim et al., 2004). Sedation was assessed immediately after each pain behavior test.

Administration of Tempol

This study consisted of two parts: (1) Assessment of the therapeutic effects of tempol on PINP, given as a single intraperitoneal injection (50, 100, or 200 mg/kg) or as intraperitoneal infusion (10 mg/day for 7 days), and (2) investigation of the preventive effects of tempol given as intraperitoneal infusion on development of PINP (**Figures 1A–C**).

Assessment of the Therapeutic Effects of Tempol

For administration of tempol as a single intraperitoneal injection, on day 20 after the first paclitaxel injection, 24 rats were divided into four groups. After the rats developed neuropathic pain behavior, they were randomly assigned to one of three treatment groups or a control group. Rats in the treatment groups (six rats per group) received 50, 100, or 200 mg/kg tempol in 5 mL/kg saline, and rats in the control group received a single 5-mL/kg injection of saline (**Figure 1C**).

For administration of tempol as a systemic intraperitoneal infusion (**Figure 1C**), on the 20th day after the first paclitaxel injection, the rats that developed neuropathic pain behavior were randomly assigned to either a treatment group (tempol, six rats) or a control group (vehicle, five rats) before the insertion of a mini-osmotic pump (Alzet model 2001; Alzet, Cupertino, CA, USA). The rats in the treatment group received an infusion of tempol at a rate of 1 μL/h for 7 days (10 mg/day). Additionally, loading doses of tempol (200 mg/kg) were administered on days 20 and 21 after the first paclitaxel injection. The rats in the control group received equivalent volumes of saline via the pump and as loading doses (5 mL/kg).

Assessment of the Preventive Effects of Tempol

Tempol (10 mg/day) was infused intraperitoneally (Alzet model 2001 mini-osmotic pump) by one of the following methods of administration. In paradigm I, a bolus of tempol was injected intraperitoneally at a dose of 200 mg/kg on days 0 and 1 and continuously infused intraperitoneally for 7 days (days 0 through 6; **Figure 1A**). In paradigm II, the same dose of tempol was given as a bolus on days 6 and 7, and continuous infusion was administered on days 6 through 13 (**Figure 1B**). Mechanical allodynia was measured on days 0, 2, 4, 6, 7, 9, 10, 11, 12, 13, 14, 16, 17, 18, 19, 20, 24, 26, 30, 34, 37, and 40. We measured the animal's body weight regularly after the aforementioned behavioral tests. There was normal increase in their body weight. Furthermore, while observing animals, we did not notice any stress.

Intraperitoneal Implantation of the Mini-Osmotic Pump

The mini-osmotic pump was implanted intraperitoneally according to the manufacturer's protocol. Briefly, a midline skin and peritoneal wall incision was made in the lower abdomen of rats that had received isoflurane anesthesia in oxygen. The pump was filled with tempol or saline and inserted into the peritoneal cavity. The musculoperitoneal layer was sutured with silk sutures, and the skin incision was closed with wound clips. Anesthesia was discontinued, and the animals were allowed to recover from anesthesia.

DRG Cell Culture

Dorsal root ganglia cells were cultured as previously described with slight modifications (Shetty et al., 2015). Briefly, under general anesthesia with isoflurane, the lumbar DRGs from L1 to L6 were removed in sterile conditions. The DRGs were then dissociated with 1.25 mg/mL collagenase (Sigma) twice for 1 h at 37°C and mechanical dissociation. Cells were plated on a 35-mm dish (Costar, Corning, NY, USA) coated with poly-*L*-lysine and laminin in Dulbecco's Modified Eagle's Medium (DMEM) with 10% fetal bovine serum (FBS), 1% penicillin/streptomycin, and 4 mM glutamine for 5 days in CO_2 incubator (5% CO_2, 37°C). DRG cells were plated in a chambered coverglass with cover No. 1.5 borosilicate sterile (four well, Thermo Fisher Scientific, Waltham, MA, USA) in a volume of 1 mL of DMEM with 5% FBS for live cell microscopy studies. The cells were stained with trypan blue, and viability was measured by a Luna automated cell counter (Logos Biosystems, Annandale, VA, USA).

Live Cell Imaging for Mitochondrial Superoxide Level

Dorsal root ganglia cells were plated in a chambered coverglass with cover No. 1.5 borosilicate sterile (four well, Thermo Fisher Scientific) in a volume of 1 mL of DMEM with 5% FBS. After 24 h incubation, cells were stained with 5 μM MitoSOX (Molecular Probes, Eugene, OR, USA) for 10 min, washed with DMEM twice, and then treated for 2 h with 1 μM paclitaxel in vehicle (0.025% dimethyl sulfoxide in DMEM). MitoSOX is a novel fluorogenic dye and produces red fluorescence by superoxide from only mitochondria in live cells. In addition, MitoSOX can permeate live cells where it selectively targets mitochondria. Red fluorescent intensity in living cells were measured using a Zeiss LSM510 Meta laser scanning confocal system (Carl Zeiss, Inc, Thornwood, NY, USA) in a box incubator (5% CO_2, 37°C, Reinach, Switzerland). Confocal scanning setting was used at the lowest laser intensity to capture pixels in the range of 0–255. The images were quantified using Volocity imaging software (Improvision, Perkin Elmer, Waltham, MA, USA). The fluorescent threshold was set at 50–255. Data represent the sum of pixels in an image by the area that produced red fluorescence.

Statistical Analyses

Data were summarized as means with standard errors of the means for the behavioral testing, Western blotting, and live cell imaging. The data were analyzed using the GraphPad Prism 6 and two-way repeated-measures analyses of variance with one repeated factor (time), followed by the Tukey *post hoc* test for behavioral testing and the Mann–Whitney *U* test for Western blotting and cell imaging. In all cases, $P < 0.05$ was considered statistically significant.

RESULTS

Tempol Did Not Produce Sedation

All rats treated with single (50, 100, 200 mg/kg) or infusion (10 mg/day) of tempol or vehicle had a score of 0 on both the posture and righting reflex scales, indicating that tempol did not produce sedation. Reviewer recommended to use positive control such as diazepam to validate the sedation experiment. At this time, we did not use positive control because we had reported several publications using this method (Devor and Zalkind, 2001; Kim et al., 2004, 2006, 2010, 2015). In addition, all rats treated with tempol without paclitaxel showed normal behavior including no sedation, no pain behavior, and normal increase in body weight.

Tempol Increased the Mechanical Threshold of PINP

Single intraperitoneal injection of tempol at doses of 50, 100, and 200 mg/kg on day 20 increased mechanical threshold in a dose-dependent manner in rats (**Figure 2A**). Moreover, the 200-mg dose significantly increased mechanical threshold from 0.9 to 9.7 g at 0.5 h after injection compared with the saline group, but the threshold returned to baseline at 2 h. We selected 50, 100, and 200 mg/kg based on our preliminary data.

To investigate the extended analgesic effects of tempol, 200 mg/kg was intraperitoneally injected on days 20 and 21, and 10 mg/day was intraperitoneally infused for 7 days (**Figure 2B**). The control group received intraperitoneal injections and infusion of saline. Mechanical threshold was measured each morning. Tempol significantly increased the mechanical

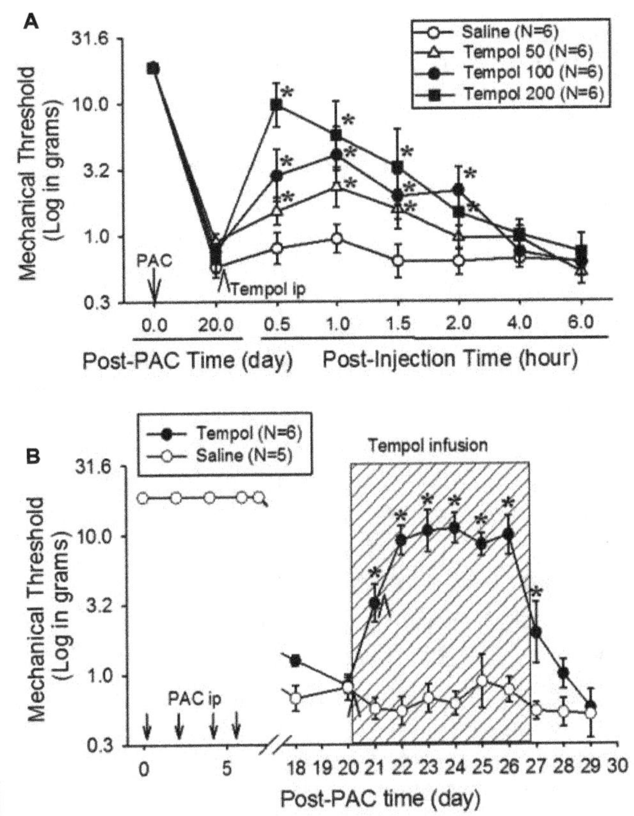

FIGURE 2 | Analgesic effects of a single systemic injection (A) or systemic infusion **(B)** of tempol on paclitaxel-induced neuropathic pain (PINP) in rats. Paclitaxel (PAC, 2 mg/kg) was injected intraperitoneally on four alternate days (days 0, 2, 4, and 6), and the mechanical threshold was measured. **(A)** On day 20 after the first paclitaxel injection, 24 rats were divided into four groups, which received an intraperitoneal injection of saline or 50, 100, or 200 mg/kg of tempol (5 mL/kg). Note that the mechanical threshold returned to more than 10 g of mechanical threshold (no pain condition in rats) at 0.5 h after the injection of 200 mg/kg of tempol. **(B)** On day 20 after the first paclitaxel injection, 11 rats were divided into two groups. In the tempol group ($N = 6$), the rats received an intraperitoneal infusion of tempol (10 mg/day) for 7 days (hatched box) in combination with intraperitoneal injections of tempol (200 mg/kg) on days 20 and 21 (arrowheads). In the saline group ($N = 5$), the rats received saline (vehicle) instead of tempol. The systemic infusion of tempol significantly increased the mechanical threshold on day 21, and the threshold remained significantly higher than the threshold in the control group for 8 days. The data are expressed as means with standard errors of the means. The asterisks indicate values that are significantly different ($P < 0.05$) from the corresponding values for the saline group as determined by a two-way repeated-measures analysis of variance with one repeated factor (time) followed by the Tukey *post hoc* test.

threshold over that of the saline group on day 21, and the threshold remained significantly higher on day 27. These data indicate that infusion of tempol produced a prolonged analgesic effect without sedation.

Tempol Prevented the Development of PINP

To examine its preventive effects, tempol (10 mg/day) was infused intraperitoneally for 7 days beginning 1 h before the first paclitaxel injection (day 0) in paradigm I or beginning on day 6 in paradigm II. The early treatment (starting on day 0) did not affect the development of pain behavior (**Figure 3A**). In contrast, the treatment beginning on day 6 completely prevented further development of pain behavior for 40 days in paradigm II (**Figure 3B**). These data indicate that tempol prevented the development of PINP when given during the development phase of mechanical hyperalgesia.

Paclitaxel Increased the Levels of p-PKC, p-NF-κB, PDE4D, IL-1β, and MCP-1 in DRGs, and Tempol Subsequently Decreased the Levels

To examine the levels of signaling molecules, paclitaxel (2 mg/kg on days 0, 2, 4, and 6) or vehicle (4% dimethyl sulfoxide and 4% Tween 80 in saline) was intraperitoneally injected, and L1-6 DRGs were collected on day 20 after the first injection of paclitaxel or vehicle for Western blot analysis. Paclitaxel significantly increased the levels of p-PKC (1.9 times), p-NF-κB (2.1 times), PDE4D (1.7 times), IL-1β (1.9 times), and MCP-1 (2.2 times) in the DRGs compared to those in the vehicle control group (**Figures 4A–F**). Subsequently, tempol was infused for 7 days (days 14–20), and lumbar DRGs were removed on day 20 for Western blot analysis. Tempol decreased the levels of p-PKC, p-NF-κB, PDE4D, IL-1β, and MCP-1 in the DRGs of paclitaxel-treated rats to the levels in the DRGs of vehicle-injected rats (**Figures 4A–F**).

Paclitaxel Increased Mitochondrial Superoxide Levels in DRG Cell Culture, and Tempol Subsequently Decreased the Levels

To examine the effects of paclitaxel and tempol on mitochondrial superoxide levels, the L1-6 DRGs were removed from a normal adult rat and DRG cells were cultured with the MitoSOX dye in a CO_2 incubator. The MitoSOX reagent produces red fluorescence by mitochondrial superoxide but not by other free radicals. Paclitaxel increased the MitoSOX-detected red fluorescence intensity (**Figures 5A–E**). The 1 μM of paclitaxel significantly increased the fluorescence intensity at 2 (126%) and 4 h (132%) compared with before the treatment with paclitaxel (**Figures 5A,D,E**). These data indicate that paclitaxel increased the mitochondrial superoxide levels in the primary DRG cell culture. The DRG cells were alive at levels of 85–95% when treated with 1 μM of paclitaxel, but treatment with 5 μM of paclitaxel decreased cell viability to 62%. Therefore, we chose 1 μM of paclitaxel and 2 h for incubation time.

Figure 6 shows that tempol decreased the MitoSOX-detected red fluorescence intensity at concentrations of 1 and 10 mM at 2 h after paclitaxel treatment. These data show that tempol decreased the mitochondrial superoxide levels in the primary DRG cell culture.

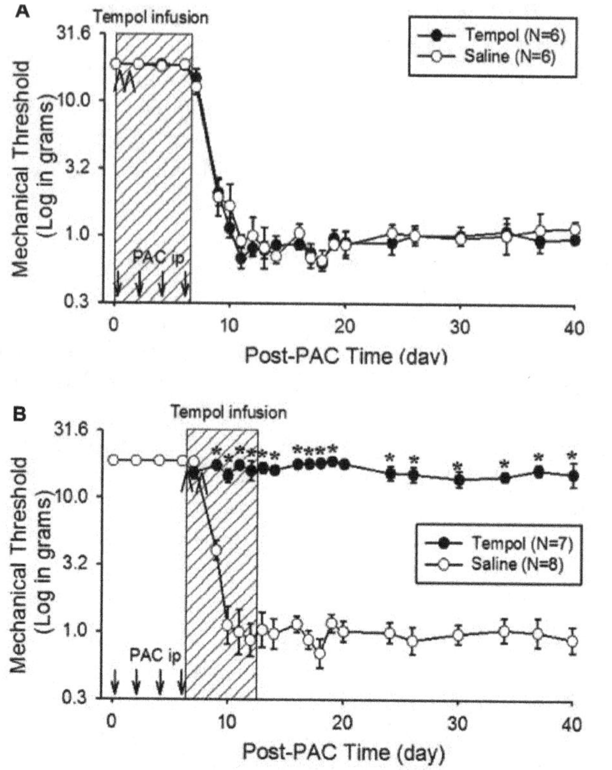

FIGURE 3 | Preventive effects of tempol on PINP in rats. Paclitaxel (PAC, 2 mg/kg) was injected intraperitoneally on four alternate days (days 0, 2, 4, and 6), and the mechanical threshold was measured. **(A)** On the day of the first paclitaxel injection, 12 rats were divided into two groups. The rats in the tempol group ($N = 6$), received an intraperitoneal infusion of tempol (10 mg/day) for 7 days (hatched box) and an intraperitoneal injection of tempol (200 mg/kg) on days 0 and 1 (arrowheads) of the infusion period. The rats in the saline group ($N = 6$) received equivalent amounts of saline. The systemic infusion of tempol did not affect the development of PINP. **(B)** On the day of the last paclitaxel injection, another 15 rats were divided into two groups. The rats in the tempol group ($N = 7$) received an intraperitoneal infusion of tempol (10 mg/day) for 7 days (hatched box) and intraperitoneal injections of tempol (200 mg/kg) on days 6 and 7 (arrowheads). The rats in the saline group ($N = 8$) received equivalent volume of saline. The systemic infusion of tempol significantly prevented the development of PINP. The data represent means with standard errors of the means. The asterisks indicate values that are significantly different ($P < 0.05$) from the corresponding values for the saline group as determined by a two-way repeated-measures analysis of variance with one repeated factor (time) followed by the Tukey *post hoc* test.

DISCUSSION

This study investigated the therapeutic and preventive effect of tempol in rats with PINP. Tempol produced analgesia

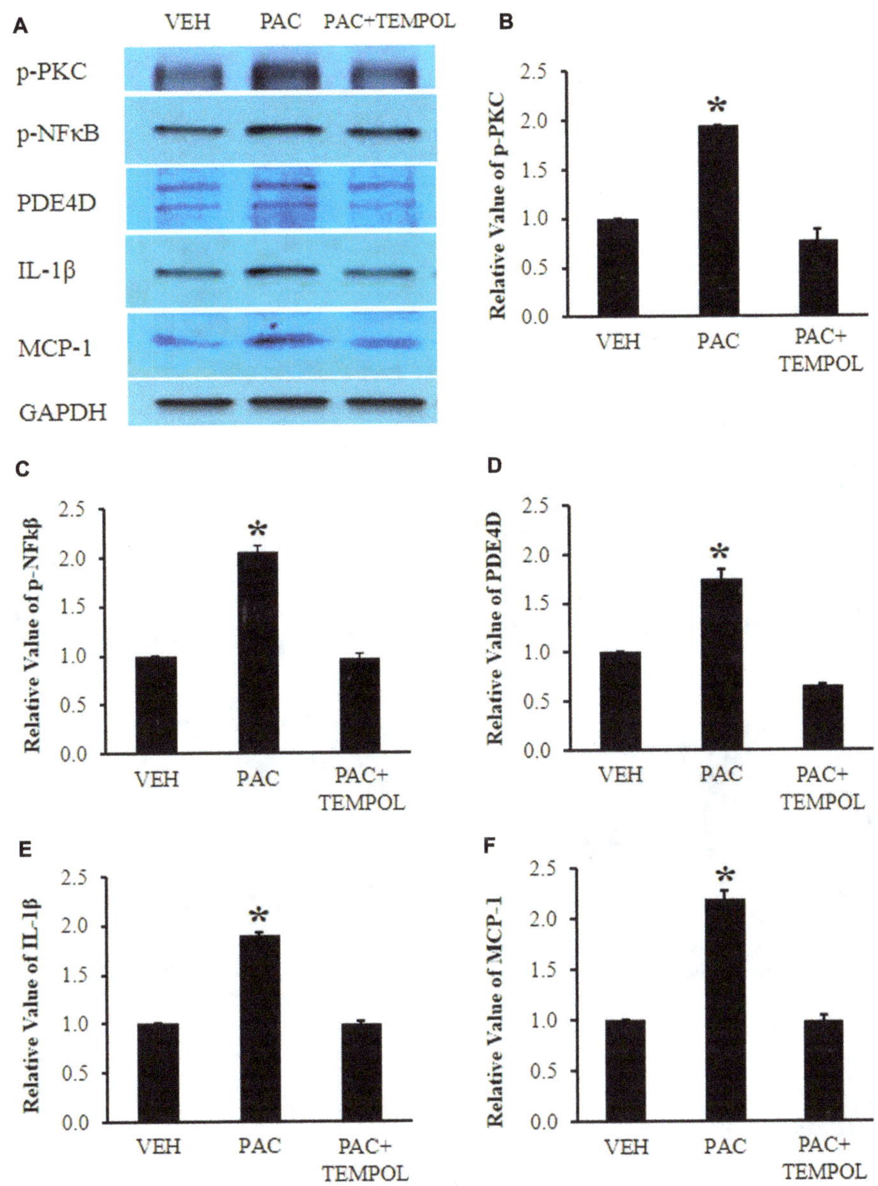

FIGURE 4 | Paclitaxel increased the levels of phosphorylated protein kinase C (p-PKC), phosphorylated nuclear factor κB (p-NF-κB), PDE4D, IL-1β, and monocyte chemoattractant protein-1 (MCP-1) in rat dorsal root ganglia (DRGs). (A) Western blot showing the expression of p-PKC, p-NF-κB, PDE4D, IL-1β, and MCP-1 in DRGs after an injection of vehicle (VEH) or paclitaxel (PAC) on day 20. Tempol was infused for 7 days (days 14–20). **(B–F)** Quantification of p-PKC, p-NF-κB, PDE4D, IL-1β, and MCP-1 in DRGs. Note that paclitaxel increased the levels of p-PKC, p-NF-κB, PDE4D, IL-1β, and MCP-1 in rat DRGs, and tempol subsequently decreased these protein levels. The data are expressed as means ± standard deviations for three rats. The asterisks indicate values that are significantly different ($P < 0.05$) from the values for the vehicle group as determined by the Mann–Whitney *U* test.

by inhibiting mitochondrial superoxide level, p-PKC, p-NF-κB, PDE4D, IL-1β, and MCP-1 in DRGs. In addition, tempol prevented the development of PINP when given during the development phase of mechanical hyperalgesia. Therefore, the results suggest that tempol has potential for the treatment and prevention of chemotherapy-induced neuropathic pain.

It is well reported that oxidative stress plays an important role in neurodegenerative diseases (Wagner et al., 1998). Free radicals (superoxide, hydroxyl radicals, hydrogen peroxide, and peroxynitrite) are derivatives of molecular oxygen and nitrogen (Lander, 1997) and are produced by both mitochondrial oxidative metabolisms and several enzymes such as phospholipase A2, cytochrome P450, monoamine oxidase, and tyrosine hydroxylase. In addition, free radicals are removed by antioxidant systems including superoxide dismutase, catalase, glutathione, and glutathione peroxidase. Pathological condition is involved in oxidative stress by the increased production of free radicals and/or

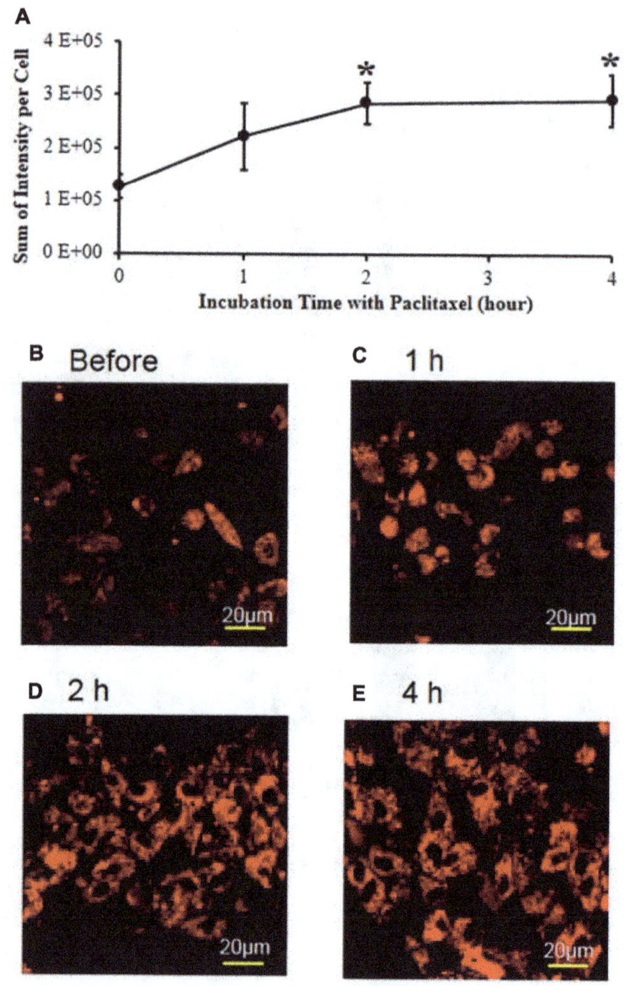

FIGURE 5 | Paclitaxel increased mitochondrial superoxide levels in the primary DRG cell culture. (A) The L1-6 DRGs were isolated from an adult male Sprague–Dawley rat. The isolated DRG cells were plated in a chambered coverglass in DMEM media for live cell imaging. Note that paclitaxel (1 μM) significantly increased the MitoSOX-detected red fluorescence intensity in the primary DRG cell cultures. The data are expressed as means ± standard deviations for three independent experiments. The asterisks indicate values that are significantly different ($P < 0.05$) from the values before treatment with paclitaxel as determined by the unpaired *t*-test. **(B–E)** The MitoSOX-detected red fluorescence intensity was measured in live cell imaging before **(B)** and 1 **(C)**, 2 **(D)**, and 4 h **(E)** after treatment with paclitaxel (1 μM). Scale bars: 20 μm.

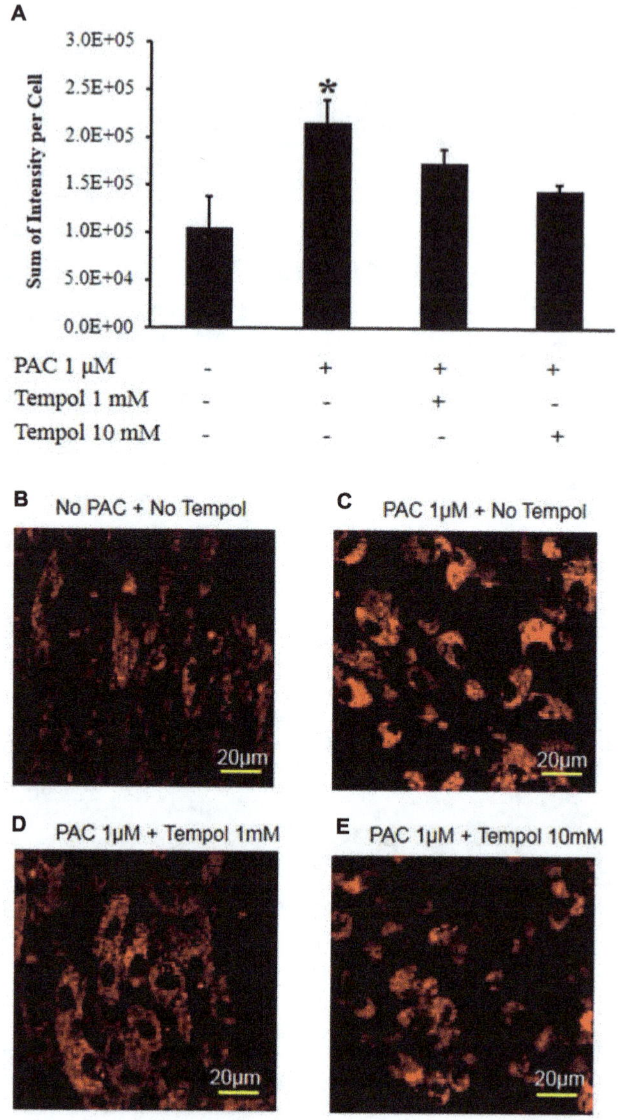

FIGURE 6 | Tempol decreased paclitaxel-induced mitochondrial superoxide levels in the primary DRG cell culture. (A) The DRG cells were cultured in a chambered cover glass in DMEM media for live cell imaging. Paclitaxel (1 μM) significantly increased the MitoSOX-detected red fluorescence intensity in the primary DRG cell cultures at 2 h. Tempol (1 and 10 mM) decreased paclitaxel-induced red fluorescence intensity. The data are expressed as means ± standard deviations for three independent experiments. The asterisks indicate values that are significantly different ($P < 0.05$) from the values before treatment with paclitaxel as determined by the unpaired *t*-test. **(B)** The MitoSOX-detected red fluorescence without paclitaxel at 2 h. **(C)** The MitoSOX-detected red fluorescence at 2 h after treatment with paclitaxel (1 μM). **(D)** The MitoSOX-detected red fluorescence of DRG cells at 2 h after treatment with paclitaxel (1 μM) and tempol (1 mM). **(E)** The MitoSOX-detected red fluorescence of DRG cells at 2 h after treatment with paclitaxel (1 μM) and tempol (10 mM). Scale bars: 20 μm.

decreased antioxidants level (Floyd, 1999; Floyd and Hensley, 2002).

Fidanboylu et al. (2011) reported that single intraperitoneal injection of 100 mg/kg of tempol had no analgesic effect at 1, 3, and 24 h after injection, but 250 mg/kg had analgesic effect on established paclitaxel-induced hypersensitivity at 1 h after injection. In addition, daily systemic injection of 100 mg/kg of tempol for 13 days did not affect the development of paclitaxel-induced hypersensitivity (Fidanboylu et al., 2011). We think daily systemic injection of 100 mg/kg tempol is too low a dose for scavenging free radicals because of the lack of analgesic effect. In our study, the 100 and 200 mg/kg doses of tempol significantly increased the mechanical threshold for only 2 h. So the prolonged effect of tempol was induced by intraperitoneal injection at 200 mg/kg as an initial dose on 2 days and an intraperitoneal infusion at a rate of 10 mg/day as a maintaining dose because of the short analgesic effect of single systemic injection. This infusion dose produced analgesic effect without sedation.

We used a PINP model in rats because paclitaxel is a first-line drug for breast cancer and damages the peripheral nervous system, including nerve endings, peripheral nerves, and DRG (Dougherty et al., 2004). Paclitaxel cannot penetrate the blood-brain barrier and thus does not accumulate located in the central nervous system (Cavaletti et al., 2000). However, this drug does accumulate in DRGs (Cavaletti et al., 2000). The drug may cause damage to the sciatic nerve, nerve endings, and DRGs during the development of pain behavior (Peters et al., 2007b). Paclitaxel induces several events in the DRGs including (1) accumulation of immune cells such as macrophage and polymorphonuclear cells; (2) an increase in calcium channel subunits in the DRG (Matsumoto et al., 2006; Peters et al., 2007a; Xiao et al., 2007); (3) an increase in the expression of phospholipase A2, chemokine ligand 21b, complement components 1 and 3, and matrix metalloproteinase 3 (Nishida et al., 2008); and (4) an increase of inflammatory cytokines such as TNF-α, IL-1, and IL-6 (Ledeboer et al., 2007). These events may be responsible for changes in pain behavior.

In our study, paclitaxel increased the mitochondrial superoxide anion level in DRG cells, and tempol subsequently decreased the level. Superoxide anion is produced by the electron transport system in the mitochondria and is decreased by superoxide dismutase (Liu et al., 1996). Mitochondrial superoxide is generated as a by-product of electron transport chain in mitochondria. MitoSOX is a cationic derivative of dihydroethidium and is reactive with superoxide to produce 2-hydroxyethidium that induces a fluorescence (Zielonka et al., 2008). In our study, paclitaxel increased the superoxide anion level in the mitochondria and then induced oxidative stress in DRGs, which may explain the pain behavior. Superoxide anion forms hydrogen peroxide in the presence of tempol, which is similar to native superoxide dismutase (Reddan et al., 1993). Further, the nitroxide structure of tempol can facilitate metabolism of a wide range of free radicals and reactive nitrogen species. Indeed, tempol can protect cells from superoxide anion, and hydrogen peroxide (Reddan et al., 1992). Therefore, tempol improved pain behavior through scavenging free radicals in the DRGs.

Furthermore, paclitaxel increased the levels of p-PKC, p-NF-κB, PDE4D, IL-1β, and MCP-1 in the DRGs (**Figures 4A–F**). PDE4D is a subgroup of PDE4 that degrades the phosphodiesterase bond of cAMP and terminates the action of cAMP (Houslay and Adams, 2003). The activation of PDE4 produces inflammatory cytokines (IL-1β) and chemokines (MCP-1) in the immune cells (Boswell-Smith et al., 2006; Kobayashi et al., 2007; Kubo et al., 2012). Recently, rolipram, a selective PDE4 inhibitor, was shown to decrease pain behavior in rat PINP models (Kim et al., 2015). Also, paclitaxel has lipopolysaccharide-like action and then accumulates immune cells in the DRGs (Manthey et al., 1992) and increases intracellular calcium levels, which promote the change from PKC to p-PKC (Peters et al., 2007b; Xiao et al., 2007). The increase in activated PKC in the DRGs was observed after treatment with paclitaxel in a mouse model of PINP (He and Wang, 2015). In addition, p-NF-κB, an activated form of NF-κB, is translocated into the nucleus and then produced various proteins including inflammatory cytokines and chemokines such as TNF-α, IL-1β, and MCP-1, thereby inducing pain behaviors (Deshpande et al., 1997). In addition, paclitaxel was reported to increase the level of TNF-α in the DRG in rats (Kim et al., 2016). In this study, tempol reduced pain behaviors by decreasing the levels of p-PKC, p-NF-κB, PDE4D, IL-1β, and MCP-1 in the DRGs (but not those of TNF-α: data not shown).

Most importantly, tempol completely prevented the development of pain behaviors when it was administered on days 6–13 after the first injection of paclitaxel but not when it was administered on days 0–6. We found that tempol decreased oxidative stress, p-PKC, p-NF-κB, PDE4D, IL-1β, and MCP-1 in the DRGs. Therefore, induction of inflammatory cytokines/chemokines and oxidative stress may have been involved in the development of pain behaviors during days 6–13 after the first injection of paclitaxel. We plan to further investigate the temporal significance in studying the pathological mechanisms of the development of chemotherapy-induced neuropathic pain.

CONCLUSION

Our study showed that systemic administration of tempol ameliorated and prevented neuropathic pain behavior in a rat model of PINP by inhibiting free radicals, p-PKC, p-NF-κB, PDE4D, IL-1β, and MCP-1 in the DRGs without inducing sedation. We conclude that oxidative stress and inflammatory processes are involved in both development and maintenance of chemotherapy-induced neuropathic pain.

AUTHOR CONTRIBUTIONS

HK contributed to conception, the design, data acquisition, analysis, interpretation, writing, and revising the manuscript. S-HH contributed to the design, data acquisition, analysis, and interpretation. SA contributed to conception, the design, data acquisition, analysis, interpretation, writing, and revising the manuscript.

FUNDING

This work was supported by grants from the Peggy and Avinash Ahuja Foundation; and the Helen Buchanan and Stanley Joseph Seeger Endowment at The University of Texas MD Anderson Cancer Center.

ACKNOWLEDGMENT

The authors thank Bryan Tutt (Department of Scientific Publications, The University of Texas MD Anderson Cancer Center) for editorial assistance.

REFERENCES

Boswell-Smith, V., Spina, D., and Page, C. P. (2006). Phosphodiesterase inhibitors. *Br. J. Pharmacol.* 147(Suppl. 1), S252–S257. doi: 10.1038/sj.bjp.0706495

Cavaletti, G., Cavalletti, E., Oggioni, N., Sottani, C., Minoia, C., D'incalci, M., et al. (2000). Distribution of paclitaxel within the nervous system of the rat after repeated intravenous administration. *Neurotoxicology* 21, 389–393.

Chaplan, S. R., Bach, F. W., Pogrel, J. W., Chung, J. M., and Yaksh, T. L. (1994). Quantitative assessment of tactile allodynia in the rat paw. *J. Neurosci. Methods* 53, 55–63. doi: 10.1016/0165-0270(94)90144-9

Deng, L., Guindon, J., Cornett, B. L., Makriyannis, A., Mackie, K., and Hohmann, A. G. (2015). Chronic cannabinoid receptor 2 activation reverses paclitaxel neuropathy without tolerance or cannabinoid receptor 1-dependent withdrawal. *Biol. Psychiatry* 77, 475–487. doi: 10.1016/j.biopsych.2014.04.009

Deng, L., Guindon, J., Vemuri, V. K., Thakur, G. A., White, F. A., Makriyannis, A., et al. (2012). The maintenance of cisplatin- and paclitaxel-induced mechanical and cold allodynia is suppressed by cannabinoid CB(2) receptor activation and independent of CXCR4 signaling in models of chemotherapy-induced peripheral neuropathy. *Mol. Pain* 8:71. doi: 10.1186/1744-8069-8-71

Deshpande, R., Khalili, H., Pergolizzi, R. G., Michael, S. D., and Chang, M. D. (1997). Estradiol down-regulates LPS-induced cytokine production and NFkB activation in murine macrophages. *Am. J. Reprod. Immunol.* 38, 46–54. doi: 10.1111/j.1600-0897.1997.tb00275.x

Devor, M., and Zalkind, V. (2001). Reversible analgesia, atonia, and loss of consciousness on bilateral intracerebral microinjection of pentobarbital. *Pain* 94, 101–112. doi: 10.1016/S0304-3959(01)00345-1

Dixon, W. J. (1980). Efficient analysis of experimental observations. *Annu. Rev. Pharmacol. Toxicol.* 20, 441–462. doi: 10.1146/annurev.pa.20.040180.002301

Dougherty, P. M., Cata, J. P., Cordella, J. V., Burton, A., and Weng, H. R. (2004). Taxol-induced sensory disturbance is characterized by preferential impairment of myelinated fiber function in cancer patients. *Pain* 109, 132–142. doi: 10.1016/j.pain.2004.01.021

Erker, L., Schubert, R., Yakushiji, H., Barlow, C., Larson, D., Mitchell, J. B., et al. (2005). Cancer chemoprevention by the antioxidant tempol acts partially via the p53 tumor suppressor. *Hum. Mol. Genet.* 14, 1699–1708. doi: 10.1093/hmg/ddi181

Fidanboylu, M., Griffiths, L. A., and Flatters, S. J. (2011). Global inhibition of reactive oxygen species (ROS) inhibits paclitaxel-induced painful peripheral neuropathy. *PLoS ONE* 6:e25212. doi: 10.1371/journal.pone.0025212

Floyd, R. A. (1999). Antioxidants, oxidative stress, and degenerative neurological disorders. *Proc. Soc. Exp. Biol. Med.* 222, 236–245. doi: 10.1046/j.1525-1373.1999.d01-140.x

Floyd, R. A., and Hensley, K. (2002). Oxidative stress in brain aging. Implications for therapeutics of neurodegenerative diseases. *Neurobiol. Aging* 23, 795–807.

Gariboldi, M. B., Ravizza, R., Petterino, C., Castagnaro, M., Finocchiaro, G., and Monti, E. (2003). Study of in vitro and in vivo effects of the piperidine nitroxide Tempol–a potential new therapeutic agent for gliomas. *Eur. J. Cancer* 39, 829–837. doi: 10.1016/S0959-8049(02)00742-6

Guindon, J., Lai, Y., Takacs, S. M., Bradshaw, H. B., and Hohmann, A. G. (2013). Alterations in endocannabinoid tone following chemotherapy-induced peripheral neuropathy: effects of endocannabinoid deactivation inhibitors targeting fatty-acid amide hydrolase and monoacylglycerol lipase in comparison to reference analgesics following cisplatin treatment. *Pharmacol. Res.* 67, 94–109. doi: 10.1016/j.phrs.2012.10.013

Hahn, S. M., Deluca, A. M., Coffin, D., Krishna, C. M., and Mitchell, J. B. (1998). In vivo radioprotection and effects on blood pressure of the stable free radical nitroxides. *Int. J. Radiat. Oncol. Biol. Phys.* 42, 839–842. doi: 10.1016/S0360-3016(98)00317-4

Harris, H. M., Sufka, K. J., Gul, W., and Elsohly, M. A. (2016). Effects of delta-9-tetrahydrocannabinol and cannabidiol on cisplatin-induced neuropathy in mice. *Planta Med.* 82, 1169–1172. doi: 10.1055/s-0042-106303

He, Y., and Wang, Z. J. (2015). Nociceptor beta II, delta, and epsilon isoforms of PKC differentially mediate paclitaxel-induced spontaneous and evoked pain. *J. Neurosci.* 35, 4614–4625. doi: 10.1523/JNEUROSCI.1580-14.2015

Hershman, D. L., Lacchetti, C., Dworkin, R. H., Lavoie Smith, E. M., Bleeker, J., Cavaletti, G., et al. (2014). Prevention and management of chemotherapy-induced peripheral neuropathy in survivors of adult cancers: american society of clinical oncology clinical practice guideline. *J. Clin. Oncol.* 32, 1941–1967. doi: 10.1200/JCO.2013.54.0914

Hewett, S. J., Csernansky, C. A., and Choi, D. W. (1994). Selective potentiation of NMDA-induced neuronal injury following induction of astrocytic iNOS. *Neuron* 13, 487–494. doi: 10.1016/0896-6273(94)90362-X

Houslay, M. D., and Adams, D. R. (2003). PDE4 cAMP phosphodiesterases: modular enzymes that orchestrate signalling cross-talk, desensitization and compartmentalization. *Biochem. J.* 370, 1–18. doi: 10.1042/bj20021698

Howard, B. J., Yatin, S., Hensley, K., Allen, K. L., Kelly, J. P., Carney, J., et al. (1996). Prevention of hyperoxia-induced alterations in synaptosomal membrane-associated proteins by N-tert-butyl-alpha-phenylnitrone and 4-hydroxy-2,2,6,6-tetramethylpiperidin-1-oxyl (Tempol). *J. Neurochem.* 67, 2045–2050. doi: 10.1046/j.1471-4159.1996.67052045.x

Ji, G., Li, Z., and Neugebauer, V. (2015). Reactive oxygen species mediate visceral pain-related amygdala plasticity and behaviors. *Pain* 156, 825–836. doi: 10.1097/j.pain.0000000000000120

Khasabova, I. A., Khasabov, S., Paz, J., Harding-Rose, C., Simone, D. A., and Seybold, V. S. (2012). Cannabinoid type-1 receptor reduces pain and neurotoxicity produced by chemotherapy. *J. Neurosci.* 32, 7091–7101. doi: 10.1523/JNEUROSCI.0403-12.2012

Khattab, M. M. (2006). TEMPOL, a membrane-permeable radical scavenger, attenuates peroxynitrite- and superoxide anion-enhanced carrageenan-induced paw edema and hyperalgesia: a key role for superoxide anion. *Eur. J. Pharmacol.* 548, 167–173. doi: 10.1016/j.ejphar.2006.08.007

Kim, H. K., Hwang, S. H., Lee, S. O., Kim, S. H., and Abdi, S. (2016). Pentoxifylline ameliorates mechanical hyperalgesia in a rat model of chemotherapy-induced neuropathic pain. *Pain Physician* 19, E589–E600.

Kim, H. K., Kim, J. H., Gao, X., Zhou, J. L., Lee, I., Chung, K., et al. (2006). Analgesic effect of vitamin E is mediated by reducing central sensitization in neuropathic pain. *Pain* 122, 53–62. doi: 10.1016/j.pain.2006.01.013

Kim, H. K., Kwon, J. Y., Yoo, C., and Abdi, S. (2015). The analgesic effect of rolipram, a phosphodiesterase 4 inhibitor, on chemotherapy-induced neuropathic pain in rats. *Anesth. Analg.* 121, 822–828. doi: 10.1213/ANE.0000000000000853

Kim, H. K., Park, S. K., Zhou, J. L., Taglialatela, G., Chung, K., Coggeshall, R. E., et al. (2004). Reactive oxygen species (ROS) play an important role in a rat model of neuropathic pain. *Pain* 111, 116–124. doi: 10.1016/j.pain.2004.06.008

Kim, H. K., Zhang, Y. P., Gwak, Y. S., and Abdi, S. (2010). Phenyl N-tert-butylnitrone, a free radical scavenger, reduces mechanical allodynia in chemotherapy-induced neuropathic pain in rats. *Anesthesiology* 112, 432–439. doi: 10.1097/ALN.0b013e3181ca31bd

Kobayashi, K., Suda, T., Manabe, H., and Miki, I. (2007). Administration of PDE4 inhibitors suppressed the pannus-like inflammation by inhibition of cytokine production by macrophages and synovial fibroblast proliferation. *Mediators Inflamm.* 2007:58901. doi: 10.1155/2007/58901

Kubo, S., Kobayashi, M., Iwata, M., Miyata, K., Takahashi, K., and Shimizu, Y. (2012). Anti-neutrophilic inflammatory activity of ASP3258, a novel phosphodiesterase type 4 inhibitor. *Int. Immunopharmacol.* 12, 59–63. doi: 10.1016/j.intimp.2011.10.011

Lander, H. M. (1997). An essential role for free radicals and derived species in signal transduction. *FASEB J.* 11, 118–124.

Ledeboer, A., Jekich, B. M., Sloane, E. M., Mahoney, J. H., Langer, S. J., Milligan, E. D., et al. (2007). Intrathecal interleukin-10 gene therapy attenuates paclitaxel-induced mechanical allodynia and proinflammatory cytokine expression in dorsal root ganglia in rats. *Brain Behav. Immun.* 21, 686–698. doi: 10.1016/j.bbi.2006.10.012

Lee, J. J., and Swain, S. M. (2006). Peripheral neuropathy induced by microtubule-stabilizing agents. *J. Clin. Oncol.* 24, 1633–1642. doi: 10.1200/JCO.2005.04.0543

Liu, S., Jiao, X., Wang, X., and Zhang, L. (1996). Interaction of electron leak and proton leak in respiratory chain of mitochondria–proton leak induced by superoxide from an electron leak pathway of univalent reduction of oxygen. *Sci. China C Life Sci.* 39, 168–178.

MacGregor, D. G., Avshalumov, M. V., and Rice, M. E. (2003). Brain edema induced by in vitro ischemia: causal factors and neuroprotection. *J. Neurochem.* 85, 1402–1411. doi: 10.1046/j.1471-4159.2003.01772.x

Manthey, C. L., Brandes, M. E., Perera, P. Y., and Vogel, S. N. (1992). Taxol increases steady-state levels of lipopolysaccharide-inducible genes and protein-tyrosine phosphorylation in murine macrophages. *J. Immunol.* 149, 2459–2465.

Matsumoto, M., Inoue, M., Hald, A., Xie, W., and Ueda, H. (2006). Inhibition of paclitaxel-induced A-fiber hypersensitization by gabapentin. *J. Pharmacol. Exp. Ther.* 318, 735–740. doi: 10.1124/jpet.106.103614

Mols, F., Beijers, T., Vreugdenhil, G., and Van De Poll-Franse, L. (2014). Chemotherapy-induced peripheral neuropathy and its association with quality of life: a systematic review. *Support Care Cancer* 22, 2261–2269. doi: 10.1007/s00520-014-2255-7

Nishida, K., Kuchiiwa, S., Oiso, S., Futagawa, T., Masuda, S., Takeda, Y., et al. (2008). Up-regulation of matrix metalloproteinase-3 in the dorsal root ganglion of rats with paclitaxel-induced neuropathy. *Cancer Sci.* 99, 1618–1625. doi: 10.1111/j.1349-7006.2008.00877.x

Peters, C. M., Jimenez-Andrade, J. M., Jonas, B. M., Sevcik, M. A., Koewler, N. J., Ghilardi, J. R., et al. (2007a). Intravenous paclitaxel administration in the rat induces a peripheral sensory neuropathy characterized by macrophage infiltration and injury to sensory neurons and their supporting cells. *Exp. Neurol.* 203, 42–54. doi: 10.1016/j.expneurol.2006.07.022

Peters, C. M., Jimenez-Andrade, J. M., Kuskowski, M. A., Ghilardi, J. R., and Mantyh, P. W. (2007b). An evolving cellular pathology occurs in dorsal root ganglia, peripheral nerve and spinal cord following intravenous administration of paclitaxel in the rat. *Brain Res.* 1168, 46–59. doi: 10.1016/j.brainres.2007.06.066

Polomano, R. C., Mannes, A. J., Clark, U. S., and Bennett, G. J. (2001). A painful peripheral neuropathy in the rat produced by the chemotherapeutic drug, paclitaxel. *Pain* 94, 293–304. doi: 10.1016/S0304-3959(01)00363-3

Reddan, J., Sevilla, M., Giblin, F., Padgaonkar, V., Dziedzic, D., and Leverenz, V. (1992). Tempol and deferoxamine protect cultured rabbit lens epithelial cells from H2O2 insult: insight into the mechanism of H2O2-induced injury. *Lens Eye Toxic. Res.* 9, 385–393.

Reddan, J. R., Sevilla, M. D., Giblin, F. J., Padgaonkar, V., Dziedzic, D. C., Leverenz, V., et al. (1993). The superoxide dismutase mimic TEMPOL protects cultured rabbit lens epithelial cells from hydrogen peroxide insult. *Exp. Eye Res.* 56, 543–554. doi: 10.1006/exer.1993.1068

Rivera, E., and Cianfrocca, M. (2015). Overview of neuropathy associated with taxanes for the treatment of metastatic breast cancer. *Cancer Chemother. Pharmacol.* 75, 659–670. doi: 10.1007/s00280-014-2607-5

Shetty, R., Deshpande, K., Ghosh, A., and Sethu, S. (2015). Management of ocular neuropathic pain with vitamin B12 supplements: a case report. *Cornea* 34, 1324–1325. doi: 10.1097/ICO.0000000000000572

Soule, B. P., Hyodo, F., Matsumoto, K., Simone, N. L., Cook, J. A., Krishna, M. C., et al. (2007). Therapeutic and clinical applications of nitroxide compounds. *Antioxid. Redox Signal.* 9, 1731–1743. doi: 10.1089/ars.2007.1722

Teichner, A., Ovadia, H., Lavie, G., and Leker, R. R. (2003). Combination of dexanabinol and tempol in focal cerebral ischemia: is there a ceiling effect? *Exp. Neurol.* 182, 353–360. doi: 10.1016/S0014-4886(03)00083-9

Vera, G., Cabezos, P. A., Martin, M. I., and Abalo, R. (2013). Characterization of cannabinoid-induced relief of neuropathic pain in a rat model of cisplatin-induced neuropathy. *Pharmacol. Biochem. Behav.* 105, 205–212. doi: 10.1016/j.pbb.2013.02.008

Wagner, R., Heckman, H. M., and Myers, R. R. (1998). Wallerian degeneration and hyperalgesia after peripheral nerve injury are glutathione-dependent. *Pain* 77, 173–179. doi: 10.1016/S0304-3959(98)00091-8

Wilcox, C. S., and Pearlman, A. (2008). Chemistry and antihypertensive effects of tempol and other nitroxides. *Pharmacol. Rev.* 60, 418–469. doi: 10.1124/pr.108.000240

Windebank, A. J., and Grisold, W. (2008). Chemotherapy-induced neuropathy. *J. Peripher. Nerv. Syst.* 13, 27–46. doi: 10.1111/j.1529-8027.2008.00156.x

Wolf, S., Barton, D., Kottschade, L., Grothey, A., and Loprinzi, C. (2008). Chemotherapy-induced peripheral neuropathy: prevention and treatment strategies. *Eur. J. Cancer* 44, 1507–1515. doi: 10.1016/j.ejca.2008.04.018

Xiao, W., Boroujerdi, A., Bennett, G. J., and Luo, Z. D. (2007). Chemotherapy-evoked painful peripheral neuropathy: analgesic effects of gabapentin and effects on expression of the alpha-2-delta type-1 calcium channel subunit. *Neuroscience* 144, 714–720. doi: 10.1016/j.neuroscience.2006.09.044

Xiao, W., Naso, L., and Bennett, G. J. (2008). Experimental studies of potential analgesics for the treatment of chemotherapy-evoked painful peripheral neuropathies. *Pain Med.* 9, 505–517. doi: 10.1111/j.1526-4637.2007.00301.x

Yazdani, S., and Abdi, S. (2014). Brief review: pain management for cancer survivors: challenges and opportunities. *Can. J. Anaesth.* 61, 745–753. doi: 10.1007/s12630-014-0170-5

Zhang, Q. S., Eaton, L., Snyder, E. R., Houghtaling, S., Mitchell, J. B., Finegold, M., et al. (2008). Tempol protects against oxidative damage and delays epithelial tumor onset in Fanconi anemia mice. *Cancer Res.* 68, 1601–1608. doi: 10.1158/0008-5472.CAN-07-5186

Zielonka, J., Vasquez-Vivar, J., and Kalyanaraman, B. (2008). Detection of 2-hydroxyethidium in cellular systems: a unique marker product of superoxide and hydroethidine. *Nat. Protoc.* 3, 8–21. doi: 10.1038/nprot.2007.473

Conflict of Interest Statement: The authors declare that the research was conducted in the absence of any commercial or financial relationships that could be construed as a potential conflict of interest.

The reviewer DP and handling Editor declared their shared affiliation, and the handling Editor states that the process nevertheless met the standards of a fair and objective review.

12

Long-Term Effects, Pathophysiological Mechanisms, and Risk Factors of Chemotherapy-Induced Peripheral Neuropathies

Nicolas Kerckhove[1], Aurore Collin[2], Sakahlé Condé[3], Carine Chaleteix[4], Denis Pezet[5] and David Balayssac[1]*

[1] INSERM U1107, NEURO-DOL, CHU Clermont-Ferrand, Délégation à la Recherche Clinique et à l'Innovation, Université Clermont Auvergne, Clermont-Ferrand, France, [2] INSERM U1107, NEURO-DOL, Université Clermont Auvergne, Clermont-Ferrand, France, [3] INSERM U1107, NEURO-DOL, CHU Clermont-Ferrand, Neurologie, Université Clermont Auvergne, Clermont-Ferrand, France, [4] CHU Clermont-Ferrand, Hématologie Clinique Adulte, Clermont-Ferrand, France, [5] INSERM U1071, CHU Clermont-Ferrand, Chirurgie et Oncologie Digestive, Université Clermont Auvergne, Clermont-Ferrand, France

Edited by:
Raquel Abalo,
King Juan Carlos University, Spain

Reviewed by:
Patrizia Gazzerro,
University of Salerno, Italy
Eva Maria Sanchez-Robles,
King Juan Carlos University, Spain
Antoinetta Beijers,
Máxima Medisch Centrum,
Netherlands
Laura Gilchrist,
St. Catherine University, USA

***Correspondence:**
David Balayssac
dbalayssac@chu-clermontferrand.fr

Neurotoxic anticancer drugs, such as platinum-based anticancer drugs, taxanes, vinca alkaloids, and proteasome/angiogenesis inhibitors are responsible for chemotherapy-induced peripheral neuropathy (CIPN). The health consequences of CIPN remain worrying as it is associated with several comorbidities and affects a specific population of patients already impacted by cancer, a strong driver for declines in older adults. The purpose of this review is to present a comprehensive overview of the long-term effects of CIPN in cancer patients and survivors. Pathophysiological mechanisms and risk factors are also presented. Neurotoxic mechanisms leading to CIPNs are not yet fully understood but involve neuronopathy and/or axonopathy, mainly associated with DNA damage, oxidative stress, mitochondria toxicity, and ion channel remodeling in the neurons of the peripheral nervous system. Classical symptoms of CIPNs are peripheral neuropathy with a "stocking and glove" distribution characterized by sensory loss, paresthesia, dysesthesia and numbness, sometimes associated with neuropathic pain in the most serious cases. Several risk factors can promote CIPN as a function of the anticancer drug considered, such as cumulative dose, treatment duration, history of neuropathy, combination of therapies and genetic polymorphisms. CIPNs are frequent in cancer patients with an overall incidence of approximately 38% (possibly up to 90% of patients treated with oxaliplatin). Finally, the long-term reversibility of these CIPNs remain questionable, notably in the case of platinum-based anticancer drugs and taxanes, for which CIPN may last several years after the end of anticancer chemotherapies. These long-term effects are associated with comorbidities such as depression, insomnia, falls and decreases of health-related quality of life in cancer patients and survivors. However, it is noteworthy that these long-term effects remain poorly studied, and only limited data are available such as in the case of bortezomib and thalidomide-induced peripheral neuropathy.

Keywords: chemotherapy-induced peripheral neuropathy, long-term effects, pathophysiological mechanisms, risk factors, anticancer drugs

INTRODUCTION

Platinum-based anticancer drugs (i.e., cisplatin, oxaliplatin), proteasome/angiogenesis inhibitors (bortezomib/thalidomide), vinca alkaloids (i.e., vincristine, vinorelbine) and taxanes (i.e., paclitaxel, docetaxel) are the most common anticancer drugs used as first-line chemotherapy for several cancers, including colorectal, gastric, breast and lung cancers, and multiple myeloma. Despite their different action mechanisms, all these anticancer drugs share a common adverse and disabling effect for patients, namely CIPN (Balayssac et al., 2011). CIPN has a considerable impact on cancer treatments and their related symptoms severely affect patients' daily activities and quality of life. Thus CIPN is often the main adverse effect leading to the reduction or discontinuation of chemotherapy. Moreover, these symptoms may continue to develop and progress for several months post-therapy (so called "coasting effect") and may persist over periods lasting from several months to years after ceasing chemotherapy (Argyriou et al., 2012). Classic clinical symptoms of CIPN involve the PNS and lead to peripheral neuropathy with a "stocking and glove" distribution characterized by sensory loss, paresthesia, dysesthesia, numbness, and tingling sometimes associated with neuropathic pain in the most serious cases (Balayssac et al., 2011; Jaggi and Singh, 2012). Today, the overall incidence of CIPN is estimated at approximately 38% (possibly up to 90% of patients treated with oxaliplatin) (Cavaletti and Zanna, 2002; Balayssac et al., 2011). Unfortunately, there is no preventive or curative treatment for CIPN at present (Hershman et al., 2014). Finally, many of these neurotoxic anticancer drugs are used in both adjuvant and palliative settings. These neurotoxic drugs raise issues in the case of adjuvant settings, because CIPN may last for a long time after the end of chemotherapy, with very negative impacts on cancer survivors. These effects are well-described for the use of adjuvant oxaliplatin-based chemotherapy for colorectal cancer, for which patients may have long life expectancy (Tofthagen, 2010; Stefansson and Nygren, 2016). The health impacts of CIPN remain worrying, because CIPN is associated with comorbidities such as psychological distress, fall risk and sleep disorders (Hong et al., 2014). Moreover, CIPN affects a specific population of patients already impacted by cancer, which is a strong driver for declines in physical functioning and increased risk of depression in older adults (Leach et al., 2016). Finally, CIPN represents a heavy economic burden. For example, in the USA, on average CIPNs increase healthcare costs by $17,344 per year per patient (Pike et al., 2012).

The purpose of this review is to present a comprehensive overview of the long-term effects of CIPN in cancer patients and survivors. Pathophysiological mechanisms and risk factors are also presented.

PLATINUM-BASED ANTICANCER DRUGS

Platinum-based anticancer drugs are composed of cisplatin, carboplatin and oxaliplatin, which are the main authorized anticancer drugs. Platinum-based anticancer drugs act through DNA platination which interferes with cell viability and division (Dilruba and Kalayda, 2016). Cisplatin and carboplatin are indicated in several solid cancers such as of the lung, ovary, testes and uterus, whereas oxaliplatin is indicated for tumors of the digestive tract, mainly in advanced colorectal cancers (Brenner et al., 2014) but also of the esophagus, stomach, liver, and pancreas (Javle and Hsueh, 2010). Cisplatin and oxaliplatin are probably more neurotoxic than carboplatin (McWhinney et al., 2009).

Pathophysiological Mechanisms of CIPN Associated to Platinum-Based Anticancer Drugs

Platinum-based anticancer drugs reach the neurons of the PNS and induce several types of toxic effects, among them nuclear and mitochondrial DNA damage, oxidative stress and ion channel disturbances. Platinum-based anticancer drugs are alkylating drugs capable of causing nuclear damage. This damage, such as to DNA cross-links, have been directly correlated to electrophysiological abnormalities in peripheral nerves (Dzagnidze et al., 2007). Such DNA damage may also affect mitochondrial DNA. Cisplatin was observed to inhibit the

Abbreviations: ABCB1, ATP binding cassette B1; AUC, area under the curve; BCRP, breast cancer resistance protein; CIPN, chemotherapy-induced peripheral neuropathy; CMT1A, Charcot-Marie-Tooth disease type 1A; DRG, dorsal root ganglia; EORTC, European Organisation for Research and Treatment of Cancer; FACT/GOG-Ntx, functional assessment of chronic illness therapy/gynecologic oncology group-neurotoxicity; GFAP, glial fibrillary acidic protein; GST, glutathione-S-transferase; GTP, guanosine triphosphate; HCN, hyperpolarization-activated cyclic nucleotide-gated; HRQOL, health-related quality of life; KCN, potassium channel; MAPK, mitogen-activated protein kinase; MyD88, myeloid differentiation primary response gene 88; NaV, voltage-gated sodium channel; NF-kB, nuclear factor kappa B; OCT2, organic cation transporter 2; PNS, peripheral nervous system; QLQ-C30, quality of life core questionnaire; QLQ-CIPN20, quality of life questionnaire to assess chemotherapy-induced peripheral neuropathy; SF-36, 36-item short form health survey; SNP, single nucleotide polymorphism; TLR, toll-like receptor; TRAAK, TWIK-related arachidonic acid activated K^+ channel; TREK1, TWIK-related K^+ channel 1; TRIF, toll/interleukin 1 receptor domain-containing adapter-inducing interferon-b; TRPM8, transient receptor potential melastatin 8; TNFα, tumor necrosis factor alpha; TWIK, tandem of P domains in a weak inward-rectifier K^+ channel; VTD, Velcade Thalidomide Dexamethasone.

replication and transcription of mitochondrial DNA, and was responsible for mitochondrial degradation (Podratz et al., 2011). Lastly, cisplatin was seen to induce pro-apoptotic changes in the sciatic nerves of cisplatin-treated mice (Sharawy et al., 2015).

Platinum derivatives are also responsible for oxidative stress in PNS neurons. Oxaliplatin treatment has been observed to increase protein carbonylation and lipid peroxidation in both the sciatic nerves and the spinal cord. This oxidative stress was reduced by antioxidants such as silibinin and α-tocopherol (Di Cesare Mannelli et al., 2012). MnL4, a superoxide dismutase mimetic compound, decreased superoxide anion production, lipid peroxidation and intracellular calcium signals induced by oxaliplatin *in vitro*. MnL4 decreased mechanical hyperalgesia, and mechanical and cold allodynia induced by oxaliplatin in rats (Di Cesare Mannelli et al., 2016). Oxidative stress has also been observed in sciatic nerves in cisplatin-treated mice, with an increase of malondialdehyde and a decrease of superoxide dismutase and glutathione (Sharawy et al., 2015).

Ion channels are also a toxic target of platinum-based anticancer drugs. These interactions with ion channels have mainly been studied for oxaliplatin. A single administration of oxaliplatin to mice induced neuronal hyperexcitability, decreasing the expression of potassium channels, TREK1, and TRAAK (TWIK refers to a tandem of P domains in a weak inward-rectifier K^+ channel), and increasing HCN channels in DRG neurons (Descoeur et al., 2011). More specifically, several ion channels act as thermal sensors which are involved with oxaliplatin-induced thermal hyperesthesia. Oxaliplatin induced cold hyperalgesia in rats through the activation of transient receptor potential ankyrin 1 and p38 MAPK (p38 mitogen-activated protein kinase) in DRG neurons (Yamamoto et al., 2015). In trigeminal ganglion neurons, the inhibition of KCNQ (potassium voltage-gated channel subfamily KQT) channels, voltage-gated K^+ channels mediating M-currents, suppressed oxaliplatin-induced orofacial cold hyperalgesia in rats (Abd-Elsayed et al., 2015). Disruption of the voltage-gated sodium channel NaV1.9 in mice suppressed oxaliplatin-induced cold allodynia and hyperalgesia (Lolignier et al., 2015). Oxaliplatin induced an increase of the cool sensor TRPM8 expression in DRG neurons in rats. Oxaliplatin-induced cold allodynia was suppressed by TRPM8 inhibition (Gauchan et al., 2009). Likewise, cisplatin seems to be able to interfere with ion channels in the DRG neurons of rats, by decreasing voltage-gated potassium and calcium channel currents (Tomaszewski and Büsselberg, 2007) (**Figure 1**).

Symptoms and Long-Term Effects of Oxaliplatin-Induced Peripheral Neuropathy

Oxaliplatin has strong neurotoxicity which is qualitatively and quantitatively different from other neurotoxic anticancer drugs (Balayssac et al., 2011). Oxaliplatin is responsible for acute neuropathic disturbances (paresthesia, dysesthesia of the hands, feet and perioral area induced by cold stimuli) occurring in the hours or days after chemotherapy infusion (Balayssac et al., 2011). At the beginning of chemotherapy cycles, this acute neuropathy usually resolved by itself within a week and disappeared for the next chemotherapy cycle. But the repetition of chemotherapy cycles induced chronic and invalidating CIPN for several patients (Balayssac et al., 2011). This chronic CIPN is associated with paresthesia, numbness, sensory ataxia and can lead to functional deficits (Zedan et al., 2014). Cold hyperesthesia is characteristic of acute oxaliplatin-induced peripheral neuropathy and may augur severe chronic neuropathy (Attal et al., 2009). This CIPN may be aggravated by cold external temperatures, such as in Nordic countries (Altaf et al., 2014; Stefansson and Nygren, 2016) (**Table 1**).

Oxaliplatin is probably the most neurotoxic anticancer drug since more than 90% of patients developed acute neuropathy and 30–50% of patients developed chronic neuropathy (Tofthagen, 2010; Beijers A.J. et al., 2014). Grade severity and symptom duration vary between studies (Beijers A.J. et al., 2014). Although symptoms decrease with time, long-term clinical studies seem to demonstrate the persistence of neuropathy after 24 months (Beijers A.J. et al., 2014): 25 months, 37.5% of grade 1, 29.2% of grade 2 and 0.7% of grade 3 (Park et al., 2011); 48 months, 11.9% of grade 1, 2.8% of grade 2 and 0.7% of grade 3 (André et al., 2009); 8 years, 30.4% of grade 2+ (Yothers et al., 2011). Consequently, the reversibility of this CIPN remains equivocal (Park et al., 2011). Moreover, some authors have suggested that oxaliplatin-induced peripheral neuropathy could be more frequent and more severe in the long-term than expected, lasting more than 12 months (Vatandoust et al., 2014); however, these patients represent a third of the population of cancer survivors (Ganz, 2003).

In colorectal cancer survivors, CIPN has a strong negative impact on HRQOL, associated with depression and sleep disorders (Mols et al., 2013; Tofthagen et al., 2013). More worrying, some cancer survivors may feel "poisoned" by chemotherapy, for more details see the patient's comments in Tofthagen (2010).

Symptoms and Long-Term Effects of Cisplatin-Induced Peripheral Neuropathy

In clinical practice, cisplatin induced neuropathy is similar to chronic oxaliplatin-induced peripheral neuropathy; it remains a sensory axonal neuropathy with abnormal nerve conduction and no remarkable vegetative disturbances (Earl et al., 1998; Balayssac et al., 2011).

The prevalence and long-term effects of this CIPN have been assessed in several studies and in different types of cancer. In the case of ovarian cancer, it has been reported that 50% of patients treated with cisplatin-based chemotherapy complained of peripheral sensory neuropathy after a median of 5.7 years (minimum: 5 months, maximum: 17 years) (Engelen et al., 2009). In the case of adolescents and young adults treated for bone and soft tissue sarcomas, approximately half of the patients presented a CIPN after an 8-month median (minimum: 1 month, maximum: 54 months) (Earl et al., 1998). In the case of testicular cancer, about 38% of patients had non-symptomatic neuropathy at a median of 15 years after cisplatin-based chemotherapy (minimum: 13, maximum: 17 years), 28% had symptomatic

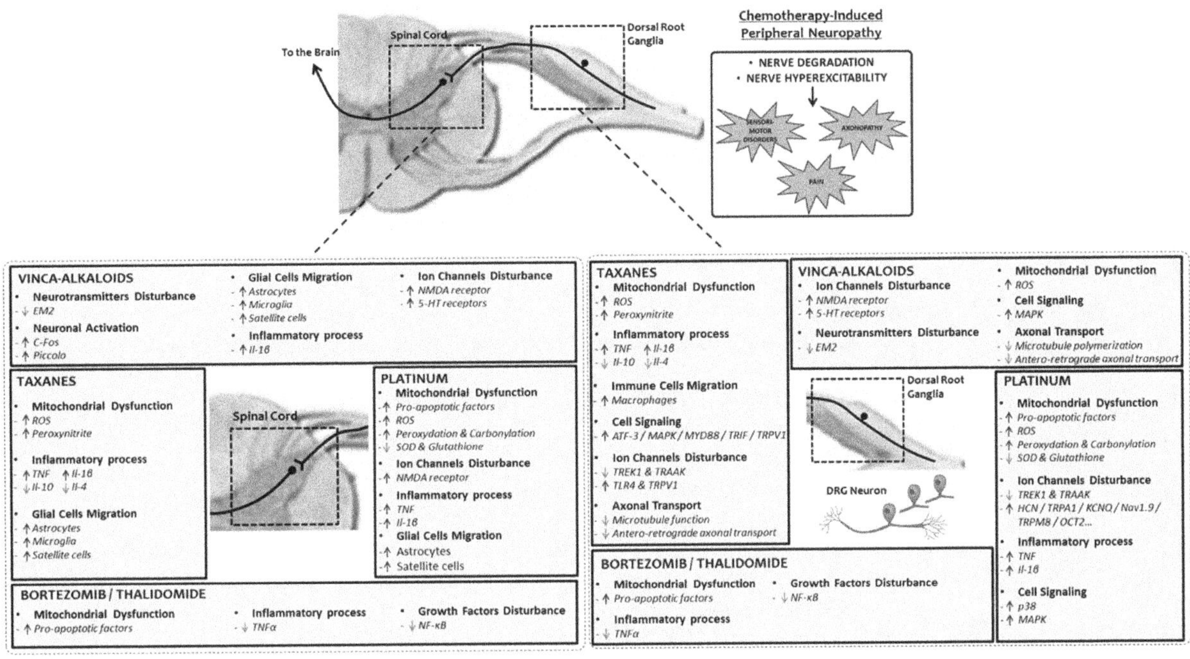

FIGURE 1 | Mechanisms of chemotherapy-induced peripheral neuropathy. Pathophysiological alterations triggered by platinum, taxanes, vinca-alkaloids, and bortezomib/thalidomide in the peripheral nervous system, dorsal root ganglia and spinal cord. 5-HT, 5-hydroxytryptamine; ATF-3, cyclic AMP-dependent transcription factor 3; EM2, endomorphin-2; HCN, potassium/sodium hyperpolarization-activated cyclic nucleotide-gated channel; Il-1β, interleukin-1β; Il-10, interleukin-10; Il-4, interleukin-4; KCNQ, potassium channel, subfamily Q; MAPK, mitogen-activated protein kinase; MYD88, myeloid differentiation primary response gene 88; Nav1.9, voltage-gated sodium channel member 1.9; NMDA, *N*-methyl-D-aspartate; NF-κB, nuclear factor-kappa B; OCT2, solute carrier family 22 member 2 (organic cation transporter); ROS, reactive oxygen species; SOD, superoxide dismutase; TLR4, toll-like receptor 4; TNF, tumor necrosis factor; TRAAK, TWIK-related arachidonic acid activated K^+ channel; TREK1, TWIK1-related K^+ channel 1; TRIF, TIR-domain-containing adapter-inducing interferon-β; TRPA1, transient receptor potential cation channel, subfamily A, member 1; TRPM8, transient receptor potential cation channel subfamily M member 8; TRPV1, transient receptor potential vanilloid 1.

neuropathy and 6% had a disabling polyneuropathy (Strumberg et al., 2002). In another study, 29% of patients had paresthesia in their hands and feet 10.7 years after the end of cisplatin-based chemotherapy (minimum: 4, maximum: 21 years) (Brydoy et al., 2009). Glendenning et al. (2010) found that after a median of 11 years (minimum: 3 years, maximum: 19 years), 21.7% of testicular cancer survivors presented a peripheral neuropathy. In adult survivors of childhood extracranial solid tumors, sensory and motor neuropathies were detected in 20 and 17.5% of patients respectively, after a median time since cancer diagnosis of 25.2 years (minimum: 10.7 years, maximum: 48.2 years). In these patients who had received several lines of different chemotherapies, motor impairment was related to vinca alkaloid whereas sensory impairment was related to platinum-based drug exposure. Sensory neuropathy was associated with a decrease of endurance and mobility (Ness et al., 2013).

CIPN Risk Factors Associated to Platinum-Based Anticancer Drugs

Several risk factors have been identified for these platinum-based anticancer drug-associated CIPN. Cumulative dose is the main risk factor for platinum-based drugs, >850 mg/m^2 for oxaliplatin (Beijers A.J. et al., 2014) and >200–300 mg/m^2 for cisplatin (Earl et al., 1998; Glendenning et al., 2010). Pre-treatment anemia, hypoalbuminemia and hypomagnesaemia and alcohol consumption have been identified as risk factors for oxaliplatin-induced peripheral neuropathy (Vincenzi et al., 2013). Gender, hypocalcaemia, diabetes, and chronic renal failure were not associated with CIPN (Vincenzi et al., 2013). Radiotherapy may increase the neurological symptoms for cisplatin-induced peripheral neuropathy (Brydoy et al., 2009).

Several studies have also assessed genetic predisposition to or protection against CIPN, mainly through polymorphisms affecting the pharmacokinetics of platinum-based anticancer drugs. Thus cisplatin-induced peripheral neuropathy was less frequent in patients with GST M1 (deletion) or GSTM3 intron 6 AGG/AGG genotypes (Khrunin et al., 2010). Conversely, SNP affecting the GSTP1 (Ile105Val) and GSTM1 (deletion) genotypes were significantly associated with a higher incidence of oxaliplatin-associated CIPN (grade > 2) (Kumamoto et al., 2013). SNPs affecting cyclin H and the BCRP were significantly associated with a higher risk of severe oxaliplatin-induced peripheral neuropathy (Custodio et al., 2014). Interestingly, NaV polymorphisms could also be associated with both the severity of acute oxaliplatin-induced neuropathy and the occurrence of chronic neuropathy (Argyriou et al., 2013). However, although several studies have been performed on this topic, the impact of SNP on platinum-based anticancer drugs remains equivocal,

TABLE 1 | Main symptoms associated with chemotherapy-induced peripheral neuropathy.

Platinum-based anticancer drugs	
Oxaliplatin	Acute CIPN (>90% of patients): paresthesia, dysesthesia of the hands, feet and perioral area induced by cold stimuli
	Chronic CIPN (30–50% of patients): paresthesia, numbness, sensory ataxia, functional deficits, and pain
	No vegetative disturbances
	Coasting effect
	Maximum duration in the literature: 8 years
Cisplatin	Sensory neuropathy similar to oxaliplatin-induced chronic neuropathy (50% of patients)
	Maximum duration in the literature: 25 years (adult survivors of childhood extracranial solid tumors)
Taxanes	
Paclitaxel	80–97% of patients
Docetaxel	Acute and chronic sensory neuropathy associated with paresthesia, numbness, tingling and burning, and mechanical and cold allodynia
	Rare motor symptoms with mild distal weakness and myalgia
	Rare vegetative disturbances
	Coasting effect
	Maximum duration in the literature: 4.75 years
Vinca alkaloids	
Vinblastine	35–45% of patients
Vinorelbine	Sensory neuropathy in the hands and feet, leading to functional disability with fine motor tasks and walking, including numbness and tingling
Vindesine	Motor neuropathy with cramps and distal muscle weakness
Vincristine	Vegetative neuropathy associated with postural hypotension, bladder and bowel disturbance
	Coasting effect
	Maximum duration in the literature: 7 years (cancer survivors of childhood hematological malignancies)
Proteasome inhibitor	
Bortezomib	31–64% of patients
	Sensory neuropathy associated with burning dysesthesia, coldness, numbness, hyperesthesia, and/or tingling in a distal stocking-and-glove distribution over the hands and feet
	Pain
	Vegetative disturbances
	Maximum duration in the literature: 2 years (little data in the literature)
Immunomodulatory	
Thalidomide	10–55% of patients
	Sensory peripheral neuropathy associated with tingling or painful paresthesia, and numbness in the lower limbs
	Mild motor impairments
	Vegetative disturbances including gastrointestinal (constipation, anorexia, and nausea) and cardiovascular (hypotension and bradycardia) manifestations
	Maximum duration in the literature: no clear information (little data in the literature)

since a meta-analysis was unable to find any association between GSTP1 IIe105Val and oxaliplatin-induced peripheral neuropathy (Peng et al., 2013). Furthermore, Terrazzino et al. (2015) did not find any association between eight selected SNPs and oxaliplatin-induced peripheral neuropathy (**Table 2**).

TAXANES

Taxane diterpenoids were isolated from the bark of the Pacific yew tree (*Taxus brevifolia* and *Taxus baccata* for paclitaxel and docetaxel, respectively) (Saloustros et al., 2008; Wani and Horwitz, 2014). Taxanes have been approved by the US Food and Drug Administration (FDA) since the mid-1990s for the treatment of several cancers: breast, ovarian, non-small cell lung, prostate, gastric, and head/neck (Qin et al., 2012).

Taxanes are microtubule-stabilizing drugs, thus preventing their depolymerization (Amos and Löwe, 1999; Zhang et al., 2014). This stabilization promotes the formation of abnormal bundles of microtubules in the cytoplasm, leading to mitotic spindle disruption. Thus cells arrest their cell cycle in the G0/G1 and G2/M phases, leading to apoptosis in dividing cells (mainly tumor cells) (Hornick et al., 2008).

Pathophysiological Mechanisms of CIPN Associated to Taxanes

The pathogenesis of peripheral neuropathy induced by taxanes has been investigated in numerous studies (Höke and Ray, 2014). Nevertheless, the primary site of pathogenesis of taxane-associated CIPN has not yet been elucidated (Gornstein and Schwarz, 2014). The increase of oxidative stress may contribute to the potent neurotoxicity of taxanes through damage to

TABLE 2 | Probable risk factors by type of anticancer drug.

Probable risk factors	Platinum-based anticancer drugs	Taxanes	Vinca alkaloids	Bortezomib thalidomide
Chemotherapy regimen	Cumulative dose >850 mg/m^2 (oxaliplatin) >200–300 mg/m^2 (cisplatin)	Dose intensity	Cumulative dose >2 mg/m^2	>1 mg/m^2 Induction therapy
Medical History	Pre-treatment anemia Hypoalbuminemia Hypomagnesaemia Radiotherapy Pre-existing neuropathy	Pre-existing neuropathy	CMT1A	Pre-existing neuropathy
Genetic factors (SNP)	GSTP1 (Ile105Val) GSTM1 (deletion) cyclin H BCRP Na_V channels	FGD4 EPHA5 FZD3 CYP2C8 CYP3A5*3 CYP3A4*22 ABCB1	CYP3A5 GLI1 CEP72	–
Demographic variables	Age	Age	Age (children)	–

Na_V, voltage-gated sodium channel; GSTP1, glutathione S-transferase pi 1; GSTM1, glutathione S-transferase mu 1; BCRP, ATP-binding cassette sub-family G member 2 (ABCG2); FGD4, FYVE, RhoGEF and PH domain containing 4; EPHA5, ephrin type-A receptor 5; FZD3, Frizzled-3; CYP2C8, cytochrome P450 2C8; CYP3A5, cytochrome P450 3A5; CYP3A4, cytochrome P450 3A4; ABCB1, ATP-binding cassette sub-family B member 1; CMT1A, Charcot-Marie-Tooth type 1A; CEP72, centrosomal protein 72.

neuronal and non-neuronal cells in the PNS, macrophage activation in the DRG and peripheral nerves, and microglial activation in the spinal cord (Jimenez-Andrade et al., 2006; Peters et al., 2007; Barrière et al., 2012; Doyle et al., 2012). Overproduction of peroxynitrite contributes to increasing neuro-excitatory and pro-inflammatory cytokines (TNF-alpha and IL-1beta) and to decreasing anti-inflammatory cytokine (IL-10 and IL-4) production (Ledeboer et al., 2007; Doyle et al., 2012).

In vitro studies highlighted that taxanes induced neuropathic symptoms by inhibiting anterograde fast axonal transport (conventional kinesin-dependent) (LaPointe et al., 2013) in the peripheral endings of sensory neurons and altering neurotransmitter release (Carozzi et al., 2010; Gracias et al., 2011; Gilardini et al., 2012). Taxane treatment revealed reversible enlargement of the nucleoli of sensory neurons after a single-dose of paclitaxel in rat (Jamieson et al., 2003). Furthermore, Jimenez-Andrade et al. (2006) reported that a cumulative dose of 36 mg/kg of paclitaxel in rat significantly increased the number of ATF-3 (a cell injury marker) neurons in trigeminal ganglia and DRG. Mitochondrial alterations caused by the production of reactive oxygen species in peripheral nerves were also shown to be closely related to neuropathic effects (Barrière et al., 2012; Xiao and Bennett, 2012). Other studies also recently reported an increase of the toll-like receptor TLR4 and its immediate downstream signaling molecules, myeloid differentiation primary response gene 88 (MyD88), and TRIF, in DRG after paclitaxel treatment in favor of a pro-inflammatory mechanism (Li et al., 2014, 2015). The activation of TLR4 was associated with the sensitization of transient receptor potential vanilloid subtype 1 (Hara et al., 2013; Li et al., 2015) known to be involved in nociception (**Figure 1**).

Symptoms and Long-Term Effects of CIPN Associated to Taxanes

Few studies have reported the increased incidence of acute and chronic toxicities with taxanes that could potentially lead to dose reductions and treatment withdrawal (Tanabe et al., 2013; Ho and Mackey, 2014). It is difficult to know whether paclitaxel or docetaxel is the most neurotoxic as the scientific literature on the topic is unclear and contradictory (Jones et al., 2005; Shimozuma et al., 2012). Neurophysiological examinations of patients with CIPN revealed a decrease in sensory nerve conduction velocity and compound action potential amplitude (Chaudhry et al., 1994; Dougherty et al., 2004). This CIPN is a typical distal sensory neuropathy with a stocking-and-glove distribution over the hands and feet. The patients can report paresthesia, dysesthesia, numbness and altered proprioception. Motor weakness of hands and feet are less frequent, such as vegetative disturbances (De Iuliis et al., 2015). Taxane-associated CIPN is considered to be a good predictor of neuropathic pain after paclitaxel treatment, as 27% of those patients with CIPN experienced neuropathic pain (Reyes-Gibby et al., 2009). These complications are often the main reason for treatment cessation (Tanabe et al., 2013). However, symptoms may aggravate after the end of the chemotherapy (De Iuliis et al., 2015) (**Table 1**).

Among patients treated with adjuvant paclitaxel chemotherapy, between 80 to 97% experienced symptoms of neuropathy with a time range to CIPN onset of 1–101 weeks (Chaudhry et al., 1994; Hershman et al., 2011; Tanabe et al., 2013). These symptoms remained during a median follow-up time of 57 months for 212 neuropathic patients (minimum: 5.3, maximum: 95.5) (Tanabe et al., 2013). In a Multicenter Italian Trial in Ovarian cancer (MITO-4), 22 out of 60 neuropathic patients (37%) treated with carboplatin and paclitaxel reported complete recovery in the first 2 months after the end of the chemotherapy (Pignata et al., 2006). Nevertheless, 15 patients (25%) recovered between 2 and 6 months, and nine patients (15%) after 6 months and more. Regarding a 46-patient cohort (ACCRU pilot trial) treated with paclitaxel alone, similar results were reported based on the sensory neuropathy scores of the QLQ-CIPN20 of the EORTC (Shinde et al., 2016). In a study conducted in the Netherlands, most of the patients complained about neurotoxicity in the upper and lower extremities 6 months after cessation of chemotherapy with oxaliplatin, paclitaxel, or docetaxel (78.8 and 89.7%, respectively) (Beijers A. et al., 2014). These neuropathies primarily included numbness and tingling in hands, feet, suffering from cold feet, and trouble distinguishing objects with the hands.

A significant correlation was found between scores on emotional well-being and neuropathy symptoms with the FACT/GOG-Ntx (Beijers A. et al., 2014). Another study demonstrated that persistent limb pain linked to docetaxel treatment was responsible for the deterioration of psychological function (Ventzel et al., 2016). More recently, breast cancer survivors with CIPN developed more severe insomnia, anxiety, and depression than those without neuropathy (Bao et al., 2016). Thornton et al. (2008) demonstrated that in the years following chemotherapy, the taxane group had significantly worse emotional distress and mental HRQOL throughout adjuvant treatment. These outcomes were also associated with rates of probable clinical depression during the first year. The taxane cohort had a significantly slower psychological recovery and required 2 years on average for emotional recovery compared with 6–12 months for patients in the no taxane comparison group (Thornton et al., 2008). Another longitudinal study monitoring HRQOL parameters in a 6-year study found similar results with a return to baseline within 2 years and no change at 6 years (Hall et al., 2014). Finally, 15% of breast cancer survivors reported CIPN with a significant impact on HRQOL scales, from 1 to 3 years after a single docetaxel containing regimen (Eckhoff et al., 2015). Interestingly, the relative tolerability of regimens according to HRQOL assessment was equivalent between the two single-agent docetaxel and paclitaxel treatments. However, the mean neurotoxicity related subscale FACT/GOG-Ntx from baseline to 1 year following the end of treatment were significantly more severe for the paclitaxel-treated group compared to the docetaxel-treated group (Shimozuma et al., 2012).

CIPN Risk Factors Associated to Taxanes

Although the severity of taxane-mediated CIPN differs as a function of several demographic variables, it is very difficult to predict which patients will develop this CIPN (Schneider et al., 2015). Demographic variables such as health status, obesity, and age are known to predispose to neuropathy (Hershman et al., 2011; Schneider et al., 2012) and influence CIPN duration (Tanabe et al., 2013). Indeed, patients with pre-existing neuropathy (related to diabetes, alcohol or even idiopathic) developed severe neuropathy after receiving taxane-based chemotherapy (Rowinsky et al., 1993; Chaudhry et al., 2003). Cumulative dose (135–1400 mg/m^2) may be a risk of CIPN, but this parameter remains a subject of debate in the literature (van Gerven et al., 1994; Tanabe et al., 2013). Tanabe et al. (2013) did not find any relation between neuropathy grade and diabetes, or with radiotherapy, dose intensity and cumulative dose. CIPN severity may differ depending on chemotherapy type and protocol (Schneider et al., 2012; Shimozuma et al., 2012; Tanabe et al., 2013). Indeed, the median time to neuropathy onset seemed to be inversely correlated with the tighter administration schedule, 35 and 21 days for weekly and tri-weekly administration, respectively (Tanabe et al., 2013). Consequently, the pharmacokinetics of taxanes impact their neurotoxicity and a pharmacokinetic-based dosing algorithm has been proposed to reduce paclitaxel-related neurotoxicity (Kraff et al., 2015).

The heterogeneity of taxane-induced neuropathy is probably not only associated with demographic variables alone, suggesting contributions of genetic variability. Investigations suggest a possible genetic predisposition to the occurrence of taxane-induced peripheral neuropathy (Frederiks et al., 2015). Recent studies examined the effect of SNP in the congenital peripheral neuropathy gene FGD4 as a genetic susceptibility to neuropathic disorders (Baldwin et al., 2012). This SNP, and markers in additional genes [including EPHA5 (rs7349683) and FZD3 (rs10771973)], were associated with the onset or severity of paclitaxel-induced peripheral neuropathy. Additional experiments examined the pharmacokinetic profiles of taxanes to establish whether exposure to them is correlated with the degree of neurotoxicity (Gréen et al., 2009; de Graan et al., 2013). The pharmacokinetic profiles of docetaxel in 50 patients with 59 different SNPs (including tag-SNSps and PXR/NR1I2, CAR/NR1I3, RXRα/NR2B1, HNF4α/NR2A1 genes) were characterized by marked interindividual variability, with approximately four- to six-fold variations observed at maximal concentration, AUC and plasma clearance (Chew et al., 2013). Another clinical study found that docetaxel clearance was also modulated in patients carrying the CYP3A*1B allele or GSTP1*A/*B and 3435TT genotypes (Tran et al., 2006). Further works demonstrated that, among 13 relevant polymorphisms in genes encoding paclitaxel metabolizing enzymes, CYP2C8 haplotype C and CYP3A5*3 were associated with neuroprotection and the clearance of paclitaxel, and conversely with an increased risk of neuropathy (Gréen et al., 2009; Leskelä et al., 2011; Hertz et al., 2013). However a recent study underlined a sexual dimorphism with CYP3A4: women carrying the CYP3A4*22 allele had increased risk of developing severe neurotoxicity during paclitaxel treatment (de Graan et al., 2013). Other studies demonstrated an involvement of ABCB1 gene polymorphisms encoding for *P*-glycoprotein, a primary protein involved in taxane elimination and distribution, with neuropathy in metastatic breast cancer patients treated with paclitaxel or docetaxel monotherapy. Patients treated with docetaxel carrying another ABCB1 2677GG genotype had a significantly longer time to neuropathy (Sissung et al., 2008). Indeed patients heterozygous for G/A in position 2677 in ABCB1 had significantly higher toxic clearance than most other ABCB1 variants (Gréen et al., 2009). Another study underlined that patients carrying two reference alleles for ABCB1 3435CT polymorphism tended toward a reduced risk of developing CIPN compared to patients carrying only one allele (Sissung et al., 2006) (**Table 2**).

VINCA ALKALOIDS

Vinca alkaloids are plant-derived microtubule assembly inhibitors originally derived from the periwinkle *Catharanthus roseus* (Liu et al., 2014). Vinca alkaloids are now produced synthetically and are used in particular in the treatment of acute lymphoblastic leukemia, Hodgkin's disease, non-Hodgkin lymphoma, and many cancers (rhabdomyosarcoma, osteosarcoma, uterus, breast, lung, etc.). They may be used in mono-chemotherapy and poly-chemotherapy treatments. The vinca alkaloid family includes vinblastine, vinorelbine, vindesine, and vincristine (Liu et al., 2014).

Pathophysiological Mechanisms of CIPN Associated to Vinca Alkaloids

Vinca alkaloids block microtubule polymerization, by binding to free tubulin dimers (β-α-tubulin heterodimers interface) close to the GTP-binding sites (vinca domain) (Jordan and Kamath, 2007), inducing an increase of microtubule depolymerization and inhibiting the hydrolysis of GTP, which stops the mitotic cycle and initiates cell apoptosis (Jordan and Wilson, 2004; Liu et al., 2014).

Due to their cytotoxic action, vinca alkaloids induce many adverse effects of which neurotoxicity remains the most frequent. This neurotoxicity affects the neuronal cytoskeleton which causes axonal degeneration and the impairment of axonal transport. For unknown reasons, the sensory fibers are reached earlier, more frequently and more severely than the motor fibers. The complete mechanism of vinca alkaloid-induced peripheral neuropathy involves several actors:

- Endogenous opioids, which play a critical role in nociception, such as endomorphin-2, are decreased in the spinal cord and DRG of animals treated with vincristine, without mu-opioid receptor expression change. This contributes to the development of neuropathic pain symptoms, leading to hypersensitivity of C-fiber nociceptors and abnormal activity of the wide dynamic range neurons (Yang et al., 2014). Oxidative stress, generated after the impairment of mitochondrial function and the overproduction of reactive oxygen species following vinca alkaloid-based treatment, influences the activity of serine protease, which inactivates endomorphins in the spinal cord, thus suggesting that oxidative stress is a key mechanism of this CIPN (Wang et al., 2008).
- Spinal synaptic plasticity involved in the maintenance of neuropathic symptoms is also related to this CIPN. C-Fos (a marker of neuronal activation) and Piccolo (maintenance of synaptic plasticity) were increased in the neurons of the spinal cord in CIPN animal models, suggesting increased neuronal activity and a structural reorganization of pre-synaptic elements (Ibi et al., 2010; Thibault et al., 2013).
- Central glia (astrocytes and microglia) plays a critical role in neuropathic symptoms and its inhibition remains a potential strategy for alleviating these symptoms (Watkins and Maier, 2005). In an animal model of vincristine-induced peripheral neuropathy, astrocyte activation participates in neuropathic symptoms through the up-regulation of interleukin-1β and NMDA sensitization (phosphorylation induced by interleukin-1β) (Ji et al., 2013).
- Serotonin transporter null mice elicit reversed neuropathic pain behavior in animal models of vincristine-associated CIPN. Considering that serotonin has an influence on pain transmission, also in CIPN animal models (Suzuki et al., 2004), this impact on neuropathic symptoms may be attributed to a lack of spinal serotonin. Furthermore, tropisetron (a selective antagonist of serotonin receptor of type 3) is able to ameliorate vincristine-induced peripheral neuropathy in rat (Barzegar-Fallah et al., 2014).
- Vinca alkaloids can alter calcium homeostasis through the dysregulation and structural modification of mitochondria, decreasing the amount and rate of calcium uptake and efflux (Tari et al., 1986). These changes induce increased neuronal excitability and impaired glial function. Moreover, neuropathic symptoms produced by vinca alkaloids are alleviated by drugs that decrease the extracellular and intracellular availability of calcium (Siau and Bennett, 2006).
- Jaggi and Singh (2012) demonstrated a link between MAPK and vincristine-induced peripheral neuropathy. In this study, the antineuropathic effects of farnesyl thiosalicylic acid (Ras inhibitor) and GW5074 (c-Raf1 kinase inhibitor) in an animal model of vincristine-induced peripheral neuropathy was demonstrated (Jaggi and Singh, 2012). This result suggests that Ras and c-Raf-1 are potential targets for preventing CIPN (**Figure 1**).

Symptoms and Long-Term Effects of CIPN Associated to Vinca Alkaloids

Vinca alkaloids induce glove-and-stocking distribution peripheral neuropathy in 35% to 45% of patients (Postma et al., 1993; Verstappen et al., 2005). Sensory neuropathy typically develops first in the hands and feet, leading to functional disability with fine motor tasks and walking, including numbness and tingling (Postma et al., 1993; Verstappen et al., 2005; Boyette-Davis et al., 2013). These symptoms often develop after several weeks of treatment but can occur after the first dose. The coasting effect was also prominent in vinca alkaloid-induced peripheral neuropathy, with 30% of patients subject to worsening symptoms after stopping treatment (Haim et al., 1994). In addition to sensory symptoms, motor and autonomic neuropathies were also prominent. Neuropathic patients experienced muscle cramps and distal muscle weakness (Haim et al., 1994). Autonomic symptoms include heart rate variability reduction (Hirvonen et al., 1989), postural hypotension, bladder and bowel disturbance, ocular palsies and vocal cord paralysis (Hancock and Naysmith, 1975; Quasthoff and Hartung, 2002). Vinca alkaloid treatment was also associated with acute motor neuropathy, similar to the Guillain–Barré syndrome (González Pérez et al., 2007). Vinca alkaloids are frequently used in pediatric hematological malignancies. Lavoie Smith et al. (2015) made an interesting assessment of the vincristine-induced peripheral neuropathy in children treated for acute lymphocytic leukemia. In these children, 78% developed a sensory-motor CIPN and 44% reported pain. Overall severity was low, but a subgroup of children developed severe forms of CIPN. The main identified symptoms were decrease of reflexes, vibration sensibility, and strength (Lavoie Smith et al., 2015). In another study on children and adolescents treated for non-CNS solid and hematological malignancies, up to 85% of vincristine-treated children suffered of CIPN during treatment and 40% at 6 months post-treatment. Higher symptoms and deficits were found for patients treated for lymphoma or solid tumors compared to acute lymphocytic leukemia (Gilchrist et al., 2017) (**Table 1**).

Neuropathy has been described to be reversible and mainly resolved within 2 months (Haim et al., 1994), although some patients report lasting dysfunction with sensory symptoms persisting longer than motor symptoms (Postma et al., 1993; Boyette-Davis et al., 2013). Nevertheless, long-term follow-up of patients who received vinca alkaloid treatment revealed that 32% had sensory symptoms which persisted from 34 to 48 months after treatment (Postma et al., 1993; Boyette-Davis et al., 2013) and 14% had disabling sensory neuropathy 9 years after treatment (Moser et al., 2005). Another study by Oerlemans et al. (2014) demonstrated that patients with diffuse large B-cell lymphoma present neuropathic symptoms for up to 5 years (tingling hands/feet are described in 30% of patients). In comparison, 30–34% of children with acute lymphoblastic leukemia had neuropathic symptoms from 3 to 7 years following vinca alkaloid chemotherapy (Ramchandren et al., 2009; Jain et al., 2014).

Only two studies assessed the impact of this CIPN on the HRQOL of patients. Both studies used either the SF-36 or the QLQ-C30 from the EORTC questionnaires to evaluate HRQOL. In the study by Kim et al. (2010) patients with sensory neuropathy following vinca alkaloid-based treatment (18 weeks) reported a lower HRQOL than those without neuropathy. The SF-36 questionnaire demonstrated that neuropathic patients had impaired physical functions and lower vitality than non-neuropathic patients. No change was observed for the other items (bodily pain, general health, social function and general mental health). In their study Liew et al. (2013) observed that global health was similar to normative data 28 months after completing vinca alkaloid-based chemotherapy, but leukemia survivors had lower cognitive and social functions and reported more financial difficulty. Fatigue and pain affected 83 and 53% of patients, respectively, and both showed significant inverse correlation with overall health and all functional scales. Nevertheless, although therapy-related symptoms were persistent, long-term survivors had a global HRQOL similar to that of the general population (Liew et al., 2013). Overall, these studies indicated that persistent neuropathy has a considerable impact on patients' lives.

CIPN Risk Factors Associated to Vinca Alkaloids

Antifungal treatment with azole-based agents may exacerbate neuropathy via the inhibition of the cytochrome CYP3A involved in vinca alkaloid metabolism (Moriyama et al., 2012). Thus the relationship between genetic factors related to CYP3A, and CIPN has been investigated by several studies. Egbelakin et al. (2011) demonstrated that CYP3A5 expression was related to CIPN in acute lymphoblastic leukemia in children. Indeed, a child with CYP3A5 genotype develops less peripheral neuropathy compared to CYP3A5 non-expressers. Another study demonstrated that acute CIPN was related to the presence of SNPs of genes involved in the cell cycle and cell proliferation, such as GLI1 (rs2228224 and rs2242578), and to the up-regulation of other genes participating in the cell cycle and cell proliferation such as aurora kinase A and the marker of proliferation Ki-67 (Broyl et al., 2010). Moreover, the chronicity of neuropathic symptoms was associated with SNPs in genes involved in absorption, distribution, metabolism, and excretion (Broyl et al., 2010). In addition, 17p11.2-12 duplication (associated with CMT1A) has been demonstrated to be a predictor of severe neurotoxicity in patients (Graf et al., 1996), and more widely, several studies have demonstrated a higher risk of inducing severe acute neurotoxicity in patients with CMT1A (Naumann et al., 2001; Orejana-García et al., 2003; Nishikawa et al., 2008). Finally, sensory neuropathy is less rare in patients expressing a variant of the gene Centrosomal Protein 72 (Diouf et al., 2015).

The occurrence of neuropathy was also strongly dose-dependent, with development at a dose of 2–6 mg/m^2 (Postma et al., 1993; Haim et al., 1994; Verstappen et al., 2005). It is noteworthy that neurotoxicity can occur with a single dose in patients receiving a 4 mg dose and demonstrating worse neurotoxicity than those receiving a 2 mg dose (Verstappen et al., 2005). Thus, total dose levels have been capped at 2 mg/m^2 regardless of body surface area (Haim et al., 1994). For vincristine treated children, older patients are at higher risk of sensory and motor CIPN. Sex is more debated, but female would be at higher risk for CIPN (Lavoie Smith et al., 2015; Gilchrist et al., 2017) (**Table 2**).

BORTEZOMIB AND THALIDOMIDE

Bortezomib, a dipeptidyl boronic acid, is the first of a new class of proteasome inhibitors approved in 2004 by both US and European authorities for the treatment of multiple myeloma and in 2006 for the treatment of mantle cell non-Hodgkin's lymphoma (Argyriou et al., 2014). Bortezomib is the cornerstone treatment for multiple myeloma, and is commonly used to treat newly diagnosed as well as relapsed/refractory multiple myeloma, either as single agent or combined with other therapies, leading to a major improvement in disease management and increasing the lifespan of patients.

Thalidomide is a glutamic acid derivative and an oral immunomodulatory and antiangiogenic agent. It was the first drug designed to treat nausea in pregnant woman in the 1960s. Widely known for its teratogenic effects, thalidomide was approved by the US Food and Drug Administration for the treatment of multiple myeloma (Richardson et al., 2002).

Pathophysiological Mechanisms of CIPN Associated to Bortezomib and Thalidomide

Both thalidomide and bortezomib exert pleiotropic actions, which complicates understanding of their neurotoxic effects (Morawska et al., 2015). Little is known at present about the mechanism underlying this neurotoxicity.

The pathogenetic hallmark of bortezomib-induced peripheral neuropathy consists of morphological alterations in the spinal cord, DRG and peripheral nerves, with specific functional alterations in Aδ and C sensory nerve fibers (Carozzi et al., 2013; Staff et al., 2013). In addition, proteasome inhibition increased a-tubulin polymerization, mitochondrial and endoplasmic reticulum damage, and dysregulation of neurotrophins through the inhibition of NF-kB (nuclear factor kappa B) activation may also significantly contribute to this CIPN genesis (Landowski et al., 2005; Staff et al., 2013). However, these findings do not explain why preferentially thin and unmyelinated nerve fibers are affected. It was recently suggested that bortezomib-induced peripheral neuropathy occurs via a proteasome-independent mechanism (Arastu-Kapur et al., 2011), possibly involving mitochondrial dysfunction (Zheng et al., 2012). By contrast with immunomodulatory drugs, a more specific neurotoxic action of bortezomib occurs through the transient release of intracellular calcium stores, leading to mitochondrial calcium influx and caspase-induced apoptosis (Landowski et al., 2005). Disruption of intracellular calcium homeostasis in nerves can promote depolarization and spontaneous discharge, causing pain and other abnormal sensations. Finally, a higher ratio of polymerized versus soluble tubulin was found in neural cells after treatment with proteasome inhibitors, suggesting a mechanism by which this neurotoxic anticancer drug could interfere with microtubular stability (Poruchynsky et al., 2008).

Thalidomide has several actions, including a role in modifying integrin receptors, altering TNFα and inhibiting angiogenesis. The mechanism of action of thalidomide on malignant cells is poorly understood but may involve both immunomodulation and antiangiogenic effects, resulting in partially irreversible damage to distal axons, DRG neurons and central projections of primary afferent neurons (Giannini et al., 2003). Because thalidomide has antiangiogenic activities, it was initially proposed that one of the mechanisms of thalidomide-induced peripheral neuropathy was capillary damage and secondary anoxemia in nerve fibers. Additionally, it was suggested that thalidomide reduces neural cell survival by downregulation of TNFα, triggering inhibition of NF-kB and subsequent acceleration of neuronal cell death (Fernyhough et al., 2005). NF-kB inhibition is one of the main effects of bortezomib and could provide a common link between the neurotoxicity of thalidomide and proteasome inhibition. A crucial event in thalidomide-induced peripheral neuropathy may be the suppression of NF-kB, a factor linked to p65 (activated by TNFα) and p75 (activated by pro-neurotrophins) receptors (Li et al., 2009). These receptors may induce both apoptosis and cell growth, depending on the circumstances (Ibáñez and Simi, 2012) (**Figure 1**).

Symptoms and Long-Term Effects of CIPN Associated to Bortezomib and Thalidomide

Although bortezomib and thalidomide represent a major advance in the treatment of multiple myeloma, they are also unfortunately accompanied by an increase of challenging treatment-related adverse events; in particular they frequently induce dose-limiting peripheral neuropathy. Bortezomib-induced peripheral neuropathy is considered to be one of the most severe, unpredictable and potentially permanent non-hematological side-effects of chemotherapy against multiple myeloma. Thus it also has a detrimental effect on the HRQOL of survivors (Argyriou et al., 2014) and compromises optimal treatment for patients with multiple myeloma. Although rare, autonomic peripheral neuropathy can be life threatening, leading to serious medical conditions such as irregular heartbeat, hypotension, and shortness of breath. The incidence of this CIPN (any grade) in large clinical studies ranges from 31 to 64% (Richardson et al., 2003, 2005; Velasco et al., 2010) for bortezomib and from 10 to 55% for thalidomide (Jongen et al., 2015). The data collected showed a higher percentage of patients developing CIPN following thalidomide at doses of 200 mg/day or higher in comparison to lower thalidomide doses (Glasmacher et al., 2006).

Bortezomib-induced peripheral neuropathy is typically a predominantly sensory axonopathy associated with burning dysesthesia, coldness, numbness, hyperesthesia, and/or tingling in a distal stocking-and-glove distribution over the hands and feet. Neuropathic pain is a prominent feature of this CIPN, occurring in 25–80% of cases (Rampen et al., 2013), characterized by shooting pain and severe cramps, due to dysfunction of all three major sensory nerve fibers (Aβ, Aδ, and C), as demonstrated in both clinical and animal models (Cata et al., 2007). Signs and symptoms of autonomic dysfunction may occur, since these are also served by unmyelinated nerve fibers. Autonomic dysfunctions are present in 12–50% of patients, with constipation and orthostatic hypotension being the most frequent symptoms (Velasco et al., 2010). Other autonomic disturbances are frequently observed and lead to adverse gastrointestinal events (Richardson et al., 2010). Motor fibers are rarely affected (Mateos, 2012). Bortezomib-induced peripheral neuropathy is an early complication when it occurs shortly after the introduction of treatment. CIPN generally occurs during the first 5 cycles of bortezomib treatment and is related to cumulative dose and reaching a plateau at cycle 5 (Richardson et al., 2009) (**Table 1**).

As with bortezomib, thalidomide-induced peripheral neuropathy causes often painful distal sensory axonal peripheral neuropathy in over half of patients if treated over a sufficiently long period of time (Cavaletti et al., 2004). Thalidomide-induced peripheral neuropathy affects large and small fibers, associated with tingling or painful paresthesia, and numbness in the lower limbs (Plasmati et al., 2007). Its onset is usually slower than for bortezomib. Mild motor impairment also appears to be present (Chaudhry et al., 2008), but is only significant in severe cases (Giannini et al., 2003). Autonomic manifestations, including gastrointestinal (constipation, anorexia, and nausea), and cardiovascular (hypotension and bradycardia) effects are commonly observed (Morawska et al., 2015). A dual role for thalidomide has been highlighted by clinical observations that suggest that thalidomide may be neuroprotective in patients receiving a combination with bortezomib, while being neurotoxic when given as a single agent (Badros et al., 2007). This might be explained by its anti-inflammatory effect in preventing excess neurotoxicity (**Table 1**).

Unfortunately, these CIPNs are not always reversible. Although reversal of bortezomib-induced peripheral neuropathy after treatment cessation is frequent, recovery in some patients may take months, up to 2 years, and some will never fully recover neurological function (Cavaletti and Jakubowiak, 2010). This CIPN has a significant impact on HRQOL, including the physical, social, and psychological effects of unrelieved pain (Tariman et al., 2008). At present, extensive reports on the long-term evolution of this CIPNs are not available. The long-term evolution of thalidomide-induced peripheral neuropathy has not yet been studied extensively, although it is suggested that this CIPN may improve after thalidomide dose-reduction or discontinuation (Argyriou et al., 2012). However, some patients may be subject to permanent damage (Mohty et al., 2010).

Maximizing the benefits of treatment while preserving HRQOL therefore requires a careful balance between achieving optimum activity and minimizing toxicity, in order to further enhance efficacy. Monitoring for signs and symptoms of peripheral neuropathy during bortezomib or thalidomide therapy, such as the Indication for Common Toxicity Criteria Grading of Peripheral Neuropathy Questionnaire, should ensure early recognition, allowing for prompt dose reduction and discontinuation which are the mainstays of preventing and managing CIPN, and increasing the probability of recovery of patients undergoing cancer treatment (Beijers et al., 2016).

CIPN Risk Factors Associated to Bortezomib and Thalidomide

Risk factors for CIPN in multiple myeloma patients include advanced age, prior neuropathy and drug combinations, but not genetic factors (García-Sanz et al., 2016). Nevertheless, in larger studies, baseline neuropathy was the only consistent risk factor for bortezomib-induced peripheral neuropathy. Age, diabetes, International Staging System stage, obesity, and creatinine clearance did not affect the overall rate of this CIPN (Dimopoulos et al., 2011; Tacchetti et al., 2014). Like almost any neurotoxic antineoplastic drug, the cumulative bortezomib dose is the most significant risk factor of CIPN development. The study by Tacchetti et al. (2014) demonstrated that the rate of grade 2 CIPN in the VTD arm was three times higher than in the thalidomide dexamethasone arm of the study. Of all the treatment phases, induction therapy was associated with the highest risk of CIPN, while the lowest risk was related to consolidation therapy (Tacchetti et al., 2014). Furthermore, lowering the dose of bortezomib to 1 mg/m^2 was associated with a reduced risk of developing severe neurological toxicity after four cycles of VTD (Moreau et al., 2011a). Since 2012, The Food and Drug Administration and the European Medicine Agency have validated the subcutaneous injection of bortezomib instead of the intravenous injection in order to limit the adverse effects and CIPN (Moreau et al., 2011b; Minarik et al., 2015). However, a recent study show that the prevalence and severity of bortezomib-induced peripheral neuropathy were not different between intravenous and subcutaneous ways (Minarik et al., 2015) (**Table 2**).

CONCLUSION

As presented in this review, CIPN represents a very problematic adverse event of certain anticancer chemotherapies. First, these CIPNs are frequent in cancer patients treated with neurotoxic anticancer drugs with an overall incidence of approximately 38% (possibly as many as 90% of patients treated with oxaliplatin). Finally, the long-term reversibility of these CIPNs remains questionable, notably in the case of platinum-based anticancer drugs and taxanes, for which CIPN may last several years after the end of anticancer chemotherapies. These CIPN are also very problematic for young patients (children, adolescents, and young adults), which may interfere with their own development and social life. As we have seen, these long-term effects are associated with comorbidities such as depression, insomnia and a decrease of HRQOL in cancer patients and survivors. However, it is noteworthy that these long-term effects remain poorly studied, and only limited data are available such as in the case of bortezomib and thalidomide-induced peripheral neuropathy, despite the shorter life expectancy of patients.

Some risk factors of CIPN have been identified for each anticancer drug. The most applicable ones are the control of cumulative doses, preexisting neuropathic disorders and age of patients. But these preventive measures have a limited effect in clinical practice because patients still suffer of CIPN. No preventive or curative pharmacological strategy has yet been acknowledged. This can be explained by the fact that the drugs chosen to treat or prevent CIPNs are the same as those used to treat common neuropathic pain conditions, such as nerve injury, post-herpetic neuralgia, polyneuropathy, and painful diabetic peripheral neuropathy. The main preclinical and clinical studies have been performed although CIPN differs from other forms of neuropathy, particularly in terms of pathophysiology and symptomatology. CIPNs are frequently associated with sensory symptoms (numbness, tingling) without severe neuropathic pain symptoms (shooting/burning pain), point that we recently debated in the literature (Kerckhove et al., 2017).

For many patients, these CIPNs are not vital adverse effects but impact greatly their quality of life, and for cancer survivors, these CIPN are reminders of the cancer disease and its treatments. Oncologists decrease or stop neurotoxic anticancer drugs, thus limiting the severity of these neurological symptoms "and that's all." However, given the major improvement of the therapeutic management of many cancers and the increasing number of cancer survivors, it is now urgent to discover new and effective strategies to prevent and/or treat these CIPNs and their long-term effects.

AUTHOR CONTRIBUTIONS

NK, AC, SC, CC, DP, and DB contributed to the design of the manuscript and the acquisition of data from the literature. All the authors participated in drafting and revising the manuscript they all approved the final version of the manuscript for submission.

ACKNOWLEDGMENT

The authors thank Accent Europe for its assistance in reading the manuscript.

REFERENCES

Abd-Elsayed, A. A., Ikeda, R., Jia, Z., Ling, J., Zuo, X., Li, M., et al. (2015). KCNQ channels in nociceptive cold-sensing trigeminal ganglion neurons as therapeutic targets for treating orofacial cold hyperalgesia. *Mol. Pain* 11:45. doi: 10.1186/s12990-015-0048-8

Altaf, R., Lund Brixen, A., Kristensen, B., and Nielsen, S. E. (2014). Incidence of cold-induced peripheral neuropathy and dose modification of adjuvant oxaliplatin-based chemotherapy for patients with colorectal cancer. *Oncology* 87, 167–172. doi: 10.1159/000362668

Amos, L. A., and Löwe, J. (1999). How Taxol stabilises microtubule structure. *Chem. Biol.* 6, R65–R69. doi: 10.1016/s1074-5521(99)89002-4

André, T., Boni, C., Navarro, M., Tabernero, J., Hickish, T., Topham, C., et al. (2009). Improved overall survival with oxaliplatin, fluorouracil, and leucovorin as adjuvant treatment in stage II or III colon cancer in the MOSAIC trial. *J. Clin. Oncol.* 27, 3109–3116. doi: 10.1200/JCO.2008.20.6771

Arastu-Kapur, S., Anderl, J. L., Kraus, M., Parlati, F., Shenk, K. D., Lee, S. J., et al. (2011). Nonproteasomal targets of the proteasome inhibitors bortezomib and carfilzomib: a link to clinical adverse events. *Clin. Cancer Res.* 17, 2734–2743. doi: 10.1158/1078-0432.CCR-10-1950

Argyriou, A. A., Bruna, J., Marmiroli, P., and Cavaletti, G. (2012). Chemotherapy-induced peripheral neurotoxicity (CIPN): an update. *Crit. Rev. Oncol. Hematol.* 82, 51–77. doi: 10.1016/j.critrevonc.2011.04.012

Argyriou, A. A., Cavaletti, G., Antonacopoulou, A., Genazzani, A. A., Briani, C., Bruna, J., et al. (2013). Voltage-gated sodium channel polymorphisms play a pivotal role in the development of oxaliplatin-induced peripheral neurotoxicity: results from a prospective multicenter study. *Cancer* 119, 3570–3577. doi: 10.1002/cncr.28234

Argyriou, A. A., Cavaletti, G., Bruna, J., Kyritsis, A. P., and Kalofonos, H. P. (2014). Bortezomib-induced peripheral neurotoxicity: an update. *Arch. Toxicol.* 88, 1669–1679. doi: 10.1007/s00204-014-1316-5

Attal, N., Bouhassira, D., Gautron, M., Vaillant, J. N., Mitry, E., Lepère, C., et al. (2009). Thermal hyperalgesia as a marker of oxaliplatin neurotoxicity: a prospective quantified sensory assessment study. *Pain* 144, 245–252. doi: 10.1016/j.pain.2009.03.024

Badros, A., Goloubeva, O., Dalal, J. S., Can, I., Thompson, J., Rapoport, A. P., et al. (2007). Neurotoxicity of bortezomib therapy in multiple myeloma: a single-center experience and review of the literature. *Cancer* 110, 1042–1049. doi: 10.1002/cncr.22921

Balayssac, D., Ferrier, J., Descoeur, J., Ling, B., Pezet, D., Eschalier, A., et al. (2011). Chemotherapy-induced peripheral neuropathies: from clinical relevance to preclinical evidence. *Expert Opin. Drug Saf.* 10, 407–417. doi: 10.1517/14740338.2011.543417

Baldwin, R. M., Owzar, K., Zembutsu, H., Chhibber, A., Kubo, M., Jiang, C., et al. (2012). A genome-wide association study identifies novel loci for paclitaxel-induced sensory peripheral neuropathy in CALGB 40101. *Am. Assoc. Cancer Res.* 18, 5099–5109. doi: 10.1158/1078-0432.CCR-12-1590

Bao, T., Basal, C., Seluzicki, C., Li, S. Q., Seidman, A. D., and Mao, J. J. (2016). Long-term chemotherapy-induced peripheral neuropathy among breast cancer survivors: prevalence, risk factors, and fall risk. *Breast Cancer Res. Treat.* 159, 327–333. doi: 10.1007/s10549-016-3939-0

Barrière, D. A., Rieusset, J., Chanteranne, D., Busserolles, J., Chauvin, M.-A., Chapuis, L., et al. (2012). Paclitaxel therapy potentiates cold hyperalgesia in streptozotocin-induced diabetic rats through enhanced mitochondrial reactive oxygen species production and TRPA1 sensitization. *Pain* 153, 553–561. doi: 10.1016/j.pain.2011.11.019

Barzegar-Fallah, A., Alimoradi, H., Mehrzadi, S., Barzegar-Fallah, N., Zendedel, A., Abbasi, A., et al. (2014). The neuroprotective effect of tropisetron on vincristine-induced neurotoxicity. *Neurotoxicology* 41, 1–8. doi: 10.1016/j.neuro.2013.12.002

Beijers, A., Mols, F., Dercksen, W., Driessen, C., and Vreugdenhil, G. (2014). Chemotherapy-induced peripheral neuropathy and impact on quality of life 6 months after treatment with chemotherapy. *J. Community Support. Oncol.* 12, 401–406. doi: 10.12788/jcso.0086

Beijers, A. J., Mols, F., and Vreugdenhil, G. (2014). A systematic review on chronic oxaliplatin-induced peripheral neuropathy and the relation with oxaliplatin administration. *Support. Care Cancer* 22, 1999–2007. doi: 10.1007/s00520-014-2242-z

Beijers, A. J., Vreugdenhil, G., Oerlemans, S., Eurelings, M., Minnema, M. C., Eeltink, C. M., et al. (2016). Chemotherapy-induced neuropathy in multiple myeloma: influence on quality of life and development of a questionnaire to compose common toxicity criteria grading for use in daily clinical practice. *Support. Care Cancer* 24, 2411–2420. doi: 10.1007/s00520-015-3032-y

Boyette-Davis, J. A., Cata, J. P., Driver, L. C., Novy, D. M., Bruel, B. M., Mooring, D. L., et al. (2013). Persistent chemoneuropathy in patients receiving the plant alkaloids paclitaxel and vincristine. *Cancer Chemother. Pharmacol.* 71, 619–626. doi: 10.1007/s00280-012-2047-z

Brenner, H., Kloor, M., and Pox, C. P. (2014). Colorectal cancer. *Lancet Lond. Engl.* 383, 1490–1502. doi: 10.1016/S0140-6736(13)61649-9

Broyl, A., Corthals, S. L., Jongen, J. L., van der Holt, B., Kuiper, R., de Knegt, Y., et al. (2010). Mechanisms of peripheral neuropathy associated with bortezomib and vincristine in patients with newly diagnosed multiple myeloma: a prospective analysis of data from the HOVON-65/GMMG-HD4 trial. *Lancet Oncol.* 11, 1057–1065. doi: 10.1016/S1470-2045(10)70206-0

Brydoy, M., Oldenburg, J., Klepp, O., Bremnes, R. M., Wist, E. A., Wentzel-Larsen, T., et al. (2009). Observational study of prevalence of long-term raynaud-like phenomena and neurological side effects in testicular cancer survivors. *J. Natl. Cancer Inst.* 101, 1682–1695. doi: 10.1093/jnci/djp413

Carozzi, V. A., Canta, A., Oggioni, N., Sala, B., Chiorazzi, A., Meregalli, C., et al. (2010). Neurophysiological and neuropathological characterization of new murine models of chemotherapy-induced chronic peripheral neuropathies. *Exp. Neurol.* 226, 301–309. doi: 10.1016/j.expneurol.2010.09.004

Carozzi, V. A., Renn, C. L., Bardini, M., Fazio, G., Chiorazzi, A., Meregalli, C., et al. (2013). Bortezomib-induced painful peripheral neuropathy: an electrophysiological, behavioral, morphological and mechanistic study in the mouse. *PLoS ONE* 8:e72995. doi: 10.1371/journal.pone.0072995

Cata, J. P., Weng, H.-R., Burton, A. W., Villareal, H., Giralt, S., and Dougherty, P. M. (2007). Quantitative sensory findings in patients with bortezomib-induced pain. *J. Pain* 8, 296–306. doi: 10.1016/j.jpain.2006.09.014

Cavaletti, G., Beronio, A., Reni, L., Ghiglione, E., Schenone, A., Briani, C., et al. (2004). Thalidomide sensory neurotoxicity: a clinical and neurophysiologic study. *Neurology* 62, 2291–2293. doi: 10.1212/WNL.62.12.2291

Cavaletti, G., and Jakubowiak, A. J. (2010). Peripheral neuropathy during bortezomib treatment of multiple myeloma: a review of recent studies. *Leuk. Lymphoma* 51, 1178–1187. doi: 10.3109/10428194.2010.483303

Cavaletti, G., and Zanna, C. (2002). Current status and future prospects for the treatment of chemotherapy-induced peripheral neurotoxicity. *Eur. J. Cancer* 1990, 1832–1837. doi: 10.1016/S0959-8049(02)00229-0

Chaudhry, V., Chaudhry, M., Crawford, T. O., Simmons-O'Brien, E., and Griffin, J. W. (2003). Toxic neuropathy in patients with pre-existing neuropathy. *Neurology* 60, 337–340. doi: 10.1212/01.WNL.0000043691.53710.53

Chaudhry, V., Cornblath, D. R., Polydefkis, M., Ferguson, A., and Borrello, I. (2008). Characteristics of bortezomib- and thalidomide-induced peripheral neuropathy. *J. Peripher. Nerv. Syst.* 13, 275–282. doi: 10.1111/j.1529-8027.2008.00193.x

Chaudhry, V., Rowinsky, E. K., Sartorius, S. E., Donehower, R. C., and Cornblath, D. R. (1994). Peripheral neuropathy from taxol and cisplatin combination chemotherapy: clinical and electrophysiological studies. *Ann. Neurol.* 35, 304–311. doi: 10.1002/ana.410350310

Chew, S.-C., Lim, J., Singh, O., Chen, X., Tan, E.-H., Lee, E.-J., et al. (2013). Pharmacogenetic effects of regulatory nuclear receptors (PXR, CAR, RXRα and HNF4α) on docetaxel disposition in Chinese nasopharyngeal cancer patients. *Eur. J. Clin. Pharmacol.* 70, 155–166. doi: 10.1007/s00228-013-1596-3

Custodio, A., Moreno-Rubio, J., Aparicio, J., Gallego-Plazas, J., Yaya, R., Maurel, J., et al. (2014). Pharmacogenetic predictors of severe peripheral neuropathy in colon cancer patients treated with oxaliplatin-based adjuvant chemotherapy: a GEMCAD group study. *Ann. Oncol.* 25, 398–403. doi: 10.1093/annonc/mdt546

de Graan, A.-J., Elens, L., Sprowl, J. A., Sparreboom, A., Friberg, L. E., van der Holt, B., et al. (2013). CYP3A4*22 genotype and systemic exposure affect paclitaxel-induced neurotoxicity. *Clin. Cancer Res.* 19, 3316–3324. doi: 10.1158/1078-0432.CCR-12-3786

De Iuliis, F., Taglieri, L., Salerno, G., Lanza, R., and Scarpa, S. (2015). Taxane induced neuropathy in patients affected by breast cancer: literature review. *Crit. Rev. Oncol. Hematol.* 96, 34–45. doi: 10.1016/j.critrevonc.2015.04.011

Descoeur, J., Pereira, V., Pizzoccaro, A., Francois, A., Ling, B., Maffre, V., et al. (2011). Oxaliplatin-induced cold hypersensitivity is due to remodelling of ion channel expression in nociceptors. *EMBO Mol. Med.* 3, 266–278. doi: 10.1002/emmm.201100134

Di Cesare Mannelli, L., Zanardelli, M., Failli, P., and Ghelardini, C. (2012). Oxaliplatin-induced neuropathy: oxidative stress as pathological mechanism. Protective effect of silibinin. *J. Pain* 13, 276–284. doi: 10.1016/j.jpain.2011.11.009

Di Cesare Mannelli, L., Zanardelli, M., Landini, I., Pacini, A., Ghelardini, C., Mini, E., et al. (2016). Effect of the SOD mimetic MnL4 on in vitro and in vivo oxaliplatin toxicity: possible aid in chemotherapy induced neuropathy. *Free Radic. Biol. Med.* 93, 67–76. doi: 10.1016/j.freeradbiomed.2016.01.023

Dilruba, S., and Kalayda, G. V. (2016). Platinum-based drugs: past, present and future. *Cancer Chemother. Pharmacol.* 77, 1103–1124. doi: 10.1007/s00280-016-2976-z

Dimopoulos, M. A., Mateos, M.-V., Richardson, P. G., Schlag, R., Khuageva, N. K., Shpilberg, O., et al. (2011). Risk factors for, and reversibility of, peripheral neuropathy associated with bortezomib-melphalan-prednisone in newly diagnosed patients with multiple myeloma: subanalysis of the phase 3 VISTA study. *Eur. J. Haematol.* 86, 23–31. doi: 10.1111/j.1600-0609.2010.01533.x

Diouf, B., Crews, K. R., Lew, G., Pei, D., Cheng, C., Bao, J., et al. (2015). Association of an inherited genetic variant with vincristine-related peripheral neuropathy in children with acute lymphoblastic leukemia. *JAMA* 313, 815–823. doi: 10.1001/jama.2015.0894

Dougherty, P. M., Cata, J. P., Cordella, J. V., Burton, A., and Weng, H.-R. (2004). Taxol-induced sensory disturbance is characterized by preferential impairment of myelinated fiber function in cancer patients. *Pain* 109, 132–142. doi: 10.1016/j.pain.2004.01.021

Doyle, T., Chen, Z., Muscoli, C., Bryant, L., Esposito, E., Cuzzocrea, S., et al. (2012). Targeting the overproduction of peroxynitrite for the prevention and reversal of paclitaxel-induced neuropathic pain. *J. Neurosci.* 32, 6149–6160. doi: 10.1523/JNEUROSCI.6343-11.2012

Dzagnidze, A., Katsarava, Z., Makhalova, J., Liedert, B., Yoon, M.-S., Kaube, H., et al. (2007). Repair capacity for platinum-DNA adducts determines the severity of cisplatin-induced peripheral neuropathy. *J. Neurosci.* 27, 9451–9457. doi: 10.1523/JNEUROSCI.0523-07.2007

Earl, H. M., Connolly, S., Latoufis, C., Eagle, K., Ash, C. M., Fowler, C., et al. (1998). Long-term neurotoxicity of chemotherapy in adolescents and young adults treated for bone and soft tissue sarcomas. *Sarcoma* 2, 97–105. doi: 10.1080/13577149878055

Eckhoff, L., Knoop, A., Jensen, M. B., and Ewertz, M. (2015). Persistence of docetaxel-induced neuropathy and impact on quality of life among breast cancer survivors. *Eur. J. Cancer* 51, 292–300. doi: 10.1016/j.ejca.2014.11.024

Egbelakin, A., Ferguson, M. J., MacGill, E. A., Lehmann, A. S., Topletz, A. R., Quinney, S. K., et al. (2011). Increased risk of vincristine neurotoxicity associated with low CYP3A5 expression genotype in children with acute lymphoblastic leukemia. *Pediatr. Blood Cancer* 56, 361–367. doi: 10.1002/pbc.22845

Engelen, M. J. A., Snel, B. J., Schaapveld, M., Pras, E., de Vries, E. G. E., Gietema, J. A., et al. (2009). Long-term morbidity of adjuvant whole abdominal radiotherapy (WART) or chemotherapy for early stage ovarian cancer. *Eur. J. Cancer* 45, 1193–1200. doi: 10.1016/j.ejca.2009.01.006

Fernyhough, P., Smith, D. R., Schapansky, J., Van Der Ploeg, R., Gardiner, N. J., Tweed, C. W., et al. (2005). Activation of nuclear factor-kappaB via endogenous tumor necrosis factor alpha regulates survival of axotomized adult sensory neurons. *J. Neurosci.* 25, 1682–1690. doi: 10.1523/JNEUROSCI.3127-04.2005

Frederiks, C. N., Lam, S. W., Guchelaar, H. J., and Boven, E. (2015). Genetic polymorphisms and paclitaxel- or docetaxel-induced toxicities: a systematic review. *Cancer Treat. Rev.* 41, 935–950. doi: 10.1016/j.ctrv.2015.10.010

Ganz, P. A. (2003). Why and how to study the fate of cancer survivors: observations from the clinic and the research laboratory. *Eur. J. Cancer* 39, 2136–2141. doi: 10.1016/S0959-8049(03)00489-1

García-Sanz, R., Corchete, L. A., Alcoceba, M., Chillon, M. C., Jiménez, C., Prieto, I., et al. (2016). Prediction of peripheral neuropathy in multiple myeloma patients receiving bortezomib and thalidomide: a genetic study based on a single nucleotide polymorphism array. *Hematol. Oncol.* doi: 10.1002/hon.2337 [Epub ahead of print] doi: 10.1002/hon.2337

Gauchan, P., Andoh, T., Kato, A., and Kuraishi, Y. (2009). Involvement of increased expression of transient receptor potential melastatin 8 in oxaliplatin-induced cold allodynia in mice. *Neurosci. Lett.* 458, 93–95. doi: 10.1016/j.neulet.2009.04.029

Giannini, F., Volpi, N., Rossi, S., Passero, S., Fimiani, M., and Cerase, A. (2003). Thalidomide-induced neuropathy: a ganglionopathy? *Neurology* 60, 877–878. doi: 10.1212/01.WNL.0000049462.03800.B1

Gilardini, A., Avila, R. L., Oggioni, N., Rodriguez-Menendez, V., Bossi, M., Canta, A., et al. (2012). Myelin structure is unaltered in chemotherapy-induced peripheral neuropathy. *Neurotoxicology* 33, 1–7. doi: 10.1016/j.neuro.2011.10.010

Gilchrist, L. S., Tanner, L. R., and Ness, K. K. (2017). Short-term recovery of chemotherapy-induced peripheral neuropathy after treatment for pediatric non-CNS cancer. *Pediatr. Blood Cancer* 64, 180–187. doi: 10.1002/pbc.26204

Glasmacher, A., Hahn, C., Hoffmann, F., Naumann, R., Goldschmidt, H., von Lilienfeld-Toal, M., et al. (2006). A systematic review of phase-II trials of thalidomide monotherapy in patients with relapsed or refractory multiple myeloma. *Br. J. Haematol.* 132, 584–593. doi: 10.1111/j.1365-2141.2005.05914.x

Glendenning, J. L., Barbachano, Y., Norman, A. R., Dearnaley, D. P., Horwich, A., and Huddart, R. A. (2010). Long-term neurologic and peripheral vascular toxicity after chemotherapy treatment of testicular cancer. *Cancer* 116, 2322–2331. doi: 10.1002/cncr.24981

González Pérez, P., Serrano-Pozo, A., Franco-Macías, E., Montes-Latorre, E., Gómez-Aranda, F., and Campos, T. (2007). Vincristine-induced acute neurotoxicity versus Guillain-Barré syndrome: a diagnostic dilemma. *Eur. J. Neurol.* 14, 826–828. doi: 10.1111/j.1468-1331.2007.01842.x

Gornstein, E., and Schwarz, T. L. (2014). The paradox of paclitaxel neurotoxicity: mechanisms and unanswered questions. *Neuropharmacology* 76(Pt A), 175–183. doi: 10.1016/j.neuropharm.2013.08.016

Gracias, N. G., Cummins, T. R., Kelley, M. R., Basile, D. P., Iqbal, T., and Vasko, M. R. (2011). Vasodilatation in the rat dorsal hindpaw induced by activation of sensory neurons is reduced by paclitaxel. *Neurotoxicology* 32, 140–149. doi: 10.1016/j.neuro.2010.09.006

Graf, W. D., Chance, P. F., Lensch, M. W., Eng, L. J., Lipe, H. P., and Bird, T. D. (1996). Severe vincristine neuropathy in Charcot-Marie-Tooth disease type 1A. *Cancer* 77, 1356–1362. doi: 10.1002/(SICI)1097-0142(19960401)77:7<1356::AID-CNCR20>3.0.CO;2-#

Gréen, H., Söderkvist, P., Rosenberg, P., Mirghani, R. A., Rymark, P., Lundqvist, E. A., et al. (2009). Pharmacogenetic studies of Paclitaxel in the treatment of ovarian cancer. *Basic Clin. Pharmacol. Toxicol.* 104, 130–137. doi: 10.1111/j.1742-7843.2008.00351.x

Haim, N., Epelbaum, R., Ben-Shahar, M., Yarnitsky, D., Simri, W., and Robinson, E. (1994). Full dose vincristine (without 2-mg dose limit) in the treatment of lymphomas. *Cancer* 73, 2515–2519. doi: 10.1002/1097-0142(19940515)73:10<2515::AID-CNCR2820731011>3.0.CO;2-G

Hall, E., Cameron, D., Waters, R., Barrett-Lee, P., Ellis, P., Russell, S., et al. (2014). Comparison of patient reported quality of life and impact of treatment side effects experienced with a taxane-containing regimen and standard anthracycline based chemotherapy for early breast cancer: 6 year results from the UK TACT trial (CRUK/01/001). *Eur. J. Cancer* 50, 2375–2389. doi: 10.1016/j.ejca.2014.06.007

Hancock, B. W., and Naysmith, A. (1975). Vincristine-induced autonomic neuropathy. *Br. Med. J.* 3, 207. doi: 10.1136/bmj.3.5977.207

Hara, T., Chiba, T., Abe, K., Makabe, A., Ikeno, S., Kawakami, K., et al. (2013). Effect of paclitaxel on transient receptor potential vanilloid 1 in rat dorsal root ganglion. *Pain* 154, 882–889. doi: 10.1016/j.pain.2013.02.023

Hershman, D. L., Lacchetti, C., Dworkin, R. H., Lavoie Smith, E. M., Bleeker, J., Cavaletti, G., et al. (2014). Prevention and management of chemotherapy-induced peripheral neuropathy in survivors of adult cancers: American Society of Clinical Oncology clinical practice guideline. *J. Clin. Oncol.* 32, 1941–1967. doi: 10.1200/JCO.2013.54.0914

Hershman, D. L., Weimer, L. H., Wang, A., Kranwinkel, G., Brafman, L., Fuentes, D., et al. (2011). Association between patient reported outcomes and quantitative sensory tests for measuring long-term neurotoxicity in breast cancer survivors treated with adjuvant paclitaxel chemotherapy. *Breast Cancer Res. Treat.* 125, 767–774. doi: 10.1007/s10549-010-1278-0

Hertz, D. L., Roy, S., Motsinger-Reif, A. A., Drobish, A., Clark, L. S., McLeod, H. L., et al. (2013). CYP2C8*3 increases risk of neuropathy in breast cancer patients treated with paclitaxel. *Ann. Oncol.* 24, 1472–1478. doi: 10.1093/annonc/mdt018

Hirvonen, H. E., Salmi, T. T., Heinonen, E., Antila, K. J., and Välimäki, I. A. (1989). Vincristine treatment of acute lymphoblastic leukemia induces transient autonomic cardioneuropathy. *Cancer* 64, 801–805. doi: 10.1002/1097-0142(19890815)64:4<801::AID-CNCR2820640406>3.0.CO;2-E

Ho, M. Y., and Mackey, J. R. (2014). Presentation and management of docetaxel-related adverse effects in patients with breast cancer. *Cancer Manag. Res.* 6, 253–259. doi: 10.2147/CMAR.S40601

Höke, A., and Ray, M. (2014). Rodent models of chemotherapy-induced peripheral neuropathy. *ILAR J.* 54, 273–281. doi: 10.1093/ilar/ilt053

Hong, J. S., Tian, J., and Wu, L. H. (2014). The influence of chemotherapy-induced neurotoxicity on psychological distress and sleep disturbance in cancer patients. *Curr. Oncol.* 21, 174–180. doi: 10.3747/co.21.1984

Hornick, J. E., Bader, J. R., Tribble, E. K., Trimble, K., Breunig, J. S., Halpin, E. S., et al. (2008). Live-cell analysis of mitotic spindle formation in taxol-treated cells. *Cell Motil. Cytoskeleton* 65, 595–613. doi: 10.1002/cm.20283

Ibáñez, C. F., and Simi, A. (2012). p75 neurotrophin receptor signaling in nervous system injury and degeneration: paradox and opportunity. *Trends Neurosci.* 35, 431–440. doi: 10.1016/j.tins.2012.03.007

Ibi, D., Nitta, A., Ishige, K., Cen, X., Ohtakara, T., Nabeshima, T., et al. (2010). Piccolo knockdown-induced impairments of spatial learning and long-term potentiation in the hippocampal CA1 region. *Neurochem. Int.* 56, 77–83. doi: 10.1016/j.neuint.2009.09.004

Jaggi, A. S., and Singh, N. (2012). Mechanisms in cancer-chemotherapeutic drugs-induced peripheral neuropathy. *Toxicology* 291, 1–9. doi: 10.1016/j.tox.2011.10.019

Jain, P., Gulati, S., Seth, R., Bakhshi, S., Toteja, G. S., and Pandey, R. M. (2014). Vincristine-induced neuropathy in childhood ALL (acute lymphoblastic leukemia) survivors: prevalence and electrophysiological characteristics. *J. Child Neurol.* 29, 932–937. doi: 10.1177/0883073813491829

Jamieson, S. M. F., Liu, J., Hsu, T., Baguley, B. C., and McKeage, M. J. (2003). Paclitaxel induces nucleolar enlargement in dorsal root ganglion neurons in vivo reducing oxaliplatin toxicity. *Br. J. Cancer* 88, 1942–1947. doi: 10.1038/sj.bjc.6601012

Javle, M., and Hsueh, C.-T. (2010). Recent advances in gastrointestinal oncology–updates and insights from the 2009 annual meeting of the American society of clinical oncology. *J. Hematol. Oncol.* 3:11. doi: 10.1186/1756-8722-3-11

Ji, X.-T., Qian, N.-S., Zhang, T., Li, J.-M., Li, X.-K., Wang, P., et al. (2013). Spinal astrocytic activation contributes to mechanical allodynia in a rat chemotherapy-induced neuropathic pain model. *PLoS ONE* 8:e60733. doi: 10.1371/journal.pone.0060733

Jimenez-Andrade, J. M., Peters, C. M., Mejia, N. A., Ghilardi, J. R., Kuskowski, M. A., and Mantyh, P. W. (2006). Sensory neurons and their supporting cells located in the trigeminal, thoracic and lumbar ganglia differentially express markers of injury following intravenous administration of paclitaxel in the rat. *Neurosci. Lett.* 405, 62–67. doi: 10.1016/j.neulet.2006.06.043

Jones, S. E., Erban, J., Overmoyer, B., Budd, G. T., Hutchins, L., Lower, E., et al. (2005). Randomized phase III study of docetaxel compared with paclitaxel in metastatic breast cancer. *J. Clin. Oncol.* 23, 5542–5551. doi: 10.1200/JCO.2005.02.027

Jongen, J. L. M., Broijl, A., and Sonneveld, P. (2015). Chemotherapy-induced peripheral neuropathies in hematological malignancies. *J. Neurooncol.* 121, 229–237. doi: 10.1007/s11060-014-1632-x

Jordan, M. A., and Kamath, K. (2007). How do microtubule-targeted drugs work? An overview. *Curr. Cancer Drug Targets* 7, 730–742. doi: 10.2174/156800907783220417

Jordan, M. A., and Wilson, L. (2004). Microtubules as a target for anticancer drugs. *Nat. Rev. Cancer* 4, 253–265. doi: 10.1038/nrc1317

Kerckhove, N., Pereira, B., Pezet, D., and Balayssac, D. (2017). Clinical assessment of new antineuropathic strategies for chemotherapy-induced peripheral neuropathy: pain should not be the principal endpoint. *Pain* 158, 180–182. doi: 10.1097/j.pain.0000000000000743

Khrunin, A. V., Moisseev, A., Gorbunova, V., and Limborska, S. (2010). Genetic polymorphisms and the efficacy and toxicity of cisplatin-based chemotherapy in ovarian cancer patients. *Pharmacogenomics J.* 10, 54–61. doi: 10.1038/tpj.2009.45

Kim, B.-J., Park, H.-R., Roh, H. J., Jeong, D.-S., Kim, B. S., Park, K.-W., et al. (2010). Chemotherapy-related polyneuropathy may deteriorate quality of life in patients with B-cell lymphoma. *Qual. Life Res.* 19, 1097–1103. doi: 10.1007/s11136-010-9670-0

Kraff, S., Nieuweboer, A. J. M., Mathijssen, R. H. J., Baty, F., de Graan, A.-J., van Schaik, R. H. N., et al. (2015). Pharmacokinetically based dosing of weekly paclitaxel to reduce drug-related neurotoxicity based on a single sample strategy. *Cancer Chemother. Pharmacol.* 75, 975–983. doi: 10.1007/s00280-015-2724-9

Kumamoto, K., Ishibashi, K., Okada, N., Tajima, Y., Kuwabara, K., Kumagai, Y., et al. (2013). Polymorphisms of GSTP1, ERCC2 and TS-3'UTR are associated with the clinical outcome of mFOLFOX6 in colorectal cancer patients. *Oncol. Lett.* 6, 648–654. doi: 10.3892/ol.2013.1467

Landowski, T. H., Megli, C. J., Nullmeyer, K. D., Lynch, R. M., and Dorr, R. T. (2005). Mitochondrial-mediated disregulation of Ca2+ is a critical determinant of Velcade (PS-341/bortezomib) cytotoxicity in myeloma cell lines. *Cancer Res.* 65, 3828–3836. doi: 10.1158/0008-5472.CAN-04-3684

LaPointe, N. E., Morfini, G., Brady, S. T., Feinstein, S. C., Wilson, L., and Jordan, M. A. (2013). Effects of eribulin, vincristine, paclitaxel and ixabepilone on fast axonal transport and kinesin-1 driven microtubule gliding: implications for chemotherapy-induced peripheral neuropathy. *Neurotoxicology* 37, 231–239. doi: 10.1016/j.neuro.2013.05.008

Lavoie Smith, E. M., Li, L., Chiang, C., Thomas, K., Hutchinson, R. J., Wells, E. M., et al. (2015). Patterns and severity of vincristine-induced peripheral neuropathy in children with acute lymphoblastic leukemia. *J. Peripher. Nerv. Syst.* 20, 37–46. doi: 10.1111/jns.12114

Leach, C. R., Bellizzi, K. M., Hurria, A., and Reeve, B. B. (2016). Is it my cancer or am I just getting older?: impact of cancer on age-related health conditions of older cancer survivors. *Cancer* 122, 1946–1953. doi: 10.1002/cncr.29914

Ledeboer, A., Jekich, B. M., Sloane, E. M., Mahoney, J. H., Langer, S. J., Milligan, E. D., et al. (2007). Intrathecal interleukin-10 gene therapy attenuates paclitaxel-induced mechanical allodynia and proinflammatory cytokine expression in dorsal root ganglia in rats. *Brain. Behav. Immun.* 21, 686–698. doi: 10.1016/j.bbi.2006.10.012

Leskelä, S., Jara, C., Leandro-García, L. J., Martínez, A., García-Donas, J., Hernando, S., et al. (2011). Polymorphisms in cytochromes P450 2C8 and 3A5 are associated with paclitaxel neurotoxicity. *Pharmacogenomics J.* 11, 121–129. doi: 10.1038/tpj.2010.13

Li, S., Xue, F., Cheng, Z., Yang, X., Wang, S., Geng, F., et al. (2009). Effect of artesunate on inhibiting proliferation and inducing apoptosis of SP2/0 myeloma cells through affecting NFkappaB p65. *Int. J. Hematol.* 90, 513–521. doi: 10.1007/s12185-009-0409-z

Li, Y., Adamek, P., Zhang, H., Tatsui, C. E., Rhines, L. D., Mrozkova, P., et al. (2015). The cancer chemotherapeutic paclitaxel increases human and rodent sensory neuron responses to TRPV1 by activation of TLR4. *J. Neurosci.* 35, 13487–13500. doi: 10.1523/JNEUROSCI.1956-15.2015

Li, Y., Zhang, H., Zhang, H., Kosturakis, A. K., Jawad, A. B., and Dougherty, P. M. (2014). Toll-like receptor 4 signaling contributes to Paclitaxel-induced peripheral neuropathy. *J. Pain* 15, 712–725. doi: 10.1016/j.jpain.2014.04.001

Liew, E., Thyagu, S., Atenafu, E. G., Alibhai, S. M. H., and Brandwein, J. M. (2013). Quality of life following completion of treatment for adult acute lymphoblastic leukemia with a pediatric-based protocol. *Leuk. Res.* 37, 1632–1635. doi: 10.1016/j.leukres.2013.09.018

Liu, Y.-M., Chen, H.-L., Lee, H.-Y., and Liou, J.-P. (2014). Tubulin inhibitors: a patent review. *Expert Opin. Ther. Pat.* 24, 69–88. doi: 10.1517/13543776.2014.859247

Lolignier, S., Bonnet, C., Gaudioso, C., Noël, J., Ruel, J., Amsalem, M., et al. (2015). The Nav1.9 channel is a key determinant of cold pain sensation and cold allodynia. *Cell Rep.* 11, 1067–1078. doi: 10.1016/j.celrep.2015.04.027

Mateos, M.-V. (2012). How to maintain patients on long-term therapy: understanding the profile and kinetics of adverse events. *Leuk. Res.* 36(Suppl. 1), S35–S43. doi: 10.1016/S0145-2126(12)70007-3

McWhinney, S. R., Goldberg, R. M., and McLeod, H. L. (2009). Platinum neurotoxicity pharmacogenetics. *Mol. Cancer Ther.* 8, 10–16. doi: 10.1158/1535-7163.MCT-08-0840

Minarik, J., Pavlicek, P., Pour, L., Pika, T., Maisnar, V., Spicka, I., et al. (2015). Subcutaneous bortezomib in multiple myeloma patients induces similar therapeutic response rates as intravenous application but it does not reduce the incidence of peripheral neuropathy. *PLoS ONE* 10:e0123866. doi: 10.1371/journal.pone.0123866

Mohty, B., El-Cheikh, J., Yakoub-Agha, I., Moreau, P., Harousseau, J.-L., and Mohty, M. (2010). Peripheral neuropathy and new treatments for multiple myeloma: background and practical recommendations. *Haematologica* 95, 311–319. doi: 10.3324/haematol.2009.012674

Mols, F., Beijers, T., Lemmens, V., van den Hurk, C. J., Vreugdenhil, G., and van de Poll-Franse, L. V. (2013). Chemotherapy-induced neuropathy and its association with quality of life among 2- to 11-year colorectal cancer survivors: results from the population-based PROFILES registry. *J. Clin. Oncol.* 31, 2699–2707. doi: 10.1200/JCO.2013.49.1514

Morawska, M., Grzasko, N., Kostyra, M., Wojciechowicz, J., and Hus, M. (2015). Therapy-related peripheral neuropathy in multiple myeloma patients. *Hematol. Oncol.* 33, 113–119. doi: 10.1002/hon.2149

Moreau, P., Avet-Loiseau, H., Facon, T., Attal, M., Tiab, M., Hulin, C., et al. (2011a). Bortezomib plus dexamethasone versus reduced-dose bortezomib, thalidomide plus dexamethasone as induction treatment before autologous stem cell transplantation in newly diagnosed multiple myeloma. *Blood* 118, 5752–5758;quiz5982. doi: 10.1182/blood-2011-05-355081

Moreau, P., Pylypenko, H., Grosicki, S., Karamanesht, I., Leleu, X., Grishunina, M., et al. (2011b). Subcutaneous versus intravenous administration of bortezomib in patients with relapsed multiple myeloma: a randomised, phase 3, non-inferiority study. *Lancet Oncol.* 12, 431–440. doi: 10.1016/S1470-2045(11)70081-X

Moriyama, B., Henning, S. A., Leung, J., Falade-Nwulia, O., Jarosinski, P., Penzak, S. R., et al. (2012). Adverse interactions between antifungal azoles and vincristine: review and analysis of cases. *Mycoses* 55, 290–297. doi: 10.1111/j.1439-0507.2011.02158.x

Moser, E. C., Noordijk, E. M., Carde, P., Tirelli, U., Baars, J. W., Thomas, J., et al. (2005). Late non-neoplastic events in patients with aggressive non-Hodgkin's lymphoma in four randomized European Organisation for Research and Treatment of Cancer trials. *Clin. Lymphoma Myeloma* 6, 122–130. doi: 10.3816/CLM.2005.n.038

Naumann, R., Mohm, J., Reuner, U., Kroschinsky, F., Rautenstrauss, B., and Ehninger, G. (2001). Early recognition of hereditary motor and sensory neuropathy type 1 can avoid life-threatening vincristine neurotoxicity. *Br. J. Haematol.* 115, 323–325. doi: 10.1046/j.1365-2141.2001.03126.x

Ness, K. K., Jones, K. E., Smith, W. A., Spunt, S. L., Wilson, C. L., Armstrong, G. T., et al. (2013). Chemotherapy-related neuropathic symptoms and functional impairment in adult survivors of extracranial solid tumors of childhood: results from the St. Jude Lifetime Cohort Study. *Arch. Phys. Med. Rehabil.* 94, 1451–1457. doi: 10.1016/j.apmr.2013.03.009

Nishikawa, T., Kawakami, K., Kumamoto, T., Tonooka, S., Abe, A., Hayasaka, K., et al. (2008). Severe neurotoxicities in a case of Charcot-Marie-Tooth disease type 2 caused by vincristine for acute lymphoblastic leukemia. *J. Pediatr. Hematol. Oncol.* 30, 519–521. doi: 10.1097/MPH.0b013e31816624a4

Oerlemans, S., Issa, D. E., van den Broek, E. C., Nijziel, M. R., Coebergh, J. W. W., Huijgens, P. C., et al. (2014). Health-related quality of life and persistent symptoms in relation to (R-)CHOP14, (R-)CHOP21, and other therapies among patients with diffuse large B-cell lymphoma: results of the population-based PHAROS-registry. *Ann. Hematol.* 93, 1705–1715. doi: 10.1007/s00277-014-2099-8

Orejana-García, A. M., Pascual-Huerta, J., and Pérez-Melero, A. (2003). Charcot-Marie-Tooth disease and vincristine. *J. Am. Podiatr. Med. Assoc.* 93, 229–233. doi: 10.7547/87507315-93-3-229

Park, S. B., Lin, C. S. Y., Krishnan, A. V., Goldstein, D., Friedlander, M. L., and Kiernan, M. C. (2011). Long-term neuropathy after oxaliplatin treatment: challenging the dictum of reversibility. *Oncologist* 16, 708–716. doi: 10.1634/theoncologist.2010-0248

Peng, Z., Wang, Q., Gao, J., Ji, Z., Yuan, J., Tian, Y., et al. (2013). Association between GSTP1 Ile105Val polymorphism and oxaliplatin-induced neuropathy: a systematic review and meta-analysis. *Cancer Chemother. Pharmacol.* 72, 305–314. doi: 10.1007/s00280-013-2194-x

Peters, C. M., Jimenez-Andrade, J. M., Jonas, B. M., Sevcik, M. A., Koewler, N. J., Ghilardi, J. R., et al. (2007). Intravenous paclitaxel administration in the rat induces a peripheral sensory neuropathy characterized by macrophage infiltration and injury to sensory neurons and their supporting cells. *Exp. Neurol.* 203, 42–54. doi: 10.1016/j.expneurol.2006.07.022

Pignata, S., De Placido, S., Biamonte, R., Scambia, G., Di Vagno, G., Colucci, G., et al. (2006). Residual neurotoxicity in ovarian cancer patients in clinical remission after first-line chemotherapy with carboplatin and paclitaxel: the Multicenter Italian Trial in Ovarian cancer (MITO-4) retrospective study. *BMC Cancer* 6:5. doi: 10.1186/1471-2407-6-5

Pike, C. T., Birnbaum, H. G., Muehlenbein, C. E., Pohl, G. M., and Natale, R. B. (2012). Healthcare costs and workloss burden of patients with chemotherapy-associated peripheral neuropathy in breast, ovarian, head and neck, and nonsmall cell lung cancer. *Chemother. Res. Pract.* 2012:913848. doi: 10.1155/2012/913848

Plasmati, R., Pastorelli, F., Cavo, M., Petracci, E., Zamagni, E., Tosi, P., et al. (2007). Neuropathy in multiple myeloma treated with thalidomide: a prospective study. *Neurology* 69, 573–581. doi: 10.1212/01.wnl.0000267271.18475.fe

Podratz, J. L., Knight, A. M., Ta, L. E., Staff, N. P., Gass, J. M., Genelin, K., et al. (2011). Cisplatin induced mitochondrial DNA damage in dorsal root ganglion neurons. *Neurobiol. Dis.* 41, 661–668. doi: 10.1016/j.nbd.2010.11.017

Poruchynsky, M. S., Sackett, D. L., Robey, R. W., Ward, Y., Annunziata, C., and Fojo, T. (2008). Proteasome inhibitors increase tubulin polymerization and stabilization in tissue culture cells: a possible mechanism contributing to peripheral neuropathy and cellular toxicity following proteasome inhibition. *Cell Cycle* 7, 940–949. doi: 10.4161/cc.7.7.5625

Postma, T. J., Benard, B. A., Huijgens, P. C., Ossenkoppele, G. J., and Heimans, J. J. (1993). Long-term effects of vincristine on the peripheral nervous system. *J. Neurooncol.* 15, 23–27. doi: 10.1007/BF01050259

Qin, H., Luo, J., Zhu, Y.-P., Xie, H.-L., Yang, W.-Q., and Lei, W.-B. (2012). Combination of taxanes, cisplatin and fluorouracil as induction chemotherapy for locally advanced head and neck cancer: a meta-analysis. *PLoS ONE* 7:e51526. doi: 10.1371/journal.pone.0051526

Quasthoff, S., and Hartung, H. P. (2002). Chemotherapy-induced peripheral neuropathy. *J. Neurol.* 249, 9–17. doi: 10.1007/PL00007853

Ramchandren, S., Leonard, M., Mody, R. J., Donohue, J. E., Moyer, J., Hutchinson, R., et al. (2009). Peripheral neuropathy in survivors of childhood acute lymphoblastic leukemia. *J. Peripher. Nerv. Syst.* 14, 184–189. doi: 10.1111/j.1529-8027.2009.00230.x

Rampen, A. J. J., Jongen, J. L. M., van Heuvel, I., Scheltens-de Boer, M., Sonneveld, P., and van den Bent, M. J. (2013). Bortezomib-induced polyneuropathy. *Neth. J. Med.* 71, 128–133.

Reyes-Gibby, C. C., Morrow, P. K., Buzdar, A., and Shete, S. (2009). Chemotherapy-induced peripheral neuropathy as a predictor of neuropathic pain in breast cancer patients previously treated with paclitaxel. *J. Pain* 10, 1146–1150. doi: 10.1016/j.jpain.2009.04.006

Richardson, P., Hideshima, T., and Anderson, K. (2002). Thalidomide in multiple myeloma. *Biomed. Pharmacother.* 56, 115–128. doi: 10.1016/S0753-3322(02)00168-3

Richardson, P. G., Barlogie, B., Berenson, J., Singhal, S., Jagannath, S., Irwin, D., et al. (2003). A phase 2 study of bortezomib in relapsed, refractory myeloma. *N. Engl. J. Med.* 348, 2609–2617. doi: 10.1056/NEJMoa030288

Richardson, P. G., Laubach, J. P., Schlossman, R. L., Mitsiades, C., and Anderson, K. (2010). Complications of multiple myeloma therapy, part 1: risk reduction and management of peripheral neuropathy and asthenia. *J. Natl. Compr. Cancer Netw.* 8 (Suppl. 1), S4–S12.

Richardson, P. G., Sonneveld, P., Schuster, M. W., Irwin, D., Stadtmauer, E. A., Facon, T., et al. (2005). Bortezomib or high-dose dexamethasone for relapsed multiple myeloma. *N. Engl. J. Med.* 352, 2487–2498. doi: 10.1056/NEJMoa043445

Richardson, P. G., Sonneveld, P., Schuster, M. W., Stadtmauer, E. A., Facon, T., Harousseau, J.-L., et al. (2009). Reversibility of symptomatic peripheral neuropathy with bortezomib in the phase III APEX trial in relapsed multiple myeloma: impact of a dose-modification guideline. *Br. J. Haematol.* 144, 895–903. doi: 10.1111/j.1365-2141.2008.07573.x

Rowinsky, E. K., Chaudhry, V., Cornblath, D. R., and Donehower, R. C. (1993). Neurotoxicity of Taxol. *J. Natl. Cancer Inst. Monogr.* 15, 107–115.

Saloustros, E., Mavroudis, D., and Georgoulias, V. (2008). Paclitaxel and docetaxel in the treatment of breast cancer. *Expert Opin. Pharmacother.* 9, 2603–2616. doi: 10.1517/14656566.9.15.2603

Schneider, B. P., Li, L., Radovich, M., Shen, F., Miller, K. D., Flockhart, D. A., et al. (2015). Genome-wide association studies for taxane-induced peripheral neuropathy in ECOG-5103 and ECOG-1199. *Clin. Cancer Res.* 21, 5082–5091. doi: 10.1158/1078-0432.CCR-15-0586

Schneider, B. P., Zhao, F., Wang, M., Stearns, V., Martino, S., Jones, V., et al. (2012). Neuropathy is not associated with clinical outcomes in patients receiving adjuvant taxane-containing therapy for operable breast cancer. *J. Clin. Oncol.* 30, 3051–3057. doi: 10.1200/JCO.2011.39.8446

Sharawy, N., Rashed, L., and Youakim, M. F. (2015). Evaluation of multi-neuroprotective effects of erythropoietin using cisplatin induced peripheral neurotoxicity model. *Exp. Toxicol. Pathol.* 67, 315–322. doi: 10.1016/j.etp.2015.02.003

Shimozuma, K., Ohashi, Y., Takeuchi, A., Aranishi, T., Morita, S., Kuroi, K., et al. (2012). Taxane-induced peripheral neuropathy and health-related quality of life in postoperative breast cancer patients undergoing adjuvant chemotherapy: N-SAS BC 02, a randomized clinical trial. *Support. Care Cancer* 20, 3355–3364. doi: 10.1007/s00520-012-1492-x

Shinde, S. S., Seisler, D., Soori, G., Atherton, P. J., Pachman, D. R., Lafky, J., et al. (2016). Can pregabalin prevent paclitaxel-associated neuropathy?–An ACCRU pilot trial. *Support. Care Cancer* 24, 547–553. doi: 10.1007/s00520-015-2807-5

Siau, C., and Bennett, G. J. (2006). Dysregulation of cellular calcium homeostasis in chemotherapy-evoked painful peripheral neuropathy. *Anesth. Analg.* 102, 1485–1490. doi: 10.1213/01.ane.0000204318.35194.ed

Sissung, T. M., Baum, C. E., Deeken, J., Price, D. K., Aragon-Ching, J., Steinberg, S. M., et al. (2008). ABCB1 genetic variation influences the toxicity and clinical outcome of patients with androgen-independent prostate cancer treated with docetaxel. *Clin. Cancer Res.* 14, 4543–4549. doi: 10.1158/1078-0432.CCR-07-4230

Sissung, T. M., Mross, K., Steinberg, S. M., Behringer, D., Figg, W. D., Sparreboom, A., et al. (2006). Association of ABCB1 genotypes with paclitaxel-mediated peripheral neuropathy and neutropenia. *Eur. J. Cancer* 42, 2893–2896. doi: 10.1016/j.ejca.2006.06.017

Staff, N. P., Podratz, J. L., Grassner, L., Bader, M., Paz, J., Knight, A. M., et al. (2013). Bortezomib alters microtubule polymerization and axonal transport in rat dorsal root ganglion neurons. *Neurotoxicology* 39, 124–131. doi: 10.1016/j.neuro.2013.09.001

Stefansson, M., and Nygren, P. (2016). Oxaliplatin added to fluoropyrimidine for adjuvant treatment of colorectal cancer is associated with long-term impairment of peripheral nerve sensory function and quality of life. *Acta Oncol.* 55, 1227–1235. doi: 10.1080/0284186X.2016.1197420

Strumberg, D., Brügge, S., Korn, M. W., Koeppen, S., Ranft, J., Scheiber, G., et al. (2002). Evaluation of long-term toxicity in patients after cisplatin-based chemotherapy for non-seminomatous testicular cancer. *Ann. Oncol.* 13, 229–236. doi: 10.1093/annonc/mdf058

Suzuki, R., Rygh, L. J., and Dickenson, A. H. (2004). Bad news from the brain: descending 5-HT pathways that control spinal pain processing. *Trends Pharmacol. Sci.* 25, 613–617. doi: 10.1016/j.tips.2004.10.002

Tacchetti, P., Terragna, C., Galli, M., Zamagni, E., Petrucci, M. T., Pezzi, A., et al. (2014). Bortezomib- and thalidomide-induced peripheral neuropathy in multiple myeloma: clinical and molecular analyses of a phase 3 study. *Am. J. Hematol.* 89, 1085–1091. doi: 10.1002/ajh.23835

Tanabe, Y., Hashimoto, K., Shimizu, C., Hirakawa, A., Harano, K., Yunokawa, M., et al. (2013). Paclitaxel-induced peripheral neuropathy in patients receiving adjuvant chemotherapy for breast cancer. *Int. J. Clin. Oncol.* 18, 132–138. doi: 10.1007/s10147-011-0352-x

Tari, C., Fournier, N., Briand, C., Ducet, G., and Crevat, A. (1986). Action of vinca alkaloides on calcium movements through mitochondrial membrane. *Pharmacol. Res. Commun.* 18, 519–528. doi: 10.1016/0031-6989(86)90147-5

Tariman, J. D., Love, G., McCullagh, E., Sandifer, S., and Imf Nurse Leadership Board (2008). Peripheral neuropathy associated with novel therapies in patients with multiple myeloma: consensus statement of the IMF Nurse Leadership Board. *Clin. J. Oncol. Nurs.* 12, 29–36. doi: 10.1188/08.CJON.S1.29-35

Terrazzino, S., Argyriou, A. A., Cargnin, S., Antonacopoulou, A. G., Briani, C., Bruna, J., et al. (2015). Genetic determinants of chronic oxaliplatin-induced peripheral neurotoxicity: a genome-wide study replication and meta-analysis. *J. Peripher. Nerv. Syst.* 20, 15–23. doi: 10.1111/jns.12110

Thibault, K., Rivals, I., M'Dahoma, S., Dubacq, S., Pezet, S., and Calvino, B. (2013). Structural and molecular alterations of primary afferent fibres in the spinal dorsal horn in vincristine-induced neuropathy in rat. *J. Mol. Neurosci.* 51, 880–892. doi: 10.1007/s12031-013-0095-4

Thornton, L. M., Carson, W. E., Shapiro, C. L., Farrar, W. B., and Andersen, B. L. (2008). Delayed emotional recovery after taxane-based chemotherapy. *Cancer* 113, 638–647. doi: 10.1002/cncr.23589

Tofthagen, C. (2010). Surviving chemotherapy for colon cancer and living with the consequences. *J. Palliat. Med.* 13, 1389–1391. doi: 10.1089/jpm.2010.0124

Tofthagen, C., Donovan, K. A., Morgan, M. A., Shibata, D., and Yeh, Y. (2013). Oxaliplatin-induced peripheral neuropathy's effects on health-related quality of life of colorectal cancer survivors. *Support. Care Cancer* 21, 3307–3313. doi: 10.1007/s00520-013-1905-5

Tomaszewski, A., and Büsselberg, D. (2007). Cisplatin modulates voltage gated channel currents of dorsal root ganglion neurons of rats. *Neurotoxicology* 28, 49–58. doi: 10.1016/j.neuro.2006.07.005

Tran, A., Jullien, V., Alexandre, J., Rey, E., Rabillon, F., Girre, V., et al. (2006). Pharmacokinetics and toxicity of docetaxel: role of CYP3A, MDR1, and GST polymorphisms. *Clin. Pharmacol. Ther.* 79, 570–580. doi: 10.1016/j.clpt.2006.02.003

van Gerven, J. M., Moll, J. W., van den Bent, M. J., Bontenbal, M., van der Burg, M. E., Verweij, J., et al. (1994). Paclitaxel (Taxol) induces cumulative mild neurotoxicity. *Eur. J. Cancer* 30A, 1074–1077. doi: 10.1016/0959-8049(94)90459-6

Vatandoust, S., Joshi, R., Pittman, K. B., Esterman, A., Broadbridge, V., Adams, J., et al. (2014). A descriptive study of persistent oxaliplatin-induced peripheral neuropathy in patients with colorectal cancer. *Support. Care Cancer* 22, 513–518. doi: 10.1007/s00520-013-2004-3

Velasco, R., Petit, J., Clapés, V., Verdú, E., Navarro, X., and Bruna, J. (2010). Neurological monitoring reduces the incidence of bortezomib-induced peripheral neuropathy in multiple myeloma patients. *J. Peripher. Nerv. Syst.* 15, 17–25. doi: 10.1111/j.1529-8027.2010.00248.x

Ventzel, L., Jensen, A. B., Jensen, A. R., Jensen, T. S., and Finnerup, N. B. (2016). Chemotherapy-induced pain and neuropathy: a prospective study in patients treated with adjuvant oxaliplatin or docetaxel. *Pain* 157, 560–568. doi: 10.1097/j.pain.0000000000000404

Verstappen, C. C. P., Koeppen, S., Heimans, J. J., Huijgens, P. C., Scheulen, M. E., Strumberg, D., et al. (2005). Dose-related vincristine-induced peripheral neuropathy with unexpected off-therapy worsening. *Neurology* 64, 1076–1077. doi: 10.1212/01.WNL.0000154642.45474.28

Vincenzi, B., Frezza, A. M., Schiavon, G., Spoto, C., Addeo, R., Catalano, V., et al. (2013). Identification of clinical predictive factors of oxaliplatin-induced

chronic peripheral neuropathy in colorectal cancer patients treated with adjuvant Folfox IV. *Support. Care Cancer* 21, 1313–1319. doi: 10.1007/s00520-012-1667-5
Wang, C.-H., Cherng, W.-J., Yang, N.-I., Hsu, C.-M., Yeh, C.-H., Lan, Y.-J., et al. (2008). Cyclosporine increases ischemia-induced endothelial progenitor cell mobilization through manipulation of the CD26 system. *Am. J. Physiol. Regul. Integr. Comp. Physiol.* 294, R811–R818. doi: 10.1152/ajpregu.00543.2007
Wani, M. C., and Horwitz, S. B. (2014). Nature as a remarkable chemist: a personal story of the discovery and development of Taxol. *Anticancer Drugs* 25, 482–487. doi: 10.1097/CAD.0000000000000063
Watkins, L. R., and Maier, S. F. (2005). Immune regulation of central nervous system functions: from sickness responses to pathological pain. *J. Intern. Med.* 257, 139–155. doi: 10.1111/j.1365-2796.2004.01443.x
Xiao, W. H., and Bennett, G. J. (2012). Effects of mitochondrial poisons on the neuropathic pain produced by the chemotherapeutic agents, paclitaxel and oxaliplatin. *Pain* 153, 704–709. doi: 10.1016/j.pain.2011.12.011
Yamamoto, K., Chiba, N., Chiba, T., Kambe, T., Abe, K., Kawakami, K., et al. (2015). Transient receptor potential ankyrin 1 that is induced in dorsal root ganglion neurons contributes to acute cold hypersensitivity after oxaliplatin administration. *Mol. Pain* 11:69. doi: 10.1186/s12990-015-0072-8
Yang, Y., Zhang, Y.-G., Lin, G.-A., Xie, H.-Q., Pan, H.-T., Huang, B.-Q., et al. (2014). Spinal changes of a newly isolated neuropeptide endomorphin-2 concomitant with vincristine-induced allodynia. *PLoS ONE* 9:e89583. doi: 10.1371/journal.pone.0089583
Yothers, G., O'Connell, M. J., Allegra, C. J., Kuebler, J. P., Colangelo, L. H., Petrelli, N. J., et al. (2011). Oxaliplatin as adjuvant therapy for colon cancer: updated results of NSABP C-07 trial, including survival and subset analyses. *J. Clin. Oncol.* 29, 3768–3774. doi: 10.1200/JCO.2011.36.4539
Zedan, A. H., Hansen, T. F., Fex Svenningsen, A., and Vilholm, O. J. (2014). Oxaliplatin-induced neuropathy in colorectal cancer: many questions with few answers. *Clin. Colorectal Cancer* 13, 73–80. doi: 10.1016/j.clcc.2013.11.004
Zhang, D., Yang, R., Wang, S., and Dong, Z. (2014). Paclitaxel: new uses for an old drug. *Drug Des. Devel. Ther.* 8, 279–284. doi: 10.2147/DDDT.S56801
Zheng, H., Xiao, W. H., and Bennett, G. J. (2012). Mitotoxicity and bortezomib-induced chronic painful peripheral neuropathy. *Exp. Neurol.* 238, 225–234. doi: 10.1016/j.expneurol.2012.08.023

Conflict of Interest Statement: The authors declare that the research was conducted in the absence of any commercial or financial relationships that could be construed as a potential conflict of interest.

The reviewer ES-R and handling Editor declared their shared affiliation, and the handling Editor states that the process nevertheless met the standards of a fair and objective review.

13

Detection of Nausea-Like Response in Rats by Monitoring Facial Expression

Kouichi Yamamoto, Soichi Tatsutani and Takayuki Ishida*

Division of Health Sciences, Department of Medical Science and Technology, Graduate School of Medicine, Osaka University, Osaka, Japan

Patients receiving cancer chemotherapy experience nausea and vomiting. They are not life-threatening symptoms, but their insufficient control reduces the patients' quality of life. To identify methods for the management of nausea and vomiting in preclinical studies, the objective evaluation of these symptoms in laboratory animals is required. Unlike vomiting, nausea is defined as a subjective feeling described as recognition of the need to vomit; thus, determination of the severity of nausea in laboratory animals is considered to be difficult. However, since we observed that rats grimace after the administration of cisplatin, we hypothesized that changes in facial expression can be used as a method to detect nausea. In this study, we monitored the changes in the facial expression of rats after the administration of cisplatin and investigated the effect of anti-emetic drugs on the prevention of cisplatin-induced changes in facial expression. Rats were housed in individual cages with free access to food and tap water, and their facial expressions were continuously recorded by infrared video camera. On the day of the experiment, rats received cisplatin (0, 3, and 6 mg/kg, i.p.) with or without a daily injection of a 5-HT_3 receptor antagonist (granisetron: 0.1 mg/kg, i.p.) or a neurokinin NK_1 receptor antagonist (fosaprepitant: 2 mg/kg, i.p.), and their eye-opening index (the ratio between longitudinal and axial lengths of the eye) in the recorded video image was calculated. Cisplatin significantly and dose-dependently induced a decrease of the eye-opening index 6 h after the cisplatin injection, and the decrease continued for 2 days. The acute phase (day 1), but not the delayed phase (day 2), of the decreased eye-opening index was inhibited by treatment with granisetron; however, fosaprepitant abolished both phases of changes. The time-course of changes in facial expression are similar to clinical evidence of cisplatin-induced nausea in humans. These findings indicate that the monitoring of facial expression has the potential to be useful for the detection of a nausea-like response in laboratory animals.

Edited by:
Raquel Abalo, Universidad Rey Juan Carlos, Spain

Reviewed by:
Gareth J. Sanger, Queen Mary University of London, UK
Linda A. Parker, University of Guelph, Canada
Gema Vera, Universidad Rey Juan Carlos, Spain

***Correspondence:**
Kouichi Yamamoto
kouichi@sahs.med.osaka-u.ac.jp

Keywords: chemotherapy-induced nausea, facial expression, infrared video camera, rats, neurokinin NK_1 receptor antagonist, serotonin 5-HT_3 receptor antagonist

INTRODUCTION

Cisplatin-based cancer chemotherapy often induces a biphasic pattern of nausea and vomiting, which are classified as the acute phase (within 24 h following drug administration) and delayed phase (24 h after drug administration) (Navari, 2015). To reduce these symptoms, serotonin 5-HT_3 receptor antagonists, neurokinin NK_1 receptor antagonists, and corticosteroids are used (Jordan et al., 2015; Natale, 2015; Einhorn et al., 2016; Navari and Aapro, 2016). This regimen proved to be significantly effective, but patients still experience nausea, especially delayed nausea (Molassiotis et al., 2008; Farrell et al., 2013). Nausea is not life-threatening, but its insufficient control is a definite factor reducing the patients' quality of life (Bloechl-Daum et al., 2006; Farrell et al., 2013; Navari, 2015).

To identify methods to manage chemotherapy-induced nausea and vomiting in preclinical studies, an objective and precise method to evaluate nausea and vomiting in laboratory animals is required. Vomiting is defined as the involuntary and forceful expulsion of the stomach contents through the mouth (Quigley et al., 2001); therefore, animal species which possess a vomiting reflex, such as ferrets, dogs, cats, and *Suncus murinus*, are used as laboratory animals for its study, because the vomiting reflex is a readily detectable behavior (Florczyk et al., 1982; Ueno et al., 1987; King, 1990). Unlike vomiting, nausea is defined as an unpleasant feeling in the upper gastrointestinal tract with an involuntary urge to vomit (Quigley et al., 2001); thus, it is difficult to recognize whether laboratory animals feel nausea even with the use of vomiting species. Rats, one of the most common laboratory animals, have been considered unsuitable for the study of nausea and vomiting because they do not show a vomiting reflex (Hatcher, 1924). We previously reported that pica behavior, a behavior seen in rats characterized by eating non-nutritive materials, such as clay (kaolin), has been considered as a model of a nausea-like response or gastrointestinal malaise because it is induced by nauseant stimuli and the amount of kaolin intake is related to the nauseant severity in humans (Yamamoto et al., 2007, 2011, 2014, 2015, 2016). However, previous studies reported that it is difficult to evaluate their nausea-like response by the amount of kaolin intake, because rats subjected to marked stimuli showed decreased feeding and locomotive behaviors due to

A

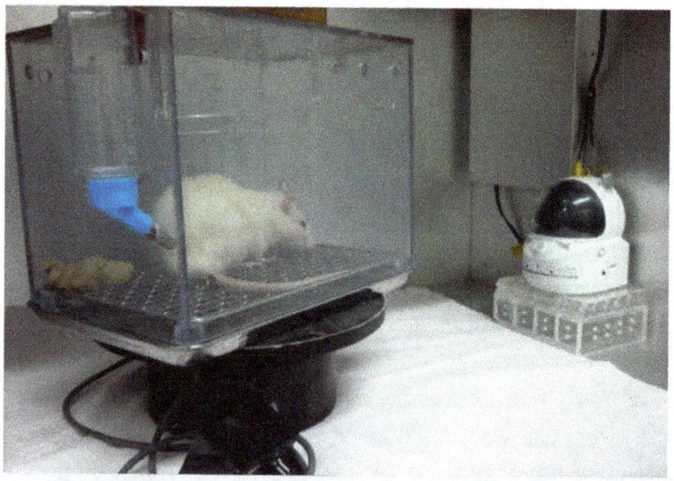

B

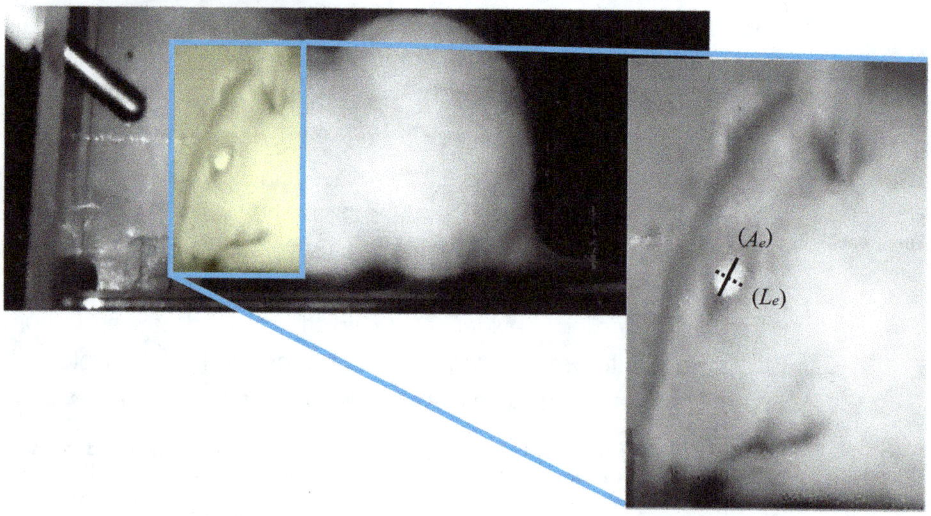

FIGURE 1 | (A) Experimental apparatus for recoding the rat's facial expression. It consists of a home cage, turntable, and infra-red camera. In order to record the facial expression continuously, the home cage was rotated in a clockwise-direction at a rate of 1 degree/sec using a turntable. **(B)** Representative image of a rat in the recorded video and method to calculate the eye-opening index. Images of the left lateral side of each rat's face were captured every 15 min. The longitudinal (L_e: dotted line) and axial (A_e: solid line) lengths of the eye in the captured images were measured, and then the ratio between longitudinal and axial lengths of the eye was calculated.

behavioral suppression (Malik et al., 2006, 2007; Cabezos et al., 2008).

Alternatively, since we observed that rats grimaced after the administration of cisplatin, we hypothesized that changes in facial expression could be used as a method to detect a nausea-like response in rats. In this study, we monitored the changes in the facial expression of rats after the administration of cisplatin and investigated the effect of anti-emetic drugs on the prevention of these cisplatin-induced changes.

MATERIALS AND METHODS

General Procedure

All experiments were approved by the Animal Care Committee of the School of Allied Health Sciences, Faculty of Medicine, Osaka University (26-05-01), and were conducted in accordance with the Animal Experiment Guidelines of Osaka University. Female Wistar/ST rats (8 weeks old, body weight: 180–210 g) were obtained from Japan SLC (Shizuoka, Japan) and housed in individual home cages (25 cm × 20 cm × 20 cm) in a room with a regular light/dark cycle (lights on 0600–1800 h) at a constant temperature (approximately 24°C) and humidity (approximately 50%). One of the risk factors of chemotherapy-induced nausea and vomiting is considered to be a female sex (du Bois et al., 1992). We previously reported that female rats are more susceptible to the induction of sevoflurane-induced pica behavior than male rats (Yamamoto et al., 2016); thus, we used only female rats in a series of experiments. They were allowed free access to tap water and commercially available standard chow (CE-2, CLEA Japan, Inc., Tokyo, Japan). During habituation and the experimental period, the home cage was rotated in a clockwise-direction at a rate of one degree per second using a turntable (S-series, Sigma Planning Corporation, Tokyo, Japan) in order to confirm the facial expression. On the day of the experiment, rats intraperitoneally (i.p.) received cisplatin (3 or 6 mg/kg) at a volume of 6 mL/kg at 1800 h and the entire home cage was continuously recorded on motion video (30 frames per second) by an infrared camera (CS-W70HD, Planex Communications, Inc., Tokyo, Japan), which was placed 30 cm away from home cage surface, for 2 days after the injection of cisplatin (see **Figure 1A**). The doses and injection time of cisplatin selected in this experiment were determined based on our previous published data (Yamamoto et al., 2014). Controls were treated with saline (6 mL/kg body weight, i.p.). At the end of the experiment, all animals were euthanized by the intraperitoneal injection of an overdose of sodium pentobarbital (150 mg/kg). There were six rats in each of the experimental groups.

Measurement of Eye-Opening Index

Frame images in the recorded motion video were analyzed by frame-by-frame playback for 5 min every 15 min, and an image of the left lateral side of each rat's face in the analyzed part

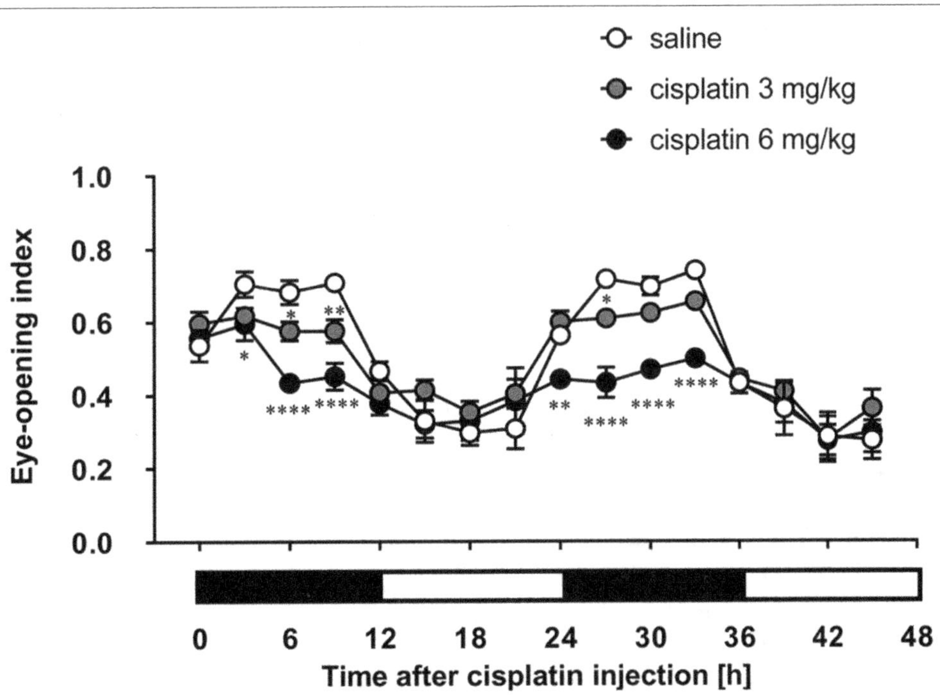

FIGURE 2 | Effects of cisplatin on the eye-opening index in rats. Cisplatin (3 and 6 mg/kg) was intraperitoneally injected and the three-hourly average eye-opening index was measured for 2 days after cisplatin administration. There were six rats in each of the experimental groups. Points and bars represent the mean ± SEM, respectively, of the index. Horizontal black and white bars represent 'lights off' and 'lights on,' respectively. Differences in the results were analyzed using the two-way repeated measure analysis of variance (ANOVA), followed by *post hoc* Bonferroni's test. *$P < 0.05$, **$P < 0.01$, and ****$P < 0.0001$ vs. saline control.

of the video was selected and captured. The longitudinal and axial lengths of the eye (**Figure 1B**) in the captured images were measured by ImageJ analysis software (Version 1.48: developed by Wayne Rasbands, National Institutes of Health, Bethesda, MD, USA), and then the ratio between the longitudinal and axial lengths of the eye (eye-opening index) was calculated, and the three-hourly average of eye-opening index was measured.

Effects of the 5-HT_3 or NK_1 Receptor Antagonist on the Cisplatin-Induced Nausea-Like Response in Rats

Rats were administered granisetron (5-HT_3 receptor antagonist, 0.1 mg/kg, i.p.) or fosaprepitant (NK_1 receptor antagonist, 2 mg/kg, i.p.) 30 min before and 24 h after the administration of cisplatin (3 or 6 mg/kg, i.p.). The doses of granisetron and fosaprepitant selected in this experiment were determined based on our previous published data (Yamamoto et al., 2014). Then, the eye-opening index was obtained using the same method as in previous experiment, and the three-hourly average of eye-opening index was analyzed. Control animals received saline (0.1 ml/100 g body weight, i.p.) as a vehicle.

Cisplatin-Induced Pica Behavior in Rats

To determine the profile of cisplatin-induced pica behavior and anorexia in female rats, we used an automatic kaolin and food intake monitoring system (FDM700SW, Melquest, Toyama, Japan) that we previously developed (Yamamoto et al., 2011). Briefly, this system is an apparatus to determine the amount of kaolin and food intakes in rats automatically consisting of an acrylic home cage (26 cm × 20 cm × 23 cm), two containers (7 cm × 4 cm × 10 cm), and a controller equipped with two load cells (weight sensor). Kaolin and food pellets (CE-2, CLEA Japan, Tokyo, Japan) were provided in their respective containers. Rats were adapted to the experimental environment for 7 days and allowed free access to tap water and both pellets throughout the experimental period. Kaolin and food intakes were monitored hourly to the nearest 0.01 g and the data were stored and analyzed using a laptop PC. Kaolin pellets were prepared according to a previously reported method (Yamamoto et al., 2011). On the day of the experiment, rats received cisplatin (3 or 6 mg/kg, i.p.) with or without granisetron or fosaprepitant, and their three hourly rates of kaolin and food consumption were measured for 2 days after the injection of cisplatin. Controls were treated with saline (i.p.). The protocol of drug administration was identical to those of experiment on measurement of eye-opening index. There were six rats in each of the experimental groups.

Drugs

Cisplatin [*cis*-Diamineplatinum(II) dichloride: Sigma-Aldrich, St. Louis, MO, USA], granisetron hydrochloride (Kytril® inj. Chugai-Roche Diagnostics Japan, Tokyo, Japan), and fosaprepitant dimeglumine (Proemend®; Ono Pharmaceutical,

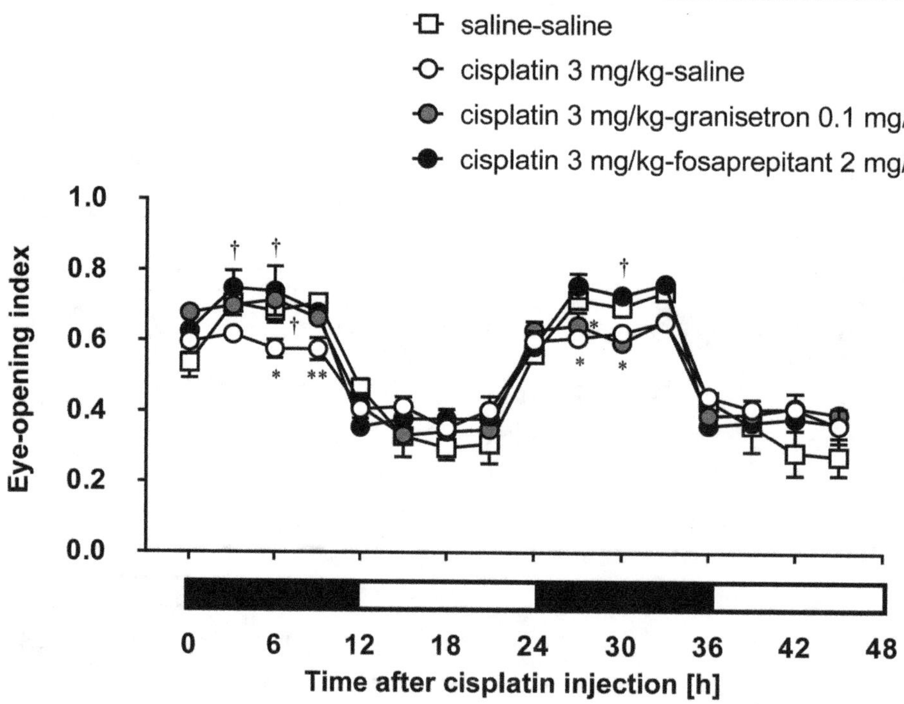

FIGURE 3 | Effects of anti-emetic drugs on the eye-opening index in rats treated with cisplatin (3 mg/kg). There were six rats in each of the experimental groups. Each anti-emetic agent (5-HT_3 antagonist: granisetron 0.1 mg/kg, and NK_1 antagonist: fosaprepitant 2 mg/kg) or saline was intraperitoneally administered 30 min before and 24 h after the administration of cisplatin. Points and bars represent the mean ± SEM, respectively, of the index. Horizontal black and white bars represent 'lights off' and 'lights on,' respectively. Differences in the results were analyzed using the two-way repeated measure ANOVA, followed by *post hoc* Bonferroni's test. *$P < 0.05$ and **$P < 0.01$ vs. saline-saline control. †$P < 0.05$ vs. cisplatin + saline group.

Osaka) were purchased through a pharmaceutical agency (Katayama Chemical Industries, Osaka, Japan) and dissolved in physiological saline. All drugs were prepared immediately before injection. Gum arabic (Sigma-Aldrich Japan, Tokyo, Japan) and kaolin (Sigma-Aldrich Japan) were also purchased through Katayama Chemical Industries. Doses are expressed as the free base.

Statistical Analysis

The data are expressed as the mean value ± SEM. Differences in the results of the eye-opening index were analyzed using the two-way repeated measure analysis of variance (ANOVA), followed by *post hoc* Bonferroni's test. Differences in the results of kaolin and food intake were analyzed using the one-way ANOVA, followed by *post hoc* Dunnett's multiple comparison test. A *P*-value of less than 0.05 was considered significant.

RESULTS

Effects of Cisplatin on Eye-Opening Index in Rats

Although rats move about in their home cage at all hours of the day and night, the rotation of the cage using a turntable allowed us to record each rat's facial expression. As shown in **Figure 2**, there was a prominent circadian variation in the eye-opening index of control rats. The values in the rats' dark-active phase were significantly higher than those in the light-inactive phase, and a similar tendency was observed on the following day. Cisplatin at doses of 3 and 6 mg/kg significantly and dose-dependently decreased the eye-opening index. These decreases were observed within 6 and 3 h after cisplatin administration, respectively. Although the decrease continued throughout the entire observation period, the values in rats treated with cisplatin at a dose of 6 mg/kg were significantly lower than those in rats treated with cisplatin at a dose of 3 mg/kg.

Effects of 5-HT$_3$ and NK$_1$ Receptor Antagonists on Cisplatin-Induced Decrease of Eye-Opening Index in Rats

Granisetron and fosaprepitant alone did not affect the eye-opening index throughout the entire period. The decrease of the eye-opening index induced within 24 h after the injection of cisplatin at a dose of 3 mg/kg was effectively inhibited by pretreatment with granisetron, but the decrease on the second day of cisplatin administration was not completely recovered by the daily administration of granisetron (**Figure 3**). On the other hand, pretreatment with fosaprepitant completely abolished both phases of cisplatin (3 mg/kg)-induced decrease of the eye-opening index.

The daily administration of granisetron did not improve the decrease of the eye-opening index induced by cisplatin at a dose of 6 mg/kg throughout the entire period (**Figure 4**). However, the administration of fosaprepitant significantly inhibited the cisplatin (6 mg/kg)-induced decrease of the eye-opening index.

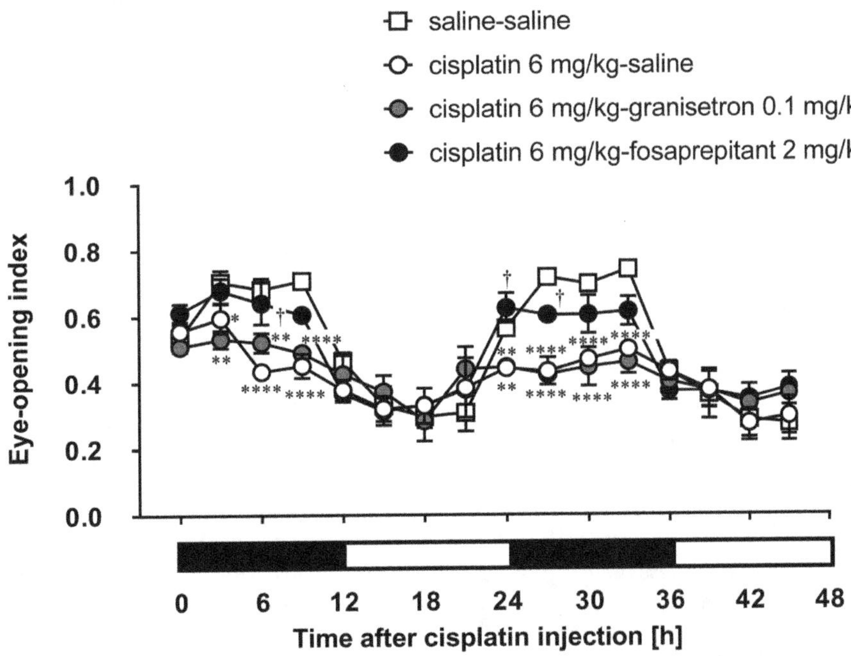

FIGURE 4 | Effects of anti-emetic drugs on the eye-opening index in rats treated with cisplatin (6 mg/kg). There were six rats in each of the experimental groups. Each anti-emetic agent (5-HT$_3$ antagonist: granisetron 0.1 mg/kg, and NK$_1$ antagonist: fosaprepitant 2 mg/kg) or saline was intraperitoneally administered 30 min before and 24 h after the administration of cisplatin. Points and bars represent the mean ± SEM, respectively, of the index. Horizontal black and white bars represent 'lights off' and 'lights on,' respectively. Differences in the results were analyzed using the two-way repeated measure ANOVA, followed by *post hoc* Bonferroni's test. *$P < 0.05$, **$P < 0.01$, and ****$P < 0.0001$ vs. saline control. †$P < 0.05$ vs. cisplatin + saline group.

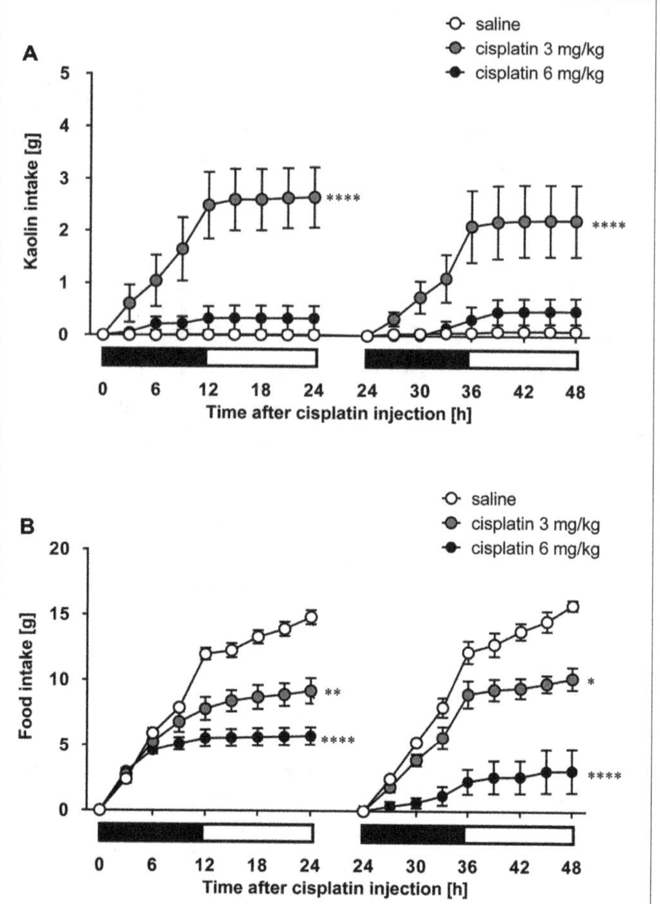

FIGURE 5 | Effect of cisplatin on (A) kaolin and (B) food intakes in rats. Cisplatin (3 and 6 mg/kg) was intraperitoneally injected and three-hourly cumulative kaolin and food intakes were measured for 2 days after cisplatin administration. There were six rats in each of the experimental groups. Points and bars represent the mean ± SEM, respectively, of each intake. Both intake values are set to zero at 24 h. Horizontal black and white bars represent 'lights off' and 'lights on,' respectively. Differences in the results were analyzed using the one-way ANOVA, followed by *post hoc* Dunnett's test. $^{*}P < 0.05$, $^{**}P < 0.01$, and $^{****}P < 0.0001$ vs. saline control.

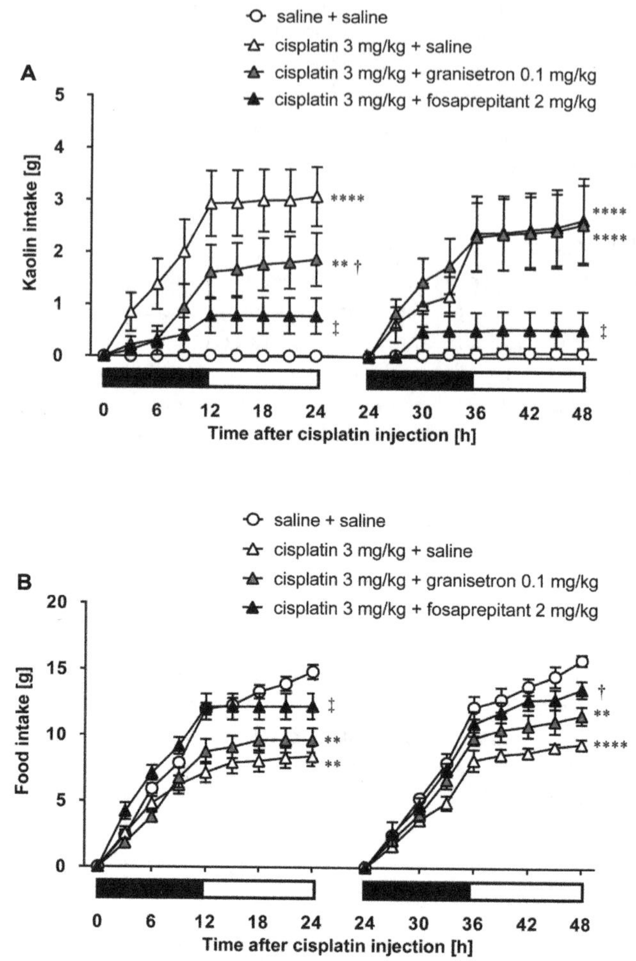

FIGURE 6 | Effects of granisetron or fosaprepitant on cisplatin (3 mg/kg)-induced (A) pica and **(B)** anorexia in rats. Granisetron (0.1 mg/kg), fosaprepitant (2 mg/kg), and saline were intraperitoneally administered 30 min before and 24 h after cisplatin administration and three-hourly cumulative kaolin and food intakes were measured for 2 days after cisplatin administration. There were six rats in each of the experimental groups. Points and bars represent the mean ± SEM, respectively, of each intake. Both intake values are set to zero at 24 h. Horizontal black and white bars represent 'lights off' and 'lights on,' respectively. Differences in the results were analyzed using the one-way ANOVA, followed by *post hoc* Dunnett's test. $^{**}P < 0.01$ and $^{****}P < 0.0001$ vs. cisplatin + saline group. $^{\dagger}P < 0.05$ and $^{\ddagger}P < 0.01$ vs. cisplatin + saline group.

Effects of Cisplatin on Pica Behavior in Rats

As shown in **Figures 5A,B**, cisplatin at a dose of 3 mg/kg induced pica behavior and anorexia, and these behaviors were continued for 2 days. These behaviors were observed within 3 and 12 h after administration, respectively. On the other hand, cisplatin at a dose of 6 mg/kg did not induce pica behavior because all rats ate a small amount of food (less than 7 g) during the observation period due to severe anorexia. Granisetron and fosaprepitant alone did not affect kaolin or food intake. The pica behavior elicited within 24 h after cisplatin (3 mg/kg) administration was effectively inhibited by pretreatment with granisetron, but the daily administration of granisetron did not inhibit pica induced beyond 24 h after cisplatin administration (**Figure 6A**) or anorexia throughout the entire observation period (**Figure 6B**). However, pretreatment with fosaprepitant abolished both phases of pica and anorexia (**Figures 6A,B**). Neither anti-emetic drug affected kaolin intake in rats treated with cisplatin at a dose of 6 mg/kg; however, pretreatment with fosaprepitant, but not granisetron, significantly improved cisplatin-induced anorexia (**Figures 7A,B**), although all rats administered cisplatin at a dose of 6 mg/kg showed severe anorexia.

DISCUSSION

Quantifying nausea in humans generally involves using a 100-mm visual analog scale (VAS), which is common in pain evaluation (Hendey et al., 2005). However, since this method is based on subjective evaluation (Wewers and Lowe, 1990), it is impossible to recognize and evaluate whether animals feel nausea with this method. Previous studies reported that salivation, conditioned taste aversion, gaping, secretion of vasopressin, and gastric stasis are closely associated with the development of nausea (Andrews and Horn, 2006; Cabezos et al., 2008; Parker, 2014; Scallan and Simon, 2016), but it is difficult to accurately measure these parameters in laboratory animals under physiological conditions. We previously suggested that pica behavior in rats can be used as a method to assess gastrointestinal malaise including nausea (Yamamoto et al., 2014, 2015, 2016). The amount of kaolin intake in rats is proportional to the emetogenicity in humans (Yamamoto et al., 2007). We also found that there are sex differences in cisplatin-induced pica in rats because cisplatin at a dose of 3 mg/kg significantly induced pica in female but not male rats (Yamamoto et al., 2014). However, we often could not evaluate their nausea by the amount of kaolin intake because rats that received severe emetic stimuli showed decrease of feeding and locomotive behavior due to behavioral suppression. We actually found that no rats administered cisplatin at a dose of 6 mg/kg ate more than 7 g of standard chow and 1 g of kaolin. Moreover, the anorexia induced by cisplatin at a dose of 6 mg/kg was resistant to premedication with anti-emetic drugs. Similar results were also observed by Malik et al. (2006, 2007) and Cabezos et al. (2008). Pain is also defined as an unpleasant sensory and emotional experience associated with potential tissue damage (Ripamonti, 2012). Since we can measure its severity from a patients' subjective report, it is also considered that the accurate evaluation of pain in animals remains impossible. Previous reports demonstrated that spontaneous pain in animals such as rats, mice, horses, and rabbits could be evaluated using the changes of facial expressions, and that patients with severe nausea change their facial expression to signify distress (Langford et al., 2010; Sotocinal et al., 2011; Hampshire and Robertson, 2015; Dalla Costa et al., 2016). We observed that rats made grimaces after the administration of cisplatin; therefore, we hypothesized that changes in facial expression can be used as a method to evaluate the nausea-like response in rats.

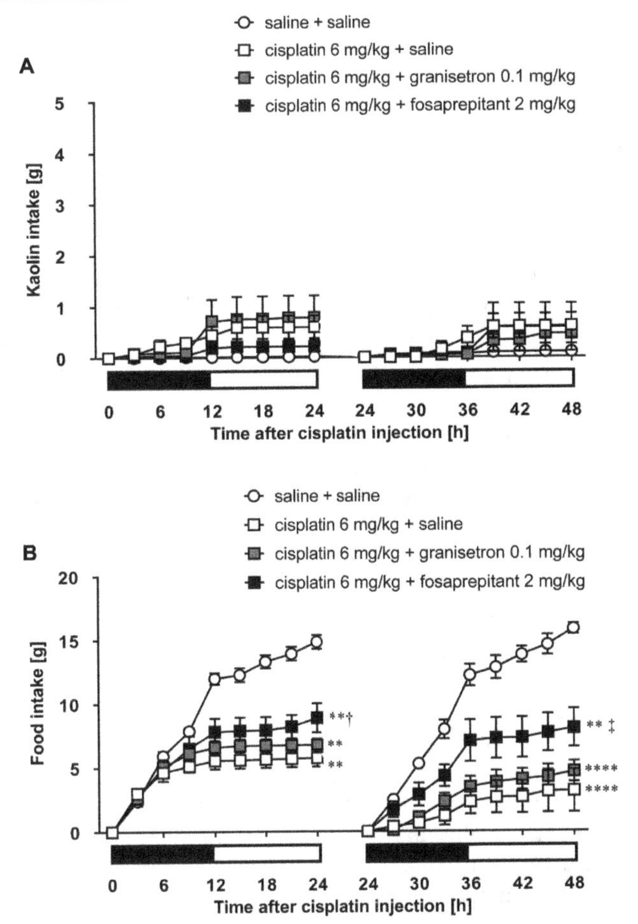

FIGURE 7 | Effects of granisetron or fosaprepitant on cisplatin (6 mg/kg)-induced (A) pica and **(B)** anorexia in rats. Granisetron (0.1 mg/kg), fosaprepitant (2 mg/kg), and saline were intraperitoneally administered 30 min before and 24 h after cisplatin administration and three-hourly cumulative kaolin and food intakes were measured for 2 days after cisplatin administration. There were six rats in each of the experimental groups. Points and bars represent the mean ± SEM, respectively, of each intake. Both intake values are set to zero at 24 h. Horizontal black and white bars represent 'lights off' and 'lights on,' respectively. Differences in the results were analyzed using the one-way ANOVA, followed by *post hoc* Dunnett's test. $^{**}P < 0.01$ and $^{****}P < 0.0001$ vs. cisplatin + saline group. $^{\dagger}P < 0.05$ and $^{\ddagger}P < 0.01$ vs. cisplatin + saline group.

Clinically, cisplatin-induced acute nausea occurs within 2 h and peaks at about 5–6 h after drug administration (Navari and Aapro, 2016). Delayed nausea begins more than 24 h after drug administration, and the intensity of this delayed nausea peaks at around 48 h and persists for about a week (Navari and Aapro, 2016). In this study, we observed that the administration of both doses of cisplatin induced a significant decrease of the eye-opening index in rats. The changes in the facial expression occurred 3 h after administration, and they were observed on the following day. The time required to induce these changes is similar to the latency of cisplatin-induced nausea in humans. Furthermore, we observed that rats pretreated with anti-emetic drugs did not show these changes and pica behavior induced by the lower dose of cisplatin. On the other hand, although we could not evaluate the effect of the higher dose of cisplatin based on pica behavior due to suppression of their behavior; we confirmed that rats treated with cisplatin at a dose of 6 mg/kg exhibited a decrease of the eye-opening index, and the decrease was significantly greater than that in rats administered cisplatin at a dose of 3 mg/kg. The therapeutic effects of anti-emetic drugs on the acute and delayed phases of the cisplatin-induced decrease of the eye-opening index in rats that received an even higher dose of cisplatin were maintained in our study. Based on these results, it is possible that the changes in the eye-opening index are also useful for assessing the nausea-like response in laboratory animals.

In this study, we found that single-treatment with fosaprepitant significantly inhibited the cisplatin-induced decrease of the eye-opening index in rats at both doses. We previously reported that substance P is predominantly involved in cisplatin-induced pica in rats, and an NK_1 receptor antagonist is considered to be the most effective treatment for a chemotherapy-induced nausea-like response in rats (Yamamoto et al., 2014); however, we recognize that NK_1 receptor antagonists are clinically used in combination with other anti-emetic drugs such as $5\text{-}HT_3$ receptor antagonists and/or corticosteroids. It will be necessary to determine the responsible etiology and establish effective treatment for the nausea-like response in laboratory animals other than rats by this method.

The administration of cisplatin is known to induce peripheral neuropathic pain (Jaggi and Singh, 2012). Since Sotocinal et al. (2011) reported that rats suffering spontaneous pain had a tendency to close their eyes, it is considered to be difficult to distinguish accurately between a nausea-like response and neuropathic pain. Seto et al. (2016) reported that rats treated with cisplatin at a dose of 4 mg/kg showed mechanical allodynia on day 6 after the administration. Joseph and Levine (2009) reported that cisplatin-induced hyperalgesia had a latency to onset of about 2 days, and it was maximal by 3–4 days. From these findings, since the results of this study are not considered to be due to the early development of neuropathy, which would probably require more time to occur, they may indicate a method for the detection of the nausea-like response in rats. We previously reported that copper sulfate, lithium chloride, and teriparatide (parathyroid hormone analog) transiently increased only kaolin consumption without affecting food consumption in rats (Yamamoto et al., 2004, 2015). Takeda et al. (1986) reported that rotation stimulation induced pica behavior in rats. Further experiments will be needed to determine the change in the eye-opening index induced by these emetogenic stimuli, that are considered to have a short latency and short-term effect, in order to distinguish between a nausea-like response and neuropathic pain.

An advantage of our developed method is that we can collect data related to a series of continuous behaviors of rats under physiological conditions because we use an infrared camera in order to record the facial expression. Furthermore, this method can be applied to other animal species such as mice, ferrets, and *Suncus murinus* as well as rats. A previous study demonstrated that automatic detection of vomiting in *Suncus murinus* (house musk shrew) was possible by the detection of contour deformation (Huang et al., 2011). Thus, it may be possible to detect nausea and vomiting simultaneously by combining these systems.

In summary, the results suggest that the changes in the facial expression have the potential to be useful for the detection of a nausea-like response in laboratory animals.

ETHICS STATEMENT

All experiments were approved by the Animal Care Committee of the School of Allied Health Sciences, Faculty of Medicine, Osaka University (26-05-01), and were conducted in accordance with the Animal Experiment Guidelines of Osaka University.

AUTHOR CONTRIBUTIONS

KY, ST, and TI designed the experiments. KY and ST performed the experiments and data analysis.

ACKNOWLEDGMENT

This study was supported by JSPS KAKENHI Grant Number JP26670268.

REFERENCES

Andrews, P. L., and Horn, C. C. (2006). Signals for nausea and emesis: implications for models of upper gastrointestinal diseases. *Auton. Neurosci.* 125, 100–115. doi: 10.1016/j.autneu.2006.01.008

Bloechl-Daum, B., Deuson, R. R., Mavros, P., Hansen, M., and Herrstedt, J. (2006). Delayed nausea and vomiting continue to reduce patients' quality of life after highly and moderately emetogenic chemotherapy despite antiemetic treatment. *J. Clin. Oncol.* 24, 4472–4478. doi: 10.1200/JCO.2006.05.6382

Cabezos, P. A., Vera, G., Castillo, M., Fernández-Pujol, R., Martín, M. I., and Abalo, R. (2008). Radiological study of gastrointestinal motor activity after acute cisplatin in the rat. Temporal relationship with pica. *Auton. Neurosci.* 141, 54–65. doi: 10.1016/j.autneu.2008.05.004

Dalla Costa, E., Stucke, D., Dai, F., Minero, M., Leach, M. C., and Lebelt, D. (2016). Using the horse grimace scale (HGS) to assess pain associated with acute laminitis in horses (Equus caballus). *Animals (Basel)* 6:E47. doi: 10.3390/ani6080047

du Bois, A., Meerpohl, H. G., Vach, W., Kommoss, F. G., Fenzl, E., and Pfleiderer, A. (1992). Course, patterns, and risk-factors for chemotherapy-induced emesis in cisplatin-pretreated patients: a study with ondansetron. *Eur. J. Cancer* 28, 450–457. doi: 10.1016/S0959-8049(05)80075-9

Einhorn, L. H., Rapoport, B., Navari, R. M., Herrstedt, J., and Brames, M. J. (2016). 2016 updated MASCC/ESMO consensus recommendations: prevention of nausea and vomiting following multiple-day chemotherapy, high-dose chemotherapy, and breakthrough nausea and vomiting. *Support Care Cancer* 25, 303–308. doi: 10.1007/s00520-016-3449-y

Farrell, C., Brearley, S. G., Pilling, M., and Molassiotis, A. (2013). The impact of chemotherapy-related nausea on patients' nutritional status, psychological distress and quality of life. *Support Care Cancer* 21, 59–66. doi: 10.1007/s00520-012-1493-9

Florczyk, A. P., Schurig, J. E., and Bradner, W. T. (1982). Cisplatin-induced emesis in the Ferret: a new animal model. *Cancer Treat. Rep.* 66, 187–189.

Hampshire, V., and Robertson, S. (2015). Using the facial grimace scale to evaluate rabbit wellness in post-procedural monitoring. *Lab. Anim. (N.Y.).* 44, 259–260. doi: 10.1038/laban.806

Hatcher, R. A. (1924). Mechanism of vomiting. *Physiol. Rev.* 4, 479–504.

Hendey, G. W., Donner, N. F., and Fuller, K. (2005). Clinically significant changes in nausea as measured on a visual analog scale. *Ann. Emerg. Med.* 45, 77–81. doi: 10.1016/j.annemergmed.2004.07.446

Huang, D., Meyers, K., Henry, S., De la Torre, F., and Horn, C. C. (2011). Computerized detection and analysis of cancer chemotherapy-induced emesis in a small animal model, musk shrew. *J. Neurosci. Methods* 197, 249–258. doi: 10.1016/j.jneumeth.2011.02.032

Jaggi, A. S., and Singh, N. (2012). Mechanisms in cancer-chemotherapeutic drugs-induced peripheral neuropathy. *Toxicology* 291, 1–9. doi: 10.1016/j.tox.2011.10.019

Jordan, K., Jahn, F., and Aapro, M. (2015). Recent developments in the prevention of chemotherapy-induced nausea and vomiting (CINV): a comprehensive review. *Ann. Oncol.* 26, 1081–1090. doi: 10.1093/annonc/mdv138

Joseph, E. K., and Levine, J. D. (2009). Comparison of oxaliplatin- and cisplatin-induced painful peripheral neuropathy in the rat. *J. Pain* 10, 534–541. doi: 10.1016/j.jpain.2008.12.003

King, G. L. (1990). Animal models in the study of vomiting. *Can. J. Physiol. Pharmacol.* 68, 260–268. doi: 10.1139/y90-040

Langford, D. J., Bailey, A. L., Chanda, M. L., Clarke, S. E., Drummond, T. E., Echols, S., et al. (2010). Coding of facial expressions of pain in the laboratory mouse. *Nat. Methods* 7, 447–479. doi: 10.1038/nmeth.1455

Malik, N. M., Liu, Y. L., Cole, N., Sanger, G. J., and Andrews, P. L. (2007). Differential effects of dexamethasone, ondansetron and a tachykinin NK1 receptor antagonist (GR205171) on cisplatin-induced changes in behaviour, food intake, pica and gastric function in rats. *Eur. J. Pharmacol.* 555, 164–173. doi: 10.1016/j.ejphar.2006.10.043

Malik, N. M., Moore, G. B., Smith, G., Liu, Y. L., Sanger, G. J., and Andrews, P. L. (2006). Behavioural and hypothalamic molecular effects of the anti-cancer agent cisplatin in the rat: a model of chemotherapy-related malaise? *Pharmacol. Biochem. Behav.* 83, 9–20. doi: 10.1016/j.pbb.2005.11.017

Molassiotis, A., Saunders, M. P., Valle, J., Wilson, G., Lorigan, P., Wardley, A., et al. (2008). A prospective observational study of chemotherapy-related nausea and vomiting in routine practice in a UK cancer centre. *Support Care Cancer* 16, 201–208. doi: 10.1007/s00520-007-0343-7

Natale, J. J. (2015). Reviewing current and emerging antiemetics for chemotherapy-induced nausea and vomiting prophylaxis. *Hosp. Pract.* 43, 226–234. doi: 10.1080/21548331.2015.1077095

Navari, R. M. (2015). Treatment of breakthrough and refractory chemotherapy-induced nausea and vomiting. *BioMed. Res. Int.* 2015:595894. doi: 10.1155/2015/595894

Navari, R. M., and Aapro, M. (2016). Antiemetic prophylaxis for chemotherapy-induced nausea and vomiting. *N. Engl. J. Med.* 374, 1356–1367. doi: 10.1056/NEJMra1515442

Parker, L. A. (2014). Conditioned flavor avoidance, and conditioned gaping: rat models of conditioned nausea. *Eur. J. Pharmacol.* 722, 122–133. doi: 10.1016/j.ejphar.2013.09.070

Quigley, E. M., Hasler, W. L., and Parkman, H. P. (2001). AGA technical review on nausea and vomiting. *Gastroenterology* 120, 263–286. doi: 10.1053/gast.2001.20516

Ripamonti, C. I. (2012). Pain management. *Ann. Oncol.* 23(Suppl. 10), x294–x301. doi: 10.1093/annonc/mds360

Scallan, E. M., and Simon, B. T. (2016). The effects of acupuncture point Pericardium 6 on hydromorphone-induced nausea and vomiting in healthy dogs. *Vet. Anaesth. Analg.* 43, 495–501. doi: 10.1111/vaa.12347

Seto, Y., Okazaki, F., Horikawa, K., Zhang, J., Sasaki, H., and To, H. (2016). Influence of dosing times on cisplatin-induced peripheral neuropathy in rats. *BMC Cancer* 16:756. doi: 10.1186/s12885-016-2777-0

Sotocinal, S. G., Sorge, R. E., Zaloum, A., Tuttle, A. H., Martin, L. J., Wieskopf, J. S., et al. (2011). The Rat grimace scale: a partially automated method for quantifying pain in the laboratory rat via facial expressions. *Mol. Pain* 7:55. doi: 10.1186/1744-8069-7-55

Takeda, N., Morita, M., Kubo, T., Yamatodani, A., Watanabe, T., Wada, H., et al. (1986). Histaminergic mechanism of motion sickness. Neurochemical and neuropharmacological studies in rats. *Acta Otolaryngol.* 101, 416–421.

Ueno, S., Matsuki, N., and Saito, H. (1987). *Suncus murinus*: a new experimental model in emesis research. *Life Sci.* 41, 513–518. doi: 10.1016/0024-3205(87)90229-3

Wewers, M. E., and Lowe, N. K. (1990). A critical review of visual analogue scales in the measurement of clinical phenomena. *Res. Nurs. Health* 13, 227–236. doi: 10.1002/nur.4770130405

Yamamoto, K., Asano, K., Matsukawa, N., Imaizumi, M., and Yamatodani, A. (2011). Time-course analysis of pica in rats using an automatic feeding monitoring system. *J. Pharmacol. Toxicol. Methods.* 63, 30–34. doi: 10.1016/j.vascn.2010.04.011

Yamamoto, K., Asano, K., Tasaka, A., Ogura, Y., Kim, S., Ito, Y., et al. (2014). Involvement of substance P in the development of cisplatin-induced acute and delayed pica in rats. *Br. J. Pharmacol.* 171, 2888–2899. doi: 10.1111/bph.12629

Yamamoto, K., Kato, N., Isogai, Y., Kuroda, T., Ishida, T., and Yamatodani, A. (2015). Induction and antagonism of pica induced by teriparatide in rats. *Eur. J. Pharmacol.* 764, 457–462. doi: 10.1016/j.ejphar.2015.07.039

Yamamoto, K., Nakai, M., Nohara, K., and Yamatodani, A. (2007). The anti-cancer drug-induced pica in rats is related to their clinical emetogenic potential. *Eur. J. Pharmacol.* 554, 34–39. doi: 10.1016/j.ejphar.2006.09.058

Yamamoto, K., Ngan, M. P., Takeda, N., Yamatodani, A., and Rudd, J. A. (2004). Differential activity of drugs to induce emesis and pica behavior in *Suncus murinus* (house musk shrew) and rats. *Physiol. Behav.* 83, 151–156. doi: 10.1016/S0031-9384(04)00332-4

Yamamoto, K., Yamamoto, E., Sugimoto, T., Sakagami, T., and Yamatodani, A. (2016). Sevoflurane-induced pica in female rats. *J. Pharmacol. Sci.* 131, 68–71. doi: 10.1016/j.jphs.2016.03.015

Conflict of Interest Statement: The authors declare that the research was conducted in the absence of any commercial or financial relationships that could be construed as a potential conflict of interest.

14

Involvement of Cannabinoid Signaling in Vincristine-Induced Gastrointestinal Dysmotility in the Rat

Gema Vera[1,2,3,4]*, Ana E. López-Pérez*[4,5]*, José A. Uranga*[3,4,6]*, Rocío Girón*[1,2,3,4]*, Mª Isabel Martín-Fontelles*[1,2,3,4] *and Raquel Abalo*[1,2,3,4*]

[1] Área de Farmacología y Nutrición, Departamento de Ciencias Básicas de la Salud, Universidad Rey Juan Carlos, Alcorcón, Spain, [2] Unidad Asociada I+D+i del Instituto de Química Médica, Consejo Superior de Investigaciones Científicas, Madrid, Spain, [3] Unidad Asociada I+D+i del Instituto de Investigación en Ciencias de la Alimentación, Consejo Superior de Investigaciones Científicas, Madrid, Spain, [4] Grupo de Excelencia Investigadora URJC-Banco de Santander-Grupo Multidisciplinar de Investigación y Tratamiento del Dolor (i+DOL), Alcorcón, Spain, [5] Unidad del Dolor, Servicio de Anestesia, Hospital General Universitario Gregorio Marañón, Madrid, Spain, [6] Área de Histología Humana y Anatomía Patológica, Departamento de Ciencias Básicas de la Salud, Universidad Rey Juan Carlos, Alcorcón, Spain

Edited by:
David A. Gewirtz, Virginia Commonwealth University, USA

Reviewed by:
Ricky Yuet-Kin Leung, University of Cincinnati, USA
Dev Prasad, Fresenius Kabi, USA

****Correspondence:***
Raquel Abalo
raquel.abalo@urjc.es

Background: In different models of paralytic ileus, cannabinoid receptors are overexpressed and endogenous cannabinoids are massively released, contributing to gastrointestinal dysmotility. The antitumoral drug vincristine depresses gastrointestinal motility and a similar mechanism could participate in this effect. Therefore, our aim was to determine, using CB_1 and CB_2 antagonists, whether an increased endocannabinoid tone is involved in vincristine-induced gastrointestinal ileus.

Methods: First, we confirmed the effects of vincristine on the gut mucosa, by conventional histological techniques, and characterized its effects on motility, by radiographic means. Conscious male Wistar rats received an intraperitoneal injection of vincristine (0.1–0.5 mg/kg), and barium sulfate (2.5 ml; 2 g/ml) was intragastrically administered 0, 24, or 48 h later. Serial X-rays were obtained at different time-points (0–8 h) after contrast. X-rays were used to build motility curves for each gastrointestinal region and determine the size of stomach and caecum. Tissue samples were taken for histology 48 h after saline or vincristine (0.5 mg/kg). Second, AM251 (a CB_1 receptor antagonist) and AM630 (a CB_2 receptor antagonist) were used to determine if CB_1 and/or CB_2 receptors are involved in vincristine-induced gastrointestinal dysmotility.

Key results: Vincristine induced damage to the mucosa of ileum and colon and reduced gastrointestinal motor function at 0.5 mg/kg. The effect on motor function was particularly evident when the study started 24 h after administration. AM251, but not AM630, significantly prevented vincristine effect, particularly in the small intestine, when administered thrice. AM251 alone did not significantly alter gastrointestinal motility.

Conclusions: The fact that AM251, but not AM630, is capable of reducing the effect of vincristine suggests that, like in other experimental models of paralytic ileus, an increased cannabinoid tone develops and is at least partially responsible for the alterations induced by the antitumoral drug on gastrointestinal motor function. Thus, CB_1 antagonists might be useful to prevent/treat ileus induced by vincristine.

Keywords: chemotherapy-induced adverse effects, cannabinoid, CB_1 receptor, gastric emptying, radiology, rat, vincristine, ileus

INTRODUCTION

Vincristine is a vinca alkaloid widely used in the treatment of hematological malignancies and solid tumors since the 1960's (Johnson et al., 1960; Bohannon et al., 1963). It is a cell cycle specific agent which blocks mitosis with metaphase arrest through disruption of the mitotic apparatus and it may affect several body systems (Rosenthal and Kaufman, 1974). The main side effect of vincristine is a dose dependent and cumulative peripheral neuropathy. Paresthesias, loss of tendon reflexes, and progressive weakness are the most common clinical features, although autonomic dysfunctions, including gastrointestinal disturbances, might occur (Rosenthal and Kaufman, 1974; Harris and Jackson, 1977; Chae et al., 1998; Wang et al., 2000). Indeed, gastrointestinal complications may be present in up to 30–40% of patients receiving vincristine and the earliest symptoms may include colicky abdominal pain, constipation, and adynamic or paralytic ileus as the major manifestations. Damage to the myenteric plexus by vinca alkaloids could be implicated in intestinal hypomotility (Smith, 1967; Kaneko et al., 2001; Peixoto Júnior et al., 2009). Since constipation is the most widely recognized manifestation, colonic motility has received the most attention. But patients treated with vincristine can also develop symptoms indicating dysmotility of the upper gastrointestinal tract, including anorexia, and nausea or even extreme symptoms such as paralytic ileus. In fact, paralytic ileus occurs in 3–12% of patients, and may be fatal in up to 30% of them (Toghill and Burke, 1970). However, the impact and mechanisms of vincristine on gastrointestinal motility have not been deeply studied in humans or animals.

The endocannabinoid system in the gastrointestinal tract has attracted much attention because both its activation and inhibition could be therapeutically useful depending on the circumstances (Abalo et al., 2012; Abalo and Martín-Fontelles, 2017; Salaga et al., 2017; Vera et al., 2017). Evidence is emerging that exogenous and endogenous cannabinoids have an important role in gastrointestinal physiopathology, such as gastrointestinal inflammation (Izzo and Camilleri, 2009). But cannabinoids mediate also other functions in the gut, such as gastroprotection and gastric secretion, gastrointestinal motility, ion transport, visceral sensation, and cell proliferation (Izzo and Sharkey, 2010). In this sense, plant-derived, endogenous, and synthetic cannabinoid receptor agonists reduced gastric emptying, upper gastrointestinal transit and colonic propulsion in rodents (Aviello et al., 2008; Izzo and Camilleri, 2009; Abalo et al., 2012; Vera et al., 2017), whereas cannabinoid receptor antagonists may increase gastrointestinal motility in experimental animals (Izzo et al., 1999) and cause diarrhea in humans (Waterlow and Chrisp, 2008).

There are functional, biochemical, and immunohistochemical evidences that alterations in the enteric endocannabinoid system contribute to causing paralytic ileus in animal models, and different strategies aimed at normalizing endocannabinoid levels were useful in these conditions. Actually, the inactivation of CB_1 (Mascolo et al., 2002) or CB_1 and CB_2 receptors (Li et al., 2010) were useful in the treatment of paralytic ileus induced by acetic acid and lipopolysaccharide (LPS), respectively. Thus, cannabinoid antagonists may be powerful tools in the treatment of adynamic ileus of different origins.

So far, we have characterized the effect of different drugs in the gastrointestinal tract of experimental animals using radiographic methods, including antitumoral drugs, like cisplatin (Cabezos et al., 2008, 2010; Vera et al., 2014) and 5-fluorouracil (Abalo et al., 2016; McQuade et al., 2016), and cannabinoids (Abalo et al., 2009, 2010, 2011, 2015). We have even performed studies of the combined effects of antitumoral drugs and cannabinoids (Abalo et al., 2013, 2016). In these regards, we showed that the non-selective cannabinoid agonist WIN 55, 212-2 was not capable of improving cisplatin-induced gastrointestinal dysmotility, and even worsened it (Abalo et al., 2013), whereas at a non-psychoactive dose, it tended to reduce diarrhea associated to 5-fluorouracil treatment (Abalo et al., 2016). Thus, these techniques might be useful to study vincristine effects on gastrointestinal motor function, and the possible role of cannabinoid agents in them.

Therefore, the aims of this work were, using radiographic means: (1) To characterize the effect of the antitumoral drug vincristine on rat gastrointestinal motor function. (2) To determine whether the motor alterations induced by vincristine might be prevented by the CB_1-selective cannabinoid antagonist AM251 and by the CB_2-selective cannabinoid antagonist AM630. Some of the present results were communicated previously in abstract form (Vera et al., 2012).

MATERIALS AND METHODS

The Ethical Committee at Universidad Rey Juan Carlos (URJC) and Hospital General Universitario Gregorio Marañón (HGUGM) approved the study. Experimental procedures were carried out in accordance with the recommendations of these Committee as well as with the EU directive for the protection of animals used for scientific purpose (2010/63/UE) and Spanish regulations (RD 109 53/2013).

Animals

Male Wistar rats (350–400 g) were obtained from the Veterinary Unit of HGUGM (Madrid, Spain) or from Envigo (Barcelona, Spain) and housed (4/cage), at the Veterinary Units of HGUGM, or URJC, in standard transparent cages (60 × 40 × 20 cm), under environmentally controlled conditions (temperature = 20°C; humidity = 60%), with a 12 h light/12 h dark cycle. Animals had free access to standard laboratory rat chow (Harlan Laboratories Inc.) and tap water.

Protocol

First, we characterized the effect of a single dose of vincristine on gastrointestinal architecture and motility by histological and radiographic means, respectively (see below). Rats received an acute intraperitoneal injection of vincristine (0.1 or 0.5 mg/kg) or saline (2–3 ml/kg). Alterations of gastrointestinal motility were measured immediately, 24 or 48 h after drug administration. Samples from ileum and colon were taken for conventional histology 48 h after saline or vincristine (0.5 mg/kg).

A second set of experiments was performed in order to determine whether the alterations induced by vincristine could be due to an increased cannabinoid tone and activation of CB_1 or CB_2 receptors. In these experiments, vincristine was administered 24 h prior to the radiographic analysis and adequate cannabinoid antagonists were tested as follows.

The cannabinoid CB_1-selective antagonist AM251 (1 mg/kg), or its vehicle (1 ml/kg), was administered once (20 min before vincristine), twice (before and 24 h after vincristine), or thrice (before, 12 and 24 h after vincristine). Thereafter (24 h after vincristine injection), the radiographic analysis of gastrointestinal motor function was performed (see below).

In the remaining experiments, the CB_2-selective antagonist AM630 (1 mg/kg), or its vehicle (1 ml/kg), was administered thrice (20 min before, and 12 and 24 h after vincristine) and gastrointestinal motor function was analyzed as described below. This group of experiments was performed at URJC, using animals from Envigo.

Histology

Forty-eight hours after vincristine, samples were obtained from terminal ileum (at least 10 cm oral to the ileocaecal junction) and colon of 4–8 animals per experimental group, fixed in buffered 10% formalin and embedded in paraffin. Sections of 5 μm were stained with hematoxylin-eosin (HE) and studied under a Zeiss Axioskop 2 microscope equipped with the image analysis software package AxioVision 4.6. Samples were studied in duplicate under a 20x objective. Histological damage was evaluated using a numerical score of 0–3 assigned to each section considering general loss of mucosal architecture (graded 0–3, absent to severe) and extent of inflammatory cell infiltrate (graded 0–3, absent to transmural). The experimenter was blind to the treatment received by the rat from which the sample under analysis was obtained.

Gastrointestinal Motility Evaluation

Gastrointestinal motor function was studied by radiographic methods as previously described (Cabezos et al., 2008). Thus, 2.5 ml of a suspension of barium sulfate (2 g/ml, temperature = 22°C) was administered *per os*. Experiments at HGUGM were performed with a Siemens (Siremobil Compact L, Erlangen, Germany) digital X-Ray apparatus (60 kV, 7 mA) and X-rays were captured with NPG Real DVD Studio II software. For the experiments at URJC, a CS2100 (Carestream Dental, Spain) digital X-ray apparatus (60 kV, 7 mA) was used, and X-rays were recorded on Carestream Dental T-MAT G/RA film (15 × 30 cm) housed in a cassette provided with regular intensifying screen; films were developed using a Kodak X-omat 2000 automatic processor. Exposure time was adjusted to 20–60 ms. Immobilization of the rats in prone position was achieved by placing them inside adjustable hand-made transparent plastic tubes, so that they could not move. Habituation to the recording chamber prior to commencement of the study did not significantly alter gastrointestinal motility (Cabezos et al., 2008). To further reduce stress, rats were released immediately after each shot (immobilization lasted for 1–2 min). X-rays were recorded at different times (immediately and 1, 2, 4, 6, and 8 h) after administration of the contrast medium. While taking the radiographs, the qualified investigator remained at least 2 m away from the X-ray source or behind a leaded wall, where radioactivity while shooting was not different from environmental readings. A trained investigator blind to the drug administered performed the analysis of the radiographs. Alterations in gut motility were semiquantitatively determined from the images by assigning a compounded value to each region of the gastrointestinal tract considering the following parameters: percentage of the gastrointestinal region filled with contrast (0–4); intensity of contrast (0–4); homogeneity of contrast (0–2); and sharpness of the gastrointestinal region profile (0–2). Each of these parameters was scored and a sum (0–12 points) was made. X-rays for characterization of vincristine and AM251 effects were obtained at HGUGM. X-rays to study the effect of AM630 were taken at URJC. Results were comparable for controls (triple administration of vehicle) obtained at both institutions.

The X-ray images were also analyzed with the aid of an image analysis system (Image J 1.38 for Windows, National Institute of Health, USA, free software: http://rsb.info.nih.gov/ij/) and the alterations of stomach size and caecum were studied.

Compounds and Drugs

Barium sulfate (Barigraf® AD, Juste SAQF, Madrid, Spain) was suspended in tap water and continuously hand-stirred until administration.

Vincristine was purchased from Sigma-Aldrich (Spain, experiments performed at HGUGM) or from Abcam (UK, experiments performed at URJC) and dissolved in saline.

N-(piperidin-1-yl)-5-(4-iodophenyl)-1-(2,4-dichlorophenyl)-4-methyl-1H-pyrazole-3-carboxamide (AM251; Gatley et al., 1996) and 6-iodo-2-methyl-1-[2-(4-morpholinyl)ethyl]-1H-indol-3-yl](4-methoxyphenyl) methanone (AM630; Hosohata et al., 1997) were purchased from Ascent Scientific Ltd (North Somerset, BS24 9 ES, UK).

Cannabinoid antagonists were dissolved in Tocrisolve, a commercially available water soluble emulsion composed of a

1:4 ratio of soya oil/water that is emulsified with the block co-polymer Pluronic F68 (Tocris, Cookson, Bristol, UK; 30 μl in 0.5 ml of saline solution).

Statistical Analysis

Data are presented as the mean values ± SEM. Differences between groups were analyzed using Student's *t*-test or two-way ANOVA followed by *post-hoc* Bonferroni multiple comparison test, as appropriate. Values of $p < 0.05$ were regarded as being significantly different.

RESULTS

Histopathological Effects of Vincristine on Intestinal Tissues

The histological pattern of the intestinal wall in HE stained sections is shown in **Figure 1**. A general and statistically significant damage was observed after vincristine administration. The epithelial layer was particularly affected, showing large areas with ulcers, and loss of normal architecture both in small (**Figures 1A,B,E**, $p < 0.01$) and large intestine (**Figures 1C,D,F**, $p < 0.01$). On the contrary, there were no differences regarding the extent of inflammatory nodules between vincristine-treated animals and controls.

Effects of Vincristine on Gastrointestinal Motor Function

In control animals, when barium was given immediately after saline, gastric emptying was complete 4 h after barium. Barium content reached its maximum in the small intestine in just 1 h and it completely emptied into the caecum by 4 h. In most animals, barium started to stain the caecum and the colorectum 2 and 4 h after barium, respectively. Both organs filled progressively until the end of the study (**Figure 2**). When barium was given 24 (**Figure 3**) or 48 h (**Figure 4**) after saline, the motility curves were very similar to those obtained immediately after saline administration.

Compared with saline, acute administration of vincristine immediately before barium administration (0 h), did not induce any significant change on gastrointestinal motility, irrespective of the dose studied. Also, the quantitative analysis of the images did not show any significant change in the stomach or caecum size (**Figure 2**).

Remarkably, vincristine intensely and significantly reduced gastrointestinal motor function when this was radiographically evaluated 24 h after administration, but only at the dose of 0.5 mg/kg. In these animals, gastric emptying was progressive but at a much lower rate than in rats treated with saline or vincristine at 0.1 mg/kg (**Figure 3A**). Intestinal transit and filling of caecum were also delayed in vincristine-treated rats at the high dose (**Figures 3B,C**). Furthermore, at the end of the experiment (8 h), contrast had not reached the colorectal region in any of those animals (**Figure 3D**). These results were confirmed in the quantitative analysis of the images. In rats treated with vincristine at 0.5 mg/kg, the stomach size at the beginning of the experiment was increased compared to saline-treated animals and remained unchanged for the rest of the experiment (**Figure 3E**). In the caecum, vincristine had a dual effect; the lower dose of vincristine increased its size and the higher one reduced it (**Figure 3F**).

When serial X-rays were obtained 48 h after vincristine, gastrointestinal motor function was still decreased, although the effect was less pronounced than in the previous experiment. Gastric emptying and intestinal transit were reduced (**Figures 4A,B**), but gastric emptying started to recover 6 h after barium (54 h after vincristine), at least in some animals, and higher levels of barium contents were reached in the small intestine at all time-points. The effect on caecum was similar to the previous experiment, but that on the colorectum was less intense and fecal pellets were seen in some animals (**Figures 4C,D**). These results were confirmed in the quantitative analysis. Thus, 0 h after contrast (48 h after vincristine), the stomach size was again comparable to that in the saline group, but not much further change was apparent in this region (**Figure 4E**). Vincristine reduced the size of the caecum at the highest dose used (**Figure 4F**).

Effect of the Cannabinoid Antagonists on Ileus Induced by Vincristine

Figure 5 shows the motility curves for controls used in this experiment. In addition to the effect of saline, the effect of injecting the cannabinoid vehicle once (20 min before saline), twice (before and 24 h after saline) and thrice (before, 12 and 24 h after saline) is shown. As can be seen, injecting the vehicle only once did not produce any effect compared to saline-treated animals. However, when it was injected twice or thrice, significant delays in gastric emptying and in filling of small intestine and caecum were seen. For the following experiments, the effects of the different drugs are compared to those of the vehicle given thrice, since it was the pattern which induced more changes compared to saline (although still very different to that found in vincristine-treated animals, see below).

Figure 6 shows that the CB_1 antagonist AM251 (1 mg/kg) improved gastrointestinal motor function compared to vincristine-treated rats and that this effect increased with the number of times it was injected ($3 > 2 > 1$). However, the normalizing effect of AM251 was different in each gastrointestinal region. Thus, in the stomach and colorectum, AM251 given thrice exerted a significant but relatively small effect. In contrast, it almost normalized the motility curve in the small intestine, and completely normalized the curve in the caecum. Efficacy of AM251 was lower in animals treated with the compound only twice and even lower when it was administered only once. AM251 given thrice did not exert any significant effect compared to its vehicle given also thrice.

Finally, the effect of the selective CB_2 antagonist AM630 was tested. For ethical reasons, and due to the fact that the CB_1 antagonist showed the best results after its triple administration, we only used this pattern of administration to test the effect of AM630. In high contrast with the effect of AM251, the triple administration of AM630 did not significantly modify the effect of vincristine (**Figure 7**).

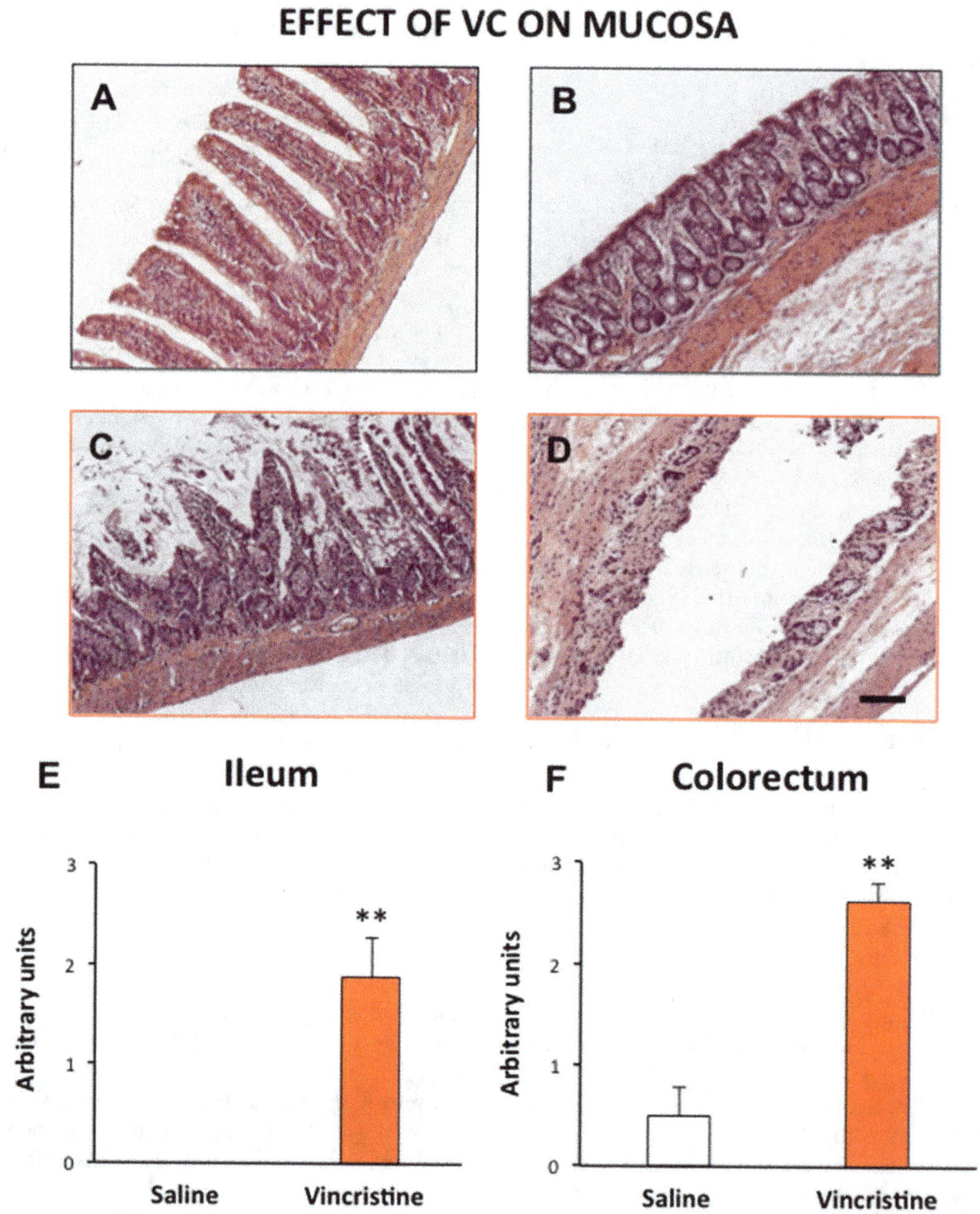

FIGURE 1 | Effect of vincristine treatment on the general structure of the rat intestine. Rats were injected intraperitoneally with vincristine (0.5 mg/kg) or saline (1–2 ml/kg). Forty-eight hours after treatment, histological samples were embedded in paraffin, and stained with HE. Left row, small intestine: tissue samples from saline **(A)** and vincristine-treated animals **(C)** showing the damaged mucosa; quantitative analysis of the histological damage **(E)**. Right row, colorectum: tissue samples from saline **(B)** and vincristine-treated animals **(D)** showing the damaged mucosa; quantitative analysis of the histological damage **(F)**. Bars show mean values ± SEM for control (white) and vincristine-treated animals (red). Each group consisted of 4–8 rats. $^{**}p < 0.01$ vs. saline; (Student's *t*-test). Scale bar: 100 μm.

DISCUSSION

This is the first work in which vincristine-induced gastrointestinal dysmotility has been characterized using radiographic methods in experimental animals. In addition, we have demonstrated that the selective CB_1 cannabinoid antagonist AM251 (but not AM630, a CB_2 selective antagonist), is capable of reducing the effect of vincristine, suggesting that an increased cannabinoid tone is, atleast partially, responsible for the alterations induced by this antitumoral drug on gastrointestinal motor function.

Vincristine Effect on Gastrointestinal Motor Function in the Rat

Gastrointestinal dysmotility associated to vinca alkaloids, including vincristine, is a known cause of drug-induced

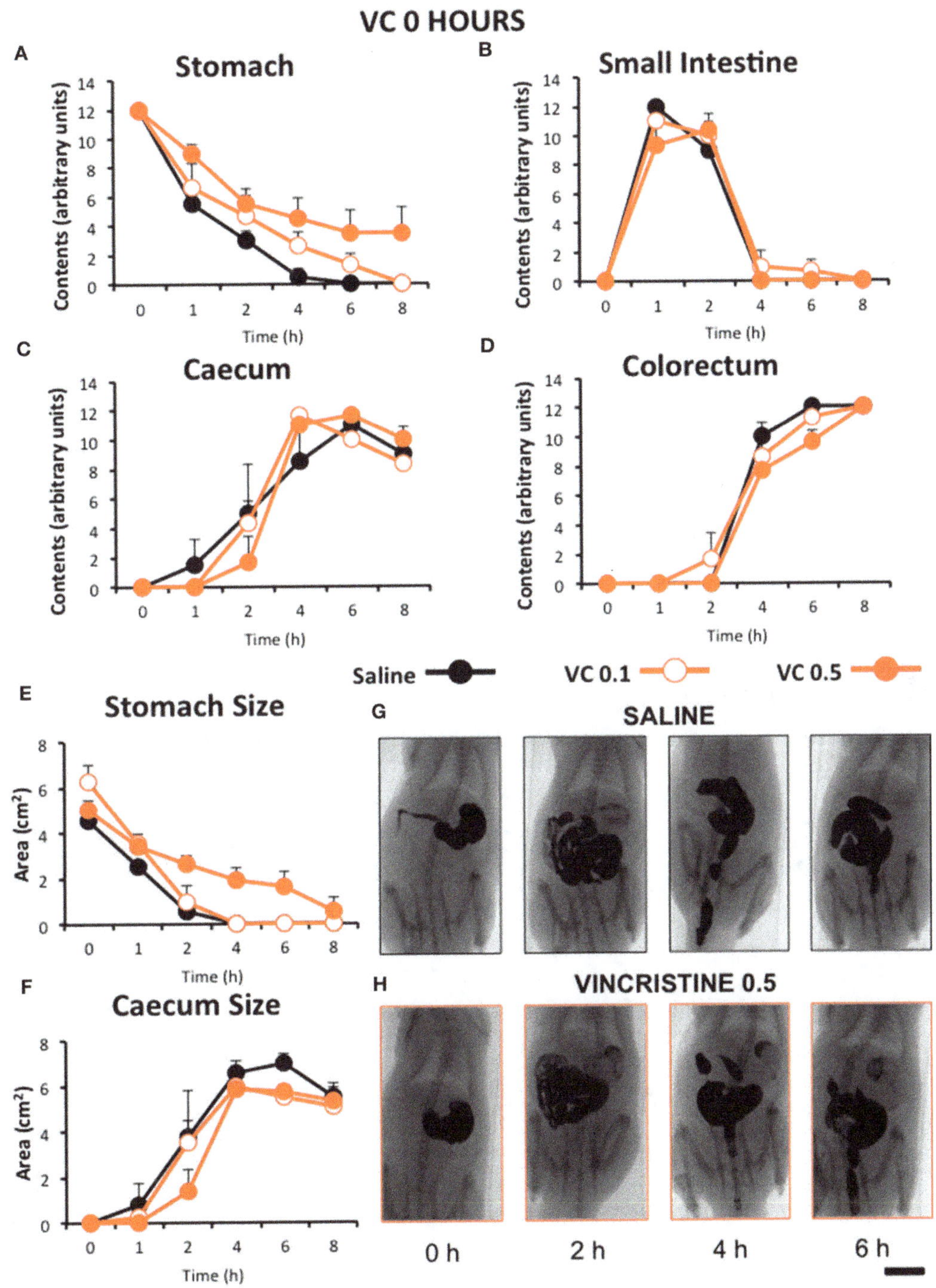

FIGURE 2 | Effect of vincristine immediately after administration on gastrointestinal motor function in the rat. Gastrointestinal motor function was evaluated by radiological methods (see text) in: **(A)** stomach (gastric emptying); **(B)** small intestine; **(C)** caecum and **(D)** colorectum. Rats were injected intraperitoneally (i.p.) with: saline (1–2 ml/kg) or vincristine at 0.1 (VC 0.1) or 0.5 mg/kg (VC 0.5). Barium sulfate (2.5 ml, 2 g/ml) was intragastrically administered immediately after drug administration and X-rays were taken 0–8 h after. The size of stomach **(E)** and caecum **(F)** was determined with Image J. Data represent mean ± SEM (two-way ANOVA followed by *post-hoc* Bonferroni multiple comparison test). **(G,H)** Representative images of animals treated with saline and VC 0.5, taken at different times throughout the experiment. $n = 8$ each group. Scale bar: 23 mm.

gastrointestinal toxicity (Bradley, 1968). Here, vincristine did not significantly alter gastrointestinal motility at a low (0.1 mg/kg) or high dose (0.5 mg/kg) when the X-ray study was performed immediately after its administration. However, when the radiographic study was carried out 24 or 48 h after the antitumoral drug at 0.5 mg/kg, an intense and significant

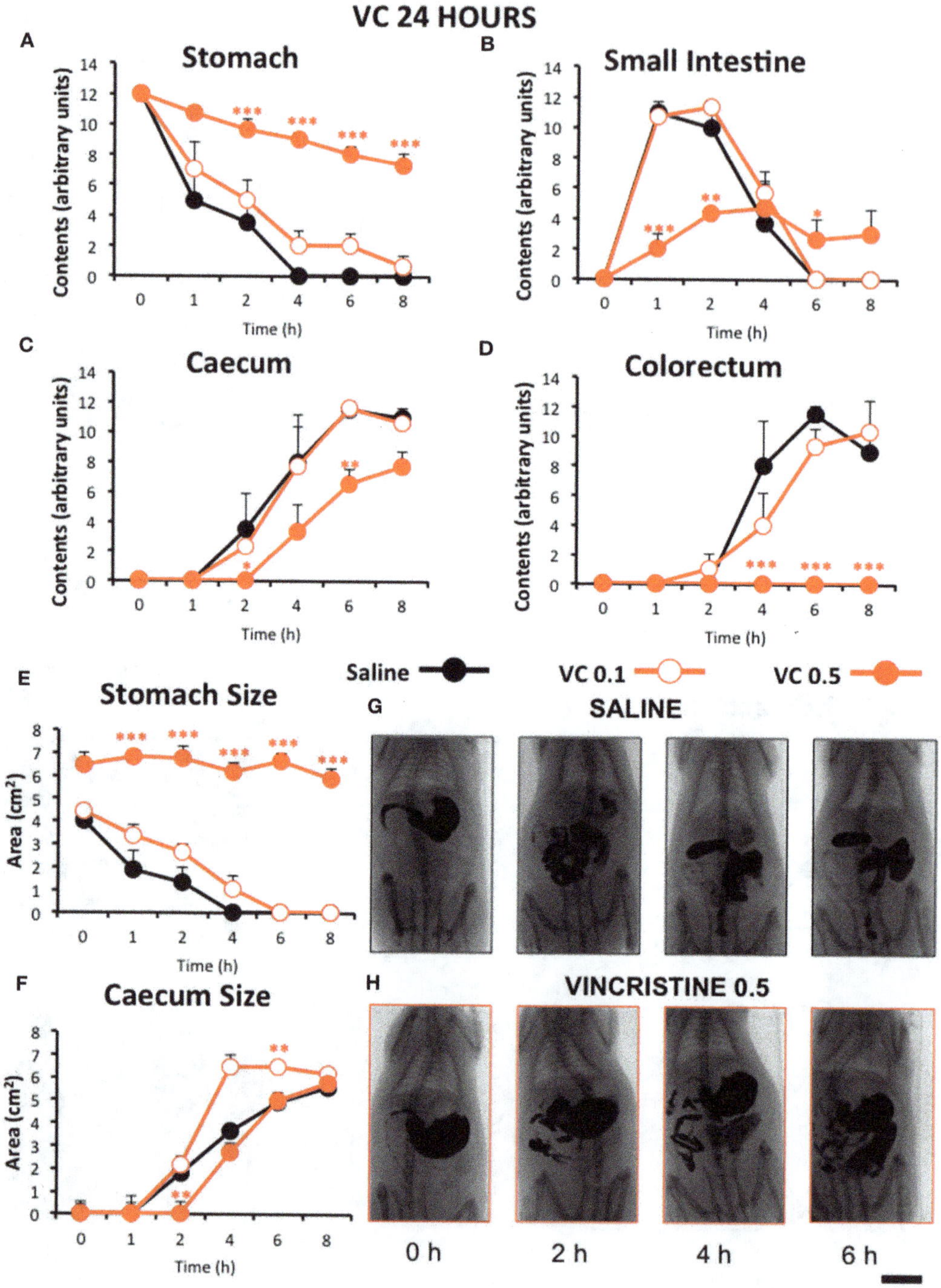

FIGURE 3 | Effect of vincristine 24 h after administration on gastrointestinal motor function in the rat. Gastrointestinal motor function was evaluated by radiological methods (see text) in: **(A)** stomach (gastric emptying); **(B)** small intestine; **(C)** caecum and **(D)** colorectum. Rats were injected intraperitoneally (i.p.) with: saline (1–2 ml/kg) or vincristine at 0.1 (VC 0.1) or 0.5 mg/kg (VC 0.5). Barium sulfate (2.5 ml, 2 g/ml) was intragastrically administered 24 h after drug administration and X-rays were taken 0–8 h after. The size of stomach **(E)** and caecum **(F)** was determined with Image J. Data represent mean ± SEM. $^{*}p < 0.05$, $^{**}p < 0.01$, $^{***}p < 0.001$ vs. saline (two-way ANOVA followed by *post-hoc* Bonferroni multiple comparison test). **(G,H)** Representative images of animals treated with saline and VC 0.5, taken at different times throughout the experiment. $n = 8$ each group. Scale bar: 23 mm.

decrease in gastric emptying and intestinal transit was observed. These results indicate that vincristine-induced dysmotility may need a relatively long time to occur or that higher doses might be needed to see early effects of this drug on gastrointestinal motor function. We did not increase the dose or the observation time because the higher dose used here

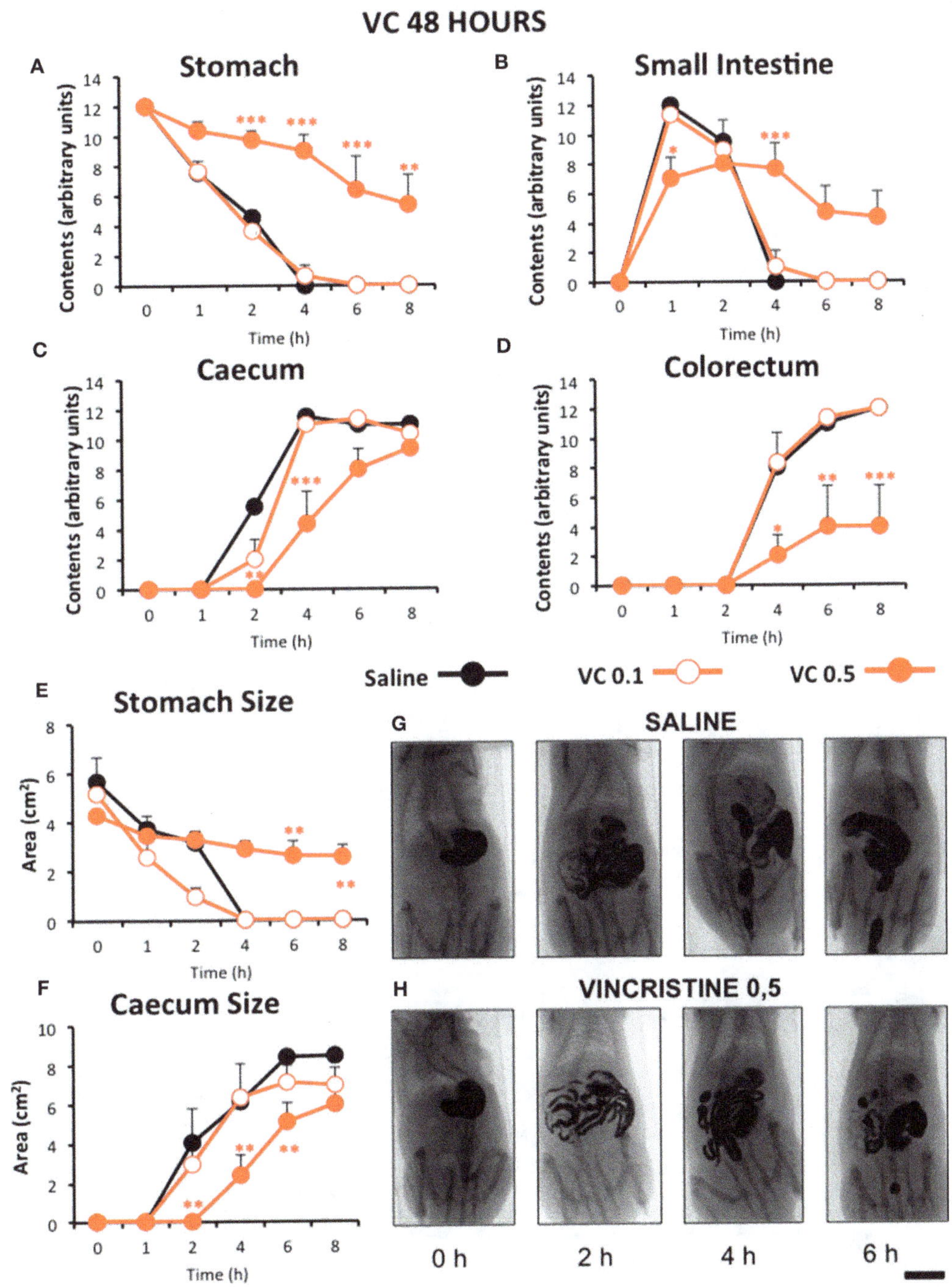

FIGURE 4 | Effect of vincristine 48 h after administration on gastrointestinal motor function in the rat. Gastrointestinal motor function was evaluated by radiological methods (see text) in: **(A)** stomach (gastric emptying); **(B)** small intestine; **(C)** caecum and **(D)** colorectum. Rats were injected intraperitoneally (i.p.) with: saline (1–2 ml/kg) or vincristine at 0.1 (VC 0.1) or 0.5 mg/kg (VC 0.5). Barium sulfate (2.5 ml, 2 g/ml) was intragastrically administered 48 h after drug administration and X-rays were taken 0–8 h after. The size of stomach **(E)** and caecum **(F)** was determined with Image J. Data represent mean ± SEM. $^{*}p < 0.05$, $^{**}p < 0.01$, $^{***}p < 0.001$ *vs*. saline (two-way ANOVA followed by *post-hoc* Bonferroni multiple comparison test). **(G,H)** Representative images of animals treated with saline and VC 0.5, taken at different times throughout the experiment. $n = 8$ each group. Scale bar: 23 mm.

was similar to the LD_{50} in rats and mortality associated to this dose may occur 4–6 days after its administration (Uy et al., 1967).

Several previous investigations have reported that vincristine-induced gastric hypomotility is not an early event (Kaneko et al., 2001; Tsukamoto et al., 2011). The delayed effect of vincristine

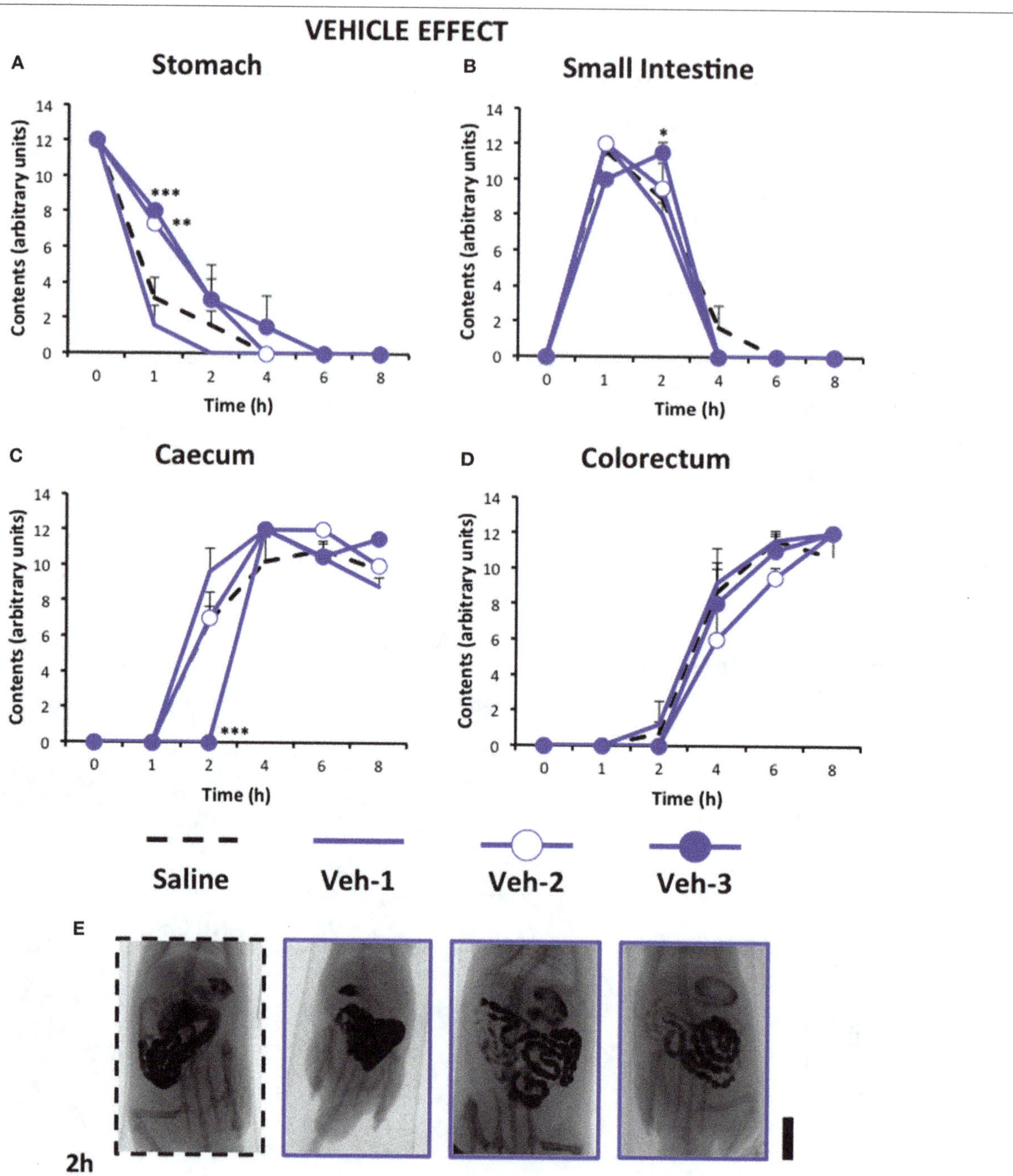

FIGURE 5 | Effect of saline or the cannabinoid vehicle on gastrointestinal motor function in the rat. Gastrointestinal motor function was evaluated by radiological methods (see text) in: **(A)** stomach (gastric emptying); **(B)** small intestine; **(C)** caecum and **(D)** colorectum. Rats were injected intraperitoneally (i.p.) with: saline (1–2 ml/kg) or the cannabinoid vehicle once (20 min before saline, Veh-1), twice (before and 24 h after saline, Veh-2), and thrice (before, 12 and 24 h after saline, Veh-3). Barium sulfate (2.5 ml, 2 g/ml) was intragastrically administered immediately or 24 h after drug administration and X-rays were taken 0–8 h after. Data represent mean ± SEM. $^{*}p < 0.05$, $^{**}p < 0.01$, $^{***}p < 0.001$ vs. saline (two-way ANOVA followed by *post-hoc* Bonferroni multiple comparison test). $n = 4$–8 animals per group. **(E)** Representative images of saline- and Veh-treated animals 2 h after contrast. Scale bar: 23 mm.

contrasts with that of other antineoplastic drugs, like cisplatin, which provokes gastric dysmotility within a much shorter time in rats (Cabezos et al., 2008, 2010; Vera et al., 2014). Cisplatin immediate (acute) effect on gastric motor function is due to serotonin release and vagal activation, through the stimulation of 5-HT$_3$ receptors (Vera et al., 2014), and underlies its intense emetogenic effect in experimental animals (Holmes et al., 2009; du Sert et al., 2011; Horn, 2014) and humans (Navari, 2013).

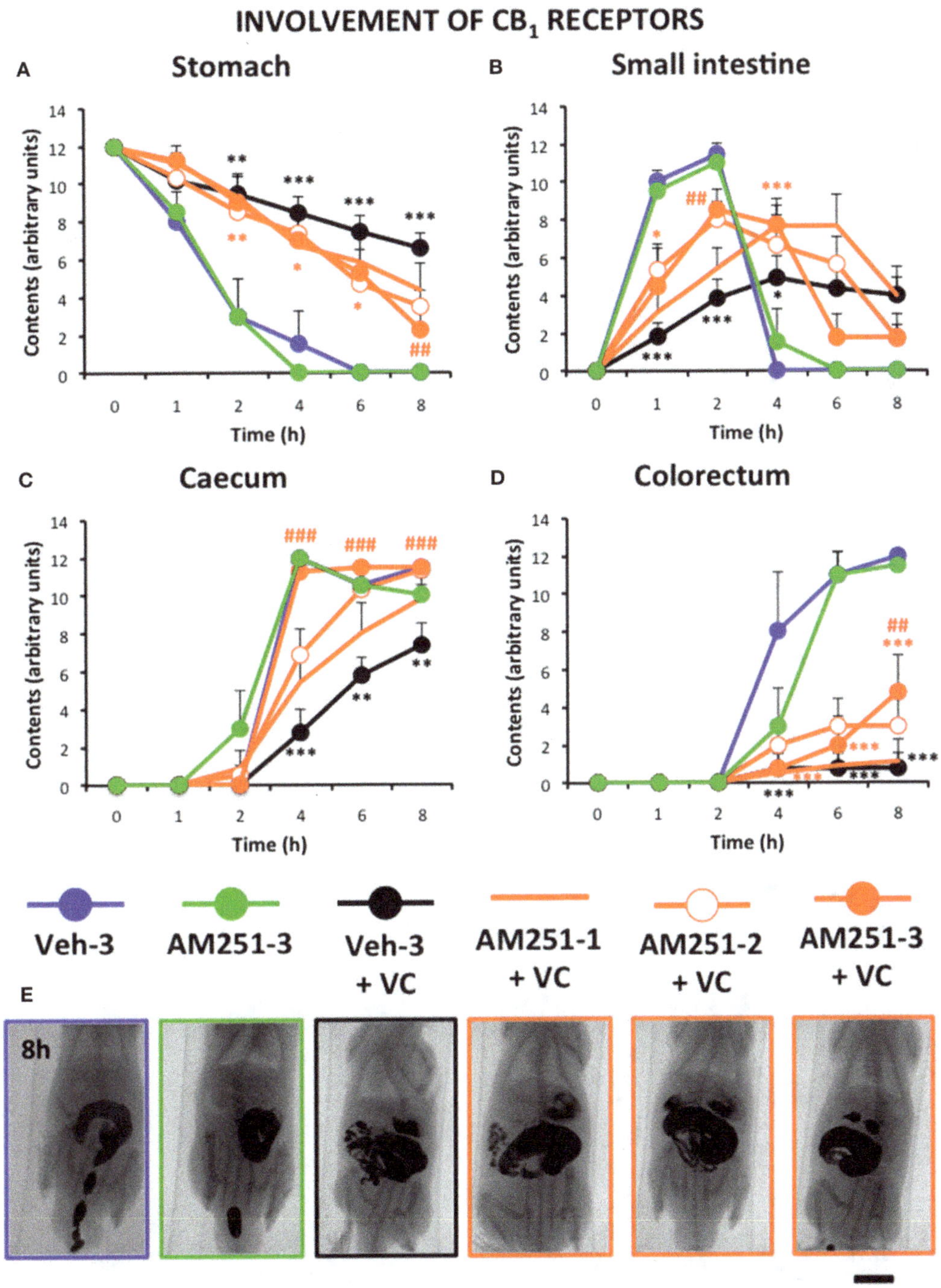

FIGURE 6 | Effect of the CB_1 antagonist AM251 on the alterations induced by vincristine on gastrointestinal motor function in the rat. Gastrointestinal motor function was evaluated by radiological methods (see text) in **(A)** stomach (gastric emptying); **(B)** small intestine; **(C)** caecum and **(D)** colorectum. Rats received two intraperitoneal injections (i.p.). One was saline (1–2 ml/kg) or vincristine at 0.5 mg/kg (VC). The other one was the cannabinoid vehicle given three times (Veh-3) or AM251 given once (20 min before saline or vincristine: AM251-1), twice (before and 24 h after saline or vincristine: AM251-2), or thrice (before, 12 and 24 h after saline or vincristine: AM251-3). Barium sulfate (2.5 ml, 2 g/ml) was intragastrically administered 24 h after saline or vincristine administration and X-rays were taken 0–8 h after. Data represent mean ± SEM. $^{*}p < 0.05$, $^{**}p < 0.01$, $^{***}p < 0.001$ vs. Veh-3; ## $p < 0.01$; ###$p < 0.001$ vs. Veh 3 + VC (two-way ANOVA followed by *post-hoc* Bonferroni multiple comparison test). $n = 4$–8 animals each group. **(E)** Representative images of the different treatments 8 h after contrast. Scale bar: 23 mm.

Cisplatin may also produce "delayed" emesis in humans, and we observed "delayed" gastric dysmotility and pica, a surrogate marker of nausea in rodents (Takeda et al., 1993), after cisplatin administration in the rat (Cabezos et al., 2008). Cisplatin-induced delayed emesis seems to be more dependent upon other mechanisms, including the activation of NK_1 receptors

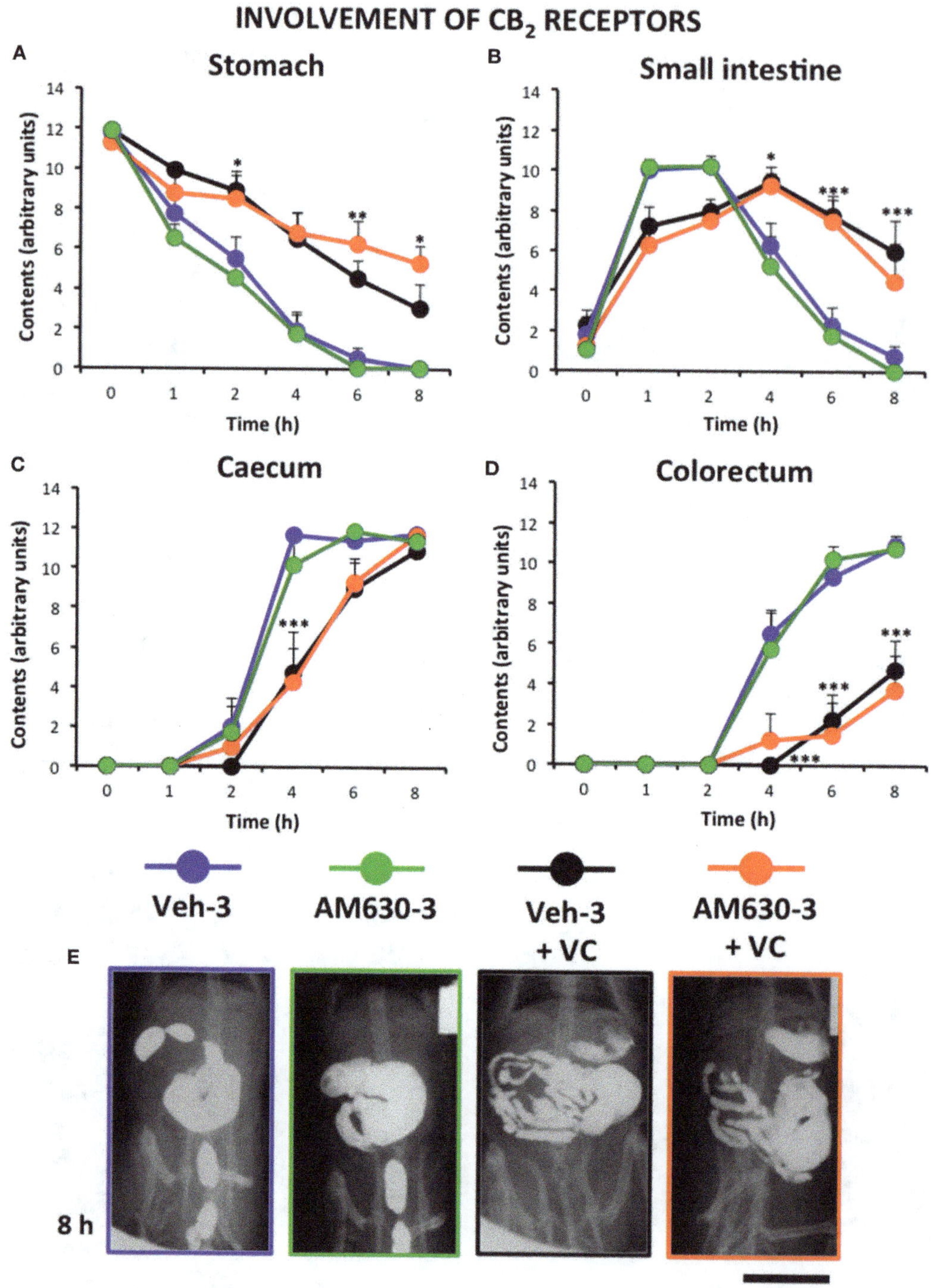

FIGURE 7 | Effect of the CB_2 antagonist AM630 on the alterations induced by vincristine on gastrointestinal motor function in the rat. Gastrointestinal motor function was evaluated by radiological methods (see text) in: **(A)** stomach (gastric emptying); **(B)** small intestine; **(C)** caecum and **(D)** colorectum. Rats received saline (1–2 ml/kg) or vincristine at 0.5 mg/kg (VC). The cannabinoid vehicle (Veh-3) or AM630 (AM630-3) were administered thrice (before, 12 and 24 h after saline or vincristine administration). Barium sulfate (2.5 ml, 2 g/ml) was intragastrically administered 24 h after saline or vincristine administration and X-rays were taken 0–8 h after. Data represent mean ± SEM. $^{*}p < 0.05$, $^{**}p < 0.01$, $^{***}p < 0.001$ vs. Veh-3 (two-way ANOVA followed by *post-hoc* Bonferroni multiple comparison test). $n = 8$ each group. **(E)** Representative images of the different treatments 8 h after contrast. Scale bar: 30 mm.

through the release of substance P (Navari, 2013; Rudd et al., 2016). These mechanisms justify the usefulness of 5-HT_3 and NK_1 antagonists for prevention of emesis associated to highly emetogenic chemotherapy in cancer patients (Navari, 2013). Vincristine may induce nausea and emesis in dogs and humans, but the incidence and intensity of these effects are much lower than with cisplatin (Navari, 2013; Mason et al., 2014) and the mechanisms might be different (see below).

The altered motility curve observed here for the small intestine 24 h after vincristine may be due, at least partly, to the delayed gastric emptying (barium reached the small intestine much later in vincristine- than in saline-treated animals). However, this would probably have produced a motility curve for the small intestine very similar in shape to that in control animals, but displaced to the right (this occurred after acute cisplatin, which only alters gastric motility; Cabezos et al., 2008). In the present study, the curve was completely distorted, suggesting that vincristine produced direct effects in this region. Direct effects of vincristine in the small intestine might include altered myoelectric activity, increased tone and spasmogenic actions, as previously suggested (Sharma, 1979, 1988; Sninsky, 1987). Small intestinal transit was accelerated in rats in the first few hours after vinblastine (Sharma, 1979), but we did not detect such an effect of vincristine in our non-invasive study. In fact, the motility curve of caecum looked very similar (parallel) to that in control animals both 24 and 48 h after vincristine (0.5 mg/kg), but displaced to the right, further suggesting that small intestinal transit was delayed. Interestingly, in spite of the fact that caecum filled adequately, there was a complete absence of stained fecal pellets in vincristine-treated rats for the whole duration of the radiologic study when it was performed 24 h after the antitumoral drug, suggesting that vincristine directly suppressed motility in colorectum, which is in accordance with the reports of constipation associated to treatment with vinca alkaloids, in both animals and humans (Harris and Jackson, 1977; Garewal and Dalton, 1985; Ikehara, 1992; Leker et al., 1997; Chae et al., 1998; Wang et al., 2000; Essa et al., 2014; Yasu et al., 2016).

Several factors may contribute to the effects found in the stomach, small intestine, caecum and colorectum 24–48 h after vincristine. Chemotherapy-induced gastrointestinal toxicity can be caused by direct damage to mucosal epithelial cells or by stimulation of the vomiting center or chemoreceptor trigger zone (Kaneko et al., 2001). Vincristine is known to induce metaphase arrest, severe villous atrophy and mucosal erosions (Beró and Jávor, 1985), which we found in our histological study. This effect would disrupt the intestinal barrier function and could contribute to dysmotility. In contrast, we did not observe evident changes in the presence of inflammatory cells within the gut wall, suggesting that these might not be determinant to acute vincristine-induced dysmotility, although this must be systematically studied. According to previous reports, direct effects on the smooth muscle layers (Kaneko et al., 2001) or the possible influence of enhanced adrenergic activity due to neuropathic pain (Peixoto Júnior et al., 2009) seem unlikely. Interestingly, due to the known neurotoxicity of the compound (whose direct effect on the vomiting center to induce gastric dysmotility and emesis cannot be discarded) and to several functional and histological evidences, the development of an autonomic neuropathy has been suggested to contribute to vincristine-induced gastrointestinal hypomotility, particularly after high doses or chronic treatments (Smith, 1967; Peixoto Júnior et al., 2009). However, a systematic analysis of the possible changes in structure and in marker expression in the enteric nervous system after vincristine treatment, as those performed with other antineoplastic drugs (Vera et al., 2011; Wafai et al., 2013; McQuade et al., 2016), is still required to define the precise role of neuropathy affecting the enteric nervous system, particularly the myenteric plexus, on gastrointestinal motor disturbances induced by vincristine. This might be particularly evident in chronic treatments.

Importantly, gastrointestinal ileus induced by vincristine, in contrast to sensory neuropathy, seems to be transient and is reverted soon after treatment discontinuation (Sharma, 1988; Chae et al., 1998; Peixoto Júnior et al., 2009). However, in addition to reducing quality of life, vincristine-induced gastrointestinal dysmotility may be problematic and even fatal, particularly under certain circumstances (liver failure, concomitant condition predisposing to constipation, drug interactions, or even accidental overdose: (Toghill and Burke, 1970; Leker et al., 1997; Bermúdez et al., 2005; Uner et al., 2005; Levêque et al., 2009; Diezi et al., 2010; Le Guellec et al., 2012; Essa et al., 2014; Yasu et al., 2016). This justifies the search for anti-ileus treatments.

Very few agents have been tested in vincristine-induced gastrointestinal ileus and most references are case reports with low numbers of subjects (Harris and Jackson, 1977; Jackson et al., 1982; Garewal and Dalton, 1985; Ikehara, 1992; Tsukamoto et al., 2011; Essa et al., 2014; Mason et al., 2014). To the best of our knowledge, the possible role of cannabinoids has never before been tested either in experimental animals or in the clinic.

Role of Cannabinoids on Gastrointestinal Ileus Induced by Vincristine

Cannabinoids have been used empirically and traditionally to treat different disorders including those of the gut, ranging from enteric infections and inflammatory conditions to motility alterations, emesis, and abdominal pain (Izzo and Camilleri, 2009; Izzo and Sharkey, 2010; Abalo et al., 2012; Abalo and Martín-Fontelles, 2017; Salaga et al., 2017; Vera et al., 2017). Central and peripheral cannabinoid receptors seem to be involved in the regulation of gastrointestinal motility. Cannabinoid CB_1 receptors are mainly found in nervous cells, including those of the myenteric plexus (Abalo et al., 2012; Vera et al., 2017), principal responsible for intestinal motility. Interestingly, these gastrointestinal CB_1 receptors appear to exert a tonic control over the enteric nervous system, and operate as a "brake" for neural over-reactivity (Schicho and Storr, 2011; Abalo et al., 2012). In fact, agonists acting at CB_1 receptors may potently depress gastrointestinal motor function even in the absence of significant central effects (Abalo et al., 2015). In contrast, CB_2 receptors are mainly found in immune cells, and have anti-inflammatory effects (Turcotte et al., 2016). Normally, CB_2 agents do not alter gastrointestinal motor function (Abalo et al., 2009, 2010, 2011, 2015). However, it has been shown that CB_2 receptors are overexpressed in the myenteric neurons under inflammatory conditions, and in such cases, they may also reduce transit and normalize intestinal motor function (Mathison et al., 2004; Duncan et al., 2008; Wright et al., 2008). Thus, selective

CB_1 and CB_2 cannabinoid receptor antagonists may be useful in situations in which gastrointestinal motor function is reduced.

The effect of CB_1 antagonists on motility in control animals is to some extent controversial, with some reports showing increased transit (Mathison et al., 2004) and others showing no effects (Landi et al., 2002), suggesting that the gastrointestinal cannabinoid tone may be sensitive to slight differences in experimental conditions (Abalo et al., 2009, 2010, 2011, 2015). In humans, diarrhea was present in some obese patients treated with rimonabant and other cannabinoid antagonists (Waterlow and Chrisp, 2008). In animal models of paralytic ileus, CB_1 receptor was overexpressed and anandamide levels were increased (Mascolo et al., 2002; de Filippis et al., 2008). Thus, an increased cannabinoid tone, due to released endocannabinoids and/or CB_1 overexpression, seem to be involved in the development of paralytic ileus and strategies aimed at normalizing endocannabinoid levels/tone could be therapeutically useful in these conditions. Consequently, the CB_1 selective antagonist AM251 (with $IC_{50} = 8$ nM, $K_i = 7.49$ nM, and 306-fold selectivity over CB_2 receptors, Lan et al., 1999) was used here to see if vincristine effects are mediated by a similar mechanism.

In our study, AM251, at a dose that lacked any significant effect on GI motility in control animals (1 m/kg), reduced the effect of vincristine on gastric emptying and intestinal transit. This was achieved when the antagonist was administered twice (once every 24 h) or thrice (once every 12 h). The gastrointestinal region most sensitive to the effect of the CB_1 antagonist was the small intestine, and transit was close to normal after its triple administration, as suggested by the motility curves for the small intestine and, even more, for the caecum, which showed normal filling. In contrast, altered gastric emptying and colorectal motility after AM251 triple administration only partially improved at the end of the study (8 h after contrast, 32 h after vincristine). Thus, an increase in cannabinoid tone affecting CB_1 receptors might underlie some of the effects of vincristine in the stomach and colorectum, but other factors may be more influential in these regions, whereas vincristine-induced small intestinal ileus seems to depend mostly, if not completely, on increased CB_1 receptor activity. Accordingly, in LPS-induced septic models of ileus, AM251 increased myoelectric activity of rat jejunum *in vitro* and upper gastrointestinal transit in mice (measured with the charcoal method; Li et al., 2010). Rimonabant (another CB_1 antagonist receptor) alleviated gastrointestinal symptoms in a murine model of paralytic ileus induced by intraperitoneal injection of acetic acid, modeling peritonitis, and an anandamide uptake inhibitor worsened motility even further (Mascolo et al., 2002). On the other hand, in a model of postoperative ileus, upper gastrointestinal transit was similarly reduced in wild type and knock-out mice for CB_1 receptors (although the inflammatory response was more intense in the latter), suggesting that altered motility in this model might not be necessarily or only due to increased CB_1 receptor activation (Li et al., 2013a).

Since AM251 (and rimonabant) is considered both an antagonist and an inverse agonist, at this stage it is not clear if our results are due to an increased basal activity of CB_1 receptors after vincristine, linked to overexpression, and/or to the release of endocannabinoids. As mentioned above, increased anandamide levels were found to occur in models of paralytic ileus (Mascolo et al., 2002), and expression of CB_1 receptors was increased in different models of ileus (Mascolo et al., 2002; de Filippis et al., 2008). Interestingly, the motility curves obtained from vincristine-treated animals here were very similar to those previously obtained from control animals treated with cannabinoids, whose effects were dependent upon CB_1 activation and much more potent on intestinal regions (particularly the small intestine) than on the stomach (Abalo et al., 2009, 2010, 2015), suggesting that the release of endogenous cannabinoids might be involved in vincristine effects.

AM630 did not significantly modify the effect of vincristine on gut motility. The involvement of CB_2 receptors in experimental models of ileus is less clear than that of CB_1 receptors. Thus, in models of septic ileus, some researchers described that inactivation of either CB_1 or CB_2 receptors normalized jejunal myoelectric activity and upper gastrointestinal transit (Li et al., 2010). In contrast, inactivation of CB_2 receptors did not normalize reduced motility associated to intraperitoneal acetic acid administration (Mascolo et al., 2002).

Finally, it cannot be discarded that AM251 exerted its effects through another mechanism. Interestingly, it has been described as a GPR55 agonist ($EC_{50} = 39$ nM; Henstridge et al., 2010). As mentioned above, when used alone in control animals, gastrointestinal motility was not significantly altered, suggesting that GPR55 receptors were not activated in these animals. O-1602, another agonist of GPR55 receptors (but 3-fold more potent than AM251 upon them: $EC_{50} = 13$ nM), did not alter upper gastrointestinal transit when used at 10 mg/kg in control or LPS-treated mice (which showed reduced transit), whereas cannabidiol, which is considered a GPR55 antagonist, counteracted O-1602, and LPS-effect (Lin et al., 2011; Li et al., 2013b). Thus, if GPR55 was overexpressed by vincristine treatment, as by LPS, it is more likely that a GPR55 antagonist was more useful to counteract GPR55 overactivation than a GPR55 agonist like AM251. The involvement of GPR55 receptors in vincristine-induced dysmotility will be specifically investigated in future work.

In conclusion, the fact that AM251 (but not AM630) is capable of reducing the effect of vincristine suggests that, like in other experimental models of paralytic ileus, an increased cannabinoid tone acting through CB_1 receptors is, at least partially, responsible for the alterations induced by vincristine on gastrointestinal motor function. The combination of different technniques, including immunohistochemistry (to locate the cells expressing the receptors) and molecular biology (to determine the levels of receptors and ligands, if appropriate), will help determine the precise mechanism of action involved in AM251 effect. Whatever this may be, ours is a clinically relevant finding and encourages the exploration of strategies aimed at reducing CB_1 receptor activity to prevent or palliate vincristine-induced ileus in the clinic.

AUTHOR CONTRIBUTIONS

RA designed the study. GV, AL, RG, and JU performed the experiments and analyzed the data. RA and GV wrote the manuscript. MM contributed financial support and essential intellectual input. All authors reviewed and approved the final version of the manuscript.

FUNDING

This work was supported by Ministerio de Ciencia e Innovación (SAF2009-12422-C02-01, SAF2012-40075-C02-01), Universidad Rey Juan Carlos—Comunidad de Madrid (URJC-CM-2006-BIO-0604) and Comunidad de Madrid (S-SAL/0261/2006; S2010/BMD-2308).

ACKNOWLEDGMENTS

The authors wish to thank R Franco, J Paredes, A Márquez, PA Cabezos, M Martínez-Villaluenga, L Blanco and C Merino for technical assistance. L Blanco has a contract by Consejería de Educación, Juventud y Deporte from Comunidad de Madrid and Fondo Social Europeo (PEJ15/BIO/TL-0580).

REFERENCES

Abalo, R., Cabezos, P. A., López-Miranda, V., Vera, G., González, C., Castillo, M., et al. (2009). Selective lack of tolerance to delayed gastric emptying after daily administration of WIN 55,212-2 in the rat. *Neurogastroenterol. Motil.* 21, e1002–e80. doi: 10.1111/j.1365-2982.2009.01315.x

Abalo, R., Cabezos, P. A., Vera, G., Fernández-Pujol, R., and Martín, M. I. (2010). The cannabinoid antagonist SR144528 enhances the acute effect of WIN 55,212-2 on gastrointestinal motility in the rat. *Neurogastroenterol. Motil.* 22, e694–e206. doi: 10.1111/j.1365-2982.2009.01466.x

Abalo, R., Cabezos, P. A., Vera, G., López-Miranda, V., Herradón, E., and Martín-Fontelles, M. I. (2011). Cannabinoid-induced delayed gastric emptying is selectively increased upon intermittent administration in the rat: role of CB1 receptors. *Neurogastroenterol. Motil.* 23:e177. doi: 10.1111/j.1365-2982.2011.01677.x

Abalo, R., Cabezos, P. A., Vera, G., López-Pérez, A. E., and Martín, M. I. (2013). Cannabinoids may worsen gastric dysmotility induced by chronic cisplatin in the rat. *Neurogastroenterol. Motil.* 25:e292. doi: 10.1111/nmo.12073

Abalo, R., Chen, C., Vera, G., Fichna, J., Thakur, G. A., López-Pérez, A. E., et al. (2015). *In vitro* and non-invasive *in vivo* effects of the cannabinoid-1 receptor agonist AM841 on gastrointestinal motor function in the rat. *Neurogastroenterol. Motil.* 27, 1721–1735. doi: 10.1111/nmo.12668

Abalo, R., and Martín-Fontelles, M. I. (2017). "Cannabis, cannabinoids, and visceral pain," in *Handbook of Cannabis and Related Pathologies*, ed V. Preedy (London: Academic Press), c0255.

Abalo, R., Uranga, J. A., Pérez-García, I., de Andrés, R., Girón, R., Vera, G., et al. (2016). May cannabinoids prevent the development of chemotherapy-induced diarrhea and intestinal mucositis? Experimental study in the rat. *Neurogastroenterol. Motil.* doi: 10.1111/nmo.12952. [Epub ahead of print].

Abalo, R., Vera, G., López-Pérez, A. E., Martínez-Villaluenga, M., and Martín-Fontelles, M. I. (2012). The gastrointestinal pharmacology of cannabinoids: focus on motility. *Pharmacology* 90, 1–10. doi: 10.1159/000339072

Aviello, G., Romano, B., and Izzo, A. A. (2008). Cannabinoids and gastrointestinal motility: animal and human studies. *Eur. Rev. Med. Pharmacol. Sci.* 12(Suppl. 1), 81–93.

Bermúdez, M., Fuster, J. L., Llinares, E., Galera, A., and Gonzalez, C. (2005). Itraconazole-related increased vincristine neurotoxicity: case report and review of literature. *J. Pediatr. Hematol. Oncol.* 27, 389–392.

Beró, T., and Jávor, T. (1985). The effect of cyclophosphamide and vincristine on intestinal protein loss in rats. *Arch. Toxicol. Suppl.* 8, 117–121.

Bohannon, R. A., Miller, D. G., and Diamond, H. D. (1963). Vincristine in the treatment of lymphomas and leukemias. *Cancer Res.* 23, 613–621.

Bradley, W. G. (1968). Side-effects of Vinca alkaloids. *Br. Med. J.* 3, 58.

Cabezos, P. A., Vera, G., Castillo, M., Fernández-Pujol, R., Martín, M. I., and Abalo, R. (2008). Radiological study of gastrointestinal motor activity after acute cisplatin in the rat. Temporal relationship with pica. *Auton Neurosci.* 141, 54–65. doi: 10.1016/j.autneu.2008.05.004

Cabezos, P. A., Vera, G., Martín-Fontelles, M. I., Fernández-Pujol, R., and Abalo, R. (2010). Cisplatin-induced gastrointestinal dysmotility is aggravated after chronic administration in the rat. Comparison with pica. *Neurogastroenterol. Motil.* 22, e224–e225. doi: 10.1111/j.1365-2982.2010.01483.x

Chae, L., Moon, H. S., and Kim, S. C. (1998). Overdose of vincristine: experience with a patient. *J. Korean Med. Sci.* 13, 334–338. doi: 10.3346/jkms.1998.13.3.33z

de Filippis, D., Iuvone, T., d'amico, A, Esposito, G., Steardo, L., Herman, A. G., et al. (2008). Effect of cannabidiol on sepsis-induced motility disturbances in mice: involvement of CB receptors and fatty acid amide hydrolase. *Neurogastroenterol. Motil.* 20, 919–927. doi: 10.1111/j.1365-2982.2008.01114.x

Diezi, M., Nydegger, A., Di Paolo, E. R., Kuchler, H., and Beck-Popovic, M. (2010). Vincristine and intestinal pseudo-obstruction in children: report of 5 cases, literature review, and suggested management. *J. Pediatr. Hematol. Oncol.* 32, e126–e130. doi: 10.1097/MPH.0b013e3181d7742f

Duncan, M., Mouihate, A., Mackie, K., Keenan, C. M., Buckley, N. E., Davison, J. S., et al. (2008). Cannabinoid CB2 receptors in the enteric nervous system modulate gastrointestinal contractility in lipopolysaccharide-treated rats. *Am. J. Physiol. Gastrointest. Liver Physiol.* 295, G78–G87. doi: 10.1152/ajpgi.90285.2008

du Sert, N. P., Rudd, J. A., Apfel, C. C., and Andrews, P. L. R. (2011). Cisplatin-induced emesis: systematic review and meta-analysis of the ferret model and the effects of 5-HT$_3$ receptor antagonists. *Cancer Chemother. Pharmacol.* 67, 667–686. doi: 10.1007/s00280-010-1339-4

Essa, M., Santo, A. E., Fleming, A., Mitchell, D., and Abish, S. (2014). Exploring the attitudes of pediatric oncologists toward the use of laxatives for the prevention of constipation in patients undergoing active treatment: a canadian perspective. *Pediatr. Hematol. Oncol.* 31, 448–457. doi: 10.3109/08880018.2013.837129

Garewal, H. S., and Dalton, W. S. (1985). Metoclopramide in vincristine-induced ileus. *Cancer Treat. Rep.* 69, 1309–1311.

Gatley, S. J., Gifford, A. N., Volkow, N. D., Lan, R., and Makriyannis, A. (1996). 123I-labeled AM251: a radioiodinated ligand which binds *in vivo* to mouse brain cannabinoid CB1 receptors. *Eur. J. Pharmacol.* 307, 331–338.

Harris, A. C., and Jackson, J. M. (1977). Lactulose in vincristine-induced constipation. *Med. J. Aust.* 2, 573–574.

Henstridge, C. M., Balenga, N. A., Schröder, R., Kargl, J. K., Platzer, W., Martini, L., et al. (2010). GPR55 ligands promote receptor coupling to multiple signalling pathways. *Br. J. Pharmacol.* 160, 604–614. doi: 10.1111/j.1476-5381.2009.00625.x

Holmes, A. M., Rudd, J. A., Tattersall, F. D., Aziz, Q., and Andrews, P. L. (2009). Opportunities for the replacement of animals in the study of nausea and vomiting. *Br. J. Pharmacol.* 157, 865–880. doi: 10.1111/j.1476-5381.2009.00176.x

Horn, C. C. (2014). Measuring the nausea-to-emesis continuum in non-human animals: refocusing on gastrointestinal vagal signaling. *Exp. Brain Res.* 232, 2471–2481. doi: 10.1007/s00221-014-3985-y

Hosohata, K., Quock, R. M., Hosohata, Y., Burkey, T. H., Makriyannis, A., Consroe, P., et al. (1997). AM630 is a competitive cannabinoid receptor antagonist in the guinea pig brain. *Life Sci.* 61, PL115–PL118.

Ikehara, O. (1992). Vincristine-induced paralytic ileus: role of fiberoptic colonoscopy and prostaglandin F2 alpha. *Am. J. Gastroenterol.* 87, 207–210.

Izzo, A. A., and Camilleri, M. (2009). Cannabinoids in intestinal inflammation and cancer. *Pharmacol. Res.* 60, 117–125. doi: 10.1016/j.phrs.2009.03.008

Izzo, A. A., Mascolo, N., Pinto, L., Capasso, R., and Capasso, F. (1999). The role of cannabinoid receptors in intestinal motility, defaecation and diarrhoea in rats. *Eur. J. Pharmacol.* 384, 37–42.

Izzo, A. A., and Sharkey, K. A. (2010). Cannabinoids and the gut: new developments and emerging concepts. *Pharmacol. Ther.* 126, 21–38. doi: 10.1016/j.pharmthera.2009.12.005

Jackson, D. V. Jr., Wu, W. C., and Spurr, C. L. (1982). Treatment of vincristine-induced ileus with sincalide, a cholecystokinin analog. *Cancer Chemother. Pharmacol.* 8, 83–85.

Johnson, I. S., Wright, H. F., Svoboda, G. H., and Vlantis, J. (1960). Antitumor principles derived from Vinca rosea Linn. I. Vincaleukoblastine and leurosine. *Cancer Res.* 20, 1016–1022.

Kaneko, H., Tomomasa, T., Watanabe, T., Takahashi, A., Tabata, M., Hussein, S., et al. (2001). Effect of vincristine on gastric motility in conscious rats. *Dig. Dis. Sci.* 46, 952–959. doi: 10.1023/A:1010785206315

Lan, R., Liu, Q., Fan, P., Lin, S., Fernando, S. R., McCallion, D., et al. (1999). Structure-activity relationships of pyrazole derivatives as cannabinoid receptor antagonists. *J. Med. Chem.* 42, 769–776.

Landi, M., Croci, T., Rinaldi-Carmona, M., Maffrand, J. P., Le Fur, G., and Manara, L. (2002). Modulation of gastric emptying and gastrointestinal transit in rats through intestinal cannabinoid CB(1) receptors. *Eur. J. Pharmacol.* 450, 77–83. doi: 10.1016/S0014-2999(02)02053-8

Le Guellec, C., Benz-de Bretagne, I., Jonville-Bera, A. P., Tarfaoui, N., Andres, C. R., Gendrot, C., et al. (2012). A case of severe toxicity during coadministration of vincristine and piperacillin: are drug transporters involved in vincristine hypersensitivity and drug-drug interactions? *J. Pediatr. Hematol. Oncol.* 34, e341–e343. doi: 10.1097/MPH.0b013e318257a4ae

Leker, R. R., Peretz, T., Hubert, A., and Lossos, A. (1997). Vincristine-induced paralytic ileus in Parkinson's disease. *Parkinsonism Relat. Disord.* 3, 109–110.

Levêque, D., Santucci, R., Pavillet, J., Herbrecht, R., and Bergerat, J. P. (2009). Paralytic ileus possibly associated with interaction between ritonavir/lopinavir and vincristine. *Pharm. World Sci.* 31, 619–621. doi: 10.1007/s11096-009-9323-y

Li, K., Fichna, J., Schicho, R., Saur, D., Bashashati, M., Mackie, K., et al. (2013b). A role for O-1602 and G protein-coupled receptor GPR55 in the control of colonic motility in mice. *Neuropharmacology* 71, 255–263. doi: 10.1016/j.neuropharm.2013.03.029

Li, Y. Y., Cao, M. H., Goetz, B., Chen, C. Q., Feng, Y. J., Chen, C. J., et al. (2013a). The dual effect of cannabinoid receptor-1 deficiency on the murine postoperative ileus. *PLoS ONE* 8:e67427. doi: 10.1371/journal.pone.0067427

Li, Y. Y., Li, Y. N., Ni, J. B., Chen, C. J., Lv, S., Chai, S. Y., et al. (2010). Involvement of cannabinoid-1 and cannabinoid-2 receptors in septic ileus. *Neurogastroenterol. Motil.* 22, e350–e88. doi: 10.1111/j.1365-2982.2009.01419.x

Lin, X. H., Yuece, B., Li, Y. Y., Feng, Y. J., Feng, J. Y., Yu, L. Y., et al. (2011). A novel CB receptor GPR55 and its ligands are involved in regulation of gut movement in rodents. *Neurogastroenterol. Motil.* 23, e862–e342. doi: 10.1111/j.1365-2982.2011.01742.x

Mascolo, N., Izzo, A. A., Ligresti, A., Costagliola, A., Pinto, L., Cascio, M. G., et al. (2002). The endocannabinoid system and the molecular basis of paralytic ileus in mice. *FASEB J.* 16, 1973–1975. doi: 10.1096/fj.02-0338fje

Mason, S. L., Grant, I. A., Elliott, J., Cripps, P., and Blackwood, L. (2014). Gastrointestinal toxicity after vincristine or cyclophosphamide administered with or without maropitant in dogs: a prospective randomised controlled study. *J. Small Anim. Pract.* 55, 391–398. doi: 10.1111/jsap.12237

Mathison, R., Ho, W., Pittman, Q. J., Davison, J. S., and Sharkey, K. A. (2004). Effects of cannabinoid receptor-2 activation on accelerated gastrointestinal transit in lipopolysaccharide-treated rats. *Br. J. Pharmacol.* 142, 1247–1254. doi: 10.1038/sj.bjp.0705889

McQuade, R. M., Stojanovska, V., Donald, E., Abalo, R., Bornstein, J. C., and Nurgali, K. (2016). Gastrointestinal dysfunction and enteric neurotoxicity following treatment with anticancer chemotherapeutic agent 5-fluorouracil. *Neurogastroenterol. Motil.* 28, 1861–1875. doi: 10.1111/nmo.12890

Navari, R. M. (2013). Management of chemotherapy-induced nausea and vomiting focus on newer agents and new uses for older agents. *Drugs* 73, 249–262. doi: 10.1007/s40265-013-0019-1

Peixoto Júnior, A. A., Teles, B. C., Castro, E. F., Santos, A. A., de Oliveira, G. R., Ribeiro, R. A., et al. (2009). Vincristine delays gastric emptying and gastrointestinal transit of liquid in awake rats. *Braz. J. Med. Biol. Res.* 42, 567–573. doi: 10.1590/S0100-879X2009000600015

Rosenthal, S., and Kaufman, S. (1974). Vincristine neurotoxicity. *Ann. Intern. Med.* 80, 733–737.

Rudd, J. A., Ngan, M. P., Lu, Z., Higgins, G. A., Giuliano, C., Lovati, E., et al. (2016). Profile of antiemetic activity of netupitant alone or in combination with palonosetron and dexamethasone in ferrets and *Suncus murinus* (House Musk Shrew). *Front. Pharmacol.* 7:263. doi: 10.3389/fphar.2016.00263

Salaga, M., Abalo, R., and Fichna, J. (2017). "Cannabis and cannabinoids and the effects on gastrointestinal function: an overview," in *Handbook of Cannabis and Related Pathologies*, ed V. Preedy (London: Academic Press), c0280.

Schicho, R., and Storr, M. (2011). Alternative targets within the endocannabinoid system for future treatment of gastrointestinal diseases. *Can. J. Gastroenterol.* 25, 377–383. doi: 10.1155/2011/953975

Sharma, R. K. (1979). A study of the effect of vinca alkaloid 'vinblastine' on gastrointestinal motility in rats. *Arch. Int. Pharmacodyn. Ther.* 239, 331–339.

Sharma, R. K. (1988). Vincristine and gastrointestinal transit. *Gastroenterology* 95, 1435–1436.

Smith, B. (1967). The myenteric plexus in drug-induced neuropathy. *J. Neurol. Neurosurg. Psychiatr.* 30, 506–510.

Sninsky, C. A. (1987). Vincristine alters myoelectric activity and transit of the small intestine in rats. *Gastroenterology* 92, 472–478.

Takeda, N., Hasegawa, S., Morita, M., and Matsunaga, T. (1993). Pica in rats is analogous to emesis: an animal model in emesis research. *Pharmacol. Biochem. Behav.* 45, 817–821.

Toghill, P. J., and Burke, J. D. (1970). Death from paralytic ileus following vincristine therapy. *Postgrad. Med. J.* 46, 330–331.

Tsukamoto, A., Ohno, K., Tsukagoshi, T., Maeda, S., Nakashima, K., Fukushima, K., et al. (2011). Ultrasonographic evaluation of vincristine-induced gastric hypomotility and the prokinetic effect of mosapride in dogs. *J. Vet. Intern. Med.* 25, 1461–1464. doi: 10.1111/j.1939-1676.2011.00795.x

Turcotte, C., Blanchet, M. R., Laviolette, M., and Flamand, N. (2016). The CB2 receptor and its role as a regulator of inflammation. *Cell. Mol. Life Sci.* 73, 4449–4470. doi: 10.1007/s00018-016-2300-4

Uner, A., Ozet, A., Arpaci, F., and Unsal, D. (2005). Long-term clinical outcome after accidental overdose of multiple chemotherapeutic agents. *Pharmacotherapy* 25, 1011–1016. doi: 10.1592/phco.2005.25.7.1011

Uy, Q. L., Moens, T. H., Johns, R. J., Owens, A. H. Jr. (1967). Vincristine neurotoxicity in rodents. *Johns Hopkins Med. J.* 121, 349–360.

Vera, G., Castillo, M., Cabezos, P. A., Chiarlone, A., Martín, M. I., Gori, A., et al. (2011). Enteric neuropathy evoked by repeated cisplatin in the rat. *Neurogastroenterol. Motil.* 23, e162–e163. doi: 10.1111/j.1365-2982.2011.01674.x

Vera, G., Fichna, J., and Abalo, R. (2017). "Cannabinoids and the effects on gastrointestinal tract: a focus on motility," in *Handbook of Cannabis and Related Pathologies*, ed V. Preedy (London: Academic Press), c0570.

Vera, G., López, A. E. M., Martínez-Villaluenga, M., Cabezos, P. A., Martín-Fontelles, M. I., and Abalo, R. (2012). The CB1-selective cannabinoid antagonist AM251 partially prevents gastrointestinal dysmotility induced by the antitumoral drug vincristine in the rat. *Neurogastroenterol. Motil.* 24(Suppl. 2), 153.

Vera, G., López-Pérez, A. E., Martínez-Villaluenga, M., Cabezos, P. A., and Abalo, R. (2014). X-ray analysis of the effect of the 5-HT3 receptor antagonist granisetron on gastrointestinal motility in rats repeatedly treated with the antitumoral drug cisplatin. *Exp. Brain Res.* 232, 2601–2612. doi: 10.1007/s00221-014-3954-5

Wafai, L., Taher, M., Jovanovska, V., Bornstein, J. C., Dass, C. R., and Nurgali, K. (2013). Effects of oxaliplatin on mouse myenteric neurons and colonic motility. *Front. Neurosci.* 7:30. doi: 10.3389/fnins.2013.00030

Wang, W. S., Chiou, T. J., Liu, J. H., Fan, F. S., Yen, C. C., Chen, P. M., et al. (2000). Vincristine-induced dysphagia suggesting esophageal motor dysfunction: a case report. *Jpn. J. Clin. Oncol.* 30, 515–518. doi: 10.1093/jjco/hyd132

Waterlow, M., and Chrisp, P. (2008). Rimonabant: the evidence for its use in the treatment of obesity and the metabolic syndrome. *Core Evid.* 2, 173–187.

Wright, K. L., Duncan, M., and Sharkey, K. A. (2008). Cannabinoid CB2 receptors in the gastrointestinal tract: a regulatory system in states of inflammation. *Br. J. Pharmacol.* 153, 263–270. doi: 10.1038/sj.bjp.0707486

Yasu, T., Ohno, N., Kawamata, T., and Kurokawa, Y. (2016). Vincristine-induced paralytic ileus during induction therapy of treatment protocols for acute lymphoblastic leukemia in adult patients. *Int. J. Clin. Pharmacol. Ther.* 54, 471–473. doi: 10.5414/CP202584

Conflict of Interest Statement: The authors declare that the research was conducted in the absence of any commercial or financial relationships that could be construed as a potential conflict of interest.

15

Characterization of Cardiovascular Alterations Induced by Different Chronic Cisplatin Treatments

*Esperanza Herradón[1,2,3], Cristina González[1,2,3], José A. Uranga[3,4], Raquel Abalo[1,2,3], Mª I. Martín[1,2,3] and Visitacion López-Miranda[1,2,3]**

[1] Área de Farmacología, Nutrición y Bromatología, Facultad Ciencias de la Salud, Departamento de Ciencias Básicas de la Salud, Universidad Rey Juan Carlos, Alcorcón, Spain, [2] Unidad Asociada I+D+i del Instituto de Química Médica, Consejo Superior de Investigaciones Científicas, Madrid, Spain, [3] Grupo Interdisciplinar de Investigación en Dolor i+Dol, Universidad Rey Juan Carlos-Banco de Santander, Alcorcón, Spain, [4] Área de Histología Humana y Anatomía Patológica, Departamento de Ciencias Básicas de la Salud, Universidad Rey Juan Carlos, Alcorcón, Spain

Edited by:
Amit K. Tiwari,
University of Toledo, USA

Reviewed by:
Enzo Spisni,
University of Bologna, Italy
Giuliano Ciarimboli,
Westfälische Wilhelms-Universität Münster, Germany
Ketan Shirish Patil,
St. John's University, USA

***Correspondence:**
Visitacion Lopez-Miranda
visitacion.lopezmiranda@urjc.es

In the last years, many clinical studies have revealed that some cisplatin-treated cancer survivors have a significantly increased risk of cardiovascular events, being cisplatin-induced cardiovascular toxicity an increasing concern. The aim of the present work was to evaluate the cardiovascular alterations induced by different chronic cisplatin treatments, and to identify some of the mechanisms involved. Direct blood pressure, basal cardiac (left ventricle and coronary arteries) and vascular (aortic and mesenteric) functions were evaluated in chronic (5 weeks) saline- or cisplatin-treated male Wistar rats. Three different doses of cisplatin were tested (1, 2, and 3 mg/kg/week). Alterations in cardiac and vascular tissues were also investigated by immunohistochemistry, Western Blot, and or quantitative RT-PCR analysis. Cisplatin treatment provoked a significant modification of arterial blood pressure, heart rate, and basal cardiac function at the maximum dose tested. However, vascular endothelial dysfunction occurred at lower doses. The expression of collagen fibers and conexin-43 were increased in cardiac tissue in cisplatin-treated rats with doses of 2 and 3 mg/kg/week. The expression of endothelial nitric oxide synthase was also modified in cardiac and vascular tissues after cisplatin treatment. In conclusion, chronic cisplatin treatment provokes cardiac and vascular toxicity in a dose-dependent manner. Besides, vascular endothelial dysfunction occurs at lower doses than cardiac and systemic cardiovascular toxicity. Moreover, some structural changes in cardiac and vascular tissues are also patent even before any systemic cardiovascular alterations.

Keywords: cisplatin, cardiac toxicity, vascular toxicity, endothelial dysfunction, autonomic neuropathy

INTRODUCTION

Cancer is among the leading causes of death worldwide. However, due to advances in early recognition and novel treatment modalities, cancer survival is improving. Unfortunately, with the improvement in morbidity and mortality rates due to cancer, the increase in long-term cardiac and vascular toxicity associated with cancer treatments has become an important concern. Cardiovascular side effects negatively impact quality of life and survival of patients. Moreover, the development of toxicity may require adjustments or discontinuation of the chemotherapy regimen, leading to worse outcomes. As such, early recognition of cardiovascular dysfunctions associated to the different chemotherapeutic agents becomes imperative (Curigliano et al., 2012; Hamo and Bloom, 2015; Denegri et al., 2016).

Cis-dichlorodiamine platinum (cisplatin) is an effective and widely used chemotherapeutic agent against various solid tumors, including those affecting the bladder, testicles, and ovaries (Mollman, 1990). Sensory neuropathy and renal damage are two of the common side effects that limit therapy with cisplatin. Neural damage provoked by cisplatin involves central, peripheral, and autonomic nerves (Boogerd et al., 1990). In relation to renal injury, it has been described that this antitumoral agent causes tubular damage and tubular dysfunction with sodium, potassium, and magnesium wasting, provoking, depending on the dose administered, a reversible or an irreversible decrease in glomerular filtration (Yao et al., 2007).

Cardiovascular alterations, such as hypertension, hyperlipidemia, and coronary artery disease or myocardial infarction are additional less frequent, but equally important, factors that have been also associated with platinum-based chemotherapy. These events do not appear to be dose dependent and they may occur during treatment, shortly after treatment, or in some cases months or years after completion of chemotherapy (Pai and Nahata, 2000).

In the past few years, cisplatin-induced vascular toxicity has become an increasing concern, affecting up to 12% of patients (Gospodarowicz, 2008; Ishioka et al., 2008; Vaughn et al., 2008). Given the efficacy of cisplatin, vascular toxicity represents a significant survivorship issue. Both endothelial dysfunction of large arteries and vascular neuropathy have been discussed as etiological factors for cisplatin-induced vascular alterations (Turlapaty and Altura, 1980; Rosenfeld and Broder, 1984; Samuels et al., 1987; Serrano-Castro et al., 2000; Pretnar-Oblak et al., 2007).

Animal models exist for cisplatin-induced sensory peripheral neuropathy (Verdú et al., 1999; Authier et al., 2003; Vera et al., 2007), or cisplatin induced-nephrotoxicity (Vickers et al., 2004) and there are experimental data about the cardiac toxicity produced by acute administration of this antitumoral agent (Al-Majed et al., 2006; Yüce et al., 2007). However, to our knowledge, no experimental data has been reported so far about the cardiovascular alterations that may be developed after chronic administration of cisplatin.

The aim of the present experimental work was to evaluate the possible cardiovascular alterations induced by different chronic cisplatin treatments (at doses at which it causes neuropathy, Vera et al., 2007). Modifications on blood pressure and heart rate (HR), basal heart function, such as conduit and resistance vascular reactivity were investigated. Besides, structural and molecular mechanisms involved in these alterations were also studied.

MATERIALS AND METHODS

The Ethical Committee at Universidad Rey Juan Carlos (URJC) approved the study. Experimental procedures were carried out in accordance with the recommendations of this Committee as well as with the EU directive for the protection of animals used for scientific purpose (2010/63/UE) and Spanish regulations (RD 109 53/2013).

Animals

Male Wistar rats [240–300 g, Harlan-Iberica (Barcelona, Spain)] were placed in cages (4–6 animals) and maintained in environmentally controlled conditions (temperature of 20°C; humidity of 60%) with a 12 h light/12 h dark cycle. Animals were allowed free access to standard laboratory rat chow (Harlan-Iberica, Barcelona, Spain) and tap water, which was refreshed every day.

Treatments

After a week of adaptation to the controlled conditions, the animals were divided into four treatment groups (10–15 animals per group), saline (0.9% NaCl) and cisplatin (1, 2, and 3 mg/kg, cumulative dose of 5, 10, and 15 mg/kg, respectively). Saline or cisplatin were administered intraperitoneally once a week for five experimental weeks. The maximum injection volume administered intraperitoneally in the animals was 0.5 ml. Before each antineoplastic drug injection, 2 ml of sterile saline solution was given subcutaneously to prevent renal damage via hyperhydration (Authier et al., 2003).

The doses of cisplatin were chosen based on those commonly used in experimental protocols in rats to induce a wide range of toxic effects caused by this anticancer agent that are also observed in humans (Authier et al., 2003; Malik et al., 2006; Vera et al., 2007; Cabezos et al., 2010).

Blood Pressure and Heart Rate Measurements in Anesthetized Rats

In all the animals of the different experimental groups, after anesthesia with sodium pentobarbital (50 mg/kg intraperitoneally), a catheter coupled to a pressure transducer was inserted into the right carotid artery of the animals for direct measurements of systolic (SBP) and diastolic arterial blood pressure (DBP) and HR using a PowerLab/4e system (PanLab S.L., Barcelona, Spain). Recording of these cardiovascular parameters lasted for 10 min (Abalo et al., 2011).

After blood pressure measurements, the animals were euthanized, and the following preparations and experiments were performed.

Isolated Heart Preparation

The hearts were removed and immersed into ice-cold modified Krebs-Henseleit buffer with the following composition: 118 mM NaCl, 4.7 mM KCl, 1.2 mM $MgSO_4$, 1.2 mM KH_2PO_4, 2.5 mM $CaCl_2$, 25 mM $NaHCO_3$, and 10 mM glucose, and 2 nM pyruvate.

Afterward, they were immediately mounted on a Langendorff set-up, the aortic stump was cannulated and the heart was retrogradely perfused with the modified Krebs-Henseleit buffer. The buffer was kept at 37°C in water-heated jacketed chambers and gassed with 95% O_2/5% CO_2. The perfusion rate was adjusted to 20 ml/min with a peristaltic pump (Gilson Inc, USA). Coronary perfusion pressure (CPP) was measured by a pressure transducer fixed on a side-port of the Langendorff set-up. Left ventricular developed pressure (LVDP) was measured by a fluid-filled balloon inserted into the left ventricle and fixed to a second pressure transducer. The volume of the balloon was adjusted once at the beginning of the experiment to obtain an end diastolic pressure (EDP) of 5–10 mm Hg. Both pressure transducers were coupled to a PowerLab 4e recording system (PanLab SA, Barcelona, Spain) to measure CPP, LVDP and EDP. HR was derived from the left ventricle pressure signals (González et al., 2011). These experiments were carried out in 10–15 isolated hearts from each experimental group.

At the end of the cardiac function experiments, a portion of the left ventricle of each heart was separated, frozen at −80°C and stored for Western Blot determinations. Another portion of the left ventricle was processed for histological analysis.

Aortic Ring Preparations

The aorta was carefully excised and placed in ice-cold Krebs-Henseleit (K-H) solution with the following composition (mM) (118 NaCl; 4.75 KCl; 1.2 $MgSO_4$; 1.19 KH_2PO_4; 2.54 $CaCl_2$; 25 $NaHCO_3$; 11 glucose). All connective and perivascular adipose tissues were removed, with care taken not to disrupt the endothelium. Transverse vascular rings 3–4 mm long were prepared. The rings were fixed vertically between two stainless steel hooks and suspended in a 5-ml jacketed glass organ bath containing K-H buffer at 37°C and continuously bubbled with 95% O_2 and 5% CO_2. The upper wire was connected to an isometric force transducer (Grass FT07) and tension measurements were recorded on a computer (PowerLab/4e program). The rings were mounted with a resting tension of 2 g. Tissues were equilibrated for 90 min, during which time the medium was replaced every 15 min.

The aorta contractile and relaxant functions from animals of all the experimental groups were tested. To assess contractile function, phenylephrine (Phe) (10^{-9} M–10^{-5} M) concentration-response curves were performed. To evaluate vascular endothelium-dependent- and independent relaxation, carbachol (10^{-9} M–10^{-4} M) or sodium nitroprusside (SNP) (10^{-9} M–10^{-6} M) concentration-response curves, respectively, were established in Phe (1 μM) (submaximal) precontracted preparations (Abboud et al., 2009). Only one concentration-response curve was carried out in each preparation. The different experiments of vascular reactivity were performed in four rings of each aorta obtained from the animals of the different experimental groups.

Contraction responses of the aorta rings are expressed as mean absolute values and relaxation responses are expressed as the percentage relaxation of the tone induced by Phe.

A portion of aorta was separated, frozen at −80°C and stored for Western Blot determinations. Another portion of aorta was processed for histological analysis.

Mesenteric Perfused Bed Preparation

The abdominal cavity was opened and the superior mesenteric artery was dissected and cannulated with a blunted hypodermic needle (21 G). The mesenteric bed was perfused with 50 ml of K-H solution containing 1000 IU of heparin and was separated from the gut by carefully cutting close to the intestinal wall. The preparation was then placed on a plate (8 cm × 8 cm) in a humid chamber and perfused with K-H at a constant flow rate of 5 ml/min, using a peristaltic pump (Gilson S.A.). The solution was maintained at 37°C and continually oxygenated (95% O_2/5% CO_2). Mesenteric vascular responses were detected as changes in perfusion pressure (mm Hg). This was monitored continuously using a pressure transducer (Transpac IV, Abbot) and recorded using a PowerLab (Powerlab 400, ADinstruments). The preparation was equilibrated for 30 min before experimentation.

The experiments were carried in intact mesenteric beds. The evaluation of functionality of the vascular bed was carried out following different procedures. Mesenteric bed contractile function (Carvalho Leone and Coelho, 2004) was evaluated by a concentration response curve of Phe (10–80 nmol). The vasorelaxant function was evaluated on precontracted bed with a concentration of Phe sufficient to increase the basal perfusion pressure by 60–100 mmHg. The endothelium-dependent vasodilatation was evaluated with a concentration-response curve of carbachol (3 × 10^{-10} mol–3 × 10^{-5} mol) and endothelium-independent vasodilatation was evaluated to a concentration-response curve of SNP (10^{-11} mol–10^{-6} mol). Doses of different drugs were injected in bolus with a Hamilton syringe (volume 50 μl) (Paniagua et al., 2016). These experiments were carried out in 10–15 isolated mesenteric beds from each experimental group.

Contraction responses of superior mesenteric artery bed are expressed as mean absolute values and relaxation responses are expressed as the percentage relaxation of the tone induced by Phe.

Histological Analysis

At the end of the experimental period, samples of heart left ventricles and aorta rings were obtained from six animals per experimental group, fixed in buffered 10% formalin and embedded in paraffin. Histological damage and fibrosis were evaluated in sections 5 μm wide stained with hematoxylin-eosin stain (HE) and Masson's trichrome stain for collagen fibers, or prepared for immunohistochemistry. Samples were studied under a Zeiss Axioskop 2 microscope equipped with the image analysis software package AxioVision 4.6. The analysis was made by triplicate in 5–8 random per section and specimen fields under a 20× or 40× objective. The experimenter was blind to the treatment received by the rat from which the sample under analysis was obtained.

For immunohistochemistry, samples were washed with phosphate buffered saline (PBS) with 0.05% Tween 20 (Calbiochem, Darmstadt, Germany). Thereafter sections were incubated for 10 min in 3% (vol vol^{-1}) in hydrogen peroxide to inhibit endogenous peroxidase activity and blocked with 1% PBS-BSA (bovine serum albumin) or calf serum for 30 min to minimize non-specific binding of the primary antibody. Pilot experiments performed to determine the optimal antibody dilution showed that some samples needed to be pretreated by boiling in 10 mM citrate buffer for 30 min. Sections were then incubated overnight at 4°C with the following antibodies: monoclonal mouse anti-human connexin-43 (1:800; Santa

Cruz Biotechnology, Santa Cruz, CA, USA); polyclonal rabbit anti-human eNOS (1:50; Novus Biologicals). After incubation, samples were washed with PBS-Tween. The peroxidase-based kit Masvision (Master Diagnostica, Granada, Spain) was used as secondary antibody. Samples were counterstained with hematoxylin and coverslips mounted with Eukitt mounting media (O. Kindler GmbH & Co., Freiburg, Germany). To determine the level of non-specific staining, the preparations were incubated without the primary antibody.

Western Blot Analysis

For protein extraction, cardiac and aorta tissues (6–8 samples from 6 to 8 animals per group) were homogenized with ice-cold RIPA buffer containing 1 mM EGTA, 1 mM Na_3VO_4, 1 mM $Na_4P_2O_7$, 10 mM NaF and a protease inhibitor cocktail (Roche, Spain). The homogenates were centrifuged (9300 × *g*, 10 min, 4°C) and the supernatant was extracted. Total protein values were quantified from all preparations using the Bradford method (Somoza et al., 2007).

Aorta (50 μg) and left ventricle (40 μg) samples were separated by electrophoresis on a 4–20% (aorta) or 10% (left ventricle tissue) Mini-protean® TGX™ Precast Gel (Bio-Rad, Spain) and transferred onto a PVDF membrane. The membranes were blocked with 3% fat-free milk at room temperature for 1 h and then incubated at 4°C overnight with primary antibody as follows: eNOS 1:250 (aorta), 1:500 (left ventricle tissue; BD Transduction Laboratories), connexin-43 (1:10000; left ventricle tissue; Santa Cruz Biotechnology, Santa Cruz, CA, USA), plasminogen activator inhibitor-1 (PAI-1) 1:500 (aorta, left ventricle tissue; Abcam, Cambridge, UK) and GAPDH 1:1000 (aorta, left ventricle tissue); Santa Cruz Biotechnology, Santa Cruz, CA, USA). These incubations were followed by incubation for 1 h at room temperature with an alkaline phosphatase-conjugated goat anti-mouse secondary antibody (1:10000) and subsequent treatment with ECF reagent (Thermo Fisher Scientific, USA). Protein bands were detected using Typhoon 9210 (GE Healthcare Life Sciences, USA) and the band intensity was assessed with ImageJ software (National Institutes of Health, USA). GAPDH was used as an internal control.

Quantitative Real-time PCR Analysis

mRNAs were evaluated by quantitative real-time PCR. Total RNA was extracted from frozen cardiac and aorta tissues in Trizol reagent according to the manufacturer's specifications (Invitrogen Life Technologies). The RNA concentrations were calculated by measuring the absorbance readings using Nanodrop Spectrophotometer ND-1000 (Nanodrop Technologies Inc., Willington, DE, USA). A total of 1 μg of RNA was reverse transcribed into cDNA using the High Capacity cDNA Archive Kit (Applied Biosystems) according to manufacturer's instructions in a 20 μl reaction. PCR was performed in duplicate for each sample using 4.5 μl of diluted cDNA as template, 0.5 μl of 20x specific primers/probe mix and 2x SSO Advanced Universal Probes Supermix (Bio-Rad) in a 10 μl reaction. The amplification was carried out in an ABI 7500 Fast System (Life Technologies) by using the following conditions: 30 s, 95°C, 40 cycles (10 s 95°C, 30 s 60°C) in fast mode. As specific oligonucleotide primers and Taqman probes to detect amplification, we used Taqman Gene Expression Assays (Life Technologies): eNOS (Rn02132634_s1) and connexin-43 (Rn01433957_m1). As normalizing internal control, we amplified ribosomal 18S RNA. These determinations were carried out in five samples from five animals per group.

Statistical Analysis

Data represent the mean ± SEM of observations obtained from 10 to 15 animals for *in vivo* and *in vitro* studies and 5–8 preparations (from different animals) for histological, Western Blot and quantitative real-time PCR analysis (*n*). Statistically significant differences were determined using by two-way or one-way analysis of variance followed by Bonferroni/Dunn *post hoc* test (Prism 4). *P*-values ≤ 0.05 were considered significant.

Drugs

Cisplatin, phenylephrine, carbachol, and sodium nitroprusside were obtained from Sigma (Sigma Chemical Company, Poole, Dorset, UK).

Phenylephrine, carbachol, and sodium nitroprusside were dissolved in distilled water. Cisplatin was dissolved in saline (0.9% NaCl).

RESULTS

Effect of Chronic Cisplatin Treatment on Blood Pressure and Heart Rate

Figure 1 shows the SBP, DBP, and HR in anesthetized rats after repeated treatment with saline or cisplatin at the three different doses evaluated.

Saline-treated rats had normotensive values for SBP (110.72 ± 8.10 mmHg, $n = 15$) and DBP (76.26 ± 5.35 mm Hg, $n = 15$) and normal HR (332.28 ± 37.82 beats/minute, $n = 15$). Cisplatin treatment caused only blood pressure alterations at the maximum dose administered (15 mg, cumulative dose), provoking, at this dose, a significant decrease in DBP (47.53 ± 11.08 mmHg, $n = 10$ $P < 0.05$ vs. control saline group) without modifying SBP (92.14 ± 14.15 mmHg, $n = 10$ $P > 0.05$ vs. control saline group) and HR (254.72 ± 20.82 beats/minute, $n = 10$ $P > 0.05$ vs. control saline group) (**Figure 1**).

Effect of Chronic Cisplatin Treatment on Heart Function

Figure 2 shows the baseline cardiac values of left ventricle function (LVDP and EDP) and coronary flow (CPP) in the different groups of rats treated with saline or cisplatin at the three doses evaluated.

In saline treated rats, the LDVP was 90.57 ± 11.10 mmHg, $n = 12$, the EDP was 8.79 ± 2.98 mmHg, $n = 12$ and the CPP was 90.91 ± 5.21 mmHg, $n = 12$. Cisplatin only caused significant cardiac alterations at the maximum dose administered (15 mg, cumulative dose), provoking at this dose, a significant decrease in contractile and relaxant function (as the increase in EDP showed) of the left ventricle (LVDP and EDP, respectively) (LVDP:

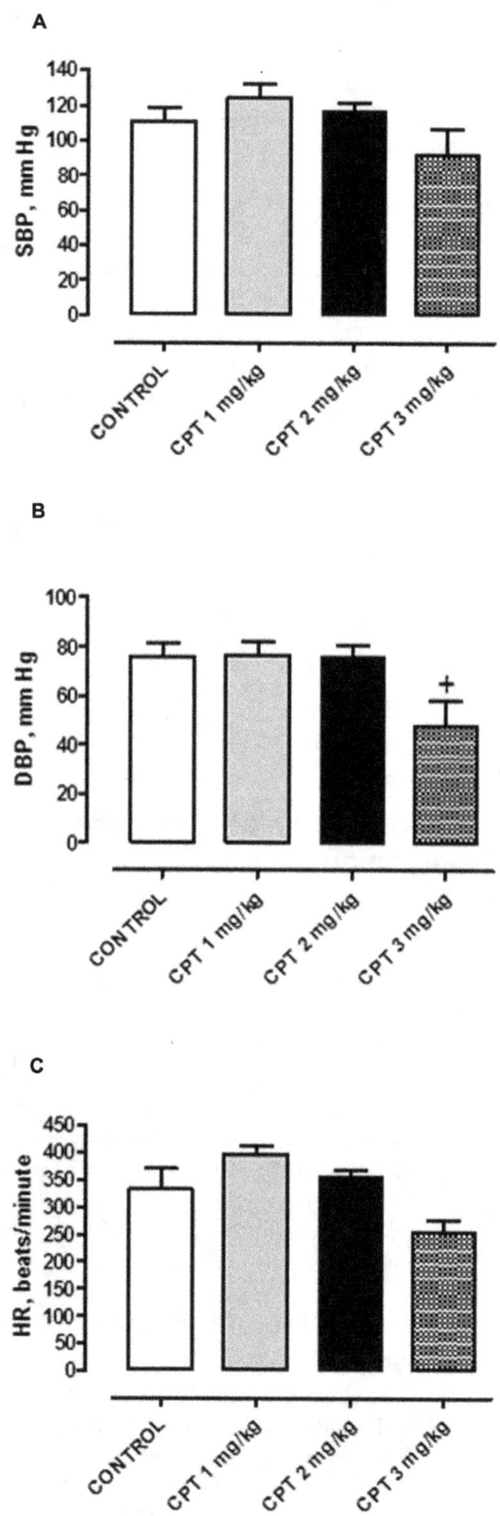

FIGURE 1 | (A) Systolic blood pressure (SBP), **(B)** diastolic blood pressure (DBP), and **(C)** heart rate (HR) of anesthetized animals chronically treated with saline (CONTROL) or cisplatin (CPT) 1 mg/kg, 2 mg/kg or 3 mg/kg. Data represent the mean ± SEM, $n = 10$–15 animals per experimental group. A one-way ANOVA followed by Bonferroni/Dunn *post hoc* test was used for statistical analysis ($^{+}P < 0.05$, CPT 3 mg/kg vs. control).

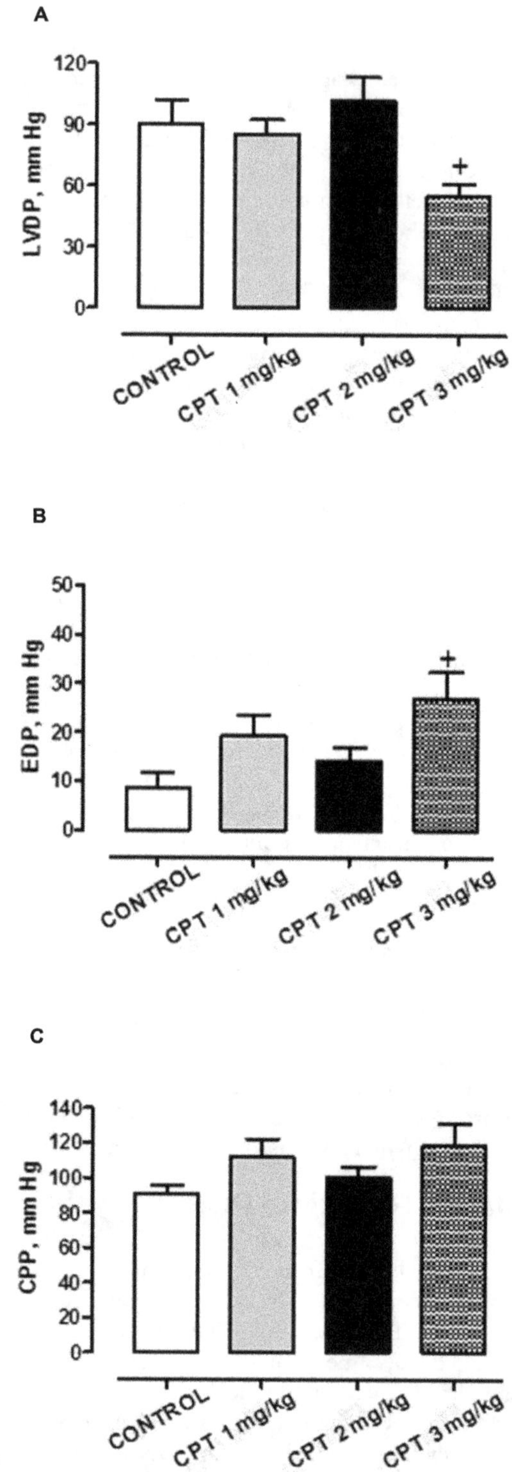

FIGURE 2 | Basal values of (A) left ventricular developed pressure (LVDP), **(B)** end diastolic pressure (EDP), and **(C)** coronary perfusion pressure (CPP) of isolated hearts from animals chronically treated with saline (CONTROL) or cisplatin (CPT) 1 mg/kg, 2 mg/kg or 3 mg/kg. Data represent the mean ± SEM, $n = 10$–15 preparations per experimental group. A one-way ANOVA followed by Bonferroni/Dunn *post hoc* test was used for statistical analysis ($^{+}P < 0.05$, CPT 3 mg/kg vs. control).

55.45 ± 6.09 mmHg, $n = 10$ $P < 0.05$; EDP: 27.03 ± 5.51 mmHg, $n = 10$ $P < 0.05$ vs. control saline group) without affecting CPP in comparison with saline treated rats (CPP: 119.17 ± 12.19 mm Hg, $n = 10$ $P > 0.05$ vs. control saline group).

Effect of Chronic Cisplatin Treatment on Aortic Vascular Function

Figure 3 shows the contractile function (measured as response to Phe), the endothelial-dependent relaxation (measured as response to carbachol) and the endothelial-independent relaxation (measured as response to SNP) in the isolated aorta (a conduit vessel) of the rats from the different groups treated with saline or cisplatin at the three doses evaluated.

In the saline-treated group, Phe provoked a concentration-dependent increase in aortic vascular tone resulting in an R_{max} value of 1.16 ± 0.05 g ($n = 15$), carbachol caused an endothelial-dependent concentration-dependent decrease in aortic vascular tone resulting in a R_{max} value of 80.70 ± 3.30% ($n = 15$), and SNP caused an endothelial-independent concentration-dependent decrease in aortic vascular tone resulting in a R_{max} value of 117.74 ± 2.01% ($n = 15$). The weekly chronic administration of cisplatin at the three doses assayed, 1, 2, and 3 mg/kg for 5 weeks (cumulative dose of 5, 10, and 15 mg, respectively) did not affect the aortic vasoconstrictor response to Phe (**Figure 3A**), but provoked a clear and significant inhibition of the carbachol-mediated vasorelaxant response at the doses of 2 and 3 mg/kg, but not at the dose of 1 mg/kg of cisplatin. It is important to mention that the inhibition of the endothelial dependent vasorelaxation was similar at the two higher cisplatin doses evaluated (2 and 3 mg/kg) (**Figure 3B**). However, the endothelial-independent vasorelaxation was only affected by chronic treatment with cisplatin at the maximum dose assayed (3 mg/kg), which showed a significant potentiation of this vasorelaxation in aorta rings from rats treated with this particular dose of the antitumoral agent (**Figure 3C**).

Effect of Chronic Cisplatin Treatment on Mesenteric Vascular Function

Figure 4 shows the contractile function (measured as response to Phe), the endothelial-dependent relaxation (measured as response to carbachol) and the endothelial-independent relaxation (measured as response to SNP) in the perfused mesenteric bed (a resistance vascular territory) of the rats from the different groups treated with saline or cisplatin at the three doses evaluated.

In the saline-treated group, Phe provoked a concentration-dependent increase in mesenteric vascular tone resulting in an R_{max} value of 99.13 ± 5.45 mm Hg ($n = 10$), carbachol caused an endothelial-dependent concentration-dependent decrease in mesenteric vascular tone resulting in a R_{max} value of 70.70 ± 4.07% ($n = 12$), and SNP caused an endothelial-independent concentration-dependent decrease in mesenteric vascular tone resulting in a R_{max} value of 83.47 ± 3.02% ($n = 10$). The results obtained in this representative resistance territory were different from those obtained in the conduit vessel, the

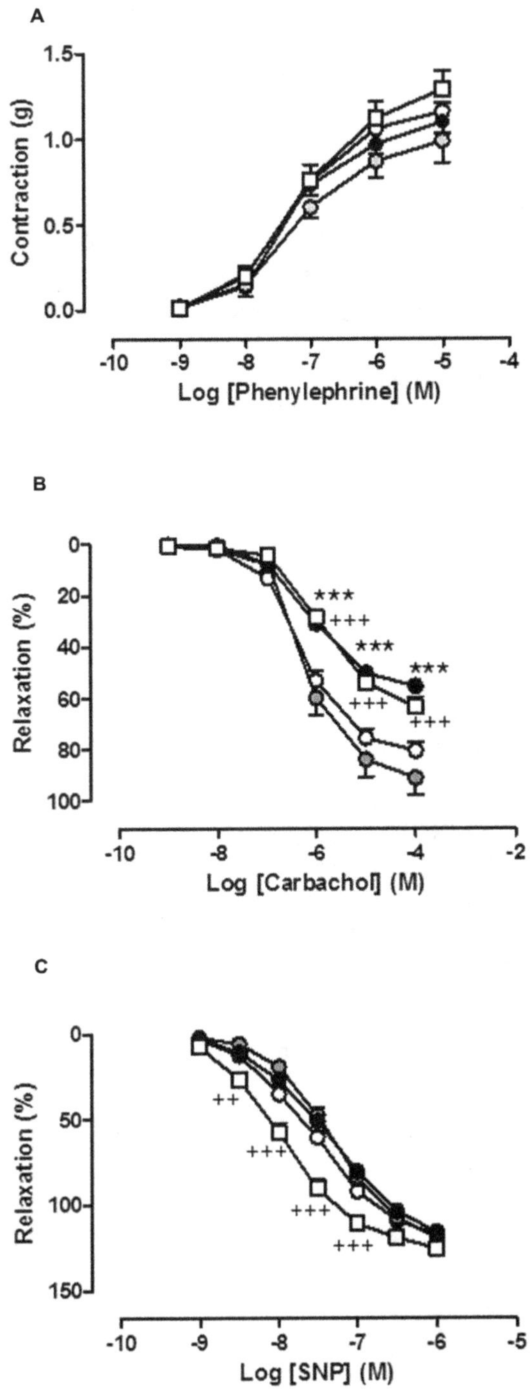

FIGURE 3 | (A) Concentration-response curve of phenylephrine (10^{-9} M–10^{-5} M), **(B)** concentration-response curve of carbachol (10^{-9} M–10^{-4} M), and **(C)** concentration-response curve of sodium nitroprusside (SNP) (10^{-9} M–10^{-6} M) in isolated rat aorta rings from animals chronically treated with saline (CONTROL, white circles) or cisplatin (CPT) 1 mg/kg (gray circles), 2 mg/kg (black circles) or 3 mg/kg (white squares). Values are expressed as mean ± SEM, $n = 10$–15 preparations per experimental group. A two-way ANOVA followed by Bonferroni/Dunn *post hoc* test was used for statistical analysis ($^{***}P < 0.001$, CPT 2 mg/kg vs. control; $^{++}P < 0.01$, $^{+++}P < 0.001$ CPT 3 mg/kg vs. control).

aorta. The weekly chronic administration of cisplatin provoked a significant decrease in the mesenteric vasoconstrictor response to Phe at the highest dose of cisplatin assayed (3 mg/kg) (**Figure 4A**), but did not provoke any modification in the endothelial-dependent or independent vasorelaxant function in mesenteric bed at any of the cisplatin doses evaluated (**Figures 4B,C**).

Cardiovascular Alterations Induced by Chronic Cisplatin Treatment: Structural and Molecular Mechanisms Involved

Cisplatin treatment evoked a clear damage in the structure of cardiac fibers (**Figures 5A,B**). Normal cardiac architecture was altered when increasing the dose of cisplatin, appearing rippled cardiomyocytes and fibrils de-arrangement. Similarly, connexin-43 expression was also modified showing a more intense and more diffused location with the higher dose of cisplatin, 3 mg/kg (**Figures 5C,D**). Western blot analysis also revealed that the expression of connexin-43 in cardiac left ventricle was significantly increased at the cisplatin doses of 2 mg/kg ($P < 0.05$) and 3 mg/kg compared with the control group ($P < 0.001$) (**Figure 6A**). Furthermore, connexin-43 expression was significantly increased in the cisplatin 3 mg/kg group in comparison with the cisplatin 2 mg/kg group ($P < 0.05$). However, no changes in connexin-43 mRNA levels were detected at the two different doses of cisplatin evaluated in comparison with control group (**Figure 6B**). On the other hand, histological preparations showed that cardiac eNOS expression was more heterogeneous after cisplatin treatment (**Figures 5E,F**). Western blot analysis showed that this eNOS expression was significantly decreased at the doses of cisplatin 2 mg/kg and 3 mg/kg compared with the control group ($P < 0.001$) (**Figure 6C**), while eNOS mRNA level was significantly decrease only at the dose of 3 mg/kg, but not at the dose of 2 mg/kg compared with the control group ($P < 0.01$) (**Figure 6D**).

An elevated level of PAI-1 is also an important diagnostic marker of cardiac fibrosis (Ghosh and Vaughan, 2012). For that, the cardiac expression of PAI-1 was analyzed in this study. There was not any change in the cardiac expression of PAI-1 in both, cisplatin 2 and 3 mg/kg treated animals with respect to the control group ($P > 0.05$) (**Figure 7**).

Regarding the aorta, the morphological analysis showed changes in the fiber arrangement in the tunica media, losing their uneven appearance (**Figures 8A,B**). eNOS staining was strongly located in endothelium with certain positive areas in tunica media that disappeared in the animals treated with cisplatin 3 mg/kg (**Figures 8C,D**). However, the cisplatin treatments did not provoke any modification either in aorta expression of eNOS or in the eNOS mRNA levels in comparison with the control group ($P > 0.05$) (**Figures 9A,B**). The expression on PAI-1 was also analyzed in aorta tissue in the different experimental groups. Aortic expression of PAI-1 was slightly, but not significantly, increased at the two different doses of cisplatin evaluated in relation to the control group (**Figure 9C**).

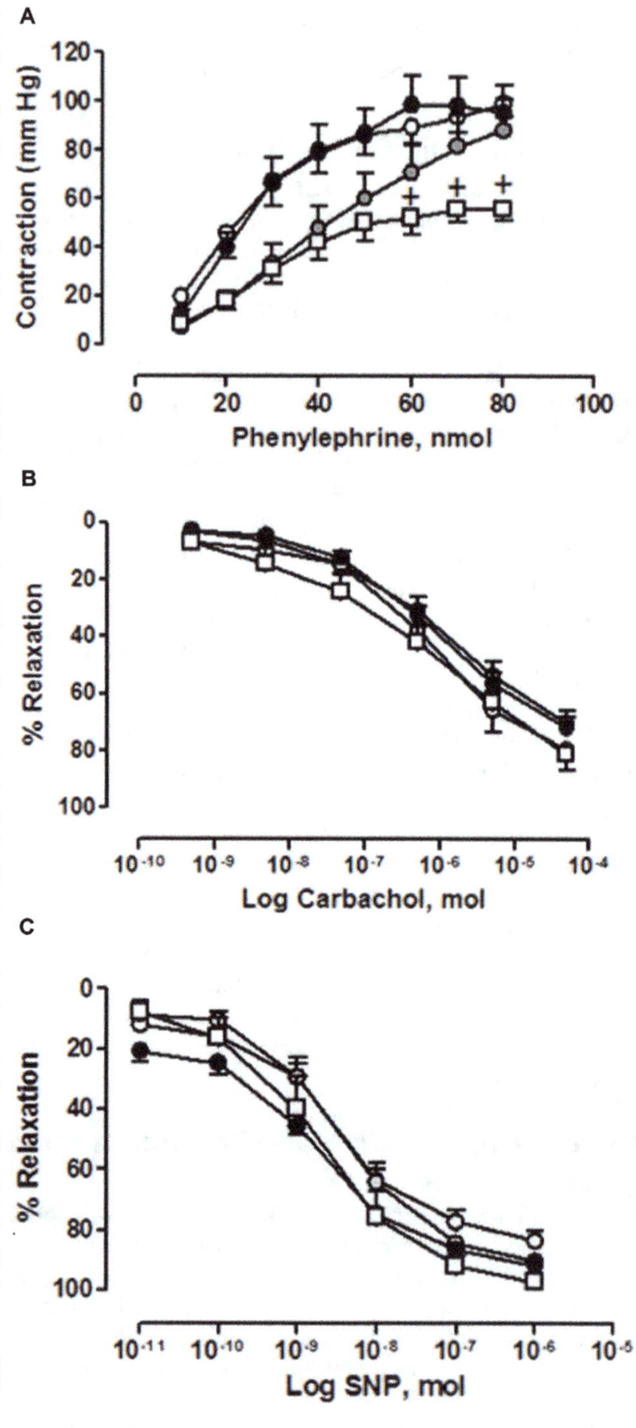

FIGURE 4 | (A) Concentration-response curve of phenylephrine (10 nmol–80 nmol), **(B)** concentration-response curve of carbachol (3×10^{-10} mol–3×10^{-5} mol) and **(C)** concentration-response curve of sodium nitroprusside (SNP) (3×10^{-11} mol–3×10^{-6} mol) in perfused mesenteric bed from animals chronically treated with saline (CONTROL, white circles) or cisplatin (CPT) at 1 mg/kg (gray circles), 2 mg/kg (black circles) or 3 mg/kg (white squares). Values are expressed as mean ± SEM, n = 10–15 preparations per experimental group. A two-way ANOVA followed by Bonferroni/Dunn *post hoc* test was used for statistical analysis ($^{+}P < 0.05$, CPT 3 mg/kg vs. control).

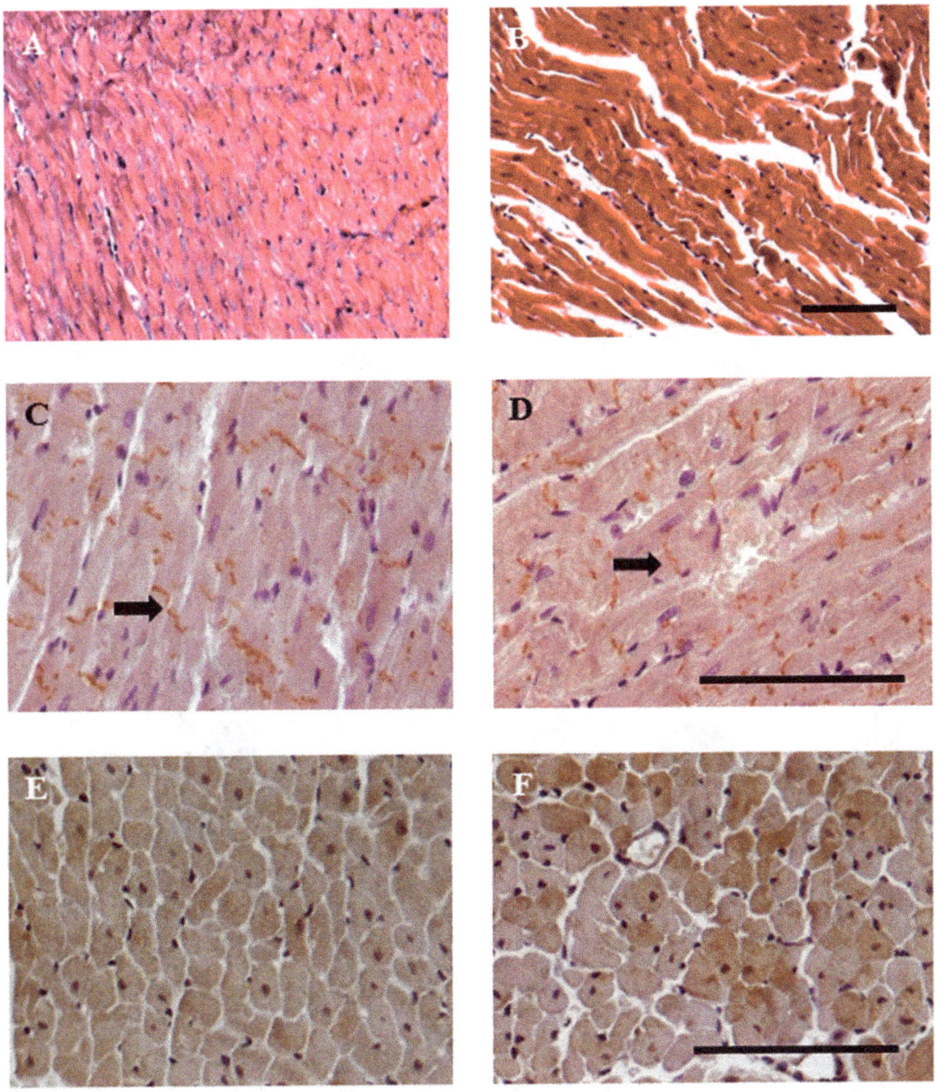

FIGURE 5 | Representative images of histology and immunohistochemistry of the effect of cisplatin treatment on rat hearts. Rats were injected intraperitoneally for 5 weeks with saline (0.9% NaCl, left column) or cisplatin (3 mg/kg week^{-1}, right column). Histological samples embedded in paraffin and stained with Masson's trichrome **(A,B)**. Samples processed for immunohistochemistry with anti connexin-43 antibody (black arrows) **(C,D)** and with anti eNOS **(E,F)**. Heterogenicity in fiber staining is clearly seen. Bar: 100 μm.

DISCUSSION

This study shows that the chronic treatment with cisplatin causes dose-dependent cardiovascular alterations. Vascular toxicity occurs at lower doses than cardiac or systemic cardiovascular alterations. The cisplatin induced-vascular toxicity could be cataloged as "silent" because it occurs even in the absence of any systemic cardiovascular modifications. At high doses of cisplatin treatment, vascular toxicity is maintained and cardiac and blood pressure alterations are present. Cisplatin treatment also produced alterations in the structure of cardiac and vascular tissue, suggesting a direct cytotoxicity. Changes in connexin-43 and eNOS expression could be related with cardiac functional alterations after cisplatin treatments.

In recent years, many clinical studies have noted that some cisplatin-treated cancer survivors have a significantly increased risk of cardiovascular events (Ishioka et al., 2008; Vaughn et al., 2008), cisplatin-induced cardiovascular toxicity being an increasing concern. Although, there are some experimental data in cardiac toxicity induced after acute administration of cisplatin (Al-Majed et al., 2006; Yüce et al., 2007), there are no experimental studies specifically evaluating cardiovascular alterations after chronic cisplatin treatment, and studying, at the same time, mechanisms involved in these particular alterations.

As a first approximation, the present study evaluated general cardiovascular parameters (blood pressure and HR) in different cisplatin chronic treatments (1, 2, and 3 mg/kg). The results show

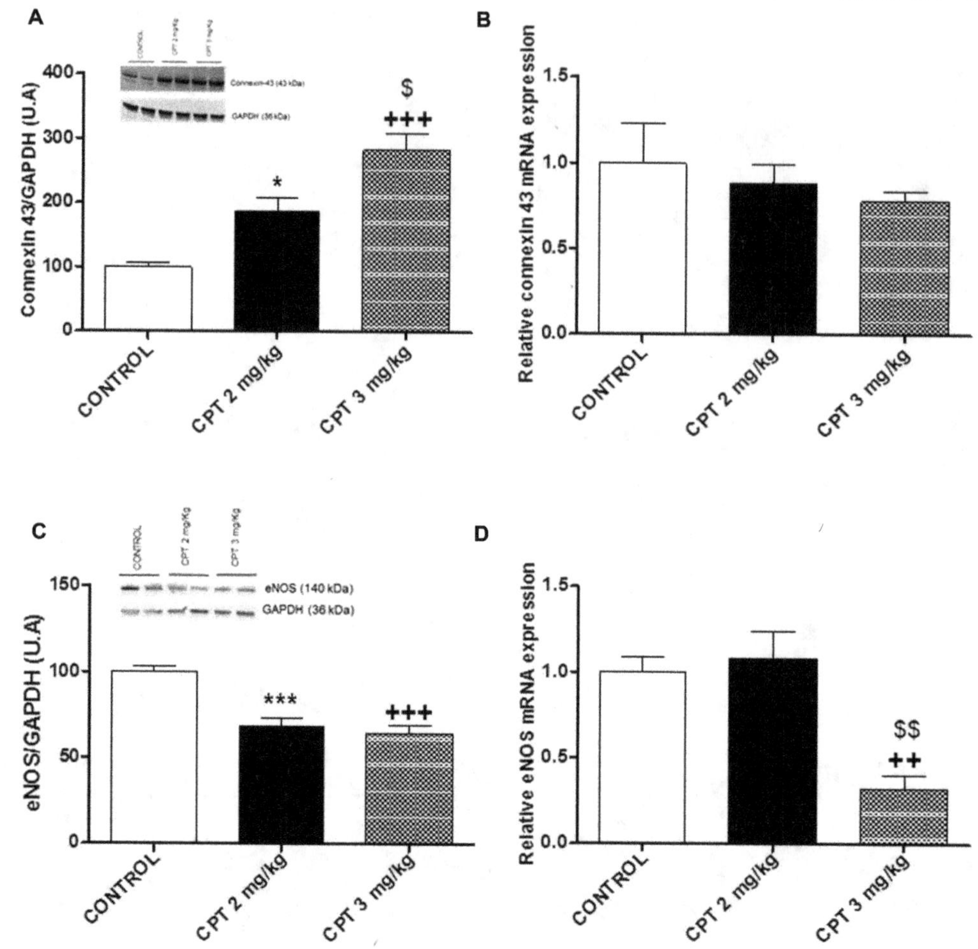

FIGURE 6 | (A) Representative immunoblots for connexin-43 protein expression in whole cardiac left ventricle. Diagram bars show the results of densitometric analysis of connexin-43 in whole cardiac left ventricle. Homogenized samples from heart show essentially the connexin-43 in its phosphorylated form (strongest bands for the quantification) **(B)** Quantitative analysis of connexin-43 mRNA levels in whole cardiac left ventricle. **(C)** Representative immunoblots for eNOS protein expression. Diagram bars show the results of densitometric analysis of eNOS in whole cardiac left ventricle. **(D)** Quantitative analysis of eNOS mRNA levels in whole cardiac left ventricle Data are presented as means ± SEM of observations obtained for 5–8 tissue samples from 5 to 8 animals per treatment. A one-way ANOVA followed by Bonferroni/Dunn *post hoc* test was used for statistical analysis ($^{*}P < 0.05$, CPT 2 mg/kg vs. control, $^{***}P < 0.001$, CPT 2 mg/kg vs. control, $^{+++}P < 0.001$, CPT 3 mg/kg vs. control, $^{\$}P < 0.05$, CPT 3 mg/kg vs. CPT 2 mg/Kg, $^{\$\$}P < 0.01$, CPT 3 mg/kg vs. CPT 2 mg/Kg).

that, at the highest dose of the antitumor drug used, a significant decrease in the DBP and a slight, although not significant bradycardia occur. SBP was not modified after treatments, and HR was not altered after low and intermediate cisplatin doses assayed. It was demonstrated that cisplatin chronic treatment at similar doses (1–3 mg/kg) than those evaluated in the present work caused peripheral sensory and enteric autonomic neuropathy (Vera et al., 2011, 2013). Our results show that cisplatin chronic treatment could also provoke an autonomic cardiovascular neuropathy resulting in a decrease in DBP and slight bradycardia, pointing out that this cardiovascular autonomic neuropathy occurs at higher doses than the sensory or enteric neuropathies that have been shown at treatment doses of cisplatin of 1 and 2 mg/kg (Vera et al., 2011, 2013). Different authors describe that cisplatin induced severe bradycardia in humans (Darling, 2015; Schlumbrecht and Hehr, 2015; Kounis et al., 2016), and other authors describe, after a single injection of cisplatin (7 mg/kg) in rats, cardiac alterations that include a decrease in blood pressure as well as a decrease in HR, due to the cardiotoxicity that cisplatin produces in the sinoatrial node, which leads to bradycardia (El-Sawalhi and Ahmed, 2014). On the other hand, cisplatin causes nephrotoxicity primarily causing tubulointerstitial lesions that provoke the urine waste of electrolytes (Vickers et al., 2004; Yao et al., 2007). Besides, it has also been demonstrated that most cisplatin-treated patients waste sodium, potassium, magnesium, and calcium in their urine and some have orthostatic hypotension (Lajer and Daugaard, 1999; Goren, 2003). In our study, renal toxicity has not been evaluated, but it is possible that both phenomena, cardiac and renal toxicities, were also related. In fact, understanding the mechanisms of cisplatin-induced renal and cardiac toxicities may help provide better treatment and preventive strategies

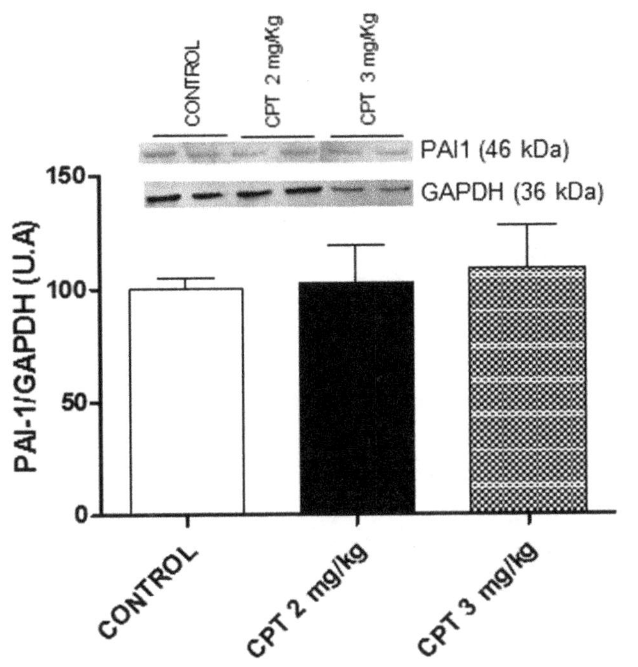

FIGURE 7 | Representative immunoblots for plasminogen activator inhibitor-1 (PAI-1) protein expression in whole cardiac left ventricle. Diagram bars show the result of densitometric analysis of PAI-1 in whole cardiac left ventricle. Data are presented as means ± SEM of observations obtained of 6–8 tissue samples from 6 to 8 animals per treatment. A one-way ANOVA followed by Bonferroni/Dunn *post hoc* test was used for statistical analysis.

(Dugbartey et al., 2016). More research is needed to investigate this aspect. It is important to note that the fact that neither SBP nor HR were modified could suggest that we detected cisplatin-induced cardiovascular neurotoxicity still at an initial developmental stage.

In cancer patients treated with chemotherapy, there is greater cardiovascular morbidity and mortality than in the general population, especially and worryingly in patients younger than 45 (van den Belt-Dusebout et al., 2006). The most evaluated cardiac toxicity is that produced by anthracyclines (Hirano et al., 1993; Soga et al., 2006; Berdichevski et al., 2010; Shaker and Sourour, 2010). However, this cardiotoxicity is not unique to this group of antineoplastic drugs, but may occur with other antitumoral agent groups (Al-Majed et al., 2006; Drimal et al., 2006; Hernández-Esquivel et al., 2006; Sudharsan et al., 2006), including cisplatin (Pai and Nahata, 2000). It was reported that treatment with a single dose of cisplatin causes left ventricular dysfunction and depression of cardiomyocyte contractility in the rat. These alterations may be related to mitochondrial function, oxidative stress and an increase in apoptosis (Ma et al., 2010; El-Sawalhi and Ahmed, 2014). The results obtained in this study confirm that chronic cisplatin produces a significant decrease in cardiac contractility, associated with a decrease in dilatory left ventricular function. Moreover, this left ventricular dysfunction could be related to the decrease in DBP observed after cisplatin at 3 mg/kg/week. Other authors, using similar or even lower doses but in an acute administration pattern, obtained similar results (Ma et al., 2010; Ciftci et al., 2011; El-Awady et al., 2011; Hussein et al., 2012; Coskun et al., 2014; El-Sawalhi and Ahmed, 2014).

In this study, it has been also evaluated the possible mechanism involved in the left ventricular dysfunction observed after cisplatin treatment. Connexins are structural proteins that bind to form gap bonds in vertebrates, and connexin-43 is a member of this family. Gap junctions allow the passage of small ions and molecules, directly connecting the cytoplasm of adjacent cells, and are of special importance in the heart, since they make possible the coordinated depolarization of the cardiac muscle. An increase in the expression of connexin-43 has been described in cisplatin-resistant tumor cell lines, which seems to be linked to the resistance of the cells to this drug (Li et al., 2006). However, the expression of this protein in cardiac tissue of animals treated with cisplatin has not been extensively studied. Our results show that cardiac architecture was altered when increasing the dose of cisplatin, with occurrence of rippled cardiomyocytes and fibrils de-arrangement. Moreover, an increase in connexin-43 expression in hearts of cisplatin-treated animals was observed with the dose of 2 mg/kg and higher. This data suggests that cisplatin can produce direct cytotoxicity in cardiac cells and that they can respond with an increase of connexin-43. Other authors have also described the cytotoxicity of acute (10 mg/kg) or chronic (4 mg/kg one a week for 4 weeks) administration of cisplatin that resulted in structural alterations in cardiac tissue in which separated cardiac muscles with interruption of myofibrils and severe interstitial hemorrhages or fibrosis were observed (Jiang et al., 2014; Saleh et al., 2015). It is important to note that connexin-43 RNAm levels were not modified after the antitumoral treatments. It is possible that alterations in some transcription and post-transcriptional factors or inhibition of connexin-43 degradation play a role in the regulation of connexin expression (Salameh et al., 2004).

It is known that an elevated level of PAI-1 is also an important profibrotic marker of cardiac fibrosis (Ghosh and Vaughan, 2012); and that an increased expression of myocardium PAI-1 contributes to ventricular remodeling and fibrosis that could be related to ventricular dysfunction (Takeshita et al., 2004; Shimizu et al., 2016). The result of the present study show that PAI-1 cardiac expression was not modified after the different cisplatin treatments, what could suggest that cardiac alterations in our experimental protocol were at an incipient stage. Other authors have described an increase of PAI-1 in cardiomyocytes treated with other chemotherapeutic agents as doxorubicin (Ghosh et al., 2016).

On the other hand, heart eNOS was heterogeneously distributed and eNOS expression and eNOS mRNA levels were diminished after cisplatin treatment at the higher doses assayed. Our data are in agreement with those showed by Saleh et al. (2015) that also described a significantly decrease in nitric oxide levels in heart homogenates after chronic cisplatin treatments. However, after acute cisplatin administration, other authors show a significant increase in the level of nitric oxide in heart (Jiang et al., 2014). It is possible that the repeated pattern of administration used in this study can ameliorate this increase. Besides, it is known that overproduction of

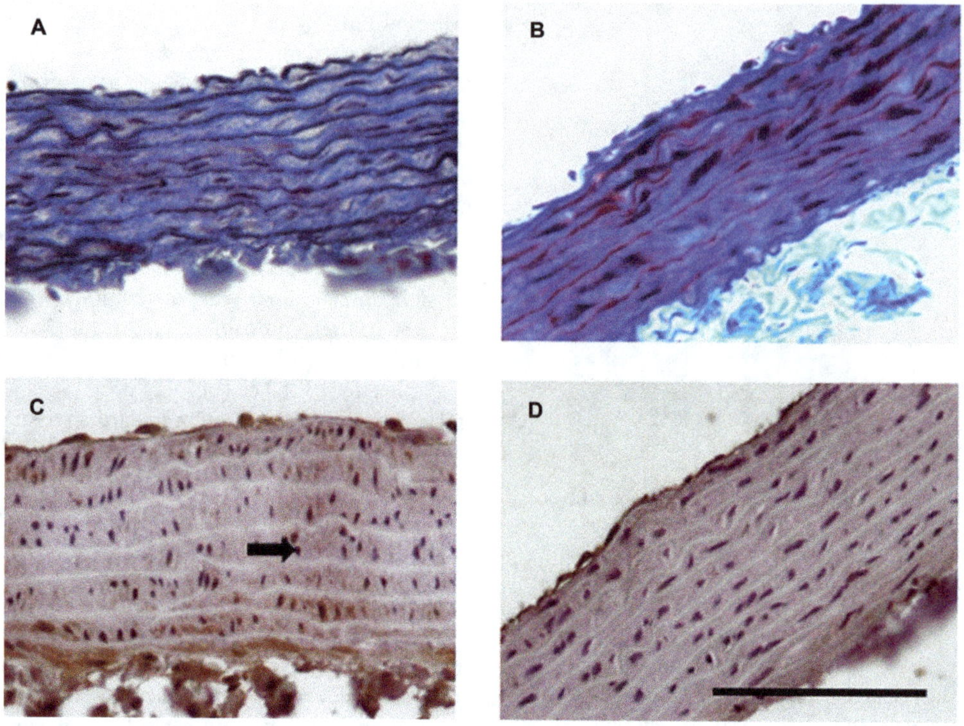

FIGURE 8 | Representative images of histology and immunohistochemistry of the effect of cisplatin treatment on rat aorta. Rats were injected intraperitoneally for 5 weeks with saline (0.9% NaCl, left column) or cisplatin (3 mg/kg week^{-1}, right column). Histological samples embedded in paraffin and stained with Masson's trichrome **(A,B)**. Samples processed for immunohistochemistry with anti eNOS antibody **(C,D)**. Bar: 100 μm.

nitric oxide was directly linked to heart damage in other models of chemotherapeutic agents-induced cardiotoxicity, as in cyclophosphamide (Mythili et al., 2004), and doxorubicin (Ghibu et al., 2012). However, our data suggest that chronic cisplatin treatment does not cause this increase. More research is needed to evaluate more deeply this alteration.

Regarding functionality of blood vessels, the results obtained showed that chronic cisplatin treatment provoked an altered vascular relaxant but not vascular contractile function in aorta, indicating the presence of a clear endothelial dysfunction in a large artery. This endothelial dysfunction did not occur at the low dose evaluated of the chemotherapeutic agent but was present at 2 and 3 mg/kg. It is important to note that the magnitude of this endothelial dysfunction is not dose-dependent since the doses of 2 and 3 mg/kg induced a similar decrease in the endothelial function. Endothelial dysfunction in large arteries has been also described in humans (Turlapaty and Altura, 1980; Rosenfeld and Broder, 1984; Samuels et al., 1987; Serrano-Castro et al., 2000; Pretnar-Oblak et al., 2007). On the other hand, endothelium-independent vasorelaxation in aorta was augmented by the maximum dose of cisplatin evaluated, which indicates a greater facility of cisplatin to produce direct relaxation in vascular smooth muscle at this dose. Recently, it has been described, in rats, that cisplatin (200 μM) decreased contractile function in thoracic aorta and that this effect was caused by a severe damage to blood vessel walls (Jiang et al., 2014). This fact could explain the potentiation of endothelial-independent vasorelaxation observed in our study in aorta after the administration of 3 mg/kg of cisplatin. However, this fact is in contrast with the endothelial dysfunction observed. The resistance vascular territory was differently affected by chronic cisplatin treatment. Thus, in the mesenteric vascular bed, cisplatin treatment did not provoke any modification in the vasorelaxant function at any of the three different cisplatin doses evaluated, but caused a significant reduction in the vasocontractile function of this vascular bed that is compatible with the existence of an autonomic neuropathy at this level. In fact, Authier and Coworkers pointed out that peripheral nerve conduction velocities were decreased in cisplatin (3 mg/kg) treated rats (Authier et al., 2003). Moreover, in cisplatin-treated patients a similar decrease in nerve conduction velocity occurred after cumulative doses of 200–400 mg/m^2 (Boogerd et al., 1990). It is possible that cumulative cisplatin doses of 10 or 15 mg/kg are not high enough to produce this altered alpha-vasoconstrictor response in large vessels, whereas resistance territories may be more sensitive to its neuronal toxicity. In the literature, there is no experimental data about cisplatin toxicity on resistance vascular vessels, to which we could compare the result obtained in the present work. More research is needed to completely establish the differences found between resistance and large vascular territories in contractile function after cisplatin treatments.

Regarding the endothelial dysfunction observed only in large but not in resistance vessels, it is possible that vascular endothelial dysfunction in large vessels occurs prior to vascular

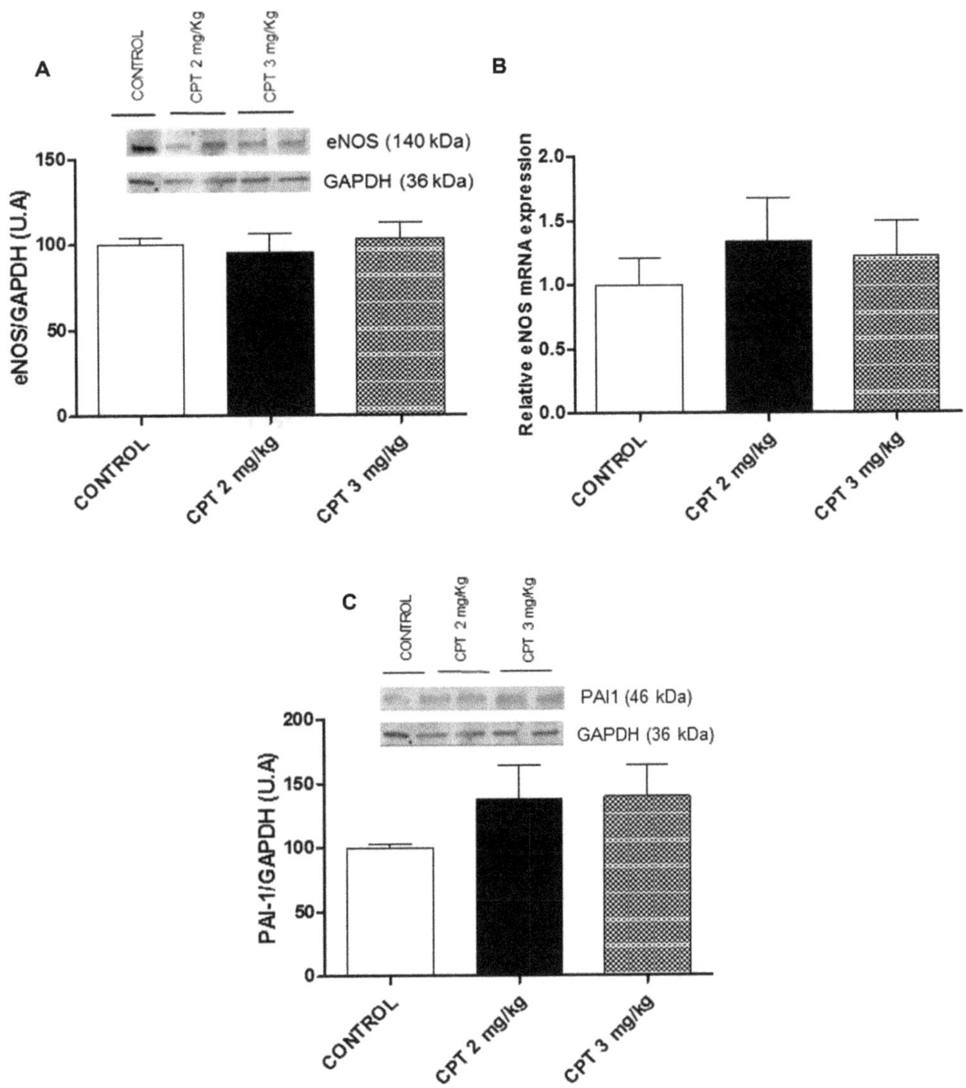

FIGURE 9 | (A) Representative immunoblots for eNOS protein expression in aorta. Diagram bars show the result of densitometric analysis of eNOS in aorta. **(B)** Quantitative analysis of eNOS mRNA levels in aorta. **(C)** Representative immunoblots for plasminogen activator inhibitor-1 (PAI-1) protein expression in aorta. Diagram bars show the result of densitometric analysis of PAI-1 in aorta. Data are presented as means ± SEM of observations obtained for 5–8 tissue samples from 5 to 8 animals per treatment. A one-way ANOVA followed by Bonferroni/Dunn *post hoc* test was used for statistical analysis.

autonomic neuropathy in cisplatin treatments. In addition, endothelial dysfunction may be more sensitive and therefore dysfunction may occur even at low doses. This pattern of events is not surprising. In fact, other authors have shown in other autonomic peripheral neuropathies, such as diabetic neuropathy, that impairment of acetylcholine-mediated vascular relaxation occurs prior to nerve blood flow and conduction deficits (Oltman et al., 2005).

Finally, in order to identify the possible molecular mechanism by which cisplatin caused the vascular toxicity described here, histological, Western Blot and quantitative PCR analyses were performed. Methodological problems have impeded us to carry out these experiments in mesenteric vessels, but they have been carried out in aorta. Structural alterations occurred in aorta after chronic cisplatin treatment. The results obtained show changes in fiber arrangement in the tunica media, losing their uneven appearance. The fundamental structural and functional unit of the aortic wall is the medial lamellar unit. The medial layer comprises elastic membrane layers between which the smooth muscle layer and a small amount of collagen and elastic fibers are encountered. The integrity of the vascular smooth muscle layer is crucial in the maintenance of normal vascular morphology and tone. Changes in arterial wall composition and function underlie all forms of vascular disease (Dabagh et al., 2008). Other authors have also described, after acute administration of cisplatin at 5 mg/kg, severe damage to the smooth muscle layer of aorta (Jiang et al., 2014). Furthermore, Saleh et al. (2015) also described an increased thickening in tunicae intima and media with an irregular luminal layer of endothelial cell linings in aorta from chronic cisplatin treated rats. In the present study, histological analysis also showed that eNOS staining disappeared in the animals treated chronically with cisplatin at 3 mg/kg. However, it was surprising that eNOs expression or eNOs RNAm levels were not altered in aorta after the different cisplatin treatments. It is possible that endothelial dysfunction also was in an incipient stage or that other mechanisms were involved in cytotoxic effect of cisplatin in blood vessels. It is known that there is a relationship between endothelial dysfunction and vascular PAI-1 upregulation (Endemann and Schiffrin, 2004; Vaughan, 2005). So, in the present work, the expression of PAI-1 was also evaluated in aorta. Cisplatin treatments induced slightly but not significant increases in PAI-1 expression in aorta tissue. More research is needed to determine the possible role of other mechanisms involved in cytotoxic effect of cisplatin in blood vessels.

CONCLUSION

In summary, the results of this study show that chronic treatment with cisplatin induces cardiovascular alterations. These cardiovascular alterations do not affect equally all cardiovascular organs/tissues and they do not occur at the same doses of the antitumor treatment. Thus, at low doses, chronic treatment with cisplatin seems safe for the cardiovascular system, since no alterations are observed. However, at intermediate doses, alterations, such as endothelial dysfunction in vessels of conductance, are apparent. At higher doses, this endothelial dysfunction is maintained, and other alterations also develop. In this sense, the autonomic neurotoxicity begins affecting resistance vessels and cardiac function, and this finally causes general symptoms such as hypotension. These functional alterations at the cardiovascular level are accompanied by structural alterations in cardiac and vascular tissue. Changes in connexin-43 and eNOS expression could be related with cardiac functional alterations after cisplatin treatments.

Both traditional and novel anticancer agents are used with curative purpose. However, limiting cardiovascular problems of these therapeutic drugs has become a priority. In this sense, experimental studies directed to the identification and understanding of the mechanisms involved in this particular toxicity could be useful to the scientific community. In the present study, the experimental conditions used provoked in the animals, cardiovascular alterations similar to those described in humans treated with cycles of cisplatin (Demkow and Stelmaszczyk-Emmel, 2013; Haugnes et al., 2015; Herrmann et al., 2016), being a useful tool for this purpose. However, further investigations are needed to identify early signs of cardiac and vascular damage in order to optimize the clinical management of cardiotoxicity in cisplatin treatments.

AUTHOR CONTRIBUTIONS

VL-M designed the study. VL-M, EH, CG, JU, and RA performed the experiments and analyzed the data. VL-M, EH, and JU wrote the manuscript. MM contributed financial support and supervised research. All authors reviewed and approved the final version of the manuscript.

FUNDING

This study was supported by grants from Ministerio de Educación y Ciencia SAF2009-12422-C02-01, MAPFRE. Ayudas a la Investigación 2011 (Promoción de la Salud: Alimentación y Ejercicio Físico) and Ministerio de Ciencia e Innovación-MICINN (SAF2012-40075-C02-01).

ACKNOWLEDGMENTS

We thank Mª Carmen Merino, Guadalupe Pablo Fernández, Raquel Franco, Julio Paredes, and Antonio Márquez for technical assistance. We thank also to José Antonio Mas Gutierrez and Mª Teresa Nuñez López and CAT of Heath Sciences for RT-PCR experiments.

REFERENCES

Abalo, R., Cabezos, P. A., Vera, G., López-Miranda, V., Herradón, E., and Martín-Fontelles, M. I. (2011). Cannabinoid-induced delayed gastric emptying is selectively increased upon intermittent administration in the rat: role of CB1 receptors. *Neurogastroenterol. Motil.* 23:e177. doi: 10.1111/j.1365-2982.2011.01677.x

Abboud, K., Bassila, J. C., Ghali-Ghoul, R., and Sabra, R. (2009). Temporal changes in vascular reactivity in early diabetes mellitus in rats: role of changes in endothelial factors and in phosphodiesterase activity. *Am. J. Physiol. Heart Circ. Physiol.* 297, H836–H845. doi: 10.1152/ajpheart.00102.2009

Al-Majed, A. A., Sayed-Ahmed, M. M., Al-Yahya, A. A., Aleisa, A. M., Al-Rejaie, S. S., and Al-Shabanah, O. A. (2006). Propionyl-L-carnitine prevents the progression of cisplatin-induced cardiomyopathy in a carnitine-depleted rat model. *Pharmacol. Res.* 53, 278–286. doi: 10.1016/j.phrs.2005.12.005

Authier, N., Gillet, J. P., Fialip, J., Eschalier, A., and Coudore, F. (2003). An animal model of nociceptive peripheral neuropathy following repeated cisplatin injections. *Exp. Neurol.* 182, 12–20. doi: 10.1016/S0014-4886(03)00003-7

Berdichevski, A., Meiry, G., Milman, F., Reiter, I., Sedan, O., Eliyahu, S., et al. (2010). TVP1022 protects neonatal rat ventricular myocytes against doxorubicin-induced functional derangements. *J. Pharmacol. Exp. Ther.* 332, 413–420. doi: 10.1124/jpet.109.161158

Boogerd, W., ten Bokkel Huinink, W. W., Dalesio, O., Hoppenbrouwers, W. J., and van der Sande, J. J. (1990). Cisplatin induced neuropathy: central, peripheral and autonomic nerve involvement. *J. Neurooncol.* 9, 255–263. doi: 10.1007/BF02341156

Cabezos, P. A., Vera, G., Martin-Fontelles, M. I., Fernández-Pujol, R., and Abalo, R. (2010). Cisplatin-induced gastrointestinal dysmotility is aggravated after chronic administration in the rat. Comparison with pica. *Neurogastroenterol. Motil.* 22, 797–805. doi: 10.1111/j.1365-2982.2010.01483.x

Carvalho Leone, A. F., and Coelho, E. B. (2004). Effects of prostanoids on phenylephrine-induced contractions in the mesenteric vascular bed of rats with streptozotocin-induced diabetes mellitus. *Life Sci.* 76, 239–247. doi: 10.1016/j.lfs.2004.06.018

Ciftci, O., Ozdemir, I., Vardi, N., and Gurbuz, N. (2011). Novel platinum-*N*-heterocyclic carbene complex is more cardiotoxic than *cis*-platin in rats. *Hum. Exp Toxicol.* 30, 1342–1349. doi: 10.1177/0960327110390064

Coskun, R., Turan, M. I., Turan, I. S., and Gulapoglu, M. (2014). The protective effect of thiamine pyrophosphate, but not thiamine, against cardiotoxicity induced with cisplatin in rats. *Drug Chem. Toxicol.* 37, 290–294. doi: 10.3109/01480545.2013.851688

Curigliano, G., Cardinale, D., Suter, T., Plataniotis, G., de Azambuja, E., Sandri, M. T., et al. (2012). Cardiovascular toxicity induced by chemotherapy, targeted agents and radiotherapy: ESMO Clinical Practice Guidelines. *Ann. Oncol.* 23(Suppl. 7), vii155–vii166. doi: 10.1093/annonc/mds293

Dabagh, M., Jalali, P., Konttinen, Y. T., and Sarkomaa, P. (2008). Distribution of shear stress over smooth muscle cells in deformable arterial wall. *Med. Biol. Eng. Comput.* 46, 649–657. doi: 10.1007/s11517-008-0338-7

Darling, H. S. (2015). Cisplatin induced bradycardia. *Int. J. Cardiol.* 182, 304–306. doi: 10.1016/j.ijcard.2015.01.013

Demkow, U., and Stelmaszczyk-Emmel, A. (2013). Cardiotoxicity of cisplatin-based chemotherapy in advanced non-small cell lung cancer patients. *Respir. Physiol. Neurobiol.* 187, 64–67. doi: 10.1016/j.resp.2013.03.013

Denegri, A., Moccetti, T., Moccetti, M., Spallarossa, P., Brunelli, C., and Ameri, P. (2016). Cardiac toxicity of trastuzumab in elderly patients with breast cancer. *J. Geriatr. Cardiol.* 13, 355–363. doi: 10.11909/j.issn.1671-5411.2016.04.003

Drimal, J., Zurova-Nedelcevova, J., Knezl, V., Sotnikova, R., and Navarova, J. (2006). Cardiovascular toxicity of the first line cancer chemotherapeutic agents: doxorubicin, cyclophosphamide, streptozotocin and bevacizumab. *Neuroendocrinol. Lett.* 27, 176–179.

Dugbartey, G. J., Pepponec, L. J., and De Graafd, I. A. M. (2016). An integrative view of cisplatin-induced renal and cardiac toxicities: molecular mechanisms, current treatment challenges and potential protective measures. *Toxicology* 371, 58–66. doi: 10.1016/j.tox.2016.10.001

El-Awady, E. E., Moustafa, Y. M., Abo-Elmatty, D. M., and Radwan, A. (2011). Cisplatin-induced cardiotoxicity: mechanisms and cardioprotective strategies. *Eur. J. Pharmacol.* 650, 335–341. doi: 10.1016/j.ejphar.2010.09.085

El-Sawalhi, M. M., and Ahmed, L. A. (2014). Exploring the protective role of apocynin, a specific NADPH oxidase inhibitor, in cisplatin-induced cardiotoxicity in rats. *Chem. Biol. Interact.* 207, 58–66. doi: 10.1016/j.cbi.2013.11.008

Endemann, D. H., and Schiffrin, E. L. (2004). Endothelial dysfunction. *J. Am. Soc. Nephrol.* 15, 1983–1992. doi: 10.1097/01.ASN.0000132474.50966.DA

Ghibu, S., Delemasure, S., Richard, C., Guilland, J. C., Martin, L., Gambert, S., et al. (2012). General oxidative stress during doxorubicin-induced cardiotoxicity in rats: absence of cardioprotection and low antioxidant efficiency of alpha-lipoic acid. *Biochimie* 94, 932–939. doi: 10.1016/j.biochi.2011.02.015

Ghosh, A. K., Rai, R., Park, K. E., Eren, M., Miyata, T., Wilsbacher, L. D., et al. (2016). A small molecule inhibitor of PAI-1 protects against doxorubicin-induced cellular senescence. *Oncotarget* 7, 72443–72457. doi: 10.18632/oncotarget.12494

Ghosh, A. K., and Vaughan, D. E. (2012). PAI-1 in tissue fibrosis. *J. Cell. Physiol.* 227, 493–507. doi: 10.1002/jcp.22783

González, C., Herradón, E., Abalo, R., Vera, G., Pérez-Nievas, B. G., Leza, J. C., et al. (2011). Cannabinoid/agonist WIN 55,212-2 reduces cardiac ischaemia-reperfusion injury in Zucker diabetic fatty rats: role of CB2 receptors and iNOS/eNOS. *Diabetes Metab. Res. Rev.* 27, 331–340. doi: 10.1002/dmrr.1176

Goren, M. P. (2003). Cisplatin nephrotoxicity affects magnesium and calcium metabolism. *Med. Pediatr. Oncol.* 41, 186–189. doi: 10.1002/mpo.10335

Gospodarowicz, M. (2008). Testicular cancer patients: considerations in long-term follow- up. *Hematol. Oncol. Clin. North. Am.* 22, 245–255. doi: 10.1016/j.hoc.2008.01.003

Hamo, C. E., and Bloom, M. W. (2015). Getting to the heart of the matter: an overview of cardiac toxicity related to cancer therapy. *Clin. Med. Insights Cardiol.* 9(Suppl. 2), 47–51. doi: 10.4137/CMC.S19704

Haugnes, H. S., Oldenburg, J., and Bremnes, R. M. (2015). Pulmonary and cardiovascular toxicity in long-term testicular cancer survivors. *Urol. Oncol.* 33, 399–406. doi: 10.1016/j.urolonc.2014.11.012

Hernández-Esquivel, L., Marín-Hernández, A., Pavón, N., Carvajal, K., and Moreno-Sánchez, R. (2006). Cardiotoxicity of copper-based antineoplastic drugs casiopeinas is related to inhibition of energy metabolism. *Toxicol. Appl. Pharmacol.* 212, 79–88. doi: 10.1016/j.taap.2005.06.023

Herrmann, J., Yang, E. H., Iliescu, C. A., Cilingiroglu, M., Charitakis, K., Hakeem, A., et al. (2016). Vascular toxicities of cancer therapies: the old and the new–an evolving avenue. *Circulation* 133, 1272–1289. doi: 10.1161/CIRCULATIONAHA.115.018347

Hirano, S., Wakazono, K., Agata, N., Iguchi, H., and Tone, H. (1993). Comparison of cardiotoxicity of pirarubicin, epirubicin and doxorubicin in the rat. *Drugs Exp. Clin. Res.* 20, 153–160.

Hussein, A., Ahmed, A. A., Shouman, S. A., and Sharawy, S. (2012). Ameliorating effect of DL-α-lipoic acid against cisplatin-induced nephrotoxicity and cardiotoxicity in experimental animals. *Drug Discov. Ther.* 6, 147–156. doi: 10.5582/ddt.2012.v6.3.147

Ishioka, J., Fujii, Y., Kageyama, Y., Fukuda, H., Higashi, Y., and Kihara, K. (2008). Cardiovascular events in survivors of high-dose chemotherapy for germ cell tumors. *Int. J. Urol.* 5, 642–645. doi: 10.1111/j.1442-2042.2008.02066.x

Jiang, Y., Shan, S., Gan, T., Zhang, X., Lu, X., Hu, H., et al. (2014). Effects of cisplatin on the contractile function of thoracic aorta of Sprague Dawley rats. *Biomed. Rep.* 2, 893–897. doi: 10.3892/Br.2014.349

Kounis, N. G., Cervellin, G., and Lippi, G. (2016). Cisplatin-induced bradycardia: cardiac toxicity or cardiac hypersensitivity and Kounis syndrome? *Int. J. Cardiol.* 202, 817–818. doi: 10.1016/j.ijcard.2015.10.027

Lajer, H., and Daugaard, G. (1999). Cisplatin and hypomagnesemia. *Cancer Treat. Rev.* 25, 47–58. doi: 10.1053/ctrv.1999.0097

Li, J., Wood, W. H. III, Becker, K. G., Weeraratna, A. T., and Morin, P. J. (2006). Gene expression response to cisplatin treatment in drug-sensitive and drug-resistant ovarian cancer cells. *Oncogene* 26, 2860–2872. doi: 10.1038/sj.onc.1210086

Ma, H., Jones, K. R., Guo, R., Xu, P., Shen, Y., and Ren, J. (2010). Cisplatin compromises myocardial contractile function and mitochondrial ultrastructure: role of endoplasmic reticulum stress. *Clin. Exp. Pharmacol. Physiol.* 37, 460–465. doi: 10.1111/j.1440-1681.2009.05323.x

Malik, N. M., Moore, G. B., Smith, G., Liu, Y. L., Sanger, G. J., and Andrews, P. L. (2006). Behavioural and hypothalamic molecular effects of the anti-cancer agent cisplatin in the rat: a model of chemotherapy-related malaise? *Pharmacol. Biochem. Behav.* 83, 9–20. doi: 10.1016/j.pbb.2005.11.017

Mollman, J. E. (1990). Cisplatin neurotoxicity. *N. Engl. J. Med.* 322, 126–127. doi: 10.1056/NEJM199001113220210

Mythili, Y., Sudharsan, P. T., Selvakumar, E., and Varalakshmi, P. (2004). Protective effect of DL-lipoic acid on cyclophosphamide induced oxidative cardiac injury. *Chem. Biol. Interact.* 151, 13–19. doi: 10.1016/j.cbi.2004.10.004

Oltman, C. L., Coppey, L. J., Gellett, J. S., Davidson, E. P., Lund, D. D., and Yorek, M. A. (2005). Progression of vascular and neural dysfunction in sciatic nerves of Zucker diabetic fatty and Zucker rats. *Am. J. Physiol. Endocrinol. Metab.* 289, E113–E122. doi: 10.1152/ajpendo.00594.2004

Pai, V., and Nahata, M. C. (2000). Cardiotoxicity of chemotherapeutic agents: incidence, treatment and prevention. *Drug Saf.* 22, 263–302. doi: 10.2165/00002018-200022040-00002

Paniagua, N., Girón, R., Goicoechea, C., López-Miranda, V., Vela, J. M., Merlos, M., et al. (2016). Blockade of sigma 1 receptors alleviates sensory signs of diabetic neuropathy in rats. *Eur. J. Pain* 21, 61–72. doi: 10.1002/ejp.897

Pretnar-Oblak, J., Zaletel, M., Jagodic, M., and Zaletel, M. (2007). Thrombosis of internal carotid artery after cisplatin-based chemotherapy. *Eur. Neurol.* 57, 109–110. doi: 10.1159/000098062

Rosenfeld, C. S., and Broder, L. E. (1984). Cisplatin-induced autonomic neuropathy. *Cancer Treat. Rep.* 68, 659–660.

Salameh, A., Schneider, P., Mühlbergm, K., Hagendorff, A., Dhein, S., and Pfeiffer, D. (2004). Chronic regulation of the expression of gap junction proteins connexin40, connexin43, and connexin45 in neonatal rat cardiomyocytes. *Eur. J. Pharmacol.* 503, 9–16. doi: 10.1016/j.ejphar.2004.09.024

Saleh, R. M., Awadin, W. F., El-Shafei, R. A., Elseady, Y. Y., Wehaish, F. E., and Elshal, M. F. (2015). Cardioprotective role of tadalafil against cisplatin-induced cardiovascular damage in rats. *Eur. J. Pharmacol.* 765, 574–581. doi: 10.1016/j.ejphar.2015.09.015

Samuels, B. L., Vogelzang, N. J., and Kennedy, B. J. (1987). Vascular toxicity following vinblastine, bleomycin, and cisplatin therapy for germ cell tumours. *Int. J. Androl.* 10, 363–369. doi: 10.1111/j.1365-2605.1987.tb00204.x

Schlumbrecht, M. P., and Hehr, K. (2015). Cisplatin-induced bradycardia and the importance of the QT interval. *J. Oncol. Pharm. Pract.* 21, 157–160. doi: 10.1177/1078155214522314

Serrano-Castro, P. J., Guardado-Santervás, P., and Olivares-Romero, J. (2000). Ischemic stroke following cisplatin and 5-fluorouracil therapy: a transcranial Doppler study. *Eur. Neurol.* 44, 63–64. doi: 10.1159/000008197

Shaker, O., and Sourour, D. A. (2010). How to protect doxorubicin-induced cardiomyopathy in male albino rats? *J. Cardiovasc. Pharmacol.* 55, 262–268. doi: 10.1097/FJC.0b013e3181cf91ac

Shimizu, T., Uematsu, M., Yoshizaki, T., Obata, J. E., Nakamura, T., Fujioka, D., et al. (2016). Myocardial production of plasminogen activator inhibitor-1 is associated with coronary endothelial and ventricular dysfunction after acute myocardial infarction. *J. Atheroscler. Thromb.* 23, 557–566. doi: 10.5551/jat.32300

Soga, M., Kamal, F. A., Watanabe, K., Ma, M., Palaniyandi, S., Prakash, P., et al. (2006). Effects of angiotensin II receptor blocker (candesartan) in daunorubicin-induced cardiomyopathic rats. *Int. J. Cardiol.* 110, 378–385. doi: 10.1016/j.ijcard.2005.08.061

Somoza, B., Guzmán, R., Cano, V., Merino, B., Ramos, P., Díez-Fernández, C., et al. (2007). Induction of cardiac uncoupling protein-2 expression and adenosine 5′-monophosphate-activated protein kinase phosphorylation during early states of diet-induced obesity in mice. *Endocrinology* 148, 924–931. doi: 10.1210/en.2006-0914

Sudharsan, P. T., Mythili, Y., Selvakumar, E., and Varalakshmi, P. (2006). Lupeol and its ester exhibit protective role against cyclophosphamide-induced cardiac mitochondrial toxicity. *J. Cardiovasc. Pharmacol.* 47, 205–210. doi: 10.1097/01.fjc.0000200658.89629.ba

Takeshita, K., Hayashi, M., Iino, S., Kondo, T., Inden, Y., Iwase, M., et al. (2004). Increased expression of plasminogen activator inhibitor-1 in cardiomyocytes contributes to cardiac fibrosis after myocardial infarction. *Am. J. Pathol.* 164, 449–456. doi: 10.1016/S0002-9440(10)63135-5

Turlapaty, P. D., and Altura, B. M. (1980). Magnesium deficiency produces spasms of coronary arteries: relationship to etiology of sudden death ischemic heart disease. *Science* 208, 198–200. doi: 10.1126/science.7361117

van den Belt-Dusebout, A. W., Nuver, J., de Wit, R., Gietema, J. A., ten Bokkel Huinink, W. W., Rodrigus, P. T., et al. (2006). Long-term risk of cardiovascular disease in 5-year survivors of testicular cancer. *J. Clin. Oncol.* 24, 467–475. doi: 10.1200/JCO.2005.02.7193

Vaughan, D. E. (2005). PAI-1 and atherothrombosis. *J. Thromb. Haemost.* 3, 1879–1883. doi: 10.1111/j.1538-7836.2005.01420.x

Vaughn, D. J., Palmer, S. C., Carver, J. R., Jacobs, L. A., and Mohler, E. R. (2008). Cardiovascular risk in long-term survivors of testicular cancer. *Cancer* 112, 1949–1953. doi: 10.1002/cncr.23389

Vera, G., Cabezos, P. A., Martín, M. I., and Abalo, R. (2013). Characterization of cannabinoid-induced relief of neuropathic pain in a rat model of cisplatin-induced neuropathy. *Pharmacol. Biochem. Behav.* 105, 205–212. doi: 10.1016/j.pbb.2013.02.008

Vera, G., Castillo, M., Cabezos, P., Chiarlone, A., Martín, M., Gori, A., et al. (2011). Enteric neuropathy evoked by repeated cisplatin in the rat. *Neurogastroenterol. Motil.* 23, 370–378, e162–e163. doi: 10.1111/j.1365-2982.2011.01674.x

Vera, G., Chiarlone, A., Cabezos, P. A., Pascual, D., Martín, M. I., and Abalo, R. (2007). WIN 55,212-2 prevents mechanical allodynia but not alterations in feeding behaviour induced by chronic cisplatin in the rat. *Life Sci.* 81, 468–479. doi: 10.1016/j.lfs.2007.06.012

Verdú, E., Vilches, J. J., Rodríguez, F. J., Ceballos, D., Valero, A., and Navarro, X. (1999). Physiological and immunohistochemical characterization of cisplatin-induced neuropathy in mice. *Muscle Nerve* 22, 329–340. doi: 10.1002/(SICI)1097-4598(199903)22:3<329::AID-MUS5>3.0.CO;2-8

Vickers, A. E., Rose, K., Fisher, R., Saulnier, M., Sahota, P., and Bentley, P. (2004). Kidney slices of human and rat to characterize cisplatin-induced injury on cellular pathways and morphology. *Toxicol. Pathol.* 32, 577–590. doi: 10.1080/01926230490508821

Yao, Y., Panichpisal, K., Kurtzman, N., and Nugent, K. (2007). Cisplatin nephrotoxicity: a review. *Am. J. Med. Sci.* 334, 115–124. doi: 10.1097/MAJ.0b013e31812dfe1e

Yüce, A., Ateahin, A., Ceribai, A. O., and Aksakal, M. (2007). Ellagic acid prevents cisplatin-induced oxidative stress in liver and heart tissue of rats. *Basic Clin. Pharmacol. Toxicol.* 101, 345–349. doi: 10.1111/j.1742-7843.2007.00129.x

Conflict of Interest Statement: The authors declare that the research was conducted in the absence of any commercial or financial relationships that could be construed as a potential conflict of interest.

16

BGP-15 Protects against Oxaliplatin-Induced Skeletal Myopathy and Mitochondrial Reactive Oxygen Species Production in Mice

James C. Sorensen[1,2], *Aaron C. Petersen*[3], *Cara A. Timpani*[1,2], *Dean G. Campelj*[1,2], *Jordan Cook*[1], *Adam J. Trewin*[3], *Vanesa Stojanovska*[1], *Mathew Stewart*[4], *Alan Hayes*[1,2,3] *and Emma Rybalka*[1,2,3]*

[1] Centre for Chronic Disease, College of Health & Biomedicine, Victoria University, Melbourne, VIC, Australia, [2] Australian Institute for Musculoskeletal Science, Melbourne, VIC, Australia, [3] Institute of Sport, Exercise & Active Living, Victoria University, Melbourne, VIC, Australia, [4] Institute of Sustainability and Innovation, Victoria University, Melbourne, VIC, Australia

Edited by:
R. Thomas Jagoe,
McGill University, Canada

Reviewed by:
Gilles Gouspillou,
Université du Québec à Montréal,
Canada
Ricky Yuet-Kin Leung,
University of Cincinnati, USA

***Correspondence:**
Emma Rybalka
emma.rybalka@vu.edu.au

Chemotherapy is a leading intervention against cancer. Albeit highly effective, chemotherapy has a multitude of deleterious side-effects including skeletal muscle wasting and fatigue, which considerably reduces patient quality of life and survivability. As such, a defense against chemotherapy-induced skeletal muscle dysfunction is required. Here we investigate the effects of oxaliplatin (OXA) treatment in mice on the skeletal muscle and mitochondria, and the capacity for the Poly ADP-ribose polymerase (PARP) inhibitor, BGP-15, to ameliorate any pathological side-effects induced by OXA. To do so, we investigated the effects of 2 weeks of OXA (3 mg/kg) treatment with and without BGP-15 (15 mg/kg). OXA induced a 15% ($p < 0.05$) reduction in lean tissue mass without significant changes in food consumption or energy expenditure. OXA treatment also altered the muscle architecture, increasing collagen deposition, neutral lipid and Ca^{2+} accumulation; all of which were ameliorated with BGP-15 adjunct therapy. Here, we are the first to show that OXA penetrates the mitochondria, and, as a possible consequence of this, increases mtROS production. These data correspond with reduced diameter of isolated FDB fibers and shift in the fiber size distribution frequency of TA to the left. There was a tendency for reduction in intramuscular protein content, albeit apparently not via Murf1 (atrophy)- or p62 (autophagy)- dependent pathways. BGP-15 adjunct therapy protected against increased ROS production and improved mitochondrial viability 4-fold and preserved fiber diameter and number. Our study highlights BGP-15 as a potential adjunct therapy to address chemotherapy-induced skeletal muscle and mitochondrial pathology.

Keywords: skeletal muscle, oxaliplatin chemotherapy, BGP-15, mitochondria, protein synthesis, muscle wasting, mitochondrial reactive oxygen species

INTRODUCTION

Cancer is a leading cause of world-wide mortality accounting for 8.2 million deaths in 2012 alone, with this figure predicted to reach 14 million by 2034 (World Health Organisation, 2015). In the majority of cases, first line treatment involves systemic chemotherapy administration. Chemotherapeutic agents target the molecular characteristics of cancerous cells, such as rapid replication, to chemically-induce cell death (de Gramont et al., 2000; Sorensen et al., 2016). However, due to its non-specific and systemic mode of action, chemotherapy also elicits effects on healthy tissues causing the classic side-effects attributable to anti-cancer therapy including nausea, vomiting, cardio-toxicity, immune disorders, peripheral and axial neuropathy, hair and weight loss and debilitative fatigue (Greene et al., 1993; Zitvogel et al., 2008; Gilliam and St Clair, 2011; National Cancer Institute, 2012; Ariaans et al., 2015). These side-effects often limit treatment tolerability, efficacy and therapeutic options, sometimes leading to the cessation of treatment all together and ultimately reducing patient quality of life and prognosis due to the development of co-morbidities (Gilliam and St Clair, 2011; Scheede-Bergdahl and Jagoe, 2013; Argilés et al., 2015; Cheregi et al., 2015). Emerging evidence suggests that the skeletal muscle is also a target of chemotherapy-induced atrophy (Pfeiffer et al., 1997), weakness and fatigue (Gilliam and St Clair, 2011), dysfunction (Scheede-Bergdahl and Jagoe, 2013; Bredahl et al., 2016) and insulin resistance (Ariaans et al., 2015). These effects appear to be more pronounced when chemotherapy is administered in childhood, due to the hyperplastic and hypertrophic nature of skeletal muscle at this early stage of life and persist well into adulthood (Ness et al., 2007; Scheede-Bergdahl and Jagoe, 2013; Ariaans et al., 2015). Since skeletal muscle has a high energy requirement, and thus a high mitochondrial density, emerging data suggests that skeletal muscle pathology may be underpinned by damage induced to the mitochondrial by chemotherapy administration (Davies and Doroshow, 1986; Doroshow and Davies, 1986; Sarosiek et al., 2013; Tabassum et al., 2015).

Oxaliplatin (OXA), a platinum (Pt)-based alkylating agent, is the leading anti-neoplastic agent against colorectal cancer (André et al., 2004; Gourdier et al., 2004; Aschele et al., 2005; Alcindor and Beauger, 2011), neuroblastoma (Tran et al., 2015) and solid tumors (Mascarenhas et al., 2013). Primarily, OXA elicits its antineoplastic effect by intercalating Pt adducts into the nuclear DNA (nDNA) causing single-stranded damage, cell cycle arrest and apoptosis (Alcindor and Beauger, 2011). In addition, it has been demonstrated that OXA has the capacity to induce a mitochondrially-driven apoptotic response that is independent of nDNA damage (Gourdier et al., 2004), implicating the mitochondria as inadvertent targets of OXA treatment. Preliminary findings by our laboratory demonstrate that OXA treatment induces significant mitochondrial dysfunction involving elevated mitochondrial (mt) reactive oxygen species (ROS) production and reduced viability of the mitochondrial pool *in vitro* (Cheregi et al., 2015). As hypothesized by us previously, these findings suggest that OXA explicitly damages the nDNA, but inadvertently hinders the mitochondria as well, by eliciting damage to either functional proteins, the mtDNA, or both (Sorensen et al., 2016). It has been established that an imbalance in the oxidant/antioxidant ratio stimulates atrophy pathways, impedes skeletal muscle growth and/or muscle turnover supressing the capacity to repair chemotherapy-induced damage (as reviewed in Sorensen et al., 2016). The net effect on the skeletal musculature would be wasting and a detrimental loss of force production capacity. While this has been increasingly established for the anthracycline chemotherapeutic, doxorubicin, which is a known pro-oxidant (Davies and Doroshow, 1986; Doroshow and Davies, 1986; Jones, 2006; Ashley and Poulton, 2009; Gilliam et al., 2012, 2013), and more recently established for combination colorectal cancer chemotherapy treatment regimens which include oxaliplatin (i.e., FOLFOX André et al., 2004; Aschele et al., 2005), there is currently no data describing the effects of OXA on the skeletal muscular system.

Here we investigate the experimental therapeutic BGP-15 (O-(3-piperidino-2-hydroxy-1-propyl)nicotinic amidoxime), which has previously been used in clinical trials for the treatment of skeletal muscle pathology associated with Type 2 Diabetes (through insulin sensitization; U.S. National Institutes of Health, 2014), Duchenne Muscular Dystrophy (DMD) and heart failure (through anti-inflammatory and anti-fibrotic mechanisms; Gehrig et al., 2012; Sapra et al., 2014). Via its action as a modulator of the cytoprotective response to cellular stress, and specifically as a poly (ADP-ribose) polymerase (PARP) inhibitor, heat shock protein-inducer (Sarszegi et al., 2012; U.S. National Institutes of Health, 2014), membrane lipid therapeutic (Salah et al., 2016) and an antioxidant inducer (Henstridge et al., 2014), BGP-15 has previously been shown to protect against skeletal muscle dysfunction, damage and wasting (Sapra et al., 2014; Kennedy et al., 2016; Salah et al., 2016). As such, it is of particular interest to us for protection against chemotherapy-induced skeletal muscle dysfunction due to its capacity to improve myopathic structural changes. Thus, we aimed to (1) investigate the effects of OXA treatment on skeletal muscle and mitochondrial function at the whole body, myocellular, and molecular level; and (2) evaluate the efficacy of BGP-15 co-treatment as a therapeutic avenue through which to protect the skeletal muscle during chemotherapy treatment. We hypothesized that OXA treatment would (1) induce skeletal muscle atrophy, wasting and/or pathology and (2) penetrate the mitochondria to induce mitochondrial pathology and dysfunction; and that (3) BGP-15 would preserve the skeletal muscle mass, as well as protect against OXA-induced perturbations in muscle morphology and mitochondrial health, thus reducing the impact of chemotherapy treatment on the skeletal muscular system.

MATERIALS AND METHODS

Ethics Approval

All experimental procedures were approved by the Victoria University Animal Ethics Experimentation Committee and conformed to the Australian Code of Practice for the Care and Use of Animals for Scientific Purposes.

Animals

Six-week old male Balb/C mice were obtained from the Australian Resource Centre (Western Australia, Australia) and were acclimatized for a minimum of 3 days before being randomly assigned to treatment groups ($n = 8$). Mice were housed in groups of 4–5 and maintained on a 12 h light/dark cycle with *ad-libitum* access to standard rodent chow and water. Prior to treatment (on day 1), mice were scanned for body composition. Mice were then treated with either vehicle (0.1% DMSO; VEH), OXA (3 mg/kg; Sigma Aldrich, Australia) or OXA with BGP-15 (15 mg/kg, kindly donated by N-gene R&D, Australia; OXAB) via intraperitoneal injection on days 1, 3, 5, 8, 10, and 12. The cumulative OXA dosage used in our study is equivalent to that given to humans, scaled for the metabolic activity of mice according to Reagan-Shaw et al. (2008). The concentrations and injection protocol for OXA have been used and published by our collaborators previously (Stojanovska et al., 2015; McQuade et al., 2016b), while the BGP-15 dosage administered has proven efficacious against murine myopathies (Chung et al., 2008; Gehrig et al., 2012; Kennedy et al., 2016). On day 14, mice were housed in the Promethion metabolic system for 24 h and on day 15, scanned again for changes in body composition, prior to being anaesthetized (sodium pentobarbitone, 60 mg/kg). When no reflexes were present, muscles and organs were harvested. Food and water consumption was monitored on treatment days.

Body Composition Analysis

Directly prior to the first treatment on Day 1 and prior to non-recovery surgery on Day 15, mice were analyzed for body composition (lean, fat and water mass) using an echo magnetic resonance imaging (echoMRI) body composition analyser (EMR-150, Echo Medical Systems, USA). Scans were conducted in triplicate at each time point and included both the standard and water phases of analysis, with a 30-s time-lapse between each scan. Data is presented as the mean of the three scans. Composition results are expressed as an index against body weight (measure/body weight) with pre-treatment data not shown since no significant differences between groups were observed.

Metabolism, Voluntary Exercise Capacity, and Behavioral Analysis

Mice were housed individually in a Promethion metabolic cage system (Sable Systems, USA) for 24 h after the cessation (day 14–15) of treatment. Respiratory gases were measured with an integrated fuel cell oxygen (O_2) analyser, spectrophotometric carbon dioxide (CO_2) analyser and capacitive water vapor partial pressure analyser (GA3, Sable Systems, USA). Gas sampling was recorded at 1 s intervals with water vapor, pressure and temperature controlled for, to assess indirect calorimetry. Gas sensors were calibrated weekly with 100% N_2 (zero reference for all other gas and vapor) and a span gas with known concentrations of O_2 and CO_2. The Promethion system utilizes a pull-mode, negative pressure system, through a multi-channel mass flow generator which measures and controls airflow (FR8, Sable Systems, USA) at an incurrent flow rate of 2,000 mL/min. Respiratory quotients (RQ) were calculated as a ratio of CO_2 production to O_2 consumption with energy expenditure calculated using the Weir equation: Kcal/hr $= 60*(0.003941*VO_2 + 0.001106*VCO_2)$ (Kaiyala et al., 2012). Mouse ambulatory activity and position (x, y, and z axis, 0.25 cm spacing) within the cages was recorded continuously (BXYZ-R Sable Systems, USA). Mice also had free access to running wheels with revolutions recorded using a magnetic reed switch. Mice were permitted *ad libitum* access to food and water hoppers which were suspended from load cells to continuously record interaction with food and water, as well as consumption. Measures of time spent during behavioral activities were derived from the ethoSCAN behavioral macro supplied by Sable Systems (USA), with short lounges identified as periods of inactivity <60s and long lounges >60s. Time spent on particular activities were calculated as a percentage of total time spent in the cage (total 24 h).

Histology

Following excision of tibialis anterior (TA) from mice, muscles were coated in OCT compound and snap frozen in liquid nitrogen-chilled isopentane (Sigma Aldrich, Australia). Frozen OCT embedded TA muscles were cryosectioned (10 μm), stained and mounted according to specific protocols as described below. Images of the whole section were captured using a Zeiss Axio Imager Z2 microscope (Carl Zeiss MicroImaging GmbH, Germany) at 10x magnification and a further magnification of 200x was used for greater detailed images.

Haematoxylin & Eosin (H&E)

Slides were stained using a standard H&E staining protocol (30 s incubation in haematoxylin and 1 m 45 s incubation in eosin; Timpani et al., 2016) and mounted with DPx (BDH, Poole, UK). To determine fiber size frequency distributions, 200 fibers per section (except for those on the periphery that were cropped) were individually circled on three images taken from the top, middle and bottom along the midline from each TA cross section. ImageJ (NIH, USA) measurement analysis was used for measurement data. Since the TA has been shown to localize different fiber types to different areas of the muscle this approach was used to limit the influence of fiber type variations within the muscle cross section (Wang and Kernell, 2001; Shortreed et al., 2009).

Oil Red O (ORO)

Air dried TA sections were fixed in 3.7% formaldehyde for 60 m before being rinsed in x3 individual deionized water baths for 30 s each. Samples were then incubated in Oil Red O working solution [5:1 Oil Red O (Sigma Aldrich, Australia) in 60% triethyl-phosphate (w/v)] for 30 min. Thereafter, samples were washed three times in individual deionized water baths for 30 s each, then rinsed in running tap water for 10 m before being mounted with 10% glycerol in PBS. Images were converted to 8bit photos and thresholded, then analyzed by assessing the intensity of black to white. The full cross section of the TA was imaged and data is expressed as the Oil Red O positive area (black) as a percentage of the total cross sectional area (black + white).

Alizarin Red

The Ca^{2+} content of TA sections was assessed using Alizarin Red (TMS-008-C, Merck Millipore), a dye which chelates with calcium to form Alizarin Red S-Ca^{2+} complexes. Slides were stained for 2 m with Alizarin Red, dipped in 100% acetone 20 times, then dipped in 1:1 acetone-xylene 20 times, before being washed in 100% xylene for 1 m. Samples were mounted with DPx then the whole cross section of the TA was photographed. Images were converted to 8bit photos then analyzed by assessing the intensity of black of the total cross-sectional area. Data is expressed as arbitrary units.

Gomori Trichrome

Gomori Trichrome (LG) stain (HT10316, Sigma Aldrich, Australia) distinguishes three muscle components: (1) muscle (red/pink), (2) nuclei (blue/black) ,and (3) collagen (green-blue). To achieve this stain, samples were bathed in hematoxylin for 1 m before being washed in tap water until the water ran clear. Samples were then stained with Gomori trichrome for 30 s and dipped in tap water 20–25 times before being dipped in a 0.2% acetic acid bath 20 times, then bathed in 0.2% acetic acid for 30 s. Samples were then bathed for 30 s increments in x4 baths containing 95% (x2) and 100% (x2) ethanol, before being bathed in xylene for 1 m. Thereafter, samples were mounted with DPx. The intensity of red (muscle), blue (nuclei) and green (collagen) pixels were assessed using ImageJ. The full cross section of the TA was imaged and data is expressed as the percentage of collagen (green) within the total cross sectional area.

Succinate Dehydrogenase (SDH)

SDH is an enzyme located in the mitochondria that oxidizes succinate to fumarate. This reaction, in the presence of nitro blue tetrazolium, is demonstrated by the formation of a blue-purple product with more intensely colored fibers indicating highly oxidative fibers with a greater mitochondrial density. Slides were incubated in working solution (0.2M sodium succinate, 0.2M PBS, 0.05% nitro blue tetrazolium, pH 7.6) for 60 min at 37°C, fixed in formal saline (0.9% NaCl, 10% formaldehyde) and mounted with glycerol jelly. Images were converted to 8bit, thresholded and SDH intensity was measured in full cross sections of the TA.

Platinum Detection in Subcellular Fractions

Subcellular Fractionation

TA muscles were homogenized in buffer (containing: 100 mM potassium chloride, 50 mM tris (hydroxymethyl)aminomethane, 5 mM magnesium chloride hexahydrate, 1.8 mM adenosine triphosphate, 0.5 mM ethylenediaminetetraacetic acid; pH 7.2). Tissue homogenates were transferred to Eppendorf tubes and centrifuged at 650G for 3 min at 4°C. The supernatant, which contains the mitochondria, was decanted into separate Eppendorf tubes. The pellet which contains the nuclear fraction was resuspended in RIPA lysis buffer (25 mM tris(hydroxymethyl)aminomethane hydrochloride, 150 mM sodium chloride, 1% sodium deoxycholate and 0.1% sodium dodecyl sulfate; pH 7.6) and further diluted to a total volume of 4 mL in MilliQ water. The mitochondrial sample was centrifuged at 15,000G for 3 min at 4°C. The supernatant was discarded and the mitochondrial pellet was resuspended in 4 mL of MilliQ water.

Atomic Absorption Spectrophotometry

Once the nuclear and mitochondrial fractions were derived, samples were aspirated into a Shimadzu AA-6300 Atomic Absorption Spectrophotometer (AAS). The specific AAS conditions used to carry out these analyses included an air-acetylene flame, with a fuel flow of 1.5 L/min and an air flow of 15 L/min. The burner height was optimized for each element. Due to the analytical wavelength used (265.9 nm for Pt), background correction was required—this was supplied by a D_2 lamp using a slit width of 0.7 nm and a current of 25 mA (Pt). Samples were aspirated, with three repeat measurements recorded following an initial 2 s pre-spray time. Individual measurements were taken by averaging the absorbance readings over 3 s, which also allowed the calculation of a relative mean square percentage (RMS%) uncertainty. These three measurements were then averaged to give a final absorbance reading for each sample. Standard calibration curves were also produced before each daily run of samples, with concentration ranges of 10-40 ppm Pt utilized. Concentration values for the unknown samples were calculated automatically by the Shimadzu AAWizard software.

Mitochondrial Viability and mtROS

Isolation of Flexor Digitorum Brevis (FDB) Fibers

FDB fibers were isolated according to procedures described by Schuh et al. (2012). Following surgical excision of the FDB from both feet, the muscles were incubated in 1 mL of pre-warmed dissociation media (DMEM, Gibco 10566016; 4.5 mg/ml glucose, 2% FBS, Bovogen Biologicals; 4 mg/mL collagenase A, Roche 10103586001; 50 μg/mL gentamycin, Sigma Aldrich, Australia G1397) for 1 h 45 min (37°C, 5% CO2). Following the incubation period, FDB muscles were removed from collagenase and placed into ~1.5 mL of incubation media [DMEM containing 4.5 mg/ml glucose, no phenol red (Gibco), 2.0% FBS, 0.1% Gentamycin solution (Sigma Aldrich, Australia G1397)] and triturated with pipette tips of decreasing bore size to yield isolated fibers. Fibers were then plated according to analysis methods described below.

Determination of Mitochondrial Viability

Mitochondrial viability was assessed using the fluorescent probes MitoTracker Green and Red (Molecular Probes, Australia). MitoTracker Green is a non-selective mitochondrial dye that labels all mitochondria irrespective of the mitochondrial membrane potential, while MitoTracker Red only permeates the mitochondrial matrix and fluoresces in the presence of an inner mitochondrial membrane potential ($\Delta\Psi$). Mitochondrial viability was calculated as the percentage ratio of active mitochondria (MitoTracker Red) to the total mitochondrial pool (MitoTracker Green).

Fifty microliters of isolated FDB fibers suspended in incubation media [DMEM containing 4.5 mg/ml glucose, no phenol red (Gibco), 2.0% FBS, 0.1% Gentamycin solution (Sigma Aldrich, Australia G1397)] was plated onto matrigel (Sigma Aldrich, Australia, E1270) coated 96 well microplates (all samples were run in triplicate) and confluency was determined using a light microscope. If ~60% of the well bottoms was not covered by isolated FDB fibers, an additional 50 μL aliquot of fibers was dispensed into the well. For wells that did not receive the additional 50 μL of fibers, 50 μL of incubation media was added and the microplate was incubated overnight.

Ten minutes prior to the addition of the MitoTracker dyes, FCCP and antimycin A (final concentration of 3 μM each, Sigma Aldrich, Australia) were added to the positive control wells. As FCCP induces the collapse of the mitochondrial membrane potential and antimycin A inhibits complex III function, mitochondrial viability decreases as evidenced by a reduction in the intensity of MitoTracker Red fluorescence. Following this, a cocktail of MitoTracker Green and Red (final concentration of 200 and 50 nM, respectively. Molecular Probes) in Flurobrite media (50 μL total, ThermoFisher, Australia) was added to each well and incubated at 37°C for 3 min. Fibers were then washed twice with Flurobrite media and imaged on an Olympus Inverted Fluorescence Microscope (IX-81, Olympus, Tokyo, Japan) using FITC and TRITC filters and a standardized exposure time. Three random images were taken of each well in a blinded fashion and with standardized exposure and brightness settings, and the average intensity of red and green fluorescence of each image analyzed using ImageJ. Relative MitoTracker Red fluorescence as a proportion of relative MitoTracker Green fluorescence was calculated to give a value of mitochondrial viability percentage. The RFU MitoTracker Green stain were also expressed as arbitrary units of mitochondrial density/population. Analyzed images were all taken using standardized imaging settings, such as ISO and exposure times.

Determination of Mitochondrial Superoxide Production

Isolated fibers suspended in incubation media were prepared as mentioned in the previous section. Fibers were labeled with MitoSOX Red mitochondrial superoxide indicator (Molecular Probes) to detect superoxide production. MitoSOX reagent stock solution (5 mM) was diluted in a HBSS/Ca/Mg buffer (10 mM HEPES, 150 mM NaCl, 5 mM KCl, 1 mM $MgCl_2$ and 1.8 mM $CaCl_2$, pH 7.4) at 37°C and added to the fibers. Fibers were incubated at 37°C in 5% CO_2 for 3 min. Following this the staining solution was removed and, as a counterstain, cells were labeled with MitoTracker Green for 30 min. After counterstaining, cells were washed twice with incubation media and live cells were photographed using an IX-81 Olympus Inverted Fluorescence Microscope. Images were quantified using ImageJ software. Data is expressed as MitoSOX Red RFU relative to the total mitochondrial pool (MitoTracker Green RFU). Three images were taken of each well in a blinded fashion and the average intensity of red and green fluorescence of each image was analyzed using ImageJ. Analyzed images were all taken using standardized imaging settings, such as ISO and exposure times.

Muscle Protein Extraction and Western Blotting

Frozen TA muscles were mechanically disrupted (TissueLyser, Qiagen, Germany) for 30 s at 30 Hz in homogenizing buffer (0.125 M Tris-HCl, 4% SDS, 10% Glycerol, 10 mM EGTA, 0.1 M DTT) containing 0.1 μL.mL^{-1} of protease and phosphatase inhibitor cocktail (Sigma Aldrich, Australia), and vortexed, followed by a freeze-thaw cycle. Protein concentration was then determined using a commercially available assay (Red 660, G-Biosciences, Astral Scientific, Gymea, Australia), and samples were diluted to equivalent concentrations (1 μg.μL^{-1}) in homogenizing buffer. Bromophenol blue (1% v/v) was then added before heating to 95°C for 5 min. Samples were loaded into pre-cast 26 well stain-free 8–16% gradient gels (Criterion™ TGX Stain-Free™ Precast, BioRad, Gladesville, Australia) at a concentration of ~8 μg protein per lane with all constituents present (i.e., no centrifugation). Molecular weight marker (PageRuler® Plus, Thermo Scientific, Australia) was loaded, along with five lanes of increasing volume of a pooled-sample to generate five-point calibration standard curves on each gel. This was used for quantification of sample blot intensities relative to the standard curve both within and between gels, and ensures sample blot intensities are within the linear range of the signal (i.e., primary antibody binding is not saturated; Murphy and Lamb, 2013). After separation by SDS PAGE, stain-free gels were activated by UV light (ChemiDoc™ MP, BioRad, Gladesville NSW, Australia) and imaged to visualize the total protein of each lane before the proteins were transferred to PVDF membranes (Trans-Blot® Turbo™, BioRad, Gladesville NSW, Australia). Membranes were then blocked in 20 mM Tris, 150 mM NaCl, and 0.1% Tween 20 (TBST) containing 5% w/v non-fat milk powder for 1 h at room temperature, then washed in TBST. After this, membranes were incubated overnight at 4°C with rocking, using the following primary antibodies diluted 1:1,000 in TBST containing 5% w/v BSA and 0.1% w/v sodium azide. Probes used: Bax total (CST #2772), MuRF1 total (ECM #MP3401), PAR total (Enzo #ALX-804-220), PARP-1 total (Santa Cruz SC-8007), PARP-2 total (Santa Cruz SC-393310), p70S6K total (CST #2708), rp-S6 total (C ST #2217), SQSTM1/p62 total (CST #5114). Membranes were subsequently washed with TBST, then probed with appropriate horseradish peroxidase-conjugated secondary antibody (PerkinElmer, Australia) diluted 1:50,000 in 5% non-fat milk TBST for 1 h at room temperature. Protein-antibody-HRP conjugates were visualized using super sensitive ECL detection (SuperSignal® West Femto, Thermo Scientific, Australia), imaged (ChemiDoc™ MP, BioRad, Australia), then analyzed using software (ImageLab v5.1, BioRad, Australia). Total protein loading was determined from stain-free gel images to measure intensity of each lane, which was expressed relative to the linear regression of the standard curve (Ashley and Poulton, 2009). These values were then used as a loading control to normalize all blot values for proteins of interest. The proteins selected were done so to cover a broad spectrum of cellular degradation pathways, including atrophy, autophagy, protein synthesis, to preliminarily investigate how OXA induces lean muscle mass loss. Further, PARP was assessed due to BGP-15's inhibitory effect on PARylation.

Statistical Analysis

Statistical analysis was performed using Graphpad Prism 7 software using one-way analysis of variance to detect treatment effects and Tukey post hoc tests for multiple group comparison.

An α value of 0.05 was considered statistically significant. Data is presented as means ± SEM.

RESULTS

Body Weight and Food Consumption

Reduced food consumption due to gastrointestinal side-effects (McQuade et al., 2016b) and nausea (Love et al., 1989; Greene et al., 1993) is associated with chemotherapy treatment in humans, and as such, body weight and food and water intake were monitored. From days 1 through 8 of treatment, there were no significant differences in body weight gain observed between groups ($p > 0.05$, **Figure 1A**), however, weight gain in OXA and OXAB treated mice plateaued at day 8 and remained significantly lower than VEH from D10 onwards ($p < 0.005$; **Figure 1A**). There were no significant differences between the groups in food (**Figure 1B**) or water (**Figure 1C**) consumption over the treatment period ($p > 0.05$).

BGP-15 Protects against OXA Induced-Lean and Fat Mass Loss but Increases Heart/Body Weight Ratio

The effects of OXA treatment on body composition, and the capacity for BGP-15 to protect against the loss of lean tissue was investigated in mice using MRI. OXA treatment induced a 15% reduction in the lean mass index ($p < 0.05$; **Figure 2A**) with this loss being completely protected against via adjunct treatment with BGP-15 ($p < 0.05$). The loss of lean tissue observed was not associated with changes in hydration status ($p > 0.05$, **Figure 2C**), however there was a trend for OXA treatment to reduce the fat mass index by 15% ($p = 0.075$; **Figure 2B**) with BGP-15 treatment affording no protection against this measure ($p > 0.05$, **Figure 2B**).

The wet weight of individual hind limb skeletal muscles, organs and the diaphragm was measured immediately after excision. There were no significant changes in wet tissue weights between treatment groups, with the exception of the liver which was reduced by 5% following OXA treatment ($p < 0.05$ from VEH, **Figure 2E**) and a further 5% following OXAB treatment ($p < 0.0001$ from VEH, **Figure 2E**). Although, there was no effect of treatments on the absolute heart weight, increased heart size when normalized to body weight was observed between OXAB and vehicle ($p < 0.005$, **Figure 2D**), however, no significant differences were observed for other collected muscles and organs when indexed against body weight.

Metabolic and Exercise Capacity Is Unaffected by OXA Treatment

To assess the impact of the effects of OXA on the skeletal muscular system at the whole body level, the metabolism, voluntary exercise capacity and participation in activities of daily living (behavioral time budgets) of mice were quantified in Promethion Metabolic cages (Sable Systems, U.S) for 24 h following the conclusion of the treatment regimen. Interestingly, no changes were noted in energy substrate utilization (**Figure 3A**), overall energy expenditure (**Figure 3B**), overall O_2 consumption (**Figure 3C**) or in exercise capacity (**Figures 3D–F**), following OXA treatment. Of note however, OXAB treatment reduced the basal energy expenditure at rest ($p < 0.05$, **Figure 3B**) and had a tendency ($p = 0.088$) to reduce the overall time spent on the running wheel, albeit the same distance was covered when compared to other groups. Furthermore, OXA treatment significantly reduced the time spent in inactivity periods longer that 60 s (long lounges), suggesting that mice were spending less time resting (**Figures 3D,F**). Interestingly though, OXA treated mice spent more time interacting with the food hoppers as seen in **Figure 3D**.

OXA Treatment Changes the Fiber Distribution of TA Sections and Reduces Isolated FDB Fiber Diameter

With previous studies showing that the oxidative stress induced by some chemotherapeutic agents potentiates skeletal muscle

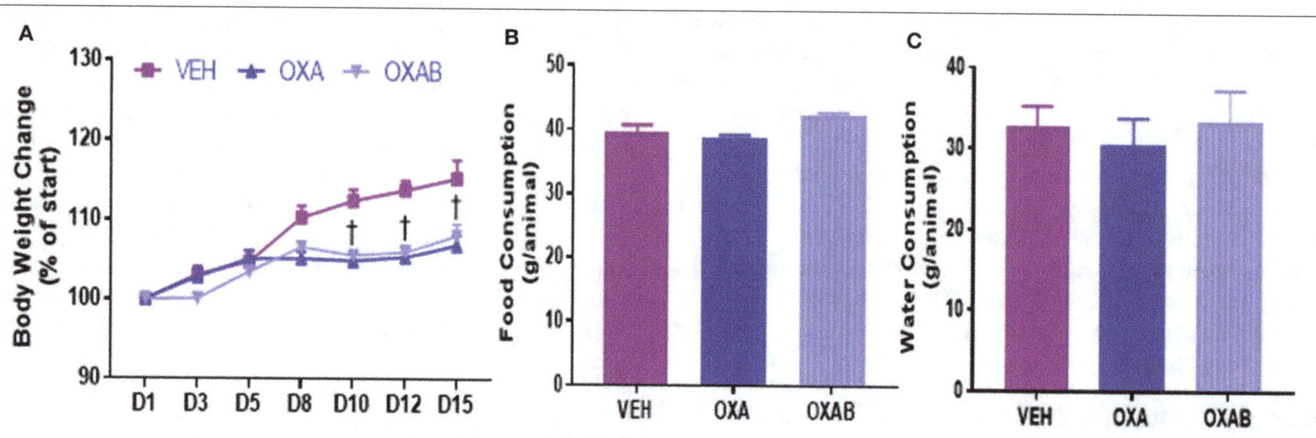

FIGURE 1 | Body weight and food consumption over the treatment period. OXA significantly reduced final post treatment body weights, with weight loss plateauing from D8 of OXA treatment **(A)**. Body weight of OXA treated mice (including OXAB) was significantly reduced from VEH from D10 onwards. No differences were detected in **(B)** Food consumption or **(C)** Water consumption between the groups. D#, treatment day number; Significance, $^{\dagger}p < 0.005$ OXA and OXAB different from VEH. $n = 6$–8.

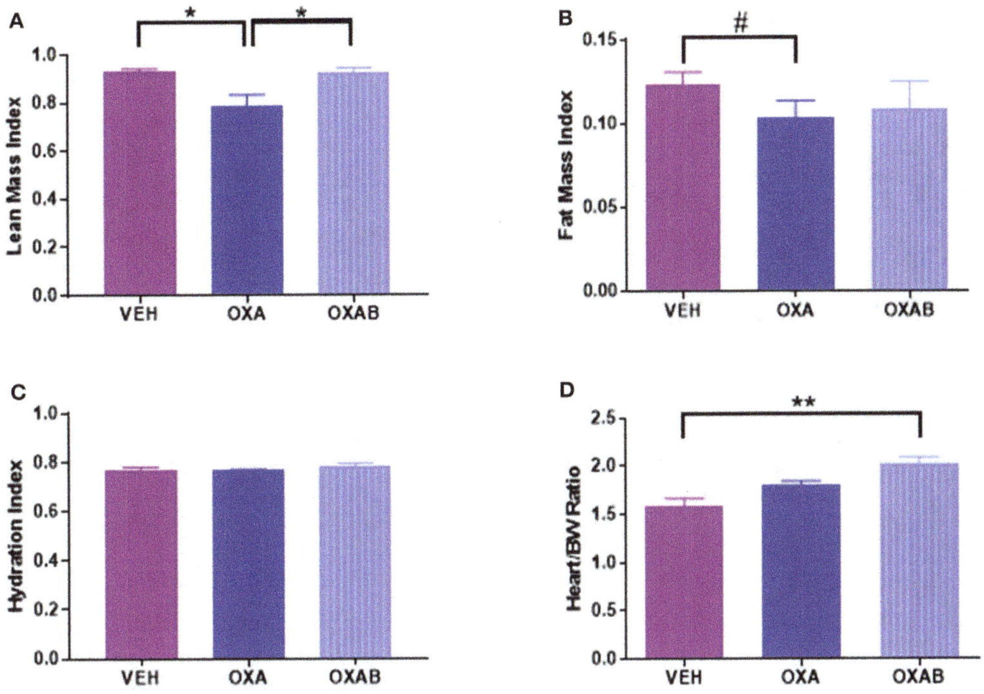

E

TISSUE	VEH	OXA	OXAB
	Mean wet tissue weight (g)		
E.D.L.	0.0118±0.0005	0.0108±0.0003	0.0103±0.0004
PLANTARIS	0.0085±0.0004	0.0086±0.0003	0.0077±0.0004
SOLEUS	0.0187±0.001	0.0186±0.0006	0.0180±0.001
TIB. ANT.	0.0484±0.004	0.0443±0.0014	0.0454±0.0035
DIAPRAGM	0.0894±0.003	0.0861±0.0043	0.0798±0.003
HEART	0.1175±0.002	0.1141±0.0034	0.1039±0.003
LUNGS	0.1722±0.005	0.1681±0.0053	0.1663±0.005
KIDNEY	0.1953±0.008	0.1802±0.0042	0.1684±0.009
LIVER	1.2489 ±0.054 AC	1.1952± 0.039 AB	1.1371 ±0.07 CB
SPLEEN	0.0882±0.003	0.0825±0.005	0.0630±0.006

FIGURE 2 | BGP-15 protects against Oxaliplatin-induced lean tissue but not fat mass loss. (A) BGP-15 protected against the OXA-induced reduction in LMI. **(B)** FMI was reduced by OXA treatment by 15% with no protection afforded by BGP-15. **(C)** Hydration Index calculated by [(echo derived total water – echo derived free water)/echo derived lean mass]. **(D)** Heart weight indexed against body weight showed OXAB treatment significantly increased heart size in relation to body weight. **(E)** Absolute wet tissue weights showed no significant difference either as raw or indexed against body weight, however OXA treatment reduced liver size with adjunct BGP-15 therapy further exacerbating this reduction (Table significance: A = $p < 0.05$ OXA to VEH. B = $p < 0.05$ OXA to OXAB. C = $p < 0.0001$ OXAB to VEH). BW, Body weight; EDL, Extensor Digitorum Longus; TID. ANT, Tibialis Anterior. Significance: *p<0.05, **p<0.005; Trend: #p = 0.076. n = 6–8.

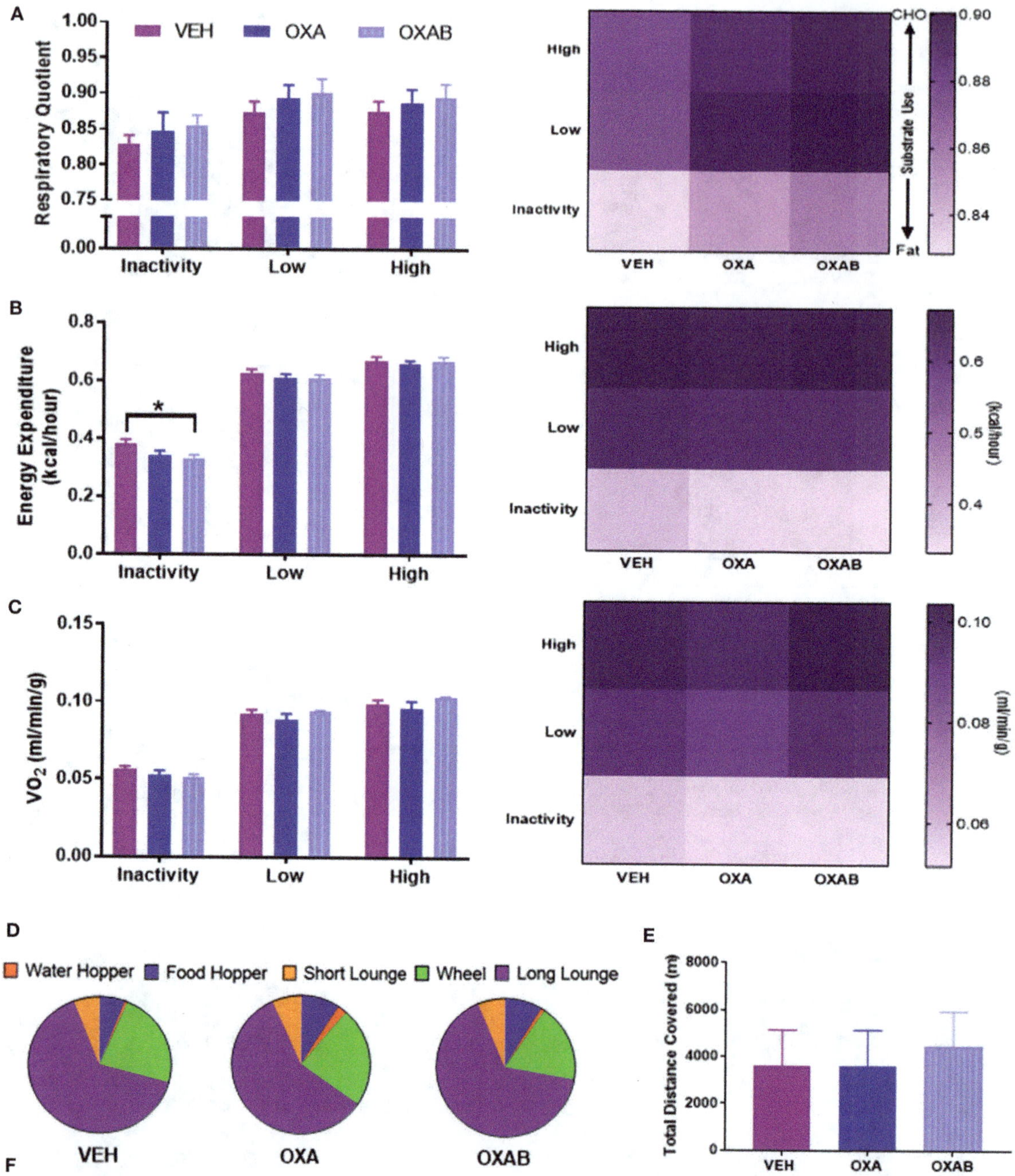

F

Interaction	VEH	OXA	OXAB
Food Hopper (%)	5.73 ± 1.29	9.18 ± 0.96 D	8.57 ± 1.22
Water Hopper (%)	0.61 ± 0.23	2.17 ± 1.12	0.88 ± 0.31
Wheel (%)	22.82 ± 7.36	23.30 ± 7.91	18.31 ± 4.84 *C*
Long Lounge (%)	64.93 ± 5.19	58.44 ± 7.15 *A*	65.81 ± 4.08 *B*
Short Lounge (%)	5.91 ± 1.47	6.90 ± 1.23	6.44 ± 0.99

FIGURE 3 | BGP-15 reduces basal energy expenditure with OXA treatment not affecting exercise capacity. (A) There was no significant effect of treatment on the respiratory quotient. **(B)** Energy expenditure at rest was reduced by BGP-15 adjunct therapy. **(C)** Oxygen consumption was not effected by treatment. **(D,F)** Time budgets of activities of daily living: OXA treatment reduced time spent engaged in long lounges ($p < 0.05$) while OXAB treatment reduced the time spent engaged in voluntary wheel running. **(E)** There was no effect of treatment on total meters covered (combination of wheel and pedestrian meters). CHO, Carbohydrate; VO_2, Volume Oxygen. Table significance: **(A)** $p < 0.05$ OXA vs. VEH, **(B)** $p < 0.05$ OXA vs. OXAB, **(C)** trend ($p = 0.088$) OXA vs. OXAB, **(D)** trend ($p = 0.057$) OXA vs. VEH. Significance: $^*p < 0.05$. $n = 6$–8.

dysfunction and atrophy (Bonifati et al., 2000; Gilliam et al., 2009), we were interested in assessing whether OXA could induce similar effects at the fiber level. OXA treatment increased the frequency of small TA fibers by 68% in the 600–899 μm bin range ($p < 0.05$), whilst reducing fiber frequency within the 1,500–1,799 μm bin range ($p < 0.005$). BGP-15 adjunct therapy offered protection exclusively against the OXA-induced fiber frequency reduction in the 1,500–1,799 μm range (**Figure 4B**). Myopathological analysis of H&E stained TA sections revealed no ultrastructural changes in nuclei location from the fiber periphery (normal) to the fiber center (pathological) and no signs of inflammatory infiltrate, which would both be indicative of damage and repair pathway activation (**Figure 4A**). In isolated FDB fibers, OXA treatment induced a 25% reduction in FDB fiber diameter ($p < 0.0001$ from VEH; **Figure 8F**). This effect was completely protected against by OXAB treatment ($p < 0.0005$ from OXA), whereby fiber diameter was comparable to VEH.

BGP-15 Protects against OXA-Induced Accumulation of Intracellular Ca^{2+}, Fat and Collagen in TA Muscle

Since intracellular Ca^{2+} dysregulation and accumulation is strongly linked with skeletal muscle pathology (Powers et al., 2007), we assessed the effect of OXA treatment on the Ca^{2+} content of TA using Alzarin Red staining (**Figure 5A**). OXA treatment increased the intracellular Ca^{2+} content by 22% from VEH ($p < 0.05$). This increase in Ca^{2+} however, could not be localized to a specific intracellular region (a limitation of the method) and did not appear to be at a concentration high enough to activate calpain-mediated damage responses as centralized nuclei were not observed in H&E stains (**Figure 4A**). Since fibrotic connective tissue and fat infiltration are also features of myopathy (Scheede-Bergdahl and Jagoe, 2013; Bredahl et al., 2016), Gomori trichrome and ORO staining were used to assess these markers, respectively. OXA treatment increased collagen deposition within TA sections by 36% ($p < 0.0005$, **Figure 5B**) and induced a 164% increase in the cross-sectional TA area infiltrated with neutral lipids ($p < 0.05$; **Figure 5C**). All OXA-induced histopathological features were completely protected against by OXAB treatment (**Figures 5A–C**).

Mitochondrial Pt Accumulation and Increased SDH following OXA Treatment

To establish whether OXA could (a) penetrate the skeletal muscle and (b) penetrate the double membrane of the mitochondria; analysis of the skeletal muscle nuclear and mitochondrial fraction was performed. We have previously hypothesized that OXA accumulation within the mitochondria could be deleterious to mitochondrial function (Sorensen et al., 2016). Pt was detected in both the nuclear (3.95 ppm) and mitochondrial (1.97 ppm) fractions compared to VEH ($p < 0.05$, **Figures 6A,B**, respectively). Of interest, there was ~50% less Pt content within the mitochondria subcellular fraction than in the nuclear fraction. To assess the impact of OXA permeation on mitochondrial capacity, we next investigated the content of the mitochondrial enzyme, SDH in TA sections (**Figure 6C**). There was a significant increase (~20%) in the SDH content of OXA treated mice compared to VEH ($p < 0.005$; **Figure 6C**), however BGP-15 had no effect on this parameter.

OXA Treatment Does Not Induce PARP Expression in Skeletal Muscle

PARP activation occurs secondary to DNA damage, and as such, we next investigated whether OXA treatment could induce PARP. Of particular interest was whether the PARP-inhibitor BGP-15 could inhibit induction of PARP activity. As such we quantified PARP1, PARP2, and total PARylation (marker of PARP activity, Gibson and Kraus, 2012, **Figure 7**) in TA muscles. Surprisingly there was no effect of OXA treatment on either PARP1 or 2 expression or total PARylation in TA. To this extent, there was no effect of BGP-15 on these parameters since PARP was not activated.

BGP-15 Adjunct Treatment Improves Mitochondrial Viability and Protects against OXA-Induced Mitochondrial Changes

mtROS are prevalent mediators of various muscle wasting mechanisms, including atrophy and apoptosis, and their production can be exacerbated if the mitochondria become dysfunctional or damaged (Kirkinezos and Moraes, 2001; Lenaz et al., 2002; Kujoth et al., 2005; Le Bras et al., 2005; Holzerová and Prokisch, 2015). At the mitochondrial level, OXA treatment induced a significant increase in mitochondrial density ($p < 0.05$, **Figure 8A**) and superoxide production ($p < 0.05$, **Figure 8B**) in FDB fibers, with OXAB treatment protecting against these effects. Interestingly, BGP-15 significantly increased mitochondrial viability 4-fold from OXA treated fibers ($p < 0.005$, **Figure 8C**) and 2-fold from VEH ($p = 0.073$) with OXA treatment alone showing a trend to decrease viability from VEH levels ($p = 0.077$).

OXA Reduces Protein Synthesis Markers

To elucidate whether the reduction in lean mass observed with OXA treatment corresponded with the activation of skeletal muscle atrophy signaling pathways, a variety of atrophy-related molecular signaling proteins were quantified via western blot. Of note, OXA treatment induced a 28% reduction of total p70S6K expression compared to VEH ($p < 0.005$, **Figure 9B**) indicating a reduced potential for protein synthesis. This was corroborated downstream by a drop in ribosomal protein S6 expression (rpS6, downstream transcription protein regulator, $p < 0.05$, **Figure 9C**) and a trend for a reduction in protein concentration within the TA ($p = 0.081$, **Figure 9A**). Of note, OXA treatment reduced BAX expression (apoptosis initiating protein, $p < 0.05$, **Figure 9E**) compared to VEH suggesting a reduced propensity for apoptosis induction. BGP-15 treatment protected against protein concentration reduction, however, had no observable effect on markers of protein synthesis.

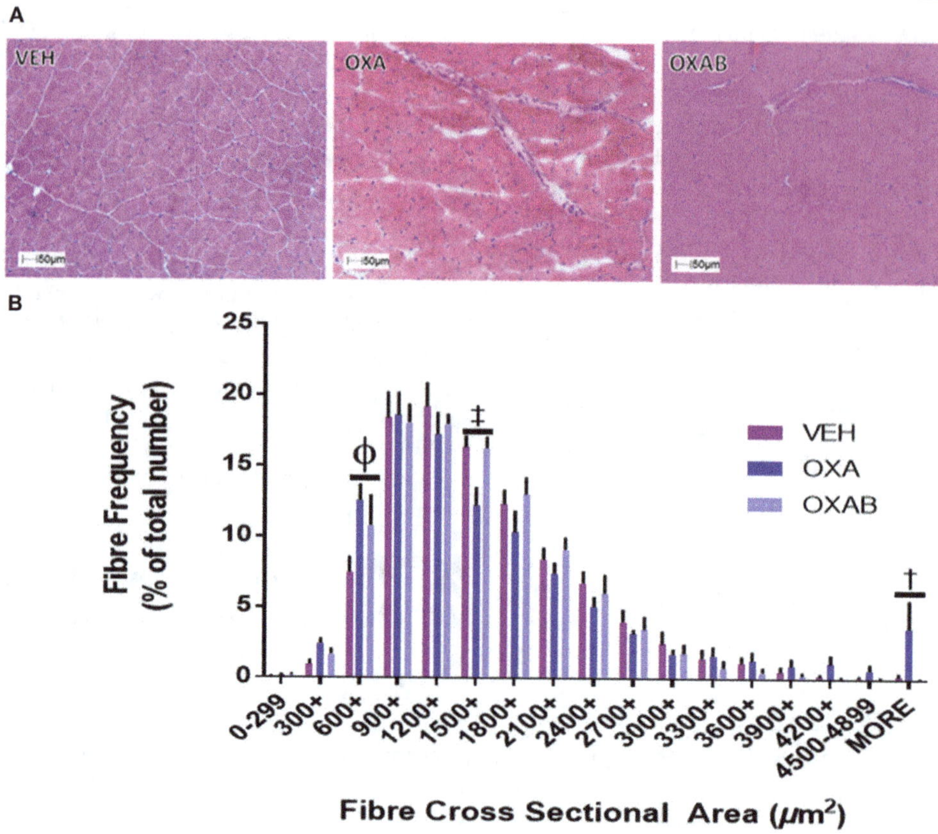

FIGURE 4 | OXA and BGP-15 treatment effect fiber size distribution in TA muscle. (A) Representative images of H&E stained TA and fiber size frequency histogram **(B)** OXA treatment significantly increased the frequency of fibers in the 600-899 μm^2 and >4,900 μm^2 size bins whilst reducing the frequency of fibers in the 1,500–1,799 μm^2 size bin. Significance: $^{\Phi}p < 0.0005$ VEH compared to OXA and $p < 0.05$ VEH from OXAB; $^{\ddagger}p < 0.005$ VEH and OXAB compared to OXA, $^{\dagger}p < 0.05$ OXA and OXAB compared to VEH. $n = 4$.

DISCUSSION

In this study we demonstrate that OXA chemotherapy: (1) significantly reduces body weight which is underpinned by a decline in lean tissue and liver mass; (2) does not impact voluntary exercise capacity, O_2 consumption or energy expenditure in mice; (3) shifts fiber size distribution to favor smaller fibers in the TA whilst increasing collagen, neutral lipid, and Ca^{2+} accumulation; (4) reduces FDB fiber diameter; (5) penetrates the mitochondria and increases mitochondrial population and superoxide (O_2^-) production in FDB fibers and SDH content/capacity in TA; and (6) reduces molecular markers of protein synthesis pathways with the tendency to reduce intramuscular protein content. Importantly, our data highlights a novel application for the pharmacological cytoprotectant, BGP-15, which when administered with OXA (OXAB) protected against the observed reductions in lean tissue mass and FDB fiber diameter and TA protein content, mitochondrial O_2^- production and histopathological features of TA sections. BGP-15 adjunct therapy also increased mitochondrial pool viability and reduced the energy expenditure of mice during inactivity.

Chemotherapeutic drugs are well described as toxic antineoplastic agents capable of causing significant side effects in healthy tissues (Davies and Doroshow, 1986; Sternberg et al., 2001; Lu, 2005; Argilés et al., 2015). In skeletal muscle, this correlates with sustained dysfunction resulting in fatigue and wasting (Mantovani et al., 2003; Gilliam and St Clair, 2011; Gilliam et al., 2012; Gouspillou et al., 2015), with wasting being traditionally attributed to an imbalance between protein degradation and synthesis (Sandri, 2008). Since a decline in muscle mass is negatively associated with patient survivability, quality of life and chemotherapeutic treatment options (Talvensaari et al., 1996; Oeffinger et al., 2006; van Brussel et al., 2006; Ness et al., 2007, 2012; Scheede-Bergdahl and Jagoe, 2013), methods to protect the skeletal muscle from dysfunction and loss is of paramount importance. Here we have investigated the effect of 2 weeks of OXA treatment in 6 week old Balb/c mice and observed, as expected, a marked reduction in body weight from D8 onwards (when compared to VEH, **Figure 1A**). Once a cumulative dose of 9 mg/kg of OXA was reached, mice ceased to accumulate body mass which was shown to be independent of caloric intake (**Figure 1B**), hydration index (**Figure 2C**) and energy expenditure (**Figure 3B**). Further

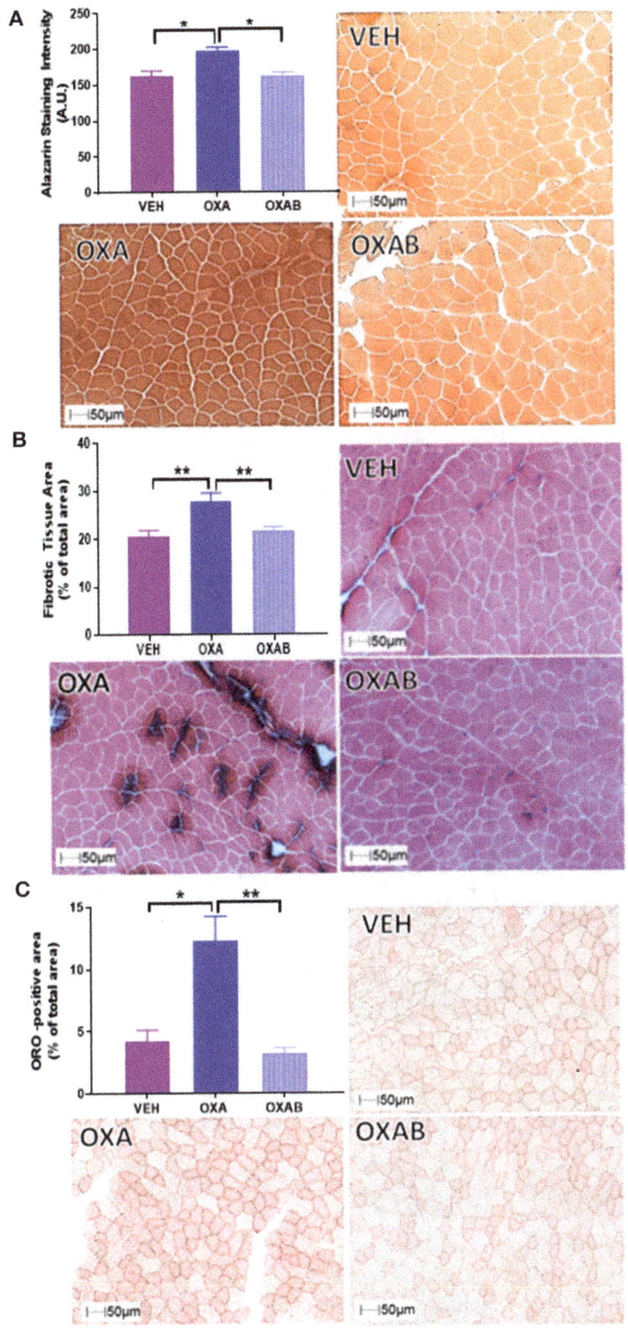

FIGURE 5 | BGP-15 protects against OXA-induced increases in intracellular Ca^{2+}, collagen deposition and fat infiltration in TA muscle. OXA treatment increased **(A)** intracellular Ca^{2+} content **(B)** fibrotic tissue and collagen deposition and **(C)** fat infiltration with OXAB protecting against all these parameters in TA muscles. A.U., Arbitrary units; ORO, Oil Red O. Significance: $^{*}p < 0.05$, $^{**}p < 0.005$.

analysis of body composition elucidated that OXA treatment depressed total lean tissue mass with a tendency for fat mass to follow the same declination when indexed against absolute body weight (**Figures 2A–C**). It is interesting to speculate that the loss of lean mass (and tendency for the loss of fat mass) might be strongly correlated with OXA-induced enteric neuropathy and gastrointestinal dysfunction which has been reported previously (Stojanovska et al., 2015; McQuade et al., 2016a) and which likely limits the capacity for nutrient absorption in the small intestine. Skeletal muscle mass is strongly associated with the nutritional status of the organism (Jeejeebhoy et al., 1990; Mithal et al., 2013; Moon, 2014), whereby in times of nutrient deprivation (i.e., starvation), skeletal muscle protein synthesis pathways are inhibited and degradation pathways are activated to liberate nutritionals stores (particularly glucose and amino acids) for key physiological functions (Thissen et al., 1994; Levine and Kroemer, 2008). Our protein analyses, although a small snapshot of a complex and dynamic system, suggests that OXA treatment reduces p70s6K (**Figure 9B**) and rpS6 expression and has the tendency to reduce intramuscular protein content, possibly via inhibition of the master hypertrophy regulator, mTOR, which is notably inhibited by nutrient deprivation in skeletal muscle (Mammucari et al., 2008; Pasiakos et al., 2010; Zoncu et al., 2011; Laplante and Sabatini, 2012). mTOR inhibition is also typically accompanied by the induction of skeletal muscle degradative pathways (Mammucari et al., 2008; Pasiakos et al., 2010). While we show no effect of OXA on MURF1 (**Figure 9F**) or the autophagy regulator p62 (**Figure 9G**), there are several other pathways implicated in nutrient-deprivation related skeletal muscle wasting that we have not investigated (such as TRAF6 Fan and Cook, 2004; Kumar et al., 2012; Paul et al., 2012) and which may be causing the loss of lean mass observed in our study.

Promisingly, adjunct BGP-15 therapy protected mice against OXA-induced changes in lean tissue mass. We have shown that BGP-15 can protect myenteric neurons against OXA-induced insult to ameliorate gastrointestinal dysfunction (McQuade et al., 2016b)—thus it is likely that BGP-15 promotes nutrient absorption and the overall nutritional status, thus protecting the muscle mass. Interestingly, we observed a marked reduction in liver weight as a result of OXA treatment which is consistent with glycogen depletion, however this effect was exacerbated by BGP-15 treatment. The effect of BGP-15 on liver mass is curious and could be a direct effect of drug metabolism that has not been reported previously. BGP-15 adjunct therapy was also observed to increase heart size to body weight ratio (**Figure 2D**). While this could be indicative of cardiac hypertrophy, previous studies have shown BGP-15 to be cardio-protective against heart failure and inflammation (Szabados et al., 2000; Sarszegi et al., 2012; Sapra et al., 2014). Indeed, our exercise and VO_2 data indicate no performance deficit following OXAB treatment, thus the increased heart weight to body weight ratio observed appears not to be detrimental to function.

Exercise therapy is an emerging treatment against chemotherapy- and cachexia-driven skeletal muscle wasting (Al-Majid and McCarthy, 2001; Smuder et al., 2011; Jarvela et al., 2012; Kavazis et al., 2014; Bredahl et al., 2016). While exercise before, during and after anti-cancer therapy is a field of research that has gained traction in the recent years, there is currently no established protocol that is prescribed in the clinic to prevent and/or treat skeletal muscle atrophy during cancer treatment (André et al., 2004; Alcindor and Beauger, 2011).

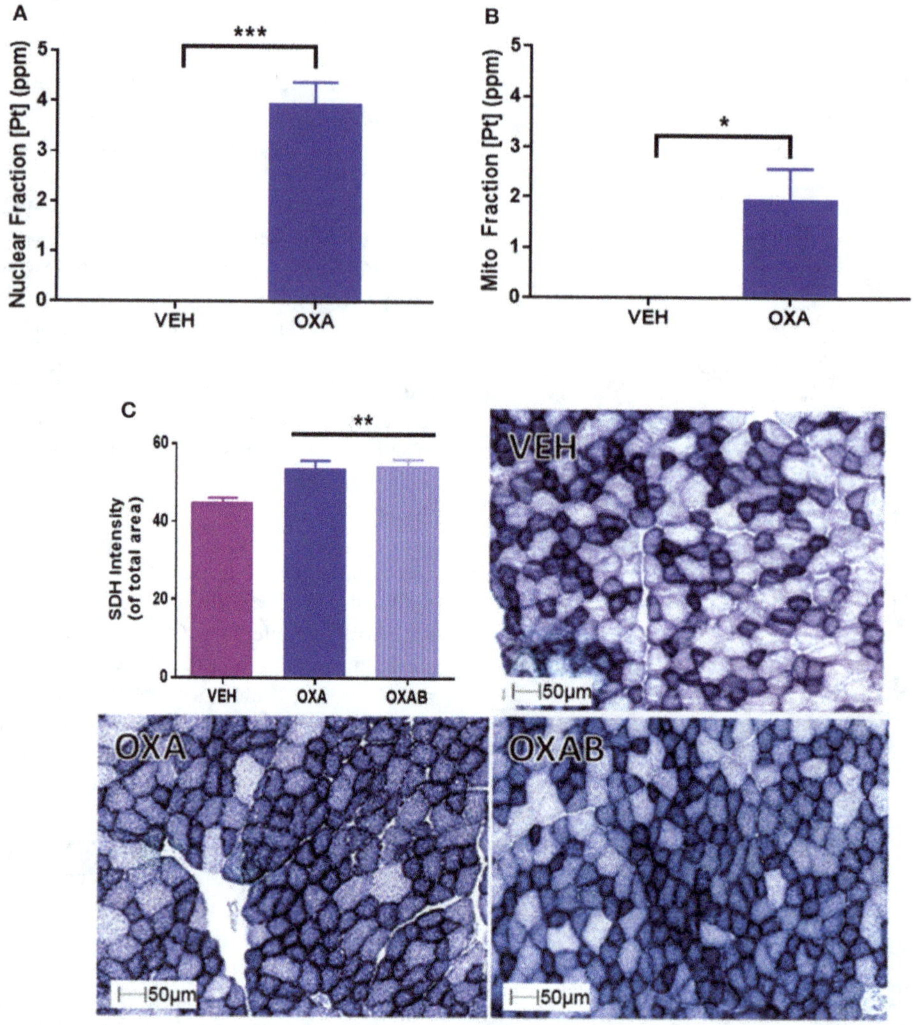

FIGURE 6 | OXA penetrates the nuclear and mitochondrial fractions of TA muscle homogenates and increases succinate dehydrogenase (SDH) content. (A) OXA penetrated the nuclear and **(B)** mitochondrial fractions as quantified by Pt detection ($n = 3$–4). **(C)** SDH staining was significantly increased with OXA treatment but OXAB had no effect on this measure ($n = 6$–8). [Pt], Platinum concentration; SDH, SDH Succinate dehydrogenase; ppm, parts per million. Significance: $^{*}p = <0.05$, $^{**}p = <0.005$, $^{***}p = <0.0005$.

For these reasons and in light of our observed reduction in lean mass, investigations into exercise tolerability and capacity were performed. Surprisingly, OXA treatment did not hinder voluntary exercise participation in mice (**Figures 3D–F**), nor did chemotherapy alter average exercise intensity (data not shown), duration or distance (**Figures 3D–F**). Interestingly though, behavioral analysis of the mice in relation to time budgeting of activities of daily living revealed that OXA-treated mice engaged in fewer long lounge periods (indicative of rest and sleep) during the 24 h analysis period, which is contradictive to the fatigue reported by chemotherapy-treated patients (Love et al., 1989; Greene et al., 1993). Given we concomitantly observed a strong trend ($p = 0.057$) for OXA-treated mice to interact with the food hopper, our data suggest that these mice might be waking more frequently to eat which is consistent with our nutrient deprivation hypothesis. As with our body composition data, BGP-15 protected against this OXA-induced behavioral change.

It is reasonable to assume that exercise could be more arduous for OXA treated mice due to the decline in lean tissue mass, however, gas exchange analysis showed comparable RQ and O_2 consumption between VEH and OXA groups at all levels of exercise intensity, and at rest. BGP-15 adjunct therapy, however, reduced basal energy expenditure at rest (**Figure 3B**) and increased mouse exercise performance (reduced time spent on wheel compared to other groups **Figures 3D,F** with same distance outcome **Figure 3E**) suggesting that BGP-15 has the capacity to improve exercise efficiency, possibly due to improved mitochondrial coupling (Conley et al., 2013). Indeed, enhanced mitochondrial efficiency is a key adaptation during nutrient deprivation to increase energy extraction from macronutrients in the form of ATP as opposed to heat (Weyer et al., 2000). While we

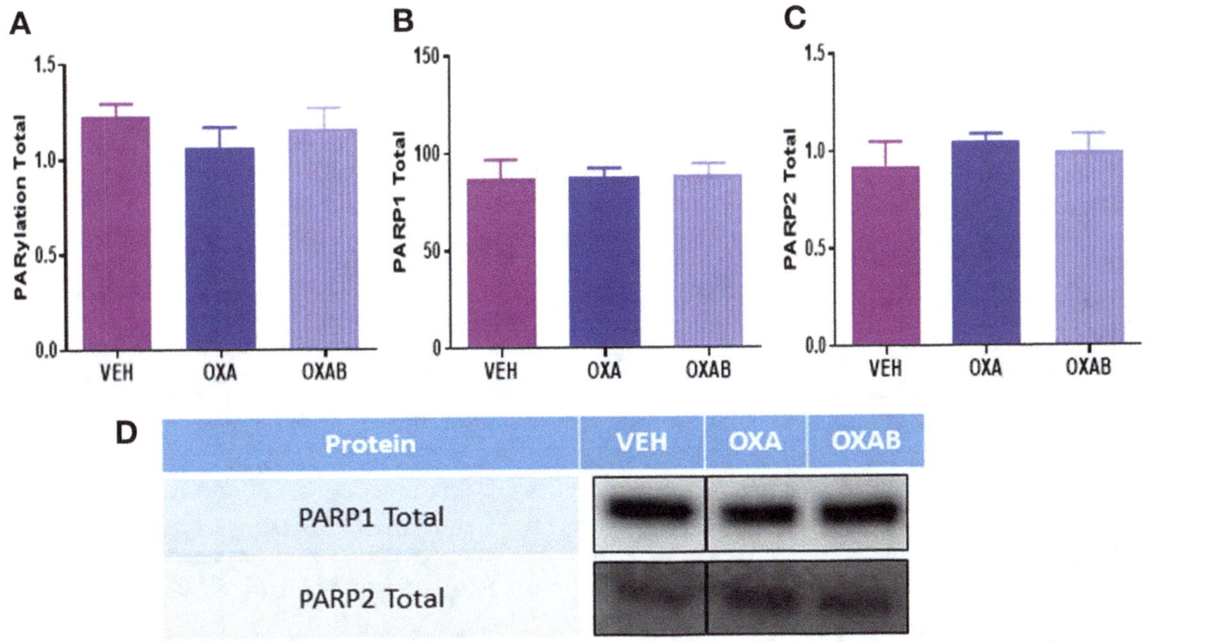

FIGURE 7 | OXA and BGP-15 treatment does not alter PARP expression in mouse TA. No changes in **(A)** total PARylation **(B)** PARP1 or **(C)** PARP2 were detected following OXA treatment. Adjunct treatment with the PARP inhibitor BGP-15 (OXAB) did not alter PARP expression. **(D)** Representative stainfree Western blot images are digitally cut together to remove blots of other chemotherapies not presented in this manuscript, no other alteration was performed.

did not measure skeletal muscle uncoupling protein expression or inducible uncoupling in our study (a noteworthy limitation), our data suggests that BGP-15 might protect the skeletal muscle from chemotherapy/nutrient-deprivation-induced wasting by enhancing mitochondrial efficiency (**Figure 8C**).

In addition to mass, muscle quality is a major contributor to the overall functional and reparative capacity of the muscle. To this effect, a reduction in quality (i.e., increased intra- and inter-muscle fat) irrespective of absolute mass would greatly impede a patients' ability to perform activities of daily living, ultimately reducing independence and quality of life. Histological analysis of TA muscles following OXA treatment highlighted features consistent with myopathy including a significant accumulation of both Ca^{2+} and neutral lipids within the TA architecture (**Figures 5A,C**). Furthermore, markedly higher levels of collagen deposition were identified in OXA-treated TA muscle. These findings, taken together with the fact that hind limb muscle weights were comparable to VEH following OXA treatment, suggest that gross measurement of muscle weight was not sensitive enough to detect changes in muscle mass, whereby increased collagen and fat would contribute to muscle weight. At the cross sectional level, OXA treatment shifted the fiber size distribution to the left, in particular, reducing the number of fibers within the 1,200–2,999 μm^2 fiber cross sectional area range, whilst increasing the number of smaller fibers within the 300–1,199 μm^2 bin ranges (**Figure 4B**). While the mechanism behind this fiber size distribution shift remains unclear, the significant increase in fibers above 4,900 μm^2 in OXA treated mice (21x greater compared to VEH) suggests that OXA treatment induced pathological changes. Pseudohypertrophic fibers are a pronounced feature of myopathy, in which healthy fibers hypertrophy to compensate for the loss of strength induced by muscle atrophy, wasting and/or replacement with non-functional tissue (such as fat and connective tissue; Briguet et al., 2004; Timpani et al., 2016). Importantly, BGP-15 adjunct therapy ameliorated all of these OXA-induced pathologies by protecting against Ca^{2+}, lipid and collagen accumulation and restoring a normal fiber distribution. These findings, albeit novel in the chemotherapy/skeletal muscle arena, align with the findings of a recent study by Salah et al. (2016) who demonstrated that BGP-15 could protect against fibrotic tissue and collagen accumulation within mechanically-ventilated diaphragm muscle. They suggested that BGP-15's efficacy was mediated via membrane lipid therapy mechanisms (Salah et al., 2016), an effect that has also been established in other myopathies (Gehrig et al., 2012). Furthermore, BGP-15 has recently been shown to improve certain myopathological aspects of DMD such as collagen deposition (Kennedy et al., 2016), which is consistent with our data.

Chemotherapy-induced oxidative stress has previously been linked, albeit almost exclusively following anthracycline treatment (Gilliam et al., 2012; Gouspillou et al., 2015), to mitochondrial-mediated cell damage pathways within skeletal muscle (Davies and Doroshow, 1986; Doroshow and Davies, 1986; Gilliam et al., 2012; Min et al., 2015). Since OXA, via the Pt component of the molecule, adducts nDNA resulting in DNA damage, impeded transcription/translation and cell death (Raymond et al., 1998; André et al., 2004; Gourdier et al., 2004; Alcindor and Beauger, 2011), we have previously hypothesized that OXA could induce the same damage to

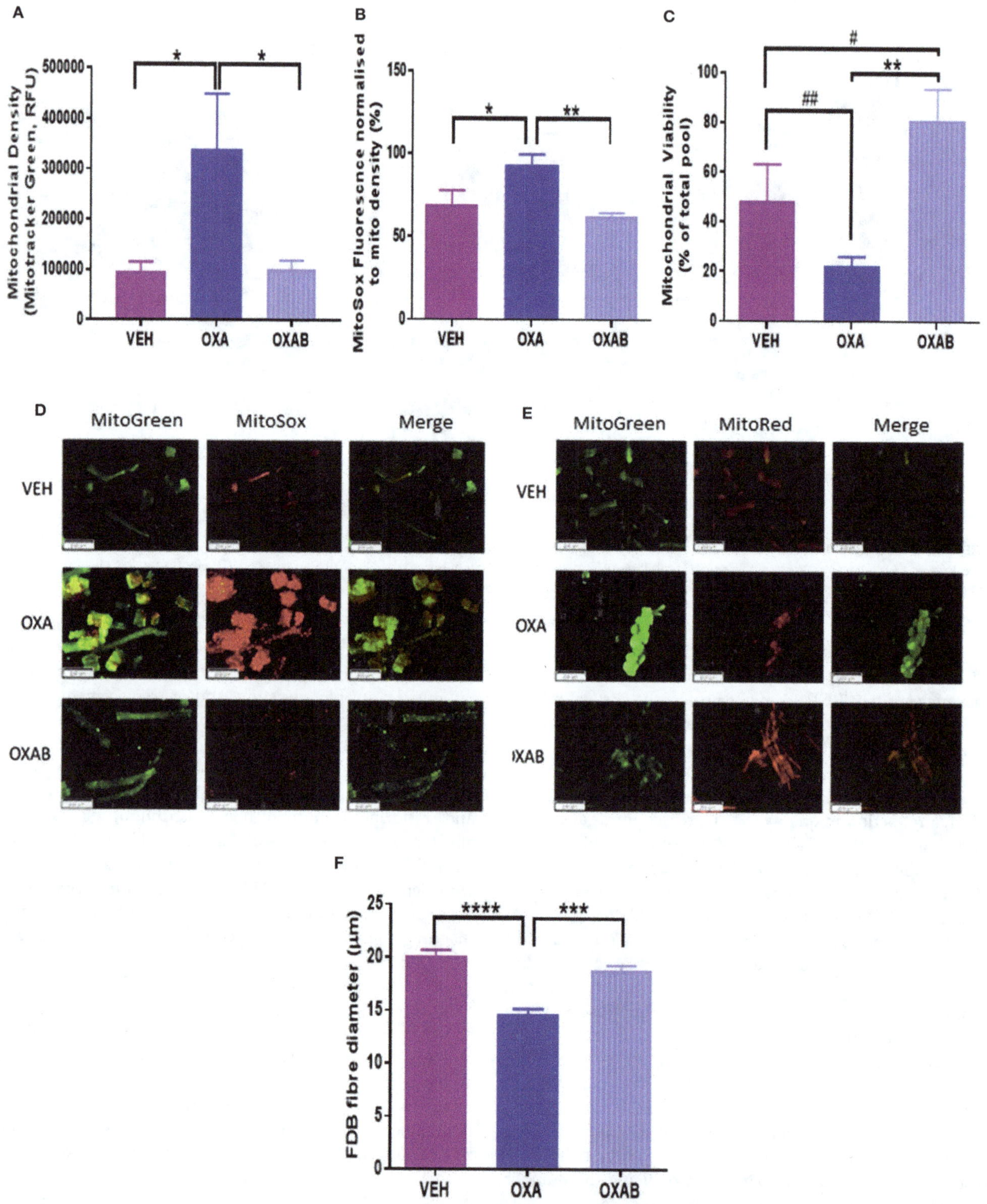

FIGURE 8 | BGP-15 protects against OXA-induced mitochondrial superoxide production and fiber diameter loss and improves mitochondrial viability in FDB fibers. OXA treatment induced **(A)** A 4-fold increase in mitochondrial density, with OXAB protecting against this increase. **(B)** OXAB protected against a 25% increase in MitoSOX fluorescence induced by OXA treatment. **(C)** OXA treatment reduced mitochondrial viability while OXAB treatment protected against the effects of OXA and improved viability 4-fold from VEH. Representative images of MitoSOX and MitoTracker stained FDB fibers **(D,E)**. OXA treatment also induced a **(F)** 25% reduction in FDB Fiber diameter with OXAB protecting against this reduction. FDB, Flexor Digitorum Longus; Mito, Mitochondria; SOX, Superoxide. Significance: *$p < 0.05$, **$p < 0.005$, ***$p < 0.0005$, ****$p < 0.0001$. Trend: $\#p = 0.073$, $\#\#p = 0.077$. n = 4–6.

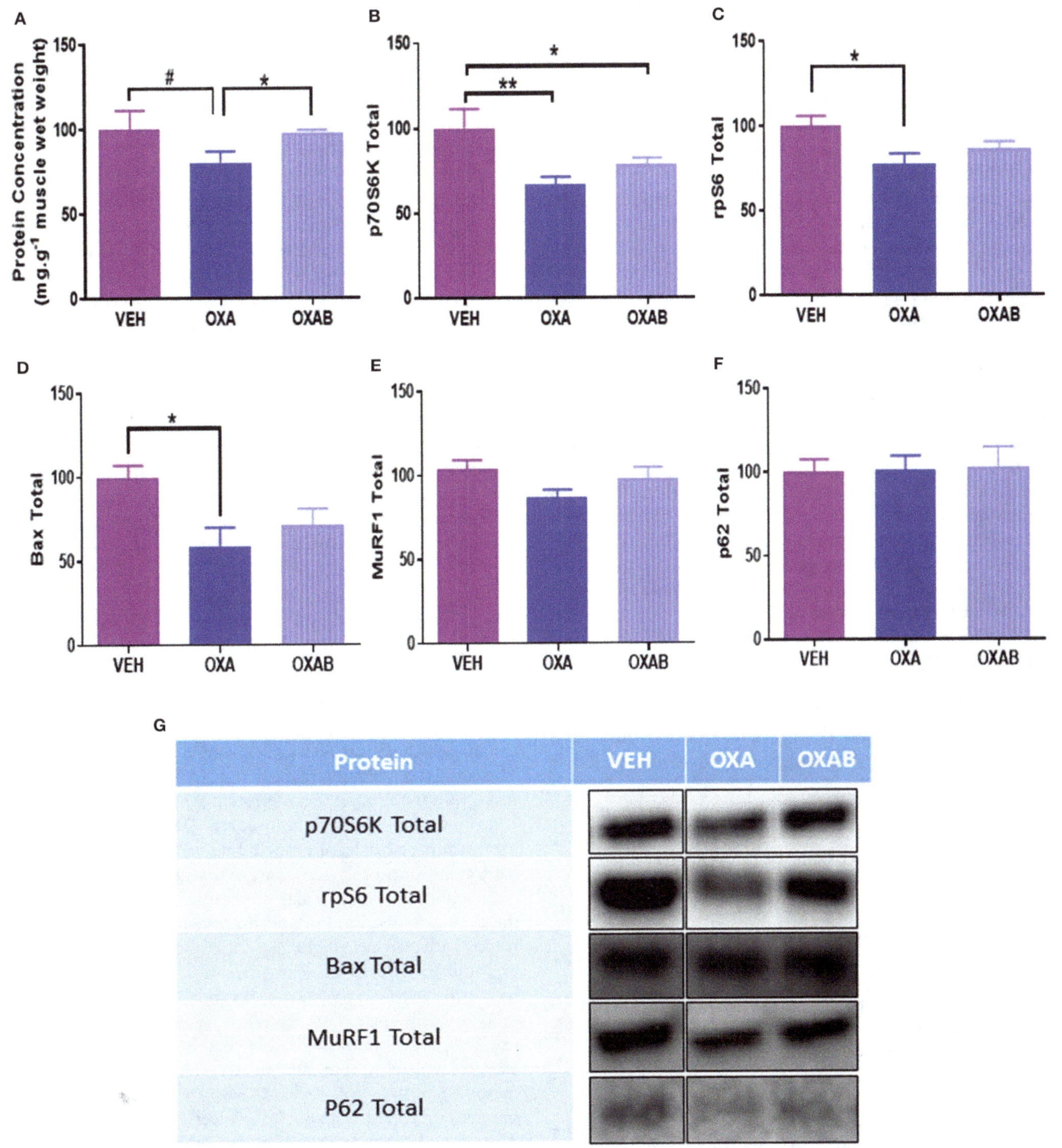

FIGURE 9 | OXA treatment reduces protein synthesis and concentration within TA muscle. (A) OXA treatment showed a trend to reduce total protein concentration, and reduced **(B)** total p70S6K and **(C)** total rpS6 when compared to VEH suggesting a suppression of protein synthesis. **(D)** Apoptosis initiation marker total Bax was also supressed in TA muscle. Contrastingly no change in **(E)** total ubiquitin-proteasome marker MuRF1 or **(F)** autophagy marker p62 expression was noted. **(G)** Western blot representative images are digitally cut together to remove blots of other chemotherapies not presented in this manuscript, no other alteration was performed. Significance: $^{*}p < 0.05$, $^{**}p < 0.005$ Trend: $^{\#}p = 0.081$. $n = 6$–8.

mtDNA (Sorensen et al., 2016). To substantiate this, atomic absorption spectrophotometry was utilized to detect Pt in the subcellular mitochondrial fraction. Pertinently, we are the first to show that OXA does in fact penetrate both the skeletal muscle and the mitochondria, suggesting that OXA could also be inducing Pt adducts into mtDNA (**Figure 6B**).

The net effect of OXA treatment at the mitochondrial level was increased succinate dehydrogenase (SDH) content within the muscle, indicative of a greater mitochondrial oxidative capacity. However, there was a trend for OXA ($p = 0.07$) to reduce mitochondrial viability relative to VEH (**Figure 8C**), highlighting that the innate response to oxidative stress and/or mitochondrial toxicity is to increase the total pool to preserve energy production capacity (Hsin-Chen et al., 2000) as indicated by more intense SDH staining (**Figure 6C**) and mitochondrial density (**Figure 8C**). Consistent with this finding, a marked increase in mtROS production was detected in FDB fibers following OXA treatment (**Figure 8B**) giving further support to our theory that mitochondrial biogenesis could be increased in order to accommodate oxidative stress and a dysfunctional mitochondrial population (Hsin-Chen et al., 2000; Kujoth et al., 2005; Stowe and Camara, 2009; Sorensen et al., 2016). Remarkably, BGP-15 completely protected against the OXA-induced increase in mtROS production and reduction in FDB fiber diameter and intramuscular protein content, however, this effect was independent from any modulation of protein synthesis, atrophy, autophagy or apoptosis markers measured in our study (**Figure 9**). Moreover, BGP-15 treatment was shown to improve mitochondrial viability by 60% from OXA- and 40% from VEH-treated groups (**Figure 8C**), which we originally hypothesized would be due to molecular inhibition of PARP and the restoration of mitochondrial substrates (NADH) to the electron transport chain (NADH is a known substrate of PARP) (Zhou et al., 2006). Unexpectedly though, we were unable to detect any changes in PARP1, PARP2, or total PARylation with OXA or OXAB treatment (**Figure 7A–C**). This suggests in the first instance that OXA treatment at the dosage administered (18 mg/kg cumulative dose) does not stimulate PARP activity in skeletal muscle; and secondly that BGP-15 improved mitochondrial viability and normalized mtROS production via an alternative mechanism. Since mtROS are key mediators of muscle maintenance pathways (Powers et al., 2005, 2011, 2012; Min et al., 2011; Smuder et al., 2011), BGP-15's capacity to reduce mtROS could be key to its therapeutic benefit. By limiting oxidative stress, BGP-15 likely affords protection to the mitochondria from protein oxidation and dysfunction, subsequently resulting in the observed increase in both mitochondrial density and viability. While not a definitive mechanism, we speculate that BGP-15 might achieve this by enhancing mitochondrial coupling efficiency, which would explain the lower resting energy expenditure observed in mice and potentially reduce electron leak (and therefore ROS production) concomitantly with proton leak. Certainly, our data highlights the therapeutic potential of BGP-15 to protect against the debilitating side-effects of OXA chemotherapy, at the whole body, organ and mitochondrial levels.

LIMITATIONS

It should be noted, that the present study is limited in its resemblance to the clinical setting in which only patients afflicted with cancer are administered chemotherapy treatment. As such, it does not take into consideration the complex interactions between tumor-mediated cachexia and chemotherapy-driven muscle wasting. Furthermore, the complexity of the pathways underlying cachexia- and chemotherapy-driven wasting have not been completely illuminated herein, with only a selection of highly investigated protein markers of molecular atrophy signaling being presented. At the organ level reductions in the liver and heart mass were observed following OXA treatment and were exacerbated with OXAB treatment. Since blood samples were not taken, we were unable to investigate markers of liver damage (such as aspartate transaminase, alanine transaminase and lactate dehydrogenase levels) which may have shed light on the underlying mechanisms behind the observed decrease in liver sizes with OXA and combination OXAB therapy. Although investigations of lower limb muscle weights showed no significant changes, this finding is limited in its interpretation as the remaining upper limb and core muscles as well as organs, such as the gastrointestinal tract and brain, were not collected. Furthermore, fiber typing of the skeletal muscle was not performed and this would be useful to determine whether the OXA-induced increases in SDH and neutral lipid density within TA sections were due to oxidative fiber type transitions. While we are currently undertaking these investigations, previous studies have shown that muscle mass loss induced by other pro-oxidant chemotherapy drugs (specifically doxorubicin) is independent of fiber type (Gilliam et al., 2009).

CONCLUSION

Chemotherapy treatment remains the foremost defense against advanced neoplastic growth, however treatment often creates and exacerbates considerable dysfunctions within the skeletal muscle system, which endure well after chemotherapy treatment ceases. This study has demonstrated that OXA-treatment reduces lean mass, with the suppression of protein synthesis pathways a likely contributing mechanism. Moreover, OXA treatment induces various myopathic features including the accumulation of Ca^{2+}, neutral lipid, and collagen tissue within the muscle architecture, a reduction in intramuscular protein content, a leftward shift in the fiber size distribution and exacerbated mtROS production. Importantly, we have highlighted the efficacy of BGP-15 therapy to combat OXA-driven lean mass loss. For the first time we have demonstrated that OXA can independently penetrate the mitochondria, and is thus a likely contributor to these myopathic features. We importantly show that BGP-15 adjunct therapy either completely or partially protects the skeletal muscle against these deleterious side effects. BGP-15 appears to modulate the cytoprotective response to protect the mitochondria from damage and enhance both pool density and viability, albeit not via PARP inhibition. Although the precise mechanism of action requires further elucidation, here we show a novel application for the small molecule, BGP-15, in the protection of skeletal muscle against platinum-based chemotherapy-induced myopathy and wasting.

AUTHOR CONTRIBUTIONS

ER, AP, and AH conceived the study and obtained funding. ER, AH, JS, and CT designed the experiments. JS, CT, DC, JC,

AT, VS, and MS contributed to the experimental acquisition of the data. ER, JS, AP, CT, DC, JC, VS, and MS contributed to the analysis of the data. All authors contributed to the interpretation of the data and the writing and editing of the manuscript. All authors approve of the final manuscript submission and agree to be accountable for all aspects of the work. The authors all contributed to the writing of this manuscript.

FUNDING

This work was supported by the Centre for Chronic Disease and the Institute of Sport, Exercise and Active Living (ISEAL) Clinical Exercise Program funding schemes (both Victoria University).

SUPPLEMENTARY MATERIAL

Supplementary Figure1 | Stain free images of western blot analysis. Representative images for PARylation and PARP1 and PARP2 total used for signal protein analysis in the range of ~250–25 kDa.

Supplementary Figure2 | Stain free images of western blot analysis. Representative images used for signal protein analysis in the range of ~250–25 kDa.

REFERENCES

Alcindor, T., and Beauger, N. (2011). Oxaliplatin: a review in the era of molecularly targeted therapy. *Curr. Oncol.* 18, 18–25. doi: 10.3747/co.v18i1.708

Al-Majid, S., and McCarthy, D. O. (2001). Cancer-induced fatigue and skeletal muscle wasting: the role of exercise. *Biol. Res. Nurs.* 2, 186–197. doi: 10.1177/109980040100200304

André, T., Boni, C., Mounedji-Boudiaf, L., Navarro, M., Tabernero, J., Hickish, T., et al. (2004). Oxaliplatin, fluorouracil, and leucovorin as adjuvant treatment for colon cancer. *New Engl. J. Med.* 350, 2343–2351. doi: 10.1056/NEJMoa032709

Argilés, J. M., López-Soriano, F. J., and Busquets, S. (2015). Muscle wasting in cancer: the role of mitochondria. *Curr. Opin. Clin. Nutr. Metab. Care* 18, 221–225. doi: 10.1097/MCO.0000000000000164

Ariaans, G., de Jong, S., Gietema, J., Lefrandt, J., de Vries, E., and Jalving, M. (2015). Cancer-drug induced insulin resistance: innocent bystander or unusual suspect. *Cancer Treat. Rev.* 41, 376–384. doi: 10.1016/j.ctrv.2015.02.007

Aschele, C., Friso, M. L., Pucciarelli, S., Lonardi, S., Sartor, L., Fabris, G., et al. (2005). A phase I–II study of weekly oxaliplatin, 5-fluorouracil continuous infusion and preoperative radiotherapy in locally advanced rectal cancer. *Ann. Oncol.* 16, 1140–1146. doi: 10.1093/annonc/mdi212

Ashley, N., and Poulton, J. (2009). Mitochondrial DNA is a direct target of anti-cancer anthracycline drugs. *Biochem. Biophys. Res. Commun.* 378, 450–455. doi: 10.1016/j.bbrc.2008.11.059

Bonifati, D. M., Ori, C., Rossi, C. R., Caira, S., Fanin, M., and Angelini, C. (2000). Neuromuscular damage after hyperthermic isolated limb perfusion in patients with melanoma or sarcoma treated with chemotherapeutic agents. *Cancer Chemother. Pharmacol.* 46, 517–522. doi: 10.1007/s002800000175

Bredahl, E. C., Pfannenstiel, K. B., Quinn, C. J., Hayward, R., and Hydock, D. S. (2016). Effects of exercise on doxorubicin-induced skeletal muscle dysfunction. *Med. Sci. Sports Exer.* 48, 1468–1473. doi: 10.1249/MSS.0000000000000926

Briguet, A., Courdier-Fruh, I., Foster, M., Meier, T., and Magyar, J. P. (2004). Histological parameters for the quantitative assessment of muscular dystrophy in the mdx-mouse. *Neuromusc. Disord.* 14, 675–682. doi: 10.1016/j.nmd.2004.06.008

Cheregi, B., Timpani, C., Nurgali, K., Hayes, A., and Rybalka, E. (2015). Chemotherapy-induced mitochondrial respiratory dysfunction, oxidant production and death in healthy skeletal muscle C2C12 myoblast and myotube models. *Neuromusc. Disord.* 25(Suppl. 2), S202. doi: 10.1016/j.nmd.2015.06.069

Chung, J., Nguyen, A.-K., Henstridge, D. C., Holmes, A. G., Chan, M. S., and Duffy, S. J. (2008). HSP72 protects against obesity-induced insulin resistance. *Proc. Natl. Acad. Sci. U.S.A.* 105, 1739–1744. doi: 10.1073/pnas.0705799105

Conley, K. E., Jubrias, S. A., Cress, M. E., and Esselman, P. C. (2013). Elevated energy coupling and aerobic capacity improves exercise performance in endurance-trained elderly subjects. *Exp. Physiol.* 98, 899–907. doi: 10.1113/expphysiol.2012.069633

Davies, K., and Doroshow, J. (1986). Redox cycling of anthracyclines by cardiac mitochondria. I. Anthracycline radical formation by NADH dehydrogenase. *J. Biol. Chem.* 261, 3060–3067.

de Gramont, A., Figer, A., Seymour, M., Homerin, M., Hmissi, A., Cassidy, J., et al. (2000). Leucovorin and fluorouracil with or without oxaliplatin as first-line treatment in advanced colorectal cancer. *J. Clin. Oncol.* 18, 2938–2947. doi: 10.1200/JCO.2000.18.16.2938

Doroshow, J., and Davies, K. (1986). Redox cycling of anthracyclines by cardiac mitochondria. II. Formation of superoxide anion, hydrogen peroxide, and hydroxyl radical. *J. Biol. Chem.* 261, 3068–3074.

Fan, H., and Cook, J. A. (2004). Review: molecular mechanisms of endotoxin tolerance. *J. Endotoxin Res.* 10, 71–84. doi: 10.1179/096805104225003997

Gehrig, S. M., C., van der Poel, Sayer, T. A., Schertzer, J. D., Henstridge, D. C., Church, J. E., et al. (2012). Hsp-72 preserves muscle function and slows progression of severe muscular dystrophy. *Nature* 484, 394–398. doi: 10.1038/nature10980

Gibson, B. A., and Kraus, W. L. (2012). New insights into the molecular and cellular functions of poly(ADP-ribose) and PARPs. *Nat. Rev. Mol. Cell Biol.* 13, 411–424. doi: 10.1038/nrm3376

Gilliam, L. A. A., and St Clair, D. K. (2011). Chemotherapy-induced weakness and fatigue in skeletal muscle: the role of oxidative stress. *Antioxid. Redox Signal.* 15, 2543–2563. doi: 10.1089/ars.2011.3965

Gilliam, L. A. A., Ferreira, L. F., Bruton, J. D., Moylan, J. S., Westerblad, H., St Clair, D. K., et al. (2009). Doxorubicin acts through tumor necrosis factor receptor subtype 1 to cause dysfunction of murine skeletal muscle. *J. Appl. Physiol.* 107, 1935–1942. doi: 10.1152/japplphysiol.00776.2009

Gilliam, L. A. A., Fisher-Wellman, K. H., Lin, C.-T., Maples, J. M., Cathey, B. L., and Neufer, P. D. (2013). The anticancer agent doxorubicin disrupts mitochondrial energy metabolism and redox balance in skeletal muscle. *Free Rad. Biol. Med.* 65, 988–996. doi: 10.1016/j.freeradbiomed.2013.08.191

Gilliam, L. A. A., Moylan, J. S., Patterson, E. W., Smith, J. D., Wilson, A. S., Rabbani, Z., et al. (2012). Doxorubicin acts via mitochondrial ROS to stimulate catabolism in C2C12 myotubes. *Am. J. Physiol. Cell Physiol.* 302, C195–C202. doi: 10.1152/ajpcell.00217.2011

Gourdier, I., Crabbe, L., Andreau, K., Pau, B., and Kroemer, G. (2004). Oxaliplatin-induced mitochondrial apoptotic response of colon carcinoma cells does not require nuclear DNA. *Oncogene* 23, 7449–7457. doi: 10.1038/sj.onc.1208047

Gouspillou, G., Scheede-Bergdahl, C., Spendiff, S., Vuda, M., Meehan, B., Mlynarski, H., et al. (2015). Anthracycline-containing chemotherapy causes long-term impairment of mitochondrial respiration and increased reactive oxygen species release in skeletal muscle. *Sci. Rep.* 5:8717. doi: 10.1038/srep08717

Greene, D., Nail, L., Fieler, V., Dudgeon, D., and Jones, L. (1993). A comparison of patient-reported side effects among three chemotherapy regimens for breast cancer. *Cancer Pract.* 2, 57–62.

Henstridge, D. C., Bruce, C. R., Drew, B. G., Tory, K., Kolonics, A., Estevez, E., et al. (2014). Activating HSP72 in rodent skeletal muscle increases mitochondrial number and oxidative capacity and decreases insulin resistance. *Diabetes* 63, 1881–1894. doi: 10.2337/db13-0967

Holzerová, E., and Prokisch, H. (2015). Mitochondria: Much ado about nothing? How dangerous is reactive oxygen species production? *Int. J. Biochem. Cell Biol.* 63, 16–20. doi: 10.1016/j.biocel.2015.01.021

Hsin-Chen, L., Pen-Hui, Y., Ching-You, L., Chin-Wen, C., and Yau-Huei, W. (2000). Increase of mitochondria and mitochondrial DNA in response to oxidative stress in human cells. *Biochem. J.* 348, 425–432. doi: 10.1042/bj3480425

Jarvela, L. S., Kemppainen, J., Niinikoski, H., Hannukainen, J. C., Lahteenmaki, P. M., Kapanen, J., et al. (2012). Effects of a home-based exercise program on metabolic risk factors and fitness in long-term survivors of childhood acute lymphoblastic leukemia. *Pediatr. Blood Cancer* 59, 155–160. doi: 10.1002/pbc.24049

Jeejeebhoy, K., Detsky, A., and Baker, J. (1990). Assessment of nutritional status. *J. Parent. Enteral Nutr.* 14(5 suppl.), 193S–196S. doi: 10.1177/014860719001400509

Jones, D. P. (2006). Disruption of mitochondrial redox circuitry in oxidative stress. *Chem. Biol. Interact.* 163, 38–53. doi: 10.1016/j.cbi.2006.07.008

Kaiyala, K. J., Morton, G. J., Thaler, J. P., Meek, T. H., Tylee, T., Ogimoto, K., et al. (2012). Acutely decreased thermoregulatory energy expenditure or decreased activity energy expenditure both acutely reduce food intake in mice. *PLoS ONE* 7:e41473. doi: 10.1371/journal.pone.0041473

Kavazis, A. N., Smuder, A. J., and Powers, S. K. (2014). Effects of short-term endurance exercise training on acute doxorubicin-induced FoxO transcription in cardiac and skeletal muscle. *J. Appl. Physiol.* 117, 223–230. doi: 10.1152/japplphysiol.00210.2014

Kennedy, T. L., Swiderski, K., Murphy, K. T., Gehrig, S. M., Curl, C. L., Chandramouli, C., et al. (2016). BGP-15 Improves Aspects of the Dystrophic Pathology in *mdx* and *dko* Mice with Differing Efficacies in Heart and Skeletal Muscle. *Am. J. Pathol.* 186, 3246–3260. doi: 10.1016/j.ajpath.2016.08.008

Kirkinezos, G. I., and Moraes, C. T. (2001). Reactive oxygen species and mitochondrial diseases. *Cell Dev. Biol.* 12, 449–457. doi: 10.1006/scdb.2001.0282

Kujoth, G., Hiona, A., Pugh, T., Someya, S., Panzer, K., Wohlgemuth, S., et al. (2005). Mitochondrial DNA mutations, oxidative stress, and apoptosis in mammalian aging. *Science* 309, 481–484. doi: 10.1126/science.1112125

Kumar, A., Bhatnagar, S., and Paul, P. K. (2012). TWEAK and TRAF6 regulate skeletal muscle atrophy. *Curr. Opin. Clin. Nutr. Metab. Care* 15:233. doi: 10.1097/MCO.0b013e328351c3fc

Laplante, M., and Sabatini, D. M. (2012). mTOR signaling in growth control and disease. *Cell* 149, 274–293. doi: 10.1016/j.cell.2012.03.017

Le Bras, M., Clement, M., Pervaiz, S., and Brenner, C. (2005). Reactive oxygen species and the mitochondrial signaling pathway of cell death. *Histol. Histopathol.* 20, 205–219.

Lenaz, G., Bovina, C., D'Aurelio, M., Fato, R., Formiggini, G., Genova, M. L., et al. (2002). Role of mitochondria in oxidative stress and aging. *Ann. N. Y. Acad. Sci.* 959, 199–213. doi: 10.1111/j.1749-6632.2002.tb02094.x

Levine, B., and Kroemer, G. (2008). Autophagy in the pathogenesis of disease. *Cell* 132, 27–42. doi: 10.1016/j.cell.2007.12.018

Love, R. R., Leventhal, H., Easterling, D. V., and Nerenz, D. R. (1989). Side effects and emotional distress during cancer chemotherapy. *Cancer* 63, 604–612. doi: 10.1002/1097-0142(19890201)63:3<604::AID-CNCR2820630334>3.0.CO;2-2

Lu, P. (2005). Monitoring Cardiac Function in Patients Receiving Doxorubicin. *Semin. Nucl. Med.* 35, 197–201. doi: 10.1053/j.semnuclmed.2005.02.005

Mammucari, C., Schiaffino, S., and Sandri, M. (2008). Downstream of Akt: FoxO3 and mTOR in the regulation of autophagy in skeletal muscle. *Autophagy* 4, 524–526. doi: 10.4161/auto.5905

Mantovani, G., Macciò, A., Madeddu, C., and Massa, E. (2003). Cancer-related cachexia and oxidative stress: beyond current therapeutic options. *Expert Rev. Anticancer Ther.* 3, 381–392. doi: 10.1586/14737140.3.3.381

Mascarenhas, L., Malogolowkin, M., Armenian, S. H., Sposto, R., and Venkatramani, R. (2013). A phase I study of oxaliplatin and doxorubicin in pediatric patients with relapsed or refractory extracranial non-hematopoietic solid tumors. *Pediatr. Blood Cancer* 60, 1103–1107. doi: 10.1002/pbc.24471

McQuade, R. M., Stojanovska, V., Petersen, A. C., Abalo, R., Bornstein, J. C., Rybalka, E., et al. (2016b). Oxaliplatin-induced enteric neuronal loss and gastrointestinal dysfunction is alleviated by co-treatment with BGP-15. *Neurogastroenterol. Motil.* 28, 52–53.

McQuade, R. M., Carbone, S. E., Stojanovska, V., Rahman, A., Gwynne, R. M., Robinson, A. M., et al. (2016a). Role of oxidative stress in oxaliplatin-induced enteric neuropathy and colonic dysmotility in mice. *Br. J. Pharmacol.* 173, 3502–3521. doi: 10.1111/bph.13646

Min, K., Kwon, O.-S., Smuder, A. J., Wiggs, M. P., Sollanek, K. J., and Powers, S. K. (2015). Increased mitochondrial emission of reactive oxygen species and calpain activation are required for doxorubicin-induced cardiac and skeletal muscle myopathy. *J. Physiol.* 593, 2017–2036. doi: 10.1113/jphysiol.2014.286518

Min, K., Smuder, A. J., Kwon, O.-S., Kavazis, A. N., Szeto, H. H., and Powers, S. K. (2011). Mitochondrial-targeted antioxidants protect skeletal muscle against immobilization-induced muscle atrophy. *J. Appl. Physiol. (1985)* 111, 1459–1466. doi: 10.1152/japplphysiol.00591.2011

Mithal, A., Bonjour, J.-P., Boonen, S., Burckhardt, P., Degens, H. E., and Rizzoli, R. (2013). Impact of nutrition on muscle mass, strength, and performance in older adults. *Osteoporos. Int.* 24, 1555–1566. doi: 10.1007/s00198-012-2236-y

Moon, S.-S. (2014). Low skeletal muscle mass is associated with insulin resistance, diabetes, and metabolic syndrome in the Korean population: the Korea National Health and Nutrition Examination Survey (KNHANES) 2009-2010. *Endocr. J.* 61, 61–70. doi: 10.1507/endocrj.EJ13-0244

Murphy, R. M., and Lamb, G. D. (2013). Important considerations for protein analyses using antibody based techniques: down-sizing Western blotting up-sizes outcomes. *J. Physiol.* 591, 5823–5831. doi: 10.1113/jphysiol.2013.263251

National Cancer Institute (2012). *Targeted Cancer Therapies.* Available online at: http://www.cancer.gov/cancertopics/treatment/types/targeted-therapies/targeted-therapies-fact-sheet

Ness, K. K., Baker, K. S., Dengel, D. R., Youngren, N., Sibley, S., Mertens, A. C., et al. (2007). Body composition, muscle strength deficits and mobility limitations in adult survivors of childhood acute lymphoblastic leukemia. *Pediatr. Blood Cancer* 49, 975–981. doi: 10.1002/pbc.21091

Ness, K. K., Hudson, M. M., Pui, C.-H., Green, D. M., Krull, K. R., and Morris, E. B. (2012). Neuromuscular impairments in adult survivors of childhood acute lymphoblastic leukemia. *Cancer* 118, 828–838. doi: 10.1002/cncr.26337

Oeffinger, K. C., Mertens, A. C., Sklar, C. A., Kawashima, T., Hudson, M. M., Meadows, A. T., et al. (2006). Chronic health conditions in adult survivors of childhood cancer. *N. Engl. J. Med.* 355, 1572–1582. doi: 10.1056/NEJMsa060185

Pasiakos, S. M., Vislocky, L. M., Carbone, J. W., Altieri, N., Konopelski, K., Freake, H. C., et al. (2010). Acute energy deprivation affects skeletal muscle protein synthesis and associated intracellular signaling proteins in physically active adults. *J. Nutr.* 140, 745–751. doi: 10.3945/jn.109.118372

Paul, P. K., Bhatnagar, S., Mishra, V., Srivastava, S., Darnay, B. G., Choi, Y., et al. (2012). The E3 ubiquitin ligase TRAF6 intercedes in starvation-induced skeletal muscle atrophy through multiple mechanisms. *Mol. Cell. Biol.* 32, 1248–1259. doi: 10.1128/MCB.06351-11

Pfeiffer, T., Krause, U., Thome, U., Rajewski, A., Skorzek, M., and Scheulen, M. (1997). Tissue toxicity of doxorubicin in first and second hyperthermic isolated limb perfusion—an experimental study in dogs. *Euro. J. Surg. Oncol.* 23, 439–444. doi: 10.1016/S0748-7983(97)93727-6

Powers, S. K., Kavazis, A. N., and DeRuisseau, K. C. (2005). Mechanisms of disuse muscle atrophy: role of oxidative stress. *Am. J. Physiol. Regul. Integr. Comp. Physiol.* 288, R337–R344.

Powers, S. K., Kavazis, A. N., and McClung, J. M. (2007). Oxidative stress and disuse muscle atrophy. *J. Appl. Physiol.* 102, 2389–2397. doi: 10.1152/japplphysiol.01202.2006

Powers, S. K., Talbert, E. E., and Adhihetty, P. J. (2011). Reactive oxygen and nitrogen species as intracellular signals in skeletal muscle. *J. Physiol. (Lond).* 589, 2129–2138. doi: 10.1113/jphysiol.2010.201327

Powers, S. K., Wiggs, M. P., Duarte, J. A., Zergeroglu, A. M., and Demirel, H. A. (2012). Mitochondrial signaling contributes to disuse muscle atrophy. *Am. J. Physiol. Endocrinol.* 303, E31–E39. doi: 10.1152/ajpendo.00609.2011

Raymond, E., Faivre, S., Woynarowski, J. M., and Chaney, S. G. (1998). Oxaliplatin: mechanism of action and antineoplastic activity. *Semin. Oncol.* 25(2 Suppl. 5), 4–12.

Reagan-Shaw, S., Nihal, M., and Ahmad, N. (2008). Dose translation from animal to human studies revisited. *FASEB J.* 22, 659–661. doi: 10.1096/fj.07-9574LSF

Salah, H., Li, M., Cacciani, N., Gastaldello, S., Ogilvie, H., Akkad, H., et al. (2016). The chaperone co-inducer BGP-15 alleviates ventilation-induced diaphragm dysfunction. *Sci. Transl. Med.* 8, 350ra103. doi: 10.1126/scitranslmed.aaf7099

Sandri, M. (2008). Signaling in muscle atrophy and hypertrophy. *Physiology* 23, 160–170. doi: 10.1152/physiol.00041.2007

Sapra, G., Tham, Y. K., Cemerlang, N., Matsumoto, A., Kiriazis, H., Bernardo, B. C., et al. (2014). The small-molecule BGP-15 protects against heart failure and atrial fibrillation in mice. *Nat. Commun.* 5:5705. doi: 10.1038/ncomms6705

Sarosiek, K. A., Ni Chonghaile, T., and Letai, A. (2013). Mitochondria: gatekeepers of response to chemotherapy. *Trends Cell Biol.* 23, 612–619. doi: 10.1016/j.tcb.2013.08.003

Sarszegi, Z., Bognar, E., Gaszner, B., Kónyi, A., Gallyas, F. Jr., Sumegi, B., et al. (2012). BGP-15, a PARP-inhibitor, prevents imatinib-induced cardiotoxicity by activating Akt and suppressing JNK and p38 MAP kinases. *Mol. Cell. Biochem.* 365, 129–137. doi: 10.1007/s11010-012-1252-8

Scheede-Bergdahl, C., and Jagoe, R. T. (2013). After the chemotherapy: potential mechanisms for chemotherapy-induced delayed skeletal muscle dysfunction in survivors of acute lymphoblastic leukaemia in childhood. *Front. Pharmacol.* 4:49. doi: 10.3389/fphar.2013.00049

Schuh, R. A., Jackson, K. C., Khairallah, R. J., Ward, C. W., and Spangenburg, E. E. (2012). Measuring mitochondrial respiration in intact single muscle fibers. *Am. J. Physiol. Regul. Integr. Comp. Physiol.* 302. R712–R719. doi: 10.1152/ajpregu.00229.2011

Shortreed, K. E., Krause, M. P., Huang, J. H., Dhanani, D., Moradi, J., Ceddia, R. B., et al. (2009). Muscle-specific adaptations, impaired oxidative capacity and maintenance of contractile function characterize diet-induced obese mouse skeletal muscle. *PLoS ONE* 4:e7293. doi: 10.1371/journal.pone.0007293

Smuder, A. J., Kavazis, A. N., Min, K., and Powers, S. K. (2011). Exercise protects against doxorubicin-induced oxidative stress and proteolysis in skeletal muscle. *J. Appl. Physiol.* 110, 935–942. doi: 10.1152/japplphysiol.00677.2010

Sorensen, J. C., Cheregi, B. D., Timpani, C. A., Nurgali, K., Hayes, A., and Rybalka, E. (2016). Mitochondria: inadvertent targets in chemotherapy-induced skeletal muscle toxicity and wasting? *Cancer Chemother Pharmacol.* 78, 673–683. doi: 10.1007/s00280-016-3045-3

Sternberg, C., De Mulder, P., Schornagel, J., Theodore, C., Fossa, S., Van Oosterom, A., et al. (2001). Randomized phase III trial of high-dose-intensity methotrexate, vinblastine, doxorubicin, and cisplatin (MVAC) chemotherapy and recombinant human granulocyte colony-stimulating factor versus classic MVAC in advanced urothelial tract tumors: European Organization for Research and Treatment of Cancer Protocol No. 30924. *J. Clin. Oncol.* 19, 2638–2646. doi: 10.1200/JCO.2001.19.10.2638

Stojanovska, V., Stewart, M., Timpani, C. A., Sorensen, J. C., Orbell, J., Rybalka, E., et al. (2015). Platinum accumulation and changes in mitochondrial function of the longitudinal muscle & myenteric plexus following oxaliplatin administration. *Proc. Aus. Physiol. Soc.* 46:91.

Stowe, D. F., and Camara, A. K. (2009). Mitochondrial reactive oxygen species production in excitable cells: modulators of mitochondrial and cell function. *Antioxid. Redox Signal.* 11, 1373–1414. doi: 10.1089/ars.2008.2331

Szabados, E., Literati-Nagy, P., Farkas, B., and Sumegi, B. (2000). BGP-15, a nicotinic amidoxime derivate protecting heart from ischemia reperfusion injury through modulation of poly (ADP-ribose) polymerase. *Biochem. Pharmacol.* 59, 937–945. doi: 10.1016/S0006-2952(99)00418-9

Tabassum, H., Waseem, M., Parvez, S., and Qureshi, M. I. (2015). Oxaliplatin-induced oxidative stress provokes toxicity in isolated rat Liver Mitochondria. *Arch. Med. Res.* 46, 597–603. doi: 10.1016/j.arcmed.2015.10.002

Talvensaari, K. K., Lanning, M., Tapanainen, P., and Knip, M. (1996). Long-term survivors of childhood cancer have an increased risk of manifesting the metabolic syndrome. *J. Clin. Endocrinol. Metab.* 81, 3051–3055.

Thissen, J.-P., Ketelslegers, J.-M., and Underwood, L. E. (1994). Nutritional Regulation of the Insulin-Like Growth Factors*. *Endocr. Rev.* 15, 80–101.

Timpani, C. A., Trewin, A. J., Stojanovska, V., Robinson, A., Goodman, C. A., Nurgali, K., et al. (2016). Attempting to compensate for reduced neuronal nitric oxide synthase protein with nitrate supplementation cannot overcome metabolic dysfunction but rather has detrimental effects in dystrophin-deficient mdx muscle. *Neurotherapeutics.* doi: 10.1007/s13311-016-0494-7. [Epub ahead of print].

Tran, H. C., Marachelian, A., Venkatramani, R., Jubran, R. F., and Mascarenhas, L. (2015). Oxaliplatin and Doxorubicin for relapsed or refractory high-risk neuroblastoma. *Pediatr. Hematol. Oncol.* 32, 26–31. doi: 10.3109/08880018.2014.983624

U.S. National Institutes of Health (2014). *Safety and Efficacy of BGP-15 in Patients With Type 2 Diabetes Mellitus,* 2016. Available online at: https://clinicaltrials.gov/ct2/show/NCT01069965

van Brussel, M., Takken, T. J., van der Net, Engelbert, R. H., Bierings, M., Schoenmakers, M. A., et al. (2006). Physical function and fitness in long-term survivors of childhood leukaemia. *Pediatr. Rehabil.* 9, 267–274. doi: 10.1080/13638490500523150

Wang, L., and Kernell, D. (2001). Fibre type regionalisation in lower hindlimb muscles of rabbit, rat and mouse: a comparative study. *J. Anat.* 199, 631–643. doi: 10.1046/j.1469-7580.2001.19960631.x

Weyer, C., Walford, R. L., Harper, I. T., Milner, M., MacCallum, T., Tataranni, P. A., et al. (2000). Energy metabolism after 2 y of energy restriction: the biosphere 2 experiment. *Am. J. Clin. Nutr.* 72, 946–953.

World Health Organisation (2015). *Cancer.* Available online at: http://www.who.int/topics/cancer/en/

Zhou, H.-Z., Swanson, R. A., Simonis, U., Ma, X., Cecchini, G., and Gray, M. O. (2006). Poly (ADP-ribose) polymerase-1 hyperactivation and impairment of mitochondrial respiratory chain complex I function in reperfused mouse hearts. *Am. J. Physiol. Heart Circul. Physiol.* 291. H714–H723. doi: 10.1152/ajpheart.00823.2005

Zitvogel, L., Apetoh, L., Ghiringhelli, F., and Kroemer, G. (2008). Immunological aspects of cancer chemotherapy. *Nat. Rev. Immunol.* 8, 59–73. doi: 10.1038/nri2216

Zoncu, R., Efeyan, A., and Sabatini, D. M. (2011). mTOR: from growth signal integration to cancer, diabetes and ageing. *Nat. Rev. Mol. Cell Biol.* 12, 21–35. doi: 10.1038/nrm3025

Conflict of Interest Statement: The authors declare that the research was conducted in the absence of any commercial or financial relationships that could be construed as a potential conflict of interest.

17

Limb Hypothermia for Preventing Paclitaxel-Induced Peripheral Neuropathy in Breast Cancer Patients

Raghav Sundar[1†], Aishwarya Bandla[2,3†], Stacey Sze Hui Tan[2], Lun-De Liao[2,4], Nesaretnam Barr Kumarakulasinghe[1], Anand D. Jeyasekharan[1], Samuel Guan Wei Ow[1], Jingshan Ho[1], David Shao Peng Tan[1], Joline Si Jing Lim[1], Joy Vijayan[5], Aravinda K. Therimadasamy[6], Zarinah Hairom[7], Emily Ang[7], Sally Ang[1], Nitish V. Thakor[2,3,8], Soo-Chin Lee[1,9] and Einar P. V. Wilder-Smith[2,5,10]*

[1]Department of Haematology-Oncology, National University Health System, Singapore, Singapore, [2]Singapore Institute for Neurotechnology, National University of Singapore, Singapore, Singapore, [3]Department of Biomedical Engineering, National University of Singapore, Singapore, Singapore, [4]Institute of Biomedical Engineering and Nanomedicine, National Health Research Institutes, Zhunan Township, Taiwan, [5]Department of Medicine, National University Health System, Singapore, Singapore, [6]Neurology Diagnostic Laboratory, National University Hospital, Singapore, Singapore, [7]National University Cancer Institute, National University Health System, Singapore, Singapore, [8]Department of Biomedical Engineering, Johns Hopkins University, Baltimore, MD, USA, [9]Cancer Science Institute of Singapore, National University of Singapore, Singapore, Singapore, [10]Department of Medicine, Yong Loo Lin School of Medicine, National University of Singapore, Singapore, Singapore

Edited by:
R. Thomas Jagoe,
McGill University, Canada

Reviewed by:
Raquel Abalo,
King Juan Carlos University, Spain
Maria Caffo,
University of Messina, Italy

***Correspondence:**
Einar P. V. Wilder-Smith
einar_wilder-smith@nuhs.edu.sg

†These authors have contributed equally to this work.

Background: Peripheral neuropathy (PN) due to paclitaxel is a common dose-limiting toxicity with no effective prevention or treatment. We hypothesize that continuous-flow limb hypothermia can reduce paclitaxel-induced PN.

Patients and methods: An internally controlled pilot trial was conducted to investigate the neuroprotective effect of continuous-flow limb hypothermia in breast cancer patients receiving weekly paclitaxel. Patients underwent limb hypothermia of one limb for a duration of 3 h with every paclitaxel infusion, with the contralateral limb used as control. PN was primarily assessed using nerve conduction studies (NCSs) before the start of chemotherapy, and after 1, 3, and 6 months. Skin temperature and tolerability to hypothermia were monitored using validated scores.

Results: Twenty patients underwent a total of 218 cycles of continuous-flow limb hypothermia at a coolant temperature of 22°C. Continuous-flow limb hypothermia achieved mean skin temperature reduction of 1.5 ± 0.7°C and was well tolerated, with no premature termination of cooling due to intolerance. Grade 3 PN occurred in 2 patients (10%), grade 2 in 2 (10%), and grade 1 in 12 (60%). Significant correlation was observed between amount of skin cooling and motor nerve amplitude preservation at 6 months ($p < 0.0005$). Sensory velocity and amplitude in the cooled limbs were less preserved

Abbreviations: AH, abductor hallucis; CIPN, chemotherapy-induced peripheral neuropathy; cMAP, compound muscle action potentials; CTS, composite tolerability score; EDB, extensor digitorum brevis; NCI-CTC, National Cancer Institute-Common Toxicity Criteria grading of neuropathy; NCSs, nerve conduction studies; PN, peripheral neuropathy; PPMC, Pearson's Product Moment Coefficient; SAS, Shivering Assessment Scale; SNAP, sensory nerve action potential; STS, subjective tolerance scale; TNS, Total Neuropathy Score; VAS, visual analog pain scale.

than in the control limbs, but the difference did not attain statistical significance. One patient with a history of diabetes mellitus had significant preservation of compound muscle action potential in the cooled limb on NCS analysis.

Conclusion: This study suggests that continuous limb hypothermia accompanying paclitaxel infusion may reduce paclitaxel-induced PN and have therapeutic potential in select patients and warrants further investigation. The method is safe and well tolerated.

Keywords: chemotherapy-induced peripheral neuropathy, limb hypothermia, paclitaxel, nerve conduction, neuroprotection

INTRODUCTION

Chemotherapy-induced peripheral neuropathy (CIPN) is a common dose-limiting toxicity of paclitaxel. At present, dose modification remains the most successful approach for the management of CIPN, and pharmacological treatment is limited to alleviating symptoms such as paresthesias, dysesthesia, and pain (1). To date, none of the potential neuroprotective agents tested in clinical trials have proven effective (2).

The mechanisms of neurotoxicity in paclitaxel-induced peripheral neuropathy (PN) have not been fully elucidated; however, disruption of microtubule dynamics has been identified. Taxanes binding to β-tubulin components of microtubule assemblies lead to microtubule stabilization, thereby causing a disruption of microtubule dynamics (3, 4). It has also been observed that paclitaxel administration produces abnormalities in axonal mitochondria (5). Additional targets of neurotoxicity include direct axonal toxicity at the distal nerve terminals (6). Patients with pre-existing conditions that are capable of inducing PN (such as diabetes, Charcot–Marie–Tooth, or kidney disease) are particularly predisposed to developing CIPN (7).

Given the dose-dependent pathophysiology of paclitaxel-induced PN, we proposed a novel strategy for prevention of paclitaxel-induced PN by employing continuous-flow limb hypothermia to reduce delivery of the toxic chemotherapeutic agents to the peripheral nerves. Our previous *in vivo* study showed that a drop in rat sciatic nerve temperature from 30 to 20°C produced a fivefold reduction of nerve blood flow (8). Furthermore, in studies of chemotherapy-induced alopecia (CIA), which is a result of toxic accumulation of chemotherapeutics in the hair follicle, there is compelling evidence that cooling of the scalp protects against the development of CIA (9, 10). The rationale behind using hypothermia in the prevention of CIA is that scalp cooling decreases the blood supply to the hair follicles, and hence, hair follicle protection is a result of reduced delivery of toxic chemotherapeutics (10). However, scalp cooling employing traditional cooling methods such as ice packs is poorly tolerated, which limits efficacy of the treatment itself (11). Hence, we employed a better-tolerated and efficient cooling technique of continuous-flow hypothermia. In a previous study in healthy subjects, we also established that continuous-flow limb hypothermia at a coolant temperature of 22°C was the lowest tolerable temperature for a duration of 3 h, matching the duration of paclitaxel infusion in cancer patients (12).

The goal of the current study was to determine if continuous-flow limb hypothermia may be neuroprotective in patients receiving paclitaxel chemotherapy, as well as assessing safety and tolerability.

PATIENTS AND METHODS

Study Design

This prospective study was carried out in accordance with the recommendations of the Institutional Review Board of the National Health Group, Singapore, with written informed consent from all subjects. All the subjects gave written informed consent in accordance with the Declaration of Helsinki. The study population comprised breast cancer patients scheduled to receive adjuvant weekly paclitaxel chemotherapy for 12 cycles following standard anthracycline-based chemotherapy (doxorubicin and cyclophosphamide). (For detailed inclusion/exclusion criteria, see supplementary material.) During every cycle of chemotherapy, premedication drugs (dexamethasone, diphenhydramine, and ranitidine) were administered 30 min prior to paclitaxel infusion. 80 mg/m^2 of paclitaxel was administered as a 1-h infusion (indicated in orange in **Figure 1A**). The chemotherapy unit ambient temperature was adjusted to 21°C *via* air-conditioning. Randomization for limb cooling was carried out and the non-cooled limb served as internal control prior to the first cycle of therapy, and the same limb underwent cooling for all subsequent cycles, while the non-cooled limb remained as control (**Figure 2A**).

Limb hypothermia sessions comprised of a pre-cooling period (1 h), continued with paclitaxel infusion and a post-cooling period (on average 30 min after the end of paclitaxel infusion) (**Figure 1A**). Overall, hypothermia was administered for no longer than 4 h. A detailed safety protocol was followed for coolant thermoregulation, if the patient found the hypothermia intolerable (Tables S1 and S2 in Supplementary Material).

Safety and tolerance of limb hypothermia were measured using three validated scales: visual analog pain scale (VAS), subjective tolerance scale, and the Shivering Assessment Scale (Figure S1 and Tables S3 and S4 in Supplementary Material) (13, 14). Skin surface temperature was continuously recorded throughout limb hypothermia *via* temperature sensors (accurate to ±0.1°C) placed at seven locations on both the legs (**Figure 2B**) (12). Body core temperature was measured over the frontal non-glabrous scalp (**Figure 1A**).

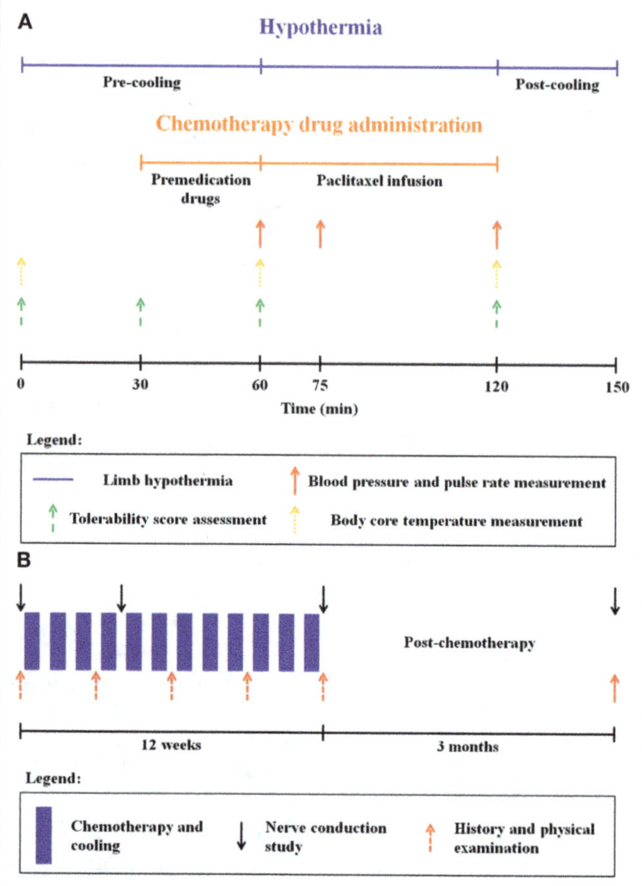

FIGURE 1 | **(A)** Limb hypothermia protocol for one chemotherapy cycle. Premedication drugs: dexamethasone, diphenhydramine, and ranitidine. **(B)** Study schema.

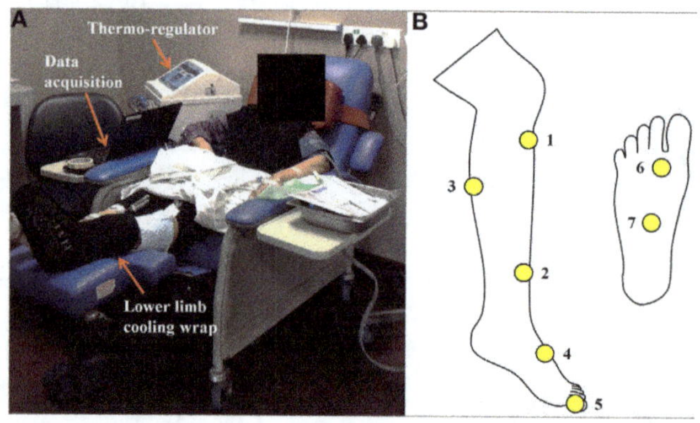

FIGURE 2 | **(A)** Continuous-flow limb hypothermia setup by means of a thermoregulator device supplying coolant (water) at a set desired temperature (22°C) to limb wraps that cool the limb. Continuous skin temperature data are acquired *via* a temperature monitoring system consisting of wireless sensors placed at seven different sensor locations on the cooled and control legs as indicated in **(B)**, which transmit data wirelessly to a receiver and recorded for analysis.

Assessment of Neuropathy

Assessment for neuropathy was performed using nerve conduction studies (NCSs) and clinical examination. NCSs are the most sensitive and specific detection method for neuropathies and superior to clinical examination or scores (15). Primary endpoint was differences in NCSs carried out at baseline ($NCS_{baseline}$), 1 month into treatment (NCS_{mid}), the end of treatment (NCS_{end}), and 3 months post-treatment (NCS_{3m}) (**Figure 1B**). Sensory nerve action potential (SNAP) amplitudes and conduction velocities were measured in the bilateral sural, superficial peroneal, saphenous, and medial and lateral plantar nerves (16). Compound motor action potential (cMAP) amplitudes and motor nerve conduction velocities were evaluated in the bilateral common peroneal and tibial nerves (17).

At the same time points, clinical evaluation using the validated Total Neuropathy Score (TNS) was performed (18).

Statistical Analysis

Temporal trend of skin temperature variation over the duration of hypothermia was summarized as an average of the recorded temperatures for all cycles of cooling for all the patients. Similarly, tolerability was analyzed as an average of all patients' tolerance scores across all cycles of cooling. Sensory and motor nerve parameters of amplitude and velocity at every NCS visit were analyzed as relative percentage changes with respect to the first NCS visit (NCS_{base}) and averaged across patients.

We assessed the effect of varying amounts of cooling on nerve conduction parameters through correlation analysis (Pearson). Limb cooling was quantified by calculating each patient's average reduction in baseline skin temperature over 12 cooling cycles. Limb cooling was correlated with mean SNAP amplitude/velocity percentage changes at the sural, superficial peroneal, and saphenous nerves. Similarly, limb cooling was correlated with mean cMAP amplitude/velocity percentage changes from all peroneal nerve stimulation points (ankle, below fibula head, and above fibula head) at the recording site of the extensor digitorum brevis (EDB) and from the tibial nerve ankle stimulation point on the abductor hallucis. This was done for values obtained at NCS_{end} and NCS_{3m}. A negative correlation shows that more cooling results in better preservation of nerve conduction parameters. Comparison of three different degrees of cooling achieved and the relation to the degree of preservation on nerve conduction parameters were also assessed.

Continuous variables are shown as mean ± SD. A parametric paired *t*-test was used to compare the changes in temperature and NCS values of the cooled and control limbs in each patient. A two-tailed *p*-value <0.05 was considered statistically significant. The Pearson's correlation coefficient was calculated to determine the correlation between amount of limb cooling and NCS preservation. All statistical analyses were performed in Microsoft Excel (V.12.0 for Windows, Microsoft Corp., Washington, DC, USA).

RESULTS

Twenty female breast cancer patients were enrolled in the study (**Table 1**). Of these 20 patients, 17 (85%) completed 12 cycles of

TABLE 1 | Baseline patient characteristics.

Variables	*N* (%) (total *N* = 20)	Mean (range)
Age (years)		53 (32–67)
Weight (kg)		60 (38–81)
Height (cm)		154 (135–167)
BSA (m²) baseline		1.6 (1.2–1.9)
Cumulative dose of paclitaxel (mg/m²)		868.0 (160.0–960.0)
Cancer stage		–
Stage 1	3 (15)	
Stage 2	11 (55)	
Stage 3	5 (25)	
Stage 4	1 (5)	
Type of surgery		–
Breast conservation	5 (25)	
Mastectomy	15 (75)	
Lymph node assessment		–
Sentinel lymph node biopsy	9 (45)	
Axillary clearance	8 (40)	
Both	3 (15)	
ER-positive	18 (90)	–
Her-2-positive	3 (15)	–
Concurrent herceptin	3 (15)	–
TNS baseline		–
0	15 (75)	
1	4 (20)	
2	1 (5)	

continuous-flow limb hypothermia and one patient developed an infected seroma after her ninth cycle and deemed not fit for further paclitaxel by the treating oncologist. The abovementioned 18 patients completed all TNS and nerve conduction assessments before and after chemotherapy and were included in the analysis of nerve conduction changes and assessment of clinical neuropathy. The remaining two patients who were enrolled in the study did not complete all assessments and hence were not included for analysis of nerve conduction changes and assessment of clinical neuropathy [one patient completed two cycles before discontinuing due to development of grade 3 PN. Another withdrew from the study after three cycles due to ineligible inclusion criteria (not adjuvant therapy, Stage IV disease)]. However, all the 20 enrolled patients were included for safety and tolerability analysis.

Safety and Tolerability

Continuous-flow limb hypothermia was well tolerated by all patients. Premature termination of cooling was never necessary and only one patient (for 2 out of a total 218 cycles) required one intra-cycle thermoregulator temperature increase of 1°C toward the end of a hypothermia session (Figure S2 in Supplementary Material). Overall, minimal discomfort was reported at the end of each limb hypothermia session. No serious or lasting adverse events as a result of hypothermia were encountered. Only temporary erythema lasting a few minutes was observed upon removal of the cooling wrap. All recorded adverse events were due to chemotherapy (Table S5 in Supplementary Material). Patients' core body temperature showed negligible changes (0.03 ± 0.18°C) across chemotherapy cycles.

Skin Temperature Changes with Limb Hypothermia

Skin temperature changes at all the seven sensor locations on the cooled and control limbs were calculated and averaged across all patients over all 218 cycles. Following the onset of hypothermia, skin temperatures of the cooled leg showed significantly lower temperatures than the control leg ($p = 0.0003$) (**Figures 3A–G**). A mean temperature drop of 1.5 ± 0.7°C was achieved across all sensor points on the cooled limb and averaged across all the patients. The largest temperature drops in the cooled limb was achieved in the shin (2.2 ± 1.1°C) (**Figure 3B**) and foot arch (2.2 ± 1.3°C) (**Figure 3G**).

Clinical Neuropathy

Assessment of neuropathy using clinical and nerve conduction parameters of 18 patients was done. The TNS grade of PN reported during all the four visits were documented (Figure S3 in Supplementary Material). Baseline TNS ranged between 0 and 2 for all patients, thereby indicating absence of any baseline neuropathy. As per the National Cancer Institute-Common Toxicity Criteria grading of neuropathy (19), sensory PN of the following grades were experienced by patients at the end of chemotherapy: grade 3 PN occurred in two patients (10%), grade 2 in two patients (10%), grade 1 in 12 patients (60%), and grade 0 in four patients (20%). One patient developed grade 3 PN after two cycles and dropped out of the study. She was included for safety analysis but not efficacy analysis. The other patient with grade 3 PN completed all 12 cycles. Both patients with grade 2 PN completed 12 cycles of limb hypothermia.

Nerve Conduction Changes

The SNAP amplitudes showed decreasing trend over time, in both cooled and control limbs (**Figures 4A–C**; Table S6 in Supplementary Material). While the sural nerve showed more preservation of SNAP amplitude in the cooled than in the control limb at NCS_{3m}, the difference was not significant [−19.9 ± 23.7% (cooled) vs. −25.8 ± 21.8% (control), $p = 0.16$]. Sensory velocities between the limbs showed no significant difference ($0.09 < p < 0.89$) (**Figures 4D–F**; Table S6 in Supplementary Material).

The cMAP amplitudes of all recorded motor nerves were more preserved in the cooled limb than the control limb (**Figures 4G–I**; Table S7 in Supplementary Material) at NCS_{3m}, without reaching significance. At NCS_{3m}, the EDB cMAP amplitudes of the cooled limb showed more preservation [stimulation below fibula head: −2.1 ± 25.3% (cooled) vs. −18.3 ± 30.0% (control), $p = 0.07$; stimulation above fibula head: −4.3 ± 23.9% (cooled) vs. −18.7 ± 32.0%, $p = 0.10$] (**Figure 4G**). Motor velocities did not show significant change between limbs (**Figures 4J–L**; Table S7 in Supplementary Material).

We identified one subject who experienced significant preservation of cMAP amplitudes (EDB) in the cooled leg,

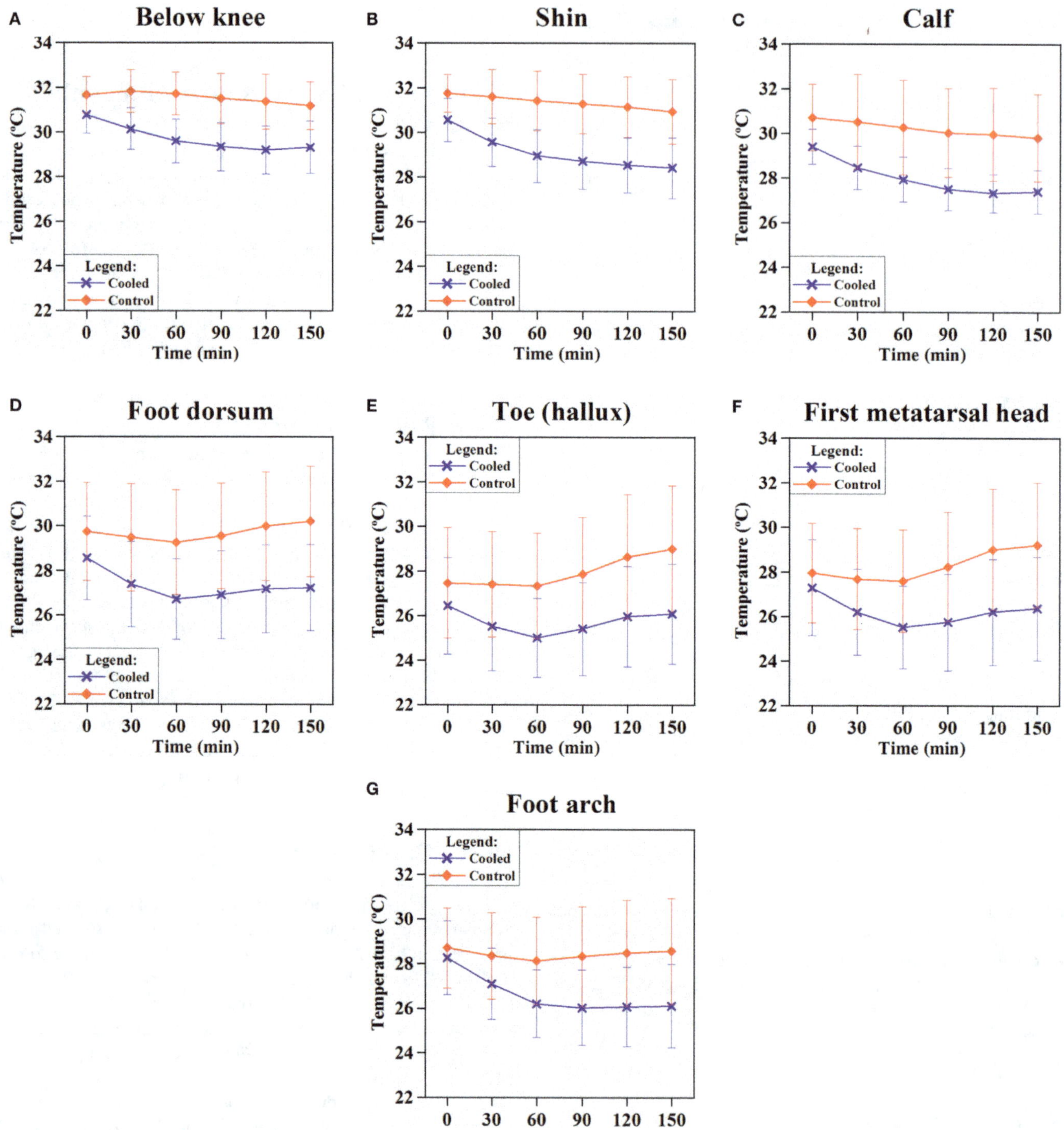

FIGURE 3 | Trend of skin temperature of the cooled (blue) vs. control (red) leg over the duration of limb hypothermia in breast cancer patients. Skin temperature was acquired continuously at various sensor locations: **(A)** below knee, **(B)** at the shin, **(C)** calf, **(D)** dorsum of the foot, **(E)** toe (hallux), **(F)** first metatarsal head, and **(G)** foot arch (foot plantar). Skin temperatures of the cooled leg showed significantly lower temperatures than the control leg at each time point ($p < 0.05$). Limb hypothermia was administered at a coolant temperature of 22°C throughout the duration of chemotherapy.

compared to the control leg (**Figure 5**). This was a 64-year-old female patient with Stage II hormone receptor-positive and Her2-positive breast cancer. She had a history of diabetes with an Hba1c of 7.3% at the time of her screening visit. She had no pre-existing neuropathy from her diabetes with a baseline TNS score of 1.

While her cMAP (EDB) amplitudes in the cooled and control legs were below baseline for NCS_{mid}, NCS_{end}, and NCS_{3m}, separation between cMAP in the cooled and control legs was shown at NCS_{end} where cMAP amplitude (EDB, ankle stimulation) was 41.8% higher in the cooled leg than the control leg. At NCS_{3m}, cMAP amplitude (EDB, ankle stimulation) was 53.2% higher in the cooled leg.

Effect of the Amount of Limb Cooling on NCS

The greatest negative correlation was between cooling and cMAP recordings over the EDB with distal stimulation at NCS_{3m} ($r = -0.55$). SNAP amplitudes and limb cooling

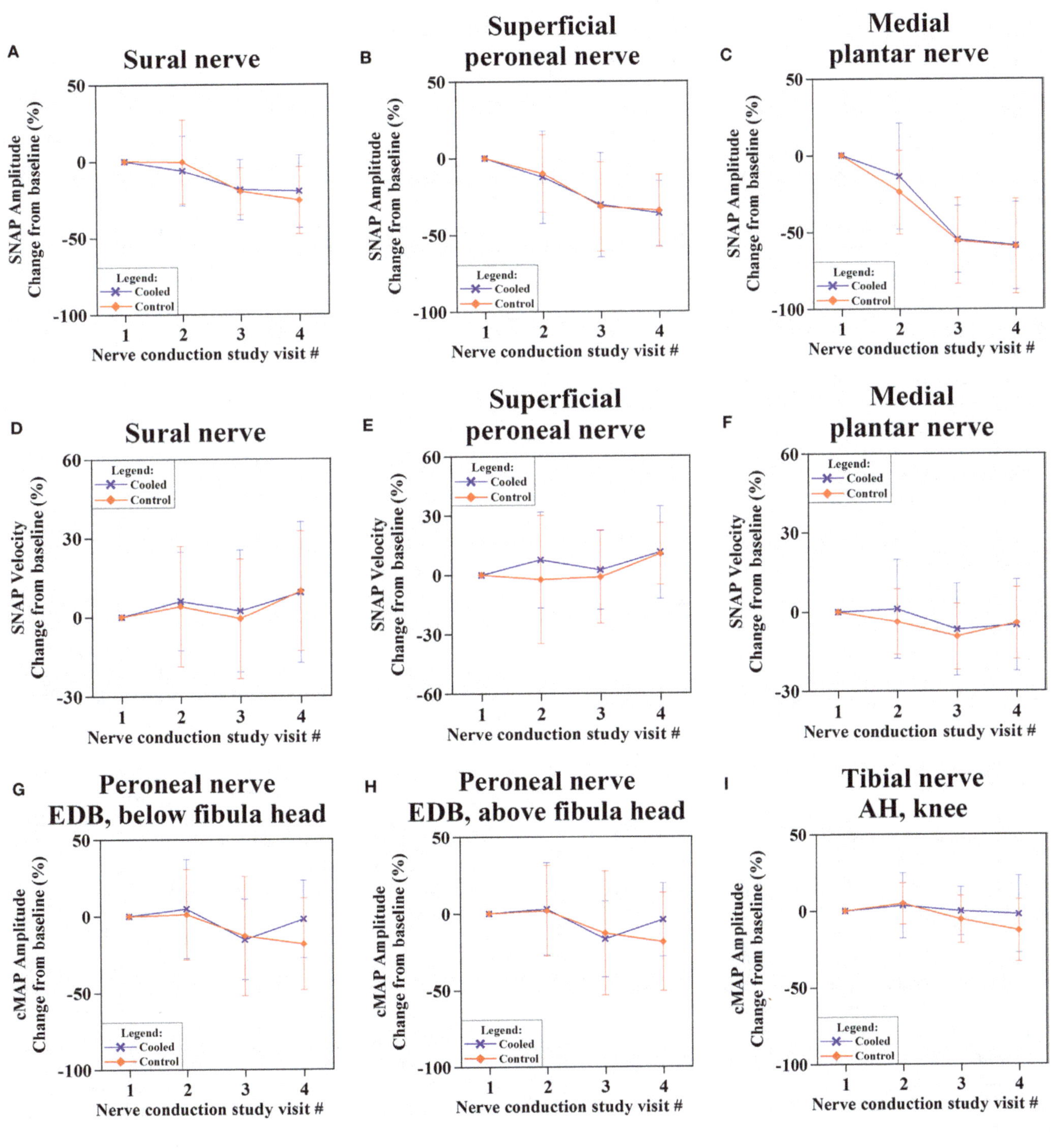

FIGURE 4 | Continued

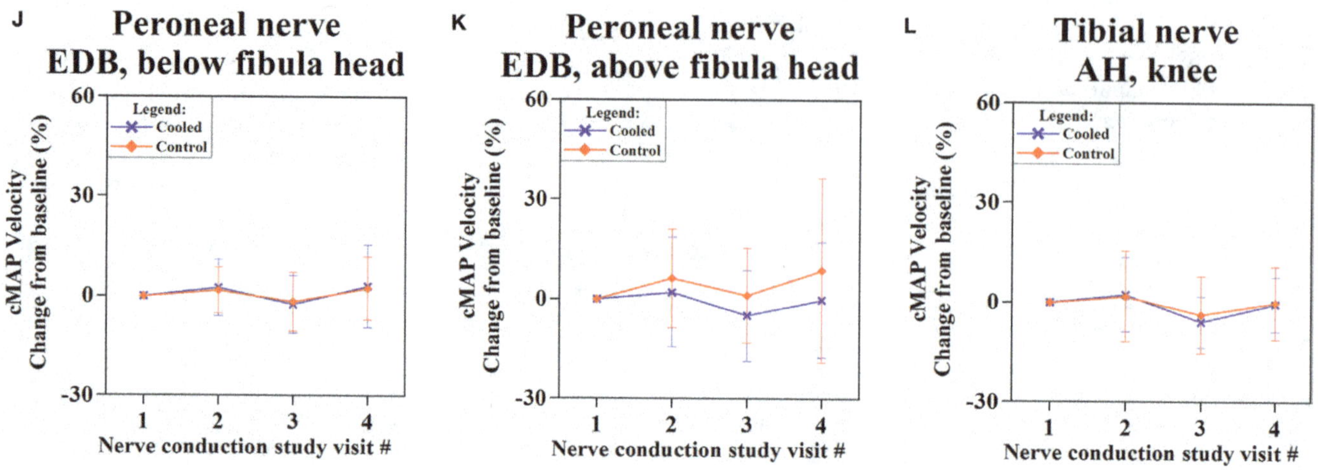

FIGURE 4 | Percentage change of sensory nerve action potential (SNAP) amplitudes (A–C) and velocities (D–F), and compound motor action potential (cMAP) amplitudes (G–I) and velocities (J–L) over four nerve conduction study visits from baseline.

did not show a large correlation at NCS_{end} ($r = -0.17$) or NCS_{3m} ($r = -0.13$).

To ascertain whether different degrees of cooling achieved different preservation of cMAP amplitude, three different degrees of cooling were plotted against the achieved preservation in cMAP. All groups showed highly significant differences: high ($\Delta t > -2.2$°C) vs. moderate cooling (Δt 2.2–1.5°C) ($p = 0.002$); moderate vs. low cooling ($\Delta t < -1.5$°C) ($p = 0.0006$) (**Figure 6**).

DISCUSSION

Our study shows that continuous-flow limb hypothermia using coolant temperatures of 22°C lasting the duration of paclitaxel chemotherapy is well tolerated and safe. Limb hypothermia with higher degrees of cooling significantly preserves selected nerve motor amplitudes at 3 months after start of chemotherapy.

Safety and Tolerability of Continuous-Flow Limb Hypothermia

Our results show good tolerability (Figure S2 in Supplementary Material) and, importantly, no early termination of cooling.

Various limb cooling modalities are used for different therapeutic interventions, most of which involve the direct application of ice or frozen gloves and cause steep cooling gradients with varied and often poor tolerability (20). Large cooling gradients permit only intermittent coolant application and are limited by significant intolerance and sometimes frostbite (21, 22). Advantages of continuous-flow limb cooling with thermoregulation features are controlled and more tolerable temperature reduction for the duration of chemotherapy infusion with better outcomes (21). Concern could be raised regarding cold-induced nerve damage, which is known to occur, depending on length and degree of cooling. The work by Jia et al. has examined in detail the required circumstances for cold-induced ischemia to occur in animal experiments (23). It is concluded that cooling the sciatic nerve for 3 h at 2°C does not result in vascular occlusions or morphological change in the nerves suggestive of ischemia from vasoconstriction. Looking at the difference in temperatures it is unlikely that 22°C cooling will be able to result in additional counteractive ischemia.

Skin Temperature and Hypothermia

Limb hypothermia caused significant decrease in skin temperature in the cooled limb across all sensor locations (**Figure 3**), while body core temperature was unaffected. The majority of cooling occurred in the first 60 min, consistent with other studies (24). Taking into consideration the objective of inducing maximal vasoconstriction before the initiation of chemotherapy, a period of pre-cooling, may be crucial (25). Hypothermia-induced vasoconstriction should be maintained throughout the duration of chemotherapy (12). All of these conditions were met by our study.

In studies of scalp cooling to prevent CIA, subcutaneous scalp temperature (depth 1–2 mm) had to be less than 22°C to prevent doxorubicin-induced alopecia (26). To achieve a subcutaneous temperature of 22°C, a surface scalp temperature of 19°C was necessary (27). Our study only achieved a mean skin surface temperature of 26.0 ± 0.8°C on the cooled limb. Although the targeted tissues are different, the temperature achieved in our study seems modest to achieve neuroprotection. We utilized a coolant temperature of 22°C based on this representing maximum tolerability for 3 h of continuous cooling (12). Future studies will need to explore techniques such as cryocompression to achieve more cooling while ensuring tolerability (28).

Although thermoregulator temperature was constant (22°C), different patients achieved different amounts of limb cooling due to varying body surface area and factors beyond experimental control, such as intermittent toilet breaks. On average, each patient took one toilet break per chemotherapy cycle typically lasting 5–7 min, during which limb wraps were removed. Toilet

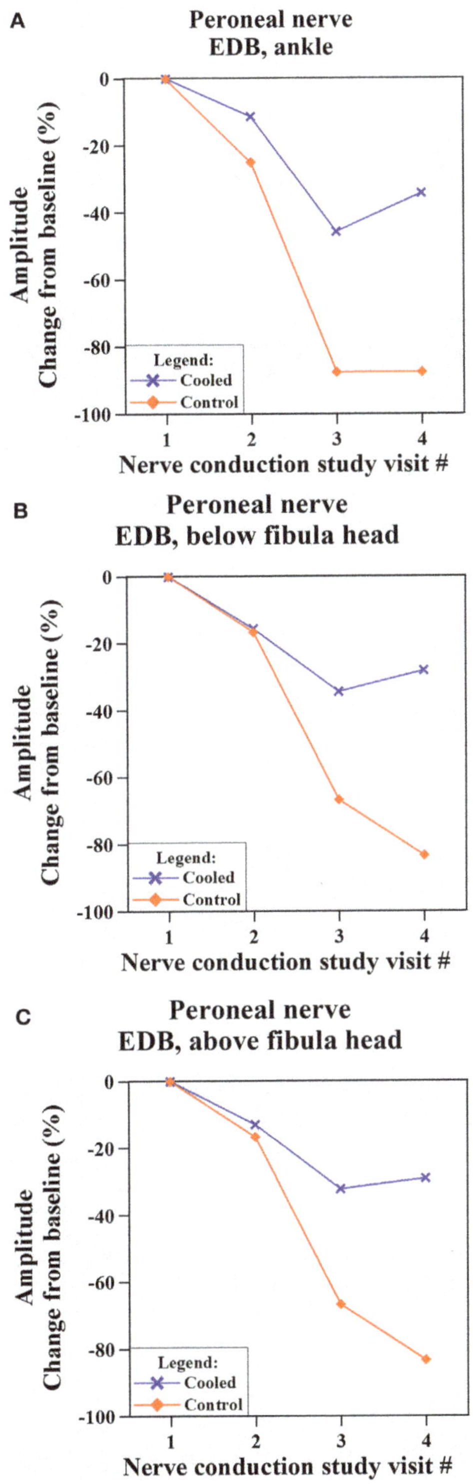

FIGURE 5 | Comparison of changes in compound motor action potential (cMAP) amplitudes in the cooled and non-cooled limb of a subject with well-preserved cMAP amplitudes in the extensor digitorum brevis (EDB) muscle on the common peroneal nerve. Over the time, the cooled leg showed consistently more preserved compound motor action potential amplitudes than the control leg at all the three stimulation points [**(A)** ankle, **(B)** below fibula head, and **(C)** above fibula head] on the EDB muscle.

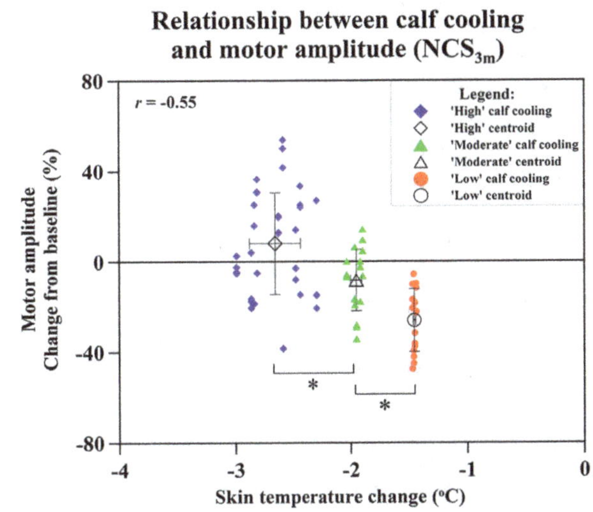

FIGURE 6 | Relation of changes of skin temperature at the calf and compound motor action potential (cMAP) amplitude percentage changes of extensor digitorum brevis (distal stimulation) cMAP at NCS_{3m}, with data grouped into "high" cooling, "moderate" cooling, and "low" cooling. Statistical significance (*$p < 0.05$).

breaks for trial subjects were similar in nature to chemotherapy patients not undergoing limb hypothermia with respect to frequency and duration and were not likely increased due to hypothermia. These breaks were mostly immediately before or after the end of paclitaxel infusion itself (**Figure 1A**).

Changes in Sensory and Motor Nerve Conduction Parameters

Both SNAP and cMAP amplitudes represent the number of functioning axons within each nerve. Lower amplitude reflects chemotherapeutic axonal damage, whereas reduction in velocity signifies nerve myelin sheath dysfunction (29, 30). Our results concur with the literature in showing paclitaxel-induced PN is predominantly axonal, length dependent, and sensory predominant (1).

Our study is the first to systematically record motor function over the course of chemotherapy using sensitive parameters (cMAP) and reveals frequent motor involvement. Clinical examination used in clinical scoring (TNS) was not able to detect motor involvement. Likely, this is because of poor sensitivity which explains the low rates of involvement in the literature (31).

It is important to consider why motor nerve parameters (cMAP) showed more effect to hypothermia than sensory parameters. cMAP amplitude, in contrast to sensory parameters, is dependent not only on nerve axonal function but additionally on muscle fiber function. Considering that paclitaxel motor neuropathy is rare (32) and myopathy is poorly identified with the TNS examination utilized, we suggest much of cMAP change could be from paclitaxel-induced myopathy. The infrequent reporting of myopathy in the literature is likely due to poor methods of detection (33).

Our hypothesis for the prevention of CIPN suggests that hypothermia reduces paclitaxel delivery to the nerve. Since hypothermia induces reduced blood flow to all exposed tissues, both motor axonal and myopathic components could underlie cMAP preservation (34). We postulate that prevention of myopathy may play a bigger role since hypothermia will affect muscle more than nerve based on the greater abundance of muscle tissue and the absence of a nerve–blood barrier.

Overall, our primary endpoint of differences in nerve conduction parameters between cooled and non-cooled limbs did not reach significance (**Figure 4**). Considering the modest degree of limb cooling achieved, we were particularly interested in assessing the effect of different degrees of cooling achieved. A good correlation ($r = -0.55$; $p < 0.001$) was found between the amount of cooling and the mean cMAP amplitude percentage changes at 3 months after the end of chemotherapy. This suggests that the degree of limb hypothermia achieved is crucial to the amount of cMAP preservation. Cluster analysis between high, moderate, and low amounts of cooling further showed significantly different amounts of cMAP amplitude preservation (**Figure 6**). This corresponds to observations suggesting a minimal threshold of temperature reduction for the prevention of alopecia (26). One patient benefited significantly from limb hypothermia, reflected through her NCS analysis. Several factors may have influenced this result including her history of diabetes, genetic predisposition, or concomitant medications. While sub-group analysis for these characteristics were not possible due to limited numbers, analysis of a larger cohort of patients undergoing limb hypothermia may identify predictive biomarkers for those who may benefit from such therapy.

Our study is adversely affected by the relatively small sample size and clinical methods that are not sensitive for assessment of mild or moderate degrees of motor dysfunction. Furthermore, only relatively modest degrees of limb cooling were achieved. While the lack of formal quality-of-life analysis in our study is a limitation, it was partially replaced by our safety scoring systems which did not reflect any concern. Future studies will also need to include more specific tests to determine the thresholds for mechanical and temperature sensitivity, or muscle strength, and to reveal alterations in sensory and motor functions related to neuropathy and myopathy (including plasma markers), as well as quality-of-life measures. A larger study using cryocompression of all four limbs is currently underway to prove efficacy. Studies to detect predictive biomarkers for paclitaxel-induced PN and to potentially identify patients from these protective therapies are also being conducted (35). Animal studies are also being performed to establish proof of reduced delivery of chemotherapy to neurons through limb hypothermia.

In summary, our results suggest that limb hypothermia, given for the duration of paclitaxel chemotherapy, preserves certain nerve conduction parameters. Preservation is directly related to the degree of limb cooling.

CONCLUSION

Our findings open up a new opportunity for more research to be conducted toward the goal of achieving neuroprotection and preventing CIPN *via* a simple, non-invasive, and non-pharmacological method. As neuropathy is an important factor leading to chemotherapy dose reduction and treatment discontinuation, this research may contribute to alleviating dose limitation and increase the likelihood of success of chemotherapy. While our results revealed some interesting findings, it must only be regarded as a pilot study and larger studies achieving well tolerated and greater limb cooling are now needed.

AUTHOR CONTRIBUTIONS

RS, AB, NT, S-CL, and EW-S developed the study concept and design. RS, NK, AJ, SO, JH, DT, and JL treated patients in this trial. AB, ST, JV, AT, ZH, EA, SA, and EW-S were involved in data acquisition. RS, AB, ST, and EW-S analyzed the data. RS, AB, ST, L-DL, and EW-S drafted the manuscript. NT, S-CL, and EW-S supervised the study. RS and AB contributed equally to this work. This manuscript has been seen, read, and agreed upon in its content by all the designated authors.

ACKNOWLEDGMENTS

The authors would like to thank all the patients who participated in this study and also the support and assistance of the physicians and nurses from the National University Hospital, Singapore. They would also like to thank the support of the Neurophotonics group under Singapore Institute for Neurotechnology.

FUNDING

The work was supported by the National Research Foundation, Singapore (NRF2013NRF-POC002-027) and the National Health Innovation Centre, Singapore (NHIC-I2D-1409031).

REFERENCES

1. Windebank AJ, Grisold W. Chemotherapy-induced neuropathy. *J Peripher Nerv Syst* (2008) 13:27–46. doi:10.1111/j.1529-8027.2008.00156.x
2. Hershman DL, Lacchetti C, Dworkin RH, Lavoie Smith EM, Bleeker J, Cavaletti G, et al. Prevention and management of chemotherapy-induced peripheral neuropathy in survivors of adult cancers: American Society of Clinical Oncology clinical practice guideline. *J Clin Oncol* (2014) 32:1941–67. doi:10.1200/JCO.2013.54.0914
3. Theiss C, Meller K. Taxol impairs anterograde axonal transport of microinjected horseradish peroxidase in dorsal root ganglia neurons in vitro. *Cell Tissue Res* (2000) 299:213–24. doi:10.1007/s004410050019
4. Nichole EL, Gerardo M, Scott TB, Stuart CF, Leslie W, Mary Ann J. Effects of eribulin, vincristine, paclitaxel and ixabepilone on fast axonal transport

and kinesin-1 driven microtubule gliding: implications for chemotherapy-induced peripheral neuropathy. *Neurotoxicology* (2013) 37:231–9. doi:10.1016/j.neuro.2013.05.008

5. Flatters SJL, Bennett GJ. Studies of peripheral sensory nerves in paclitaxel-induced painful peripheral neuropathy: evidence for mitochondrial dysfunction. *Pain* (2006) 122:245–57. doi:10.1016/j.pain.2006.01.037
6. Melli G, Jack C, Lambrinos GL, Ringkamp M, Höke A. Erythropoietin protects sensory axons against paclitaxel-induced distal degeneration. *Neurobiol Dis* (2006) 24:525–30. doi:10.1016/j.nbd.2006.08.014
7. Scripture CD, Figg WD, Sparreboom A. Peripheral neuropathy induced by paclitaxel: recent insights and future perspectives. *Curr Neuropharmacol* (2006) 4:165. doi:10.2174/157015906776359568
8. Liao LD, Orellana J, Liu YH, Lin YR, Vipin A, Thakor NV, et al. Imaging of temperature dependent hemodynamics in the rat sciatic nerve by functional photoacoustic microscopy. *Biomed Eng Online* (2013) 12:120–32. doi:10.1186/1475-925X-12-120
9. Massey CS. A multicentre study to determine the efficacy and patient acceptability of the Paxman scalp cooler to prevent hair loss in patients receiving chemotherapy. *Eur J Oncol Nurs* (2004) 8:121–30. doi:10.1016/j.ejon.2003.10.006
10. Grevelman EG, Breed WP. Prevention of chemotherapy-induced hair loss by scalp cooling. *Ann Oncol* (2005) 16:352–8. doi:10.1093/annonc/mdi088
11. Barber FA. A comparison of crushed ice and continuous flow cold therapy. *Am J Knee Surg* (2000) 13:97–101.
12. Bandla A, Sundar R, Liao L-D, Tan S, Lee SC, Thakor N, et al. Hypothermia for preventing chemotherapy-induced neuropathy – a pilot study on safety and tolerability in healthy controls. *Acta Oncol* (2016) 55:430–6. doi:10.3109/0284186X.2015.1075664
13. Hawker GA, Mian S, Kendzerska T, French M. Measures of adult pain: visual analog scale for pain (VAS pain), numeric rating scale for pain (NRS pain), McGill pain questionnaire (MPQ), short-form McGill pain questionnaire (SF-MPQ), chronic pain grade scale (CPGS), short form-36 bodily pain scale (SF-36 BPS), and measure of intermittent and constant osteoarthritis pain (ICOAP). *Arthritis Care Res (Hoboken)* (2011) 63:S240–52. doi:10.1002/acr.20543
14. Presciutti M, Bader MK, Hepburn M. Shivering management during therapeutic temperature modulation: nurses' perspective. *Crit Care Nurse* (2012) 32:33–42. doi:10.4037/ccn2012189
15. Kong X, Lesser EA, Potts FA, Gozani SN. Utilization of nerve conduction studies for the diagnosis of polyneuropathy in patients with diabetes: a retrospective analysis of a large patient series. *J Diabetes Sci Technol* (2008) 2:268–74. doi:10.1177/193229680800200217
16. Karandreas N, Papatheodorou A, Triantaphilos I, Mavridis M, Lygidakis C. Sensory nerve conduction studies of the less frequently examined nerves. *Electromyogr Clin Neurophysiol* (1995) 35:169–73.
17. Ping Ng KW, Ong JJ, Nyein Nyein TD, Liang S, Chan YC, Lee KO, et al. EMLA-induced skin wrinkling for the detection of diabetic neuropathy. *Front Neurol* (2013) 4:126. doi:10.3389/fneur.2013.00126
18. Wampler MA, Miaskowski C, Hamel K, Byl N, Rugo H, Topp KS. The modified total neuropathy score: a clinically feasible and valid measure of taxane-induced peripheral neuropathy in women with breast cancer. *J Support Oncol* (2006) 4:W9–16.
19. Cavaletti G, Frigeni B, Lanzani F, Piatti M, Rota S, Briani C, et al. The total neuropathy score as an assessment tool for grading the course of chemotherapy-induced peripheral neurotoxicity: comparison with the National Cancer Institute-common toxicity scale. *J Peripher Nerv Syst* (2007) 23:210–5. doi:10.1111/j.1529-8027.2007.00141.x
20. Scotté F, Tourani J-M, Banu E, Peyromaure M, Levy E, Marsan S, et al. Multicenter study of a frozen glove to prevent docetaxel-induced onycholysis and cutaneous toxicity of the hand. *J Clin Oncol* (2005) 23:4424–9. doi:10.1200/JCO.2005.15.651
21. Hochberg J. A randomized prospective study to assess the efficacy of two cold-therapy treatments following carpal tunnel release. *J Hand Ther* (2001) 14:208–15. doi:10.1016/S0894-1130(01)80055-7
22. McGuire DA, Hendricks SD. Incidences of frostbite in arthroscopic knee surgery postoperative cryotherapy rehabilitation. *Arthroscopy* (2006) 22:1141.e1–6. doi:10.1016/j.arthro.2005.06.027
23. Jia J, Pollock M. The pathogenesis of non-freezing cold nerve injury. Observations in the rat. *Brain* (1997) 120:631–46. doi:10.1093/brain/120.4.631
24. Tikuisis P. Heat balance precedes stabilization of body temperatures during cold water immersion. *J Appl Physiol* (2003) 95:89–96. doi:10.1152/japplphysiol.01195.2002
25. Komen MM, Smorenburg CH, Van Den Hurk CJ, Nortier JW. Factors influencing the effectiveness of scalp cooling in the prevention of chemotherapy-induced alopecia. *Oncologist* (2013) 18:885–91. doi:10.1634/theoncologist.2012-0332
26. Gregory R, Cooke T, Middleton J, Buchanan R, Williams C. Prevention of doxorubicin-induced alopecia by scalp hypothermia: relation to degree of cooling. *Br Med J (Clin Res Ed)* (1982) 284:1674. doi:10.1136/bmj.284.6330.1674
27. Bülow J, Friberg L, Gaardsting O, Hansen M. Frontal subcutaneous blood flow, and epi- and subcutaneous temperatures during scalp cooling in normal man. *Scand J Clin Lab Invest* (1985) 45:505–8. doi:10.3109/00365518509155250
28. Block JE. Cold and compression in the management of musculoskeletal injuries and orthopedic operative procedures: a narrative review.
29. Veves A, Malik RA, Lye RH, Masson EA, Sharma AK, Schady W, et al. The relationship between sural nerve morphometric findings and measures of peripheral nerve function in mild diabetic neuropathy. *Diabet Med* (1991) 8:917–21. doi:10.1111/j.1464-5491.1991.tb01530.x
30. Mallik A, Weir AI. Nerve conduction studies: essentials and pitfalls in practice. *J Neurol Neurosurg Psychiatry* (2005) 76(Suppl 2):ii23–31. doi:10.1136/jnnp.2005.069138
31. Rowinsky E, Chaudhry V, Cornblath D, Donehower R. Neurotoxicity of taxol. *J Natl Cancer Inst Monogr* (1992) 15:107–15.
32. Freilich RJ, Balmaceda C, Seidman AD, Rubin M, Deangelis LM. Motor neuropathy due to docetaxel and paclitaxel. *Neurology* (1996) 47:115–8. doi:10.1212/WNL.47.1.115
33. Gilliam LA, St Clair DK. Chemotherapy-induced weakness and fatigue in skeletal muscle: the role of oxidative stress. *Antioxid Redox Signal* (2011) 15:2543–63. doi:10.1089/ars.2011.3965
34. Franssen H, van den Bergh P. Nerve conduction studies in polyneuropathy: practical physiology and patterns of abnormality. *Acta Neurol Belg* (2006) 106:73–81.
35. Sundar R, Jeyasekharan AD, Pang B, Soong RC, Kumarakulasinghe NB, Ow SG, et al. Low levels of NDRG1 in nerve tissue are predictive of severe paclitaxel-induced neuropathy. *PLoS One* (2016) 11:e0164319. doi:10.1371/journal.pone.0164319

Conflict of Interest Statement: The authors declare that the research was conducted in the absence of any commercial or financial relationships that could be construed as a potential conflict of interest.

18

Therapeutic Potential and Molecular Mechanisms of *Emblica officinalis* Gaertn in Countering Nephrotoxicity in Rats Induced by the Chemotherapeutic Agent Cisplatin

Salma Malik[1†], Kapil Suchal[1†], Jagriti Bhatia[1*], Sana I. Khan[1], Swati Vasisth[1], Ameesha Tomar[1], Sameer Goyal[2], Rajeev Kumar[1], Dharamvir S. Arya[1] and Shreesh K. Ojha[3*]

[1] Cardiovascular Research Laboratory, Department of Pharmacology, All India Institute of Medical Sciences, New Delhi, India, [2] Department of Pharmacology, R. C. Patel Institute of Pharmaceutical Education and Research, Shirpur, India, [3] Department of Pharmacology and Therapeutics, College of Medicine and Health Sciences, United Arab Emirates University, Al Ain, UAE

Edited by:
Raquel Abalo,
King Juan Carlos University, Spain

Reviewed by:
Sachin Kumar Gupta,
Baylor College of Medicine, USA
Jose Uranga,
King Juan Carlos University, Spain
Adriana Izquierdo,
King Juan Carlos University, Spain

***Correspondence:**
Jagriti Bhatia
jagriti2012@rediffmail.com
Shreesh K. Ojha
shreeshojha@uaeu.ac.ae

† These authors have contributed equally to this work.

Emblica officinalis Gaertn. belonging to family Euphorbiaceae is commonly known as Indian gooseberry or "Amla" in India. It is used as a 'rejuvenating herb' in traditional system of Indian medicine. It has been shown to possess antioxidant, anti-inflammatory and anti-apoptotic effects. Thus, on the basis of its biological effects, the present study was undertaken to evaluate the protective effect of the dried fruit extract of the *E. Officinalis* (EO) in cisplatin-induced nephrotoxicity in rats and also to evaluate the mechanism of its nephroprotection. The study was done on male albino Wistar rats. They were divided into six groups ($n = 6$) viz. control, cisplatin-control, cisplatin and EO (150, 300, and 600 mg/kg; p.o. respectively in different groups) and EO only (600 mg/kg; p.o. only). EO was administered orally to the rats for a period of 10 days and on the 7th day, a single injection of cisplatin (8 mg/kg; i.p.) was administered to the cisplatin-control and EO treatment groups. The rats were sacrificed on the 10th day. Cisplatin-control rats had deranged renal function parameters and the kidney histology confirmed the presence of acute tubular necrosis. Furthermore, there were increased oxidative stress, apoptosis and inflammation along with higher expression of MAPK pathway proteins in the rat kidney from the cisplatin-control group. Contrary to this, EO (600 mg/kg) significantly normalized renal function, bolstered antioxidant status and ameliorated histological alterations. The inflammation and apoptosis were markedly lower in comparison to cisplatin-control rats. Furthermore, EO (600 mg/kg) inhibited MAPK phosphorylation which was instrumental in preserving renal function and morphology. In conclusion, the results of our study demonstrated that EO attenuated cisplatin-induced nephrotoxicity in rats through suppression of MAPK induced inflammation and apoptosis.

Keywords: inflammation, apoptosis, oxidative stress, *Emblica officinalis,* cisplatin, nephrotoxicity

INTRODUCTION

Cisplatin (*cis*-diamminedichloroplatinum II or CDDP) is a platinum compound which has a broad role in the management of various solid malignancies such as head and neck, bladder, lung, ovaries, testicles, and uterus (Oh et al., 2016). However, during the course of chemotherapy, cisplatin may cause ototoxicity, nephrotoxicity, myelosuppression, and peripheral neuropathy (Oh et al., 2014). Among these undesirable effects, nephrotoxicity is the most important dose limiting adverse effect of cisplatin therapy, which primarily affects the S3 segment of the proximal tubules (Bolisetty et al., 2016). It accounts for up to 60% of acute kidney injury cases acquired from the hospital and is associated with remarkably high morbidity and mortality and approximately one fourth of patients initiated on high-dose cisplatin have severe renal dysfunction while one third experience kidney injury within few days of receiving cisplatin (Oh et al., 2016). Clinically, cisplatin induced renal dysfunction manifests as decline in renal plasma flow and glomerular filtration rate with an increase in serum creatinine and blood urea nitrogen (Miller et al., 2010). The proposed molecular mechanisms underlying cisplatin nephrotoxicity involve oxidative stress, DNA damage, apoptosis and exaggerated inflammatory response (Pabla and Dong, 2008).

The oxidative stress has emerged as the main mechanism in cisplatin-induced nephrotoxicity (dos Santos et al., 2012; Oh et al., 2016). It has been reported that excess reactive oxygen species (ROS) production as well as antioxidant system depletions are consequent to cisplatin administration (Domitrović et al., 2013). The likely sources of ROS during cisplatin administration include the mitochondrial electron transport chain system (Pan et al., 2015), xanthine oxidase (Yousef and Hussien, 2015), cytochrome P450 enzymes (Pabla and Dong, 2008), and NADPH oxidase (Wang et al., 2015). Since, ROS are highly reactive and unstable; they may attack and modify cellular components such as lipids, proteins, and DNA, resulting in cellular stress (Jaiman et al., 2013). ROS accumulation also activates important signaling pathways, including apoptotic pathway, which leads to cell death in the event of cisplatin-induced nephrotoxicity (Song et al., 2015). Cisplatin mediated oxidative stress provokes the stimulation of a cascade of signaling proteins, including MAPKs and NF-κB (Malik et al., 2015). This abnormal activation of MAPK and NF-κB leads to release of inflammatory cytokines subsequently aggravating the renal damage (Sahu et al., 2014). The renal damage induced by cisplatin is managed using hydration/diuretics, renal function monitoring and adjustment of the cisplatin dose. However, renal toxicity still occurs despite the use of these measures. Therefore, taking the molecular pathways of cisplatin nephrotoxicity in consideration, exploration of more effective nephroprotective therapeutic options which would not affect the tumoricidal activity of cisplatin is essential.

Several strategies have been evaluated to minimize the nephrotoxicity caused by cisplatin. Recently, plant derived natural compounds and their active constituents are being evaluated for their beneficial effects in various pathophysiological conditions (Athira et al., 2016). *Emblica officinalis* (*E. Officinalis*) also known as Amla or Indian Gooseberry is a natural fruit that serves as a rich source of vitamin C (Krishnaveni and Mirunalini, 2010). It also contains flavonoids, tannins, terpenoids and alkaloids which possess various biological activities (Kim et al., 2005). The active extracts of *E. Officinalis* have been demonstrated to exert a wide range of activities such as antioxidant in alcohol-induced oxidative damage in rat liver microsomes (Reddy et al., 2014), anti-apoptotic in arsenic-induced apoptosis in thymocytes of mice (Singh et al., 2013), anti-inflammatory in rodent models of acute and chronic inflammation (Golechha et al., 2014), anti-diabetic in type 2 diabetes in rats (Nain et al., 2012), anti-hypertensive in DOCA salt induced hypertension in rats (Bhatia et al., 2011) and anticancer in cervical cancer cells (Mahata et al., 2013). Several studies have also been conducted to investigate its beneficial effect in kidney injury including cyclophosphamide induced renal injury (Haque et al., 2001) and mycotoxin induced renal toxicity (Verma and Chakraborty, 2008). Thus, the present study was designed to investigate the beneficial effect of the dried fruit extract of *E. officinalis* (EO) on cisplatin mediated kidney injury by assessing its antioxidant, anti-apoptotic, and anti-inflammatory properties on the kidney and further to evaluate whether MAPK pathway is involved in mediating this renoprotection.

MATERIALS AND METHODS

Plant Extract

The dried fruit extract of *E. officinalis* (EO) was obtained from Sanat Products Limited, India (a WHO-GMP and ISO 9001 Accredited Herbal Extract Manufacturer Company). The batch number of EO was 048001. The extract contained 31.58% w/w of hydrolysable tannins emblicanin A and emblicanin B on dried weight basis.

Chemicals

Cisplatin was obtained from Pfizer Products Pvt. Ltd., India. Blood urea nitrogen (BUN) and serum creatinine kits were procured from Transasia Bio-Medicals Ltd., India. Kits for Terminal deoxynucleotide transferase dUTP nick end labeling (TUNEL) assay (ApoBrduDNA fragmentation assay kit) (Biovision Inc. California), tumor necrosis factor-α (TNF-α) (Diaclone Tepnel Company, UK) and IL-6 (Ray Biotech, Inc. Norcross, GA, USA) were used. Primary antibodies against extracellular signal-regulated kinase 1/2 (ERK1/2), phospho-ERK1/2 (p-ERK1/2), c-Jun N-terminal kinase (JNK), phospho-JNK (p-JNK), Caspase-3, NF-κBp65, and β-actin were procured from cell signaling technology, USA. Antibodies for Bcl-2, Bax and p-38 were purchased from Abcam, UK. Phospho-p38 (p-p38) antibody was obtained from Santa Cruz biotechnology, USA. Secondary antibodies were from Merck Genei Pvt. Ltd., India. All other chemicals used were of analytical grade.

Experimental Animals

Adult male albino Wistar rats aged 10–12 weeks old (weighing 150–200 g) were used for the study. All experimental procedures were conducted after approval by Institutional Animal Ethics Committee of All India Institute of Medical Sciences, New Delhi (IAEC no. 604/IAEC/2011) and conformed to the Indian National Science Academy Guidelines for care and use of animals in research. During the study period, animals were kept in polypropylene cages under conditions of ambient temperature (25 ± 2°C), relative humidity (60 ± 5%) and 12 h light/dark cycle and provided food pellets (Ashirwad Industries Ltd, Chandigarh, India) and tap water *ad libitum*.

A total of 36 male albino Wistar rats were randomly divided into six groups containing six rats per group. The test drug, EO, was dissolved in distilled water for administration to rats.

Group 1 (Control)

Rats received distilled water (2 ml/kg; p.o.) for the period of 10 days.

Group 2 (Cisplatin-Control)

Rats received distilled water (2 ml/kg; p.o.) for the period of 10 days and on the 7th day, a single injection of cisplatin (8 mg/kg; i.p.) was administered to induce nephrotoxicity (Malik et al., 2015).

Groups 3–5 (Treatment Groups)

Rats received EO (150–600 mg/kg; p.o.) daily for the period of 10 days and on the 7th day, a single injection of cisplatin (8 mg/kg; i.p.) was administered to induce nephrotoxicity.

Group 6 (EO Only)

Rats received EO (600 mg/kg; p.o.) for the period of 10 days.

On the 10th day, rats were anaesthetized with pentobarbitone sodium (60 mg/kg; i.p.) and chest cavity was opened. Blood was drawn *via* cardiac puncture, and centrifuged at 4000 rpm to separate serum which was stored at −20°C for measurement of BUN, serum creatinine, TNF-α and IL-6 levels. After sacrificing, one kidney from 6 rats per group was snap frozen in liquid nitrogen and preserved in −80°C and used for biochemical estimation. The second kidney from 3 rats per group was removed and preserved in 10% neutral buffered formalin for histopatholgical and TUNEL assay and kidney from the other 3 rats per group were snap frozen in liquid nitrogen and stored in −80°C for western blot analysis.

Assessment of Kidney Function Parameters

Serum creatinine and BUN levels were measured using respective commercially available kits.

Measurement of Renal Oxidant–Antioxidant Parameters

Kidney sample was removed from −80°C, thawed, weighed and 10% homogenate was prepared in ice-chilled phosphate buffer (0.1 M, pH 7.4). The tissue homogenate was divided into two parts. One part of this homogenate was used for the estimation of malondialdehyde (MDA) level and reduced glutathione (GSH) content. The other part of this tissue homogenate was centrifuged at 5000 rpm and supernatant thus obtained was used for the estimation of superoxide dismutase (SOD), catalase (CAT) enzyme activities and protein content.

Estimation of MDA Level

MDA level was estimated by the method described by Ohkawa et al. (1979). To the 0.1 ml tissue homogenate, 0.5 ml of 8.1% sodium dodecyl sulfate, 1.5 ml of 20% acetic acid and 1.5 ml of 0.8% thiobarbituric acid was added, vortexed and heated at 95°C for 60 min. After cooling, 5 ml of butanol:pyridine (15:1) mixture was added to extract pink color complex. The pink organic layer was separated and absorbance read at 532 nm. The amount of MDA was calculated by extrapolation from the MDA standard curve and expressed as nmole/g tissue.

Estimation of GSH Content

GSH was measured by the method described by Moron et al. (1979). Firstly, homogenate was centrifuged with an equal volume of 10% trichloroacetic acid. To the 0.1 ml of supernatant, 3 ml Na_2HPO_4 (0.3 M; pH 8.0) and 0.5 ml of 5,5′-dithiobis (2-nitrobenzoic acid) prepared in 1% trisodium citrate were added and mixed thoroughly. The absorbance of yellow color formed was read at 412 nm. The amount of GSH was determined by extrapolation from standard curve and expressed as μmole/g tissue.

Estimation of SOD

Superoxide dismutase enzyme activity was determined by the method described by Marklund and Marklund (1974). To the 0.1 ml supernatant, 2.95 ml of phosphate buffer (0.1 M; pH 8.4) and 0.05 ml of pyrogallol (7.5 mM) was added and the change in absorbance was recorded at an interval of 60 s for 2 min at 420 nm. One unit of enzyme activity was defined as the amount of enzyme required to produce 50% inhibition of pyrogallol autoxidation under assay conditions and expressed as U/mg protein.

Estimation of CAT

CAT enzyme activity was estimated by the method described by Aebi (1984). To the 0.05 ml of supernatant, 1 ml of phosphate buffer (50 mM; pH 7.0) and 1.0 ml of hydrogen peroxide (H_2O_2) was added. Immediately, thereafter, change in the absorbance was recorded for 30 s at an interval of 5 s at 240 nm. One unit of CAT enzyme activity is equal to 1 μmol of H_2O_2 decomposed per min and expressed as U/mg protein.

Estimation of Protein Content

Protein was measured by a method described by Bradford (1976). To the supernatant, Bradford reagent was added and vortexed. Blue color formed was measured at 595 nm. The amount of protein was determined by standard curve and expressed as mg/ml.

Measurement of Serum Pro-inflammatory Cytokines Level

TNF-α and IL-6 levels were assessed in serum using commercially available ELISA kits as per manufacturer instructions.

Histopathological Examination

For histopathological evaluation, paraffin blocks were made from kidney tissue preserved in formalin. The tissue sections of 5-μm thickness were cut using microtome (Leica RM 2125, Germany). These sections were stained with hematoxylin and eosin (H&E) and studied under light microscope (Dewinter Technologies, Italy).

TUNEL Assay

TUNEL assay was performed for detection of apoptosis in the renal tissue. TUNEL assay was performed according to the method described by Malik et al. (2015). Briefly, sections were incubated with Proteinase K for 30 min to enhance tissue permeability and then treated with 30% H_2O_2 in methanol for 15 min to diminish any endogenous peroxidase activity. Later, sections were incubated with complete labeling reaction buffer and antibody solution, each for 1 h and 30 min. Following this, 3,3′-diaminobenzidine (DAB) solution was added and at least five fields in each slide were checked for any TUNEL positive cells in each group.

The pathologist evaluating histopathological and TUNEL slides was blinded to the treatment groups.

Western Blot Analysis

For western blot analysis, kidneys were removed from −80°C, thawed and weighed. Then tissues were homogenized in Radioimmunoprecipitation assay (RIPA) buffer (150 mM NaCl, 10% Triton X-100, 0.5% Sodium deoxycholate, 0.1% Sodium dodecyl sulfate, 50 mM Tris base), along with protease inhibitor (Sigma Aldrich, USA). The homogenate was centrifuged at 12000 rpm for 20 min at 4°C and supernatant was used for measurement of protein concentration by using the method described by Bradford (1976). Protein equivalent to 40 μg was separated by the sodium dodecyl sulfate polyacrylamide gel electrophoresis (SDS-PAGE). Separated proteins were then transferred to a nitrocellulose membrane and then blocked with 3% bovine serum albumin (BSA) for 1 h. After that, membrane was blocked with primary antibodies for ERK1/2, p-ERK1/2, JNK, p-JNK, p38, p-p38, Bcl-2, Bax, Caspase-3, NF-κBp65 and β-actin (1:3000) overnight at 4°C. The primary antibodies were detected with HRP-conjugated secondary antibodies (1:5000) for 2 h at room temperature. The antigen-antibody reaction was then visualized with enhanced chemiluminscence (ECL) kit according to manufacturer's instructions. The band intensity was measured using image-j software.

Statistical Analysis

Data of all experimental groups were analyzed by one way analysis of variance (ANOVA) followed by *post hoc* Tukey-Kramer multiple comparison test using the Graph Pad InStat software. Data are expressed as mean ± SEM and values for $P < 0.05$ were considered as statistically significant.

RESULTS

Effect of EO on Kidney Function Parameters

The kidney function parameters such as serum creatinine and BUN levels were measured in all treatment groups to assess renal function. Cisplatin injection resulted in significant increase in serum creatinine ($P < 0.001$) and BUN levels ($P < 0.001$) in comparison to control group. This elevation in serum creatinine and BUN levels suggests significant kidney damage and confirmed the induction of nephrotoxicity in cisplatin control group. EO (600 mg/kg) pretreatment significantly ($P < 0.01$) normalized serum creatinine and BUN levels as compared to cisplatin-control group. However, no significant effect was observed at two lower doses (150 and 300 mg/kg) (**Table 1**).

Effect of EO on Renal Oxidant–Antioxidant Parameters

In cisplatin-control rats, there was a significant ($P < 0.001$) increase in the level of MDA, a marker of lipid peroxidation, along with reduction in the level of antioxidants GSH ($P < 0.001$), SOD ($P < 0.01$), and CAT ($P < 0.01$) in comparison to control group. Interestingly, EO (600 mg/kg) pretreatment significantly restored the kidney antioxidant status. This is depicted by increase in the activities of GSH ($P < 0.01$), SOD ($P < 0.05$) and CAT ($P < 0.05$) and decrease in the level of MDA ($P < 0.05$) as

TABLE 1 | Effect of EO on renal function tests (serum creatinine and BUN) and biochemical parameters.

Groups	Sr. Creatinine (mg/dl)	BUN (mg/dl)	MDA (nmol/g tissue)	GSH (μmol/g tissue)	SOD (U/mg protein)	CAT (U/mg protein)
Control	0.57 ± 0.028	28.59 ± 1.62	60.50 ± 3.44	0.29 ± 0.012	3.98 ± 0.41	4.73 ± 0.42
Cis-C	1.45 ± 0.052***	53.95 ± 2.67***	109.81 ± 3.75***	0.16 ± 0.014***	2.42 ± 0.33**	2.36 ± 0.65**
EO 150+Cis	1.37 ± 0.075†††	50.35 ± 1.72†††	102.94 ± 4.54†††	0.18 ± 0.015†††	2.91 ± 0.18	3.61 ± 0.53
EO 300+Cis	1.29 ± 0.048†††	46.01 ± 2.05†††	96.63 ± 4.63†††	0.21 ± 0.012††	3.02 ± 0.19	4.13 ± 0.30
EO 600+Cis	1.18 ± 0.057†††##	42.46 ± 1.66†††##	91.66 ± 3.38†#	0.24 ± 0.014##	3.57 ± 0.15#	4.42 ± 0.26#
EO 600 only	0.62 ± 0.031	31.65 ± 1.35	71.01 ± 3.71	0.32 ± 0.012	3.96 ± 0.18	4.92 ± 0.33

*BUN, blood urea nitrogen; MDA, malondialdehyde; GSH, reduced glutathione; SOD, superoxide dismutase; CAT, catalase. Data are expressed as mean ± SEM of 6 rats per group. **$P < 0.01$, ***$P < 0.001$ versus control group; †$P < 0.05$, ††$P < 0.01$, †††$P < 0.001$ versus control group; #$P < 0.05$, ##$P < 0.01$ versus Cis-C group.*

compared to the cisplatin-control rats. Moreover, the two lower doses (150 and 300 mg/kg) of EO failed to exert any beneficial effect on the kidney antioxidant status (**Table 1**).

Effect of EO on Serum Inflammatory Cytokines Level

Cisplatin administration is known to release pro-inflammatory cytokines in serum. Thus, there was a significant ($P < 0.001$) increase in serum pro-inflammatory cytokines level (TNF-α and IL-6) in the cisplatin-control group as compared to the rats in the control group. EO (600 mg/kg) pretreatment significantly ($P < 0.01$) prevented the increase in the serum cytokines level as compared to the cisplatin-control group. However, no significant difference in the levels of these cytokines was observed with the lower doses of EO (150 and 300 mg/kg) (**Table 2**).

Effect of EO on Renal Histopathology

The histopathological evaluation of control and EO only groups demonstrated normal architecture of tubules with no evidence of inflammation (**Figures 1A,F**). The kidney sections from the cisplatin-control rats showed tubular atrophy, denudation of epithelium and infiltration of inflammatory cells (**Figure 1B**). In the groups, pretreated with 150 and 300 mg/kg dose of EO, there was marked and moderate tubular damage and inflammation respectively (**Figures 1C,D**). However, the highest dose of EO i.e., 600 mg/kg exerted significant nephroprotection and a marked absence of tubular necrosis and inflammation in the kidneys was observed (**Figure 1E**).

Thus, on the basis of results of the above mentioned parameters, EO at the dose of 600 mg/kg was found to exert maximum nephroprotection. Hence, this dose was used for further TUNEL and western blot analysis.

Effect of EO on Apoptosis and Inflammation

The apoptosis in the renal tissue was assessed by detecting the expression of apoptotic proteins in all groups. In cisplatin-control group, there was significantly increased expression of pro-apoptotic proteins [Bax ($P < 0.001$) and Caspase-3 ($P < 0.001$)] and decreased expression of Bcl-2 ($P < 0.001$), an anti-apoptotic protein. Furthermore, there was increased DNA fragmentation and increased number of TUNEL positive cells in the cisplatin-control group as compared to the control group. However, EO (600 mg/kg) treatment group reduced the apoptosis as there was significantly ($P < 0.05$) increased expression of Bcl-2 and decreased expression of Bax, Caspase-3 along with decreased DNA fragmentation as compared to cisplatin-control group. This confirms the anti-apoptotic effect of EO in renal tissue (**Figures 2** and **3**).

Further, western blot analysis was performed to determine the expression of NF-κBp65 in the renal tissue. Cisplatin-control rats demonstrated significantly ($P < 0.01$) increased level of NF-κBp65 whereas treatment with EO (600 mg/kg) attenuated this effect ($P < 0.05$) (**Figure 3**).

TABLE 2 | Effect of EO on serum pro-inflammatory cytokines level.

Groups	TNF-α (pg/ml)	IL-6 (pg/ml)
Control	37.35 ± 1.49	9.5 ± 0.46
Cis-C	58.17 ± 2.38***	17.92 ± 0.91***
EO 150+Cis	54.95 ± 2.92†††	16 ± 0.90†††
EO 300+Cis	50.07 ± 1.87††	14.21 ± 0.94††
EO 600+Cis	46.46 ± 1.84†##	12.62 ± 0.65†##
EO 600 only	38.51 ± 1.64	10.29 ± 0.65

*TNF-α, tumor necrosis factor-α; IL-6, interleukin-6. Data are expressed as mean ± SEM of 6 rats per group. ***P < 0.001 versus control group; †P < 0.05, ††P < 0.01, †††P < 0.001 versus control group; ##P < 0.01 versus Cis-C group.*

Effect of EO on MAPK Signaling Pathway

In cisplatin-control group, there was increased phosphorylation of ERK1/2, JNK and p38 proteins as compared to control rats. The increased phosphorylation of these proteins mediated apoptosis and inflammation in the cisplatin-control group. Contrary to this, EO (600 mg/kg) treatment halted the activation of this pathway and prevented apoptosis and inflammation in the renal tissue (**Figure 4**).

DISCUSSION

The current study has demonstrated the renoprotective effect of EO in cisplatin-induced acute renal toxicity in rats. The administration of EO virtually ameliorated most of the deleterious effects of cisplatin. This renoprotection was evident from improved functional as well as structural renal profiles, blunting of oxidative stress, inflammation, and apoptosis. Our results further provided evidence that this improvement was mediated by suppression of the MAPK signaling cascade.

Cisplatin's chemotherapeutic applicability is limited by renal toxicity and the latter occurs due to accumulation of cisplatin into the renal tubular cells which subsequently leads to renal tubular cell injury and renal cell death which appears histologically as tubular atrophy (Pabla et al., 2009). Many studies have proposed that cisplatin is also injurious to renal vasculature which results in decreased blood flow leading to ischemic injury of the kidneys, appearing as a decline in the glomerular filtration rate which is reflected as increased serum creatinine and BUN levels (Xu et al., 2015). In our study, we observed increased levels of serum creatinine and BUN suggesting renal damage due to cisplatin. Serum creatinine is the waste metabolic product and is formed due to breakdown of creatine phosphate in muscle. Normally, it is excreted by the kidneys, primarily by glomerular filtration but also by proximal tubular secretion with little or no reabsorption. If there is deterioration in kidney function, serum level of creatinine rises (El-Naga, 2014; Changizi-Ashtiyani et al., 2016; El-Naga and Mahran, 2016). Also, concomitant decline in urinary creatinine clearance is observed vis a vis raised serum creatinine levels. Infact, decrease in urinary creatinine clearance due to cisplatin-induced kidney injury has been reported by other researchers (Quesada et al., 2012; Nojiri et al., 2015). Although, we have not measured the urinary creatinine clearance in this

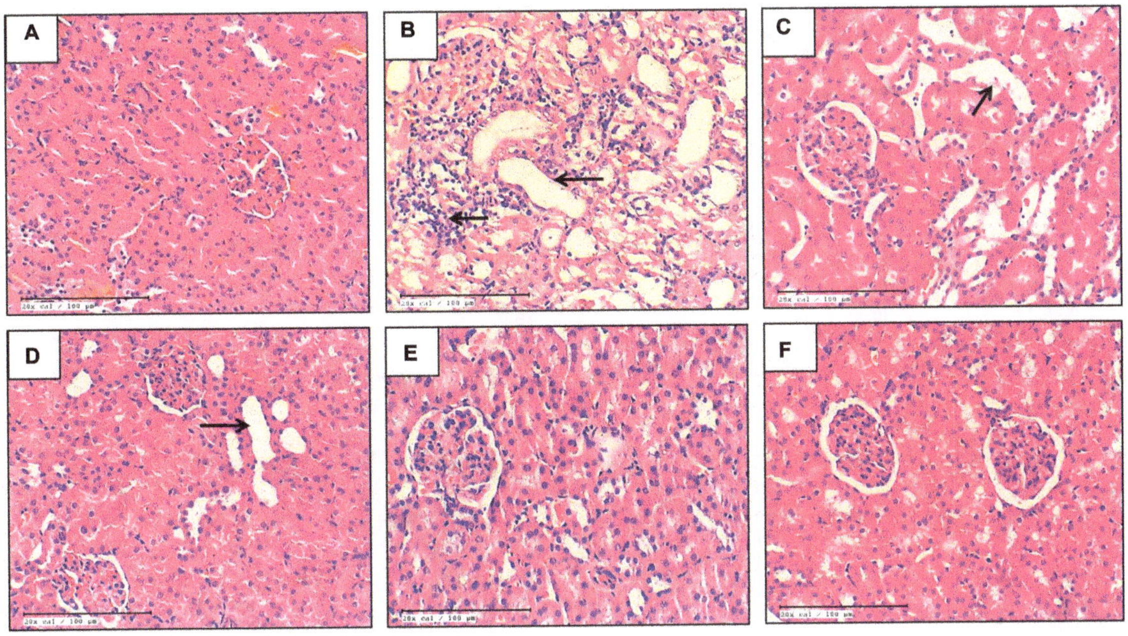

FIGURE 1 | Light microscopic study (H&E) of renal tissue in various experimental groups. (A) Control; **(B)** Cis-C; **(C–E)** EO 150, 300, 600 mg/kg+Cis respectively; **(F)** EO 600 mg/kg only. (→): acute tubular necrosis; (n = 3; 20X; scale bar 100 μm).

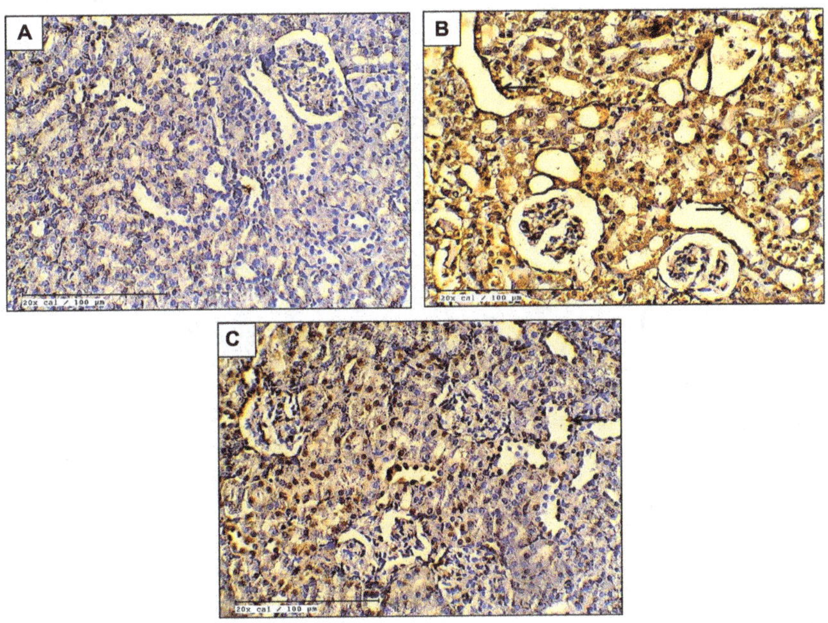

FIGURE 2 | Effect of EO on TUNEL positivity (A–C; 20X; scale bar 100 μm) in various experimental groups. (A) Control; **(B)** Cis-C; **(C)** EO 600 mg/kg+Cis. (→): tubular cell apoptosis.

particular study, the changes in serum creatinine and BUN levels observed here were clearly accompanied by changes in renal histology, further suggesting renal function deterioration in cisplatin-treated animals. There was marked renal tubular atrophy and denudation of epithelium following intraperitoneal administration of 8 mg/kg cisplatin. Administration of EO 600 mg/kg, significantly normalized serum creatinine and BUN levels and also preserved the histology of renal tubular cells.

Numerous studies have depicted the key role of oxidative stress in the pathophysiology of cisplatin-induced renal cell death (Song et al., 2015). Once cisplatin reaches the tubular cells, it rapidly reacts with thiol-containing molecules including

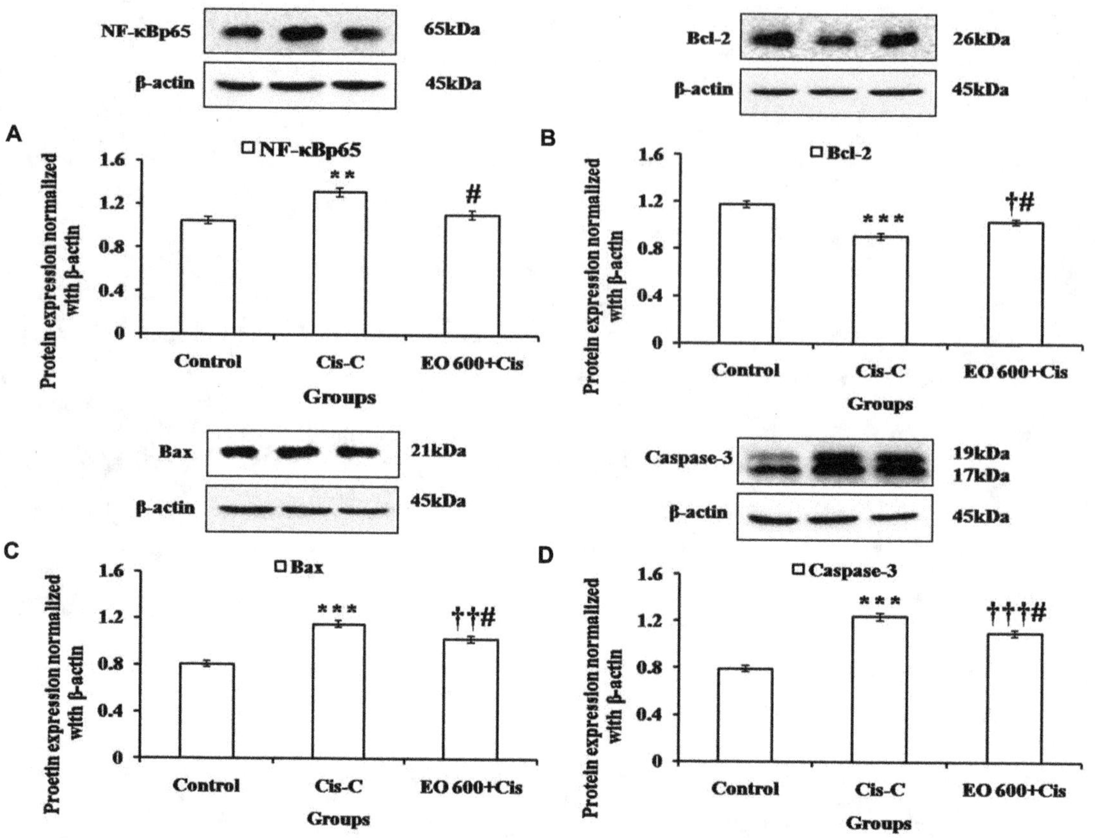

FIGURE 3 | Effect of EO on (A): NF-κBp65; (B) Bcl-2; (C) Bax; (D) Caspase-3 levels in various experimental groups. Data are expressed as mean ± SEM of 3 rats per group. $^{**}P < 0.01$, $^{***}P < 0.001$ versus control group; $^{\dagger}P < 0.05$, $^{\dagger\dagger}P < 0.01$, $^{\dagger\dagger\dagger}P < 0.001$ versus control group; $^{\#}P < 0.05$ versus Cis-C group.

glutathione by being converted to a highly reactive electrophile. This positively charged electrophile is generated by replacement of the chloride ligands of cisplatin with water molecules. Cisplatin also increases ROS synthesis by inducing mitochondrial dysfunction and disrupting the electron transport chain. Due to their unstable configuration, ROS reacts with membrane lipids, cellular proteins and DNA resulting in their modification leading to cellular stress (Pabla and Dong, 2008). Lipid peroxidation is a consequence of excessive ROS production. It leads to increased level of MDA (a lipid peroxidation marker). The rise in MDA levels following cisplatin administration *in vivo* has been observed in our study and has also been reported by other workers (Yüce et al., 2007). Excessive ROS is tackled by endogenous antioxidants. However, when the synthesis of ROS overrides its destruction, there is overconsumption of these antioxidants. This consumption has also been demonstrated previously in cisplatin nephrotoxicity models (Al-Majed et al., 2006). Similarly, there was consumption of glutathione and other endogenous antioxidants such as SOD and CAT in the cisplatin-control group of our study. However, pretreatment with EO maintained glutathione and other antioxidants at near normal levels in the renal tissue. This supports the antioxidant activity of EO which has been documented in the past (Golechha et al., 2012; Dutta and Sahu, 2013; Singh et al., 2014). Previous studies have shown that active constituents such as emblicanins A and B, gallic acid, and ellagic acids present in *E. officinalis* are responsible for its antioxidant activity (Feeney, 2004). Furthermore, free radical scavenging property of *E. officinalis* has been reported to be near to that of L-ascorbic acid, a well known antioxidant (Muthuraman et al., 2011).

Though oxidative stress is a known promoter of apoptosis, cisplatin itself directly induces apoptotic cell death which has been shown by *in vitro* and *in vivo* studies (Tsuruya et al., 2003; Seth et al., 2005; Zhou et al., 2013). According to past reports, renal tubular epithelial cell apoptosis induced by cisplatin is primarily *via* the mitochondrial pathway (Liu et al., 2014). Cisplatin induced apoptosis has been shown to be regulated by the pro-apoptotic protein Bax and the anti-apoptotic protein Bcl-2 (Jiang et al., 2009). It has been shown that cisplatin induces activation of Bax genes (Wei et al., 2007). Bax protein eventually undergoes a conformational change and binds to mitochondrial membrane and subsequently causes the release of cytochrome c from mitochondria leading to apoptosis (Tayem et al., 2006). In contrast, the anti-apoptotic protein Bcl-2 stabilizes the mitochondrial membrane potential thereby inhibiting cytochrome c release and inhibiting apoptosis (Cummings and Schnellmann, 2002). Therefore, Bax and Bcl-2 are crucial in regulating apoptosis. In our experiment,

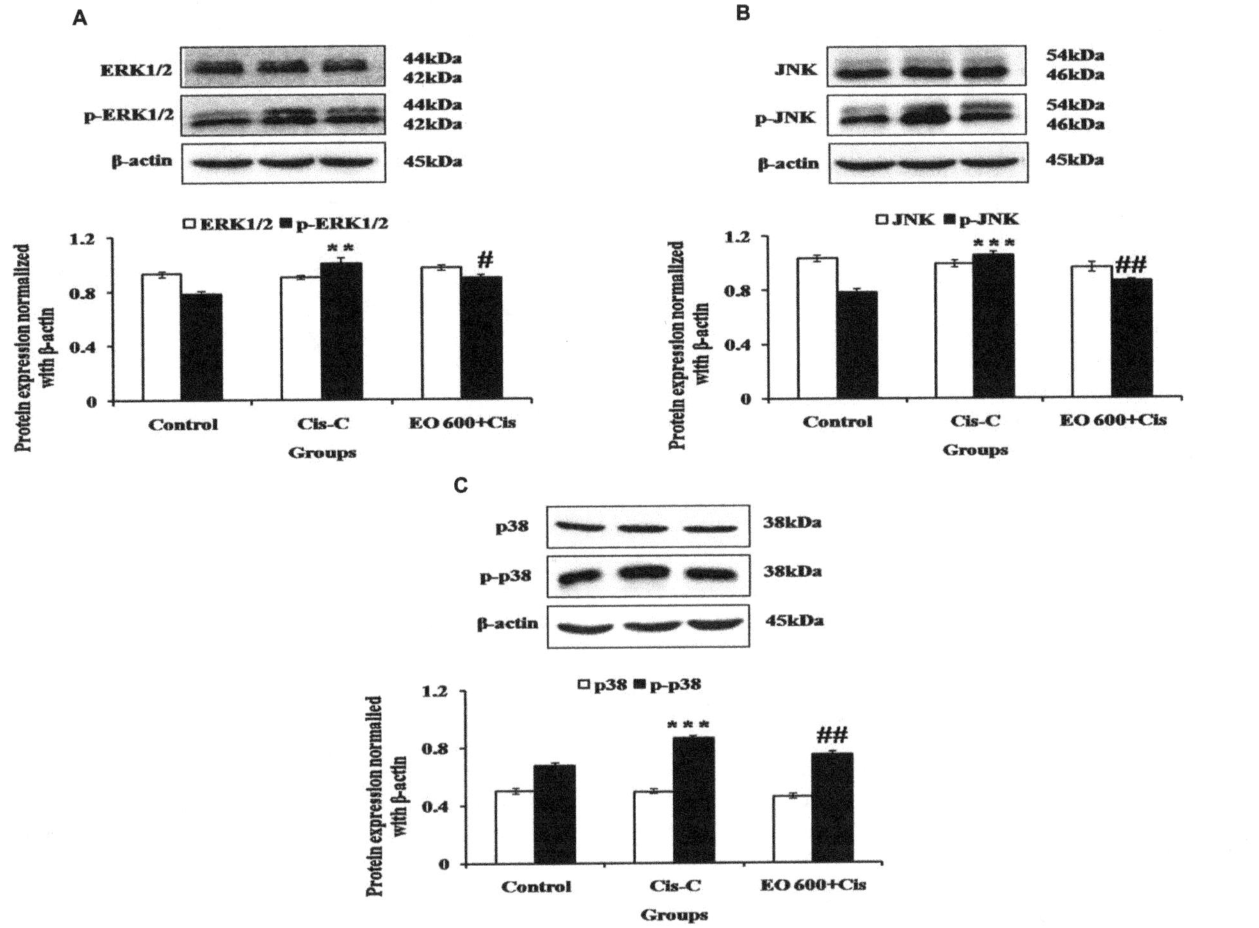

FIGURE 4 | Effect of EO on (A) ERK1/2 and p-ERK1/2; (B) JNK and p-JNK; (C) p38 and p-p38 in various experimental groups. Data are expressed as mean ± SEM of 3 rats per group. $^{**}P < 0.01$, $^{***}P < 0.001$ versus control group; $^{\#}P < 0.05$, $^{\#\#}P < 0.01$ versus Cis-C group.

significantly higher Bax and Caspase-3 and lower Bcl-2 levels were observed in cisplatin-control group. This shows that cisplatin increases Bax and Caspase-3 while lowering Bcl-2 expression of renal tissues whereas pretreatment with EO (600 mg/kg) decreased the Bax and Caspase-3 and increased Bcl-2 levels. TUNEL assay was performed to assess the DNA fragmentation. The TUNEL positivity was observed to be high in cisplatin treated rats and significantly reduced in EO pretreated group. These findings support the previously documented anti-apoptotic activity of *E. Officinalis* (Singh et al., 2013, 2014). Thus, it can be proposed that the renoprotection of EO is mediated by its antioxidant and anti-apoptotic properties.

Strong evidence suggests that the pathogenesis of cisplatin induced renal cell apoptosis is associated with the release of inflammatory cytokines and mediators, including IL-1, IL-6, and TNF-α (Zhang et al., 2007; Guerrero-Beltrán et al., 2012; Zirak et al., 2014). Additionally, NF-κB which is a transcription factor regulating the modulation of inflammatory and immunomodulatory genes, is associated with the process of cisplatin induced renal inflammation (Benedetti et al., 2013). NF-κB activity is inhibited by the specific IκB in the cytoplasm, the latter being rapidly cleared by IKKβ upon activation of NF-κB. NF-κB is released and then translocates to the nucleus, where it activates the transcription of target genes (Ma et al., 2015). Our study has shown that cisplatin-control group has a higher expression of activated NF-κB, IL-6 and TNF-α in comparison to the control rats. Interestingly, EO significantly attenuated the levels of inflammatory cytokines and also blunted the expression of NF-κB. The polyphenol rich components of ethanolic extract of *E. officinalis* have previously been demonstrated to reduce expression of NF-κB in a similar fashion (Kim et al., 2010). Therefore, the attenuation of cisplatin induced nephrotoxicity with EO in our study may also be mediated by the anti-inflammatory property of EO.

Based on the ability of EO to suppress the phosphorylation of members of the NF-κB cascade pathway and inflammation, we further investigated the effect of EO on the upstream signaling components of NF-κB, the MAPK family. MAPK family comprises of three major serine/threonine kinase proteins such as ERK 1/2, JNK and p38 which are associated with cell growth and differentiation, and are extensively linked to inflammation, apoptosis and cell death. Several *in vitro* and *in vivo* studies have demonstrated the role of p38 and JNK in cisplatin-induced nephrotoxicity (Ramesh and Reeves, 2005, 2006; Francescato et al., 2007). ERK1/2 promotes apoptosis by decreasing the production of cytochrome c, phosphorylation of caspase-3, and accelerating the translocation of Bax from cytosol to mitochondria during cisplatin-induced renal cell death (Kim et al., 2014). Cisplatin-induced phosphorylation of JNK induces inflammation of the kidney tubules, apoptosis, and kidney dysfunction (Ma et al., 2015). As anticipated, in our study, cisplatin injection increased the phosphorylation of p38, ERK1/2 and JNK. Pre-treatment with EO, however, ameliorated this increase. Our results are also in line with our study which has demonstrated ERK1/2 modulated effect of *E. officinalis* (Sumitra et al., 2009). Hence, we can convincingly propose that EO mediates its nephroprotective action by regulating MAPK signaling pathway.

In summary, our findings demonstrate that EO treatment alleviates the cisplatin-induced cytotoxicity in kidney through suppressing the ROS mediated activation of MAPKs and NF-κB signaling cascades. Furthermore, EO treatment inhibits the synthesis of intracellular inflammatory cytokines and mediators. Our study suggests that EO has good potential and may be further evaluated clinically for treating cisplatin-induced nephrotoxicity.

AUTHOR CONTRIBUTIONS

SM, KS, and RK: Perform and analyze all the experiments. SK, SV, AT, and SG: Writing of the manuscript. JB, DA, and SO: Designed the study.

ACKNOWLEDGMENT

The authors are thankful to Mr. B.M. Sharma for its technical assistance.

REFERENCES

Aebi, H. (1984). Catalase in vitro. *Methods Enzymol.* 105, 121–126. doi: 10.1016/S0076-6879(84)05016-3

Al-Majed, A. A., Sayed-Ahmed, M. M., Al-Yahya, A. A., Aleisa, A. M., Al-Rejaie, S. S., and Al-Shabanah, O. A. (2006). Propionyl-L-carnitine prevents the progression of cisplatin-induced cardiomyopathy in a carnitine-depleted rat model. *Pharmacol. Res.* 53, 278–286. doi: 10.1016/j.phrs.2005.12.005

Athira, K. V., Madhana, R. M., and Lahkar, M. (2016). Flavonoids, the emerging dietary supplement against cisplatin-induced nephrotoxicity. *Chem. Biol. Interact.* 248, 18–20. doi: 10.1016/j.cbi.2016.02.005

Benedetti, G., Fredriksson, L., Herpers, B., Meerman, J., van de Water, B., and de Graauw, M. (2013). TNF-α-mediated NF-κB survival signaling impairment by cisplatin enhances JNK activation allowing synergistic apoptosis of renal proximal tubular cells. *Biochem. Pharmacol.* 85, 274–286. doi: 10.1016/j.bcp.2012.10.012

Bhatia, J., Tabassum, F., Sharma, A. K., Bharti, S., Golechha, M., Joshi, S., et al. (2011). *Emblica officinalis* exerts antihypertensive effect in a rat model of DOCA-salt-induced hypertension: role of (p) eNOS, NO and oxidative stress. *Cardiovasc. Toxicol.* 11, 272–279. doi: 10.1007/s12012-011-9122-2

Bolisetty, S., Traylor, A., Joseph, R., Zarjou, A., and Agarwal, A. (2016). Proximal tubule-targeted heme oxygenase-1 in cisplatin-induced acute kidney injury. *Am. J. Physiol. Renal Physiol.* 310, F385–F394. doi: 10.1152/ajprenal.00335.2015

Bradford, M. M. (1976). A rapid and sensitive method for the quantitation of microgram quantities of protein utilizing the principle of protein-dye binding. *Anal. Biochem.* 72, 248–254. doi: 10.1016/0003-2697(76)90527-3

Changizi-Ashtiyani, S., Alizadeh, M., Najafi, H., Babaei, S., Khazaei, M., Jafari, M., et al. (2016). Physalis alkekengi and *Alhagi maurorum* ameliorate the side effect of cisplatin-induced nephrotoxicity. *Cancer Gene Ther.* 23, 235–240. doi: 10.1038/cgt.2016.24

Cummings, B. S., and Schnellmann, R. G. (2002). Cisplatin-induced renal cell apoptosis: caspase 3-dependent and -independent pathways. *J. Pharmacol. Exp. Ther.* 302, 8–17. doi: 10.1124/jpet.302.1.8

Domitrović, R., Cvijanović, O., Pernjak-Pugel, E., Skoda, M., Mikelić, L., Crnčević-Orlić, Z., et al. (2013). Berberine exerts nephroprotective effect against cisplatin-induced kidney damage through inhibition of oxidative/nitrosative stress, inflammation, autophagy and apoptosis. *Food Chem. Toxicol.* 62, 397–406. doi: 10.1016/j.fct.2013.09.003

dos Santos, N. A., Carvalho Rodrigues, M. A., Martins, N. M., and dos Santos, A. C. (2012). Cisplatin-induced nephrotoxicity and targets of nephroprotection: an update. *Arch. Toxicol.* 86, 1233–1250. doi: 10.1007/s00204-012-0821-7

Dutta, A. L., and Sahu, C. R. (2013). *Emblica officinalis* Garten fruits extract ameliorates reproductive injury and oxidative testicular toxicity induced by chlorpyrifos in male rats. *Springerplus* 2:541. doi: 10.1186/2193-1801-2-541

El-Naga, R. N. (2014). Pre-treatment with cardamonin protects against cisplatin-induced nephrotoxicity in rats: impact on NOX-1, inflammation and apoptosis. *Toxicol Appl. Pharmacol.* 274, 87–95. doi: 10.1016/j.taap.2013.10.031

El-Naga, R. N., and Mahran, Y. F. (2016). Indole-3-carbinol protects against cisplatin-induced acute nephrotoxicity: role of calcitonin gene-related peptide and insulin-like growth factor-1. *Sci. Rep.* 6:29857. doi: 10.1038/srep29857

Feeney, M. J. (2004). Fruits and the prevention of lifestyle-related diseases. *Clin. Exp. Pharmacol. Physiol.* 31, S11–S13. doi: 10.1111/j.1440-1681.2004.04104.x

Francescato, H. D., Costa, R. S., Júnior, F. B., and Coimbra, T. M. (2007). Effect of JNK inhibition on cisplatin-induced renal damage. *Nephrol. Dial. Transplant.* 22, 2138–2148. doi: 10.1093/ndt/gfm144

Golechha, M., Bhatia, J., and Arya, D. S. (2012). Studies on effects of *Emblica officinalis* (Amla) on oxidative stress and cholinergic function in scopolamine induced amnesia in mice. *J. Environ. Biol.* 33, 95–100.

Golechha, M., Sarangal, V., Ojha, S., Bhatia, J., and Arya, D. S. (2014). Anti-inflammatory effect of *emblica officinalis* in rodent models of acute and chronic inflammation: involvement of possible mechanisms. *Int. J. Inflam.* 2014:178408. doi: 10.1155/2014/178408

Guerrero-Beltrán, C. E., Mukhopadhyay, P., Horváth, B., Rajesh, M., Tapia, E., García-Torres, I., et al. (2012). Sulforaphane, a natural constituent of broccoli, prevents cell death and inflammation in nephropathy. *J. Nutr. Biochem.* 23, 494–500. doi: 10.1016/j.jnutbio.2011.02.004

Haque, R., Bin-Hafeez, B., Ahmad, I., Parvez, S., Pandey, S., and Raisuddin, S. (2001). Protective effects of *Emblica officinalis* Gaertn. in cyclophosphamide-treated mice. *Hum. Exp. Toxicol.* 20, 643–650. doi: 10.1191/096032701718890568

Jaiman, S., Sharma, A. K., Singh, K., and Khanna, D. (2013). Signalling mechanisms involved in renal pathological changes during cisplatin-induced nephropathy. *Eur. J. Clin. Pharmacol.* 69, 1863–1874. doi: 10.1007/s00228-013-1568-7

Jiang, M., Wang, C. Y., Huang, S., Yang, T., and Dong, Z. (2009). Cisplatin-induced apoptosis in p53-deficient renal cells via the intrinsic mitochondrial pathway. *Am. J. Physiol. Renal Physiol.* 296, F983–F993. doi: 10.1152/ajprenal.90579.2008

Kim, H. J., Ravichandran, K., Ozkok, A., Wang, Q., He, Z., Jani, A., et al. (2014). The water-soluble triptolide derivative PG490-88 protects against cisplatin-induced acute kidney injury. *J. Pharmacol. Exp. Ther.* 349, 518–525. doi: 10.1124/jpet.114.213769

Kim, H. J., Yokozawa, T., Kim, H. Y., Tohda, C., Rao, T. P., and Juneja, L. R. (2005). Influence of amla (*Emblica officinalis* Gaertn.) on hypercholesterolemia and lipid peroxidation in cholesterol-fed rats. *J. Nutr. Sci. Vitaminol.* 51, 413–418. doi: 10.3177/jnsv.51.413

Kim, H. Y., Okubo, T., Juneja, L. R., and Yokozawa, T. (2010). The protective role of amla (*Emblica officinalis* Gaertn.) against fructose-induced metabolic syndrome in a rat model. *Br. J. Nutr.* 103, 502–512. doi: 10.1017/S0007114509991978

Krishnaveni, M., and Mirunalini, S. (2010). Therapeutic potential of *Phyllanthus emblica* (amla): the ayurvedic wonder. *J. Basic Clin. Physiol. Pharmacol.* 21, 93–105.

Liu, X., Huang, Z., Zou, X., Yang, Y., Qiu, Y., and Wen, Y. (2014). Panax notoginseng saponins attenuates cisplatin-induced nephrotoxicity via inhibiting the mitochondrial pathway of apoptosis. *Int. J. Clin. Exp. Pathol.* 7, 8391–8400.

Ma, X., Dang, C., Kang, H., Dai, Z., Lin, S., Guan, H., et al. (2015). Saikosaponin-D reduces cisplatin-induced nephrotoxicity by repressing ROS-mediated activation of MAPK and NF-κB signalling pathways. *Int. Immunopharmacol.* 28, 399–408. doi: 10.1016/j.intimp.2015.06.020

Mahata, S., Pandey, A., Shukla, S., Tyagi, A., Husain, S. A., Das, B. C., et al. (2013). Anticancer activity of *Phyllanthus emblica* Linn. (Indian gooseberry): inhibition of transcription factor AP-1 and HPV gene expression in cervical cancer cells. *Nutr. Cancer* 65(Suppl. 1), 88–97. doi: 10.1080/01635581.2013.785008

Malik, S., Suchal, K., Gamad, N., Dinda, A. K., Arya, D. S., and Bhatia, J. (2015). Telmisartan ameliorates cisplatin-induced nephrotoxicity by inhibiting MAPK mediated inflammation and apoptosis. *Eur. J. Pharmacol.* 748, 54–60. doi: 10.1016/j.ejphar.2014.12.008

Marklund, S., and Marklund, G. (1974). Involvement of the superoxide anion radical in the autoxidation of pyrogallol and a convenient assay for superoxide dismutase. *Eur. J. Biochem.* 47, 469–474. doi: 10.1111/j.1432-1033.1974.tb03714.x

Miller, R. P., Tadagavadi, R. K., Ramesh, G., and Reeves, W. B. (2010). Mechanisms of Cisplatin nephrotoxicity. *Toxins (Basel).* 2, 2490–2518. doi: 10.3390/toxins2112490

Moron, M. S., Depierre, J. W., and Mannervik, B. (1979). Levels of glutathione, glutathione reductase and glutathione S-transferase activities in rat lung and liver. *Biochim. Biophys. Acta* 582, 67–78. doi: 10.1016/0304-4165(79)90289-7

Muthuraman, A., Sood, S., and Singla, A. K. (2011). The antiinflammatory potential of phenolic compounds from *Emblica officinalis* L. in rat. *Inflammopharmacology* 19, 327–334. doi: 10.1007/s10787-010-0041-9

Nain, P., Saini, V., Sharma, S., and Nain, J. (2012). Antidiabetic and antioxidant potential of *Emblica officinalis* Gaertn. leaves extract in streptozotocin-induced type-2 diabetes mellitus (T2DM) rats. *J. Ethnopharmacol.* 142, 65–71. doi: 10.1016/j.jep.2012.04.014

Nojiri, T., Hosoda, H., Kimura, T., Miura, K., Ishikane, S., Tokudome, T., et al. (2015). Atrial natriuretic peptide protects against cisplatin-induced acute kidney injury. *Cancer Chemother. Pharmacol.* 75, 123–129. doi: 10.1007/s00280-014-2624-4

Oh, G. S., Kim, H. J., Shen, A., Lee, S. B., Khadka, D., Pandit, A., et al. (2014). Cisplatin-induced kidney dysfunction and perspectives on improving treatment strategies. *Electrolyte Blood Press.* 12, 55–65. doi: 10.5049/EBP.2014.12.2.55

Oh, G. S., Kim, H. J., Shen, A., Lee, S. B., Yang, S. H., Shim, H., et al. (2016). New therapeutic concept of NAD redox balance for cisplatin nephrotoxicity. *Biomed. Res. Int.* 2016:4048390. doi: 10.1155/2016/4048390

Ohkawa, H., Ohishi, N., and Yagi, K. (1979). Assay for lipid peroxides in animal tissues by thiobarbituric acid reaction. *Anal. Biochem.* 95, 351–358. doi: 10.1016/0003-2697(79)90738-3

Pabla, N., and Dong, Z. (2008). Cisplatin nephrotoxicity: mechanisms and renoprotective strategies. *Kidney Int.* 73, 994–1007. doi: 10.1038/sj.ki.5002786

Pabla, N., Murphy, R. F., Liu, K., and Dong, Z. (2009). The copper transporter Ctr1 contributes to cisplatin uptake by renal tubular cells during cisplatin nephrotoxicity. *Am. J. Physiol. Renal Physiol.* 296, 505–511. doi: 10.1152/ajprenal.90545.2008

Pan, H., Chen, J., Shen, K., Wang, X., Wang, P., Fu, G., et al. (2015). Mitochondrial modulation by Epigallocatechin 3-Gallate ameliorates cisplatin induced renal injury through decreasing oxidative/nitrative stress, inflammation and NF-kB in mice. *PLoS ONE* 10:e0124775. doi: 10.1371/journal.pone.0124775

Quesada, A., Vargas, F., Montoro-Molina, S., O'Valle, F., Rodríguez-Martínez, M. D., Osuna, A., et al. (2012). Urinary aminopeptidase activities as early and predictive biomarkers of renal dysfunction in cisplatin-treated rats. *PLoS ONE* 7:e40402. doi: 10.1371/journal.pone.0040402

Ramesh, G., and Reeves, W. B. (2005). p38MAP kinase inhibition ameliorates cisplatin nephrotoxicity in mice. *Am. J. Physiol. Renal. Physiol.* 289, F166–F174. doi: 10.1152/ajprenal.00401.2004

Ramesh, G., and Reeves, W. B. (2006). Cisplatin increases TNF-alpha mRNA stability in kidney proximal tubule cells. *Ren. Fail.* 28, 583–592. doi: 10.1080/08860220600843839

Reddy, V. D., Padmavathi, P., Hymavathi, R., Maturu, P., and Varadacharyulu, N. Ch (2014). Alcohol-induced oxidative stress in rat liver microsomes: Protective effect of *Emblica officinalis*. *Pathophysiology* 21, 153–159. doi: 10.1016/j.pathophys.2013.12.001

Sahu, B. D., Kalvala, A. K., Koneru, M., Mahesh, Kumar J, Kuncha, M., Rachamalla, S. S., et al. (2014). Ameliorative effect of fisetin on cisplatin-induced nephrotoxicity in rats via modulation of NF-kappaB activation and antioxidant defence. *PLoS ONE* 9:e105070. doi: 10.1371/journal.pone.0105070

Seth, R., Yang, C., Kaushal, V., Shah, S. V., and Kaushal, G. P. (2005). p53-dependent caspase-2 activation in mitochondrial release of apoptosis-inducing factor and its role in renal tubular epithelial cell injury. *J. Biol. Chem.* 280, 31230–31239. doi: 10.1074/jbc.M503305200

Singh, M. K., Yadav, S. S., Gupta, V., and Khattri, S. (2013). Immunomodulatory role of *Emblica officinalis* in arsenic induced oxidative damage and apoptosis in thymocytes of mice. *BMC Complement. Altern. Med.* 13:193. doi: 10.1186/1472-6882-13-193

Singh, M. K., Yadav, S. S., Yadav, R. S., Singh, U. S., Shukla, Y., Pant, K. K., et al. (2014). Efficacy of crude extract of *Emblica officinalis* (amla) in arsenic-induced oxidative damage and apoptosis in splenocytes of mice. *Toxicol. Int.* 21, 8–17. doi: 10.4103/0971-6580.128784

Song, K. I., Park, J. Y., Lee, S., Lee, D., Jang, H. J., Kim, S. N., et al. (2015). Protective effect of tetrahydrocurcumin against cisplatin-induced renal damage: in vitro and in vivo studies. *Planta Med.* 81, 286–291. doi: 10.1055/s-0035-154 5696

Sumitra, M., Manikandan, P., Gayathri, V. S., Mahendran, P., and Suguna, L. (2009). *Emblica officinalis* exerts wound healing action through up-regulation of collagen and extracellular signal-regulated kinases (ERK1/2). *Wound Repair Regen.* 17, 99–107. doi: 10.1111/j.1524-475X.2008.00446.x

Tayem, Y., Johnson, T. R., Mann, B. E., Green, C. J., and Motterlini, R. (2006). Protection against cisplatin-induced nephrotoxicity by a carbon monoxide-releasing molecule. *Am. J. Physiol. Renal Physiol.* 290, F789–F794. doi: 10.1152/ajprenal.00363.2005

Tsuruya, K., Ninomiya, T., Tokumoto, M.,. Hirakawa, M., Masutani, K., Taniguchi, M., et al. (2003). Direct involvement of the receptor-mediated apoptotic pathways in cisplatin-induced renal tubular cell death. *Kidney Int.* 63, 72–82. doi: 10.1046/j.1523-1755.2003.00709.x

Verma, R., and Chakraborty, D. (2008). Alterations in DNA, RNA and protein contents in liver and kidney of mice treated with ochratoxin and their amelioration by *Emblica officinalis* aqueous extract. *Acta Pol. Pharm.* 65, 3–9.

Wang, Y., Luo, X., Pan, H., Huang, W., Wang, X., Wen, H., et al. (2015). Pharmacological inhibition of NADPH oxidase protects against cisplatin induced nephrotoxicity in mice by two step mechanism. *Food Chem. Toxicol.* 83, 251–260. doi: 10.1016/j.fct.2015.05.007

Wei, Q., Dong, G., Franklin, J., and Dong, Z. (2007). The pathological role of Bax in cisplatin nephrotoxicity. *Kidney Int.* 72, 53–62. doi: 10.1038/sj.ki.5002256

Xu, Y., Ma, H., Shao, J., Wu, J., Zhou, L., Zhang, Z., et al. (2015). A role for tubular necroptosis in cisplatin-induced AKI. *J. Am. Soc. Nephrol.* 26, 2647–2658. doi: 10.1681/ASN.2014080741

Yousef, M. I., and Hussien, H. M. (2015). Cisplatin-induced renal toxicity via tumor necrosis factor-α, interleukin 6, tumor suppressor P53, DNA damage, xanthine oxidase, histological changes, oxidative stress and nitric oxide in rats: protective effect of ginseng. *Food Chem. Toxicol.* 78, 17–25. doi: 10.1016/j.fct.2015.01.014

Yüce, A., Ateşşahin, A., Ceribaşi, A. O., and Aksakal, M. (2007). Ellagic acid prevents cisplatin-induced oxidative stress in liver and heart tissue of rats. *Basic Clin. Pharmacol. Toxicol.* 101, 345–349. doi: 10.1111/j.1742-7843.2007.00129.x

Zhang, B., Ramesh, G., Norbury, C. C., and Reeves, W. B. (2007). Cisplatin-induced nephrotoxicity is mediated by tumor necrosis factor-alpha produced by renal parenchymal cells. *Kidney Int.* 72, 37–44. doi: 10.1038/sj.ki.5002242

Zhou, Y., Xu, H., Xu, W., Wang, B., Wu, H., Tao, Y., et al. (2013). Exosomes released by human umbilical cord mesenchymal stem cells protect against cisplatin-induced renal oxidative stress and apoptosis in vivo and in vitro. *Stem Cell Res. Ther.* 4:34. doi: 10.1186/scrt194

Zirak, M. R., Rahimian, R., Ghazi-Khansari, M., Abbasi, A., Razmi, A., Mehr, S. E., et al. (2014). Tropisetron attenuates cisplatin-induced nephrotoxicity in mice. *Eur. J. Pharmacol.* 738, 222–229. doi: 10.1016/j.ejphar.2014.05.050

Conflict of Interest Statement: The authors declare that the research was conducted in the absence of any commercial or financial relationships that could be construed as a potential conflict of interest.

The reviewers AI and JU and handling Editor declared their shared affiliation, and the handling Editor states that the process nevertheless met the standards of a fair and objective review.

Permissions

All chapters in this book were first published in AECCANITRS, by Frontiers Media SA; hereby published with permission under the Creative Commons Attribution License or equivalent. Every chapter published in this book has been scrutinized by our experts. Their significance has been extensively debated. The topics covered herein carry significant findings which will fuel the growth of the discipline. They may even be implemented as practical applications or may be referred to as a beginning point for another development.

The contributors of this book come from diverse backgrounds, making this book a truly international effort. This book will bring forth new frontiers with its revolutionizing research information and detailed analysis of the nascent developments around the world.

We would like to thank all the contributing authors for lending their expertise to make the book truly unique. They have played a crucial role in the development of this book. Without their invaluable contributions this book wouldn't have been possible. They have made vital efforts to compile up to date information on the varied aspects of this subject to make this book a valuable addition to the collection of many professionals and students.

This book was conceptualized with the vision of imparting up-to-date information and advanced data in this field. To ensure the same, a matchless editorial board was set up. Every individual on the board went through rigorous rounds of assessment to prove their worth. After which they invested a large part of their time researching and compiling the most relevant data for our readers.

The editorial board has been involved in producing this book since its inception. They have spent rigorous hours researching and exploring the diverse topics which have resulted in the successful publishing of this book. They have passed on their knowledge of decades through this book. To expedite this challenging task, the publisher supported the team at every step. A small team of assistant editors was also appointed to further simplify the editing procedure and attain best results for the readers.

Apart from the editorial board, the designing team has also invested a significant amount of their time in understanding the subject and creating the most relevant covers. They scrutinized every image to scout for the most suitable representation of the subject and create an appropriate cover for the book.

The publishing team has been an ardent support to the editorial, designing and production team. Their endless efforts to recruit the best for this project, has resulted in the accomplishment of this book. They are a veteran in the field of academics and their pool of knowledge is as vast as their experience in printing. Their expertise and guidance has proved useful at every step. Their uncompromising quality standards have made this book an exceptional effort. Their encouragement from time to time has been an inspiration for everyone.

The publisher and the editorial board hope that this book will prove to be a valuable piece of knowledge for researchers, students, practitioners and scholars across the globe.

List of Contributors

Antonio Ruggiero, Daniela Rizzo, Martina Catalano, Giorgio Attinà and Riccardo Riccardi
Division of Pediatric Oncology, Catholic University of Rome, Rome, Italy

Vivek Kumar, Mohit Garg, Charalampos S. Floudas and Parita Soni
Department of Medicine, Maimonides Medical Center, Brooklyn, NY, USA

Neha Chaudhary
Department of Pediatrics, Maimonides Medical Center, Brooklyn, NY, USA

Abhinav B. Chandra
Medical Director, Yuma Regional Cancer Center, Yuma, AZ, USA

Rachel M. McQuade, Vanesa Stojanovska and Kulmira Nurgali
Centre for Chronic Disease, College of Health and Biomedicine, Victoria University, Melbourne, VIC, Australia

Raquel Abalo
Área de Farmacología y Nutrición, Universidad Rey Juan Carlos, Madrid, Spain
Grupo de Excelencia Investigadora URJC, Banco de Santander Grupo Multidisciplinar de Investigación y Tratamiento del Dolor, Universidad Rey Juan Carlos, Madrid, Spain
Unidad Asociada al Instituto de Química Médica del Consejo Superior de Investigaciones Científicas, Madrid, Spain
Unidad Asociada al Instituto de Investigación en Ciencias de la Alimentación del Consejo Superior de Investigaciones Científicas, Madrid, Spain

Joel C. Bornstein
Department of Physiology, University of Melbourne, Melbourne, VIC, Australia

Martin Uhl and Stefan Schwab
Department of Neurology, University of Erlangen-Nuremberg, Erlangen, Germany

Thomas Efferth
Institute of Pharmacy and Biochemistry, Johannes Gutenberg University, Mainz, Germany

Bernardo L. Rapoport
The Medical Oncology Centre of Rosebank, Johannesburg, South Africa

Marika Cinausero, Paola Ermacora, Debora Basile, Maria G. Vitale, Valentina Fanotto and Giuseppe Parisi
Department of Oncology, University and General Hospital, Udine, Italy

Giuseppe Aprile
Department of Oncology, University and General Hospital, Udine, Italy
Department of Oncology, San Bortolo General Hospital, Vicenza, Italy

Lorenzo Calvetti
Department of Oncology, San Bortolo General Hospital, Vicenza, Italy

Stephen T. Sonis
Divisions of Oral Medicine, Brigham and Women's Hospital, Boston, MA, United States
Dana-Farber Cancer Institute, Boston, MA, United States
Biomodels LLC, Watertown, MA, United States

Paula Mosińska, Agata Gabryelska and Jakub Fichna
Department of Biochemistry, Faculty of Medicine, Medical University of Łódź, Łódź, Poland

Malwina Zasada
Department of Biochemistry, Faculty of Medicine, Medical University of Łódź, Łódź, Poland
Department of Cosmetic Raw Materials Chemistry, Faculty of Pharmacy, Medical University of Łódź, Łódź, Poland

Hélène Castel, Marie-Christine Tonon and Martine Dubois
Laboratory of Neuronal and Neuroendocrine Differentiation and Communication, Institut National de la Santé et de la Recherche Médicale, DC2N, Normandie University, Rouen, France
Institute for Research and Innovation in Biomedicine, Rouen, France
Cancer and Cognition Platform, Ligue Nationale Contre le Cancer, Caen, France

Angeline Denouel
Institut National de la Santé et de la Recherche Médicale, U1086, Caen, France

Marie Lange
Institut National de la Santé et de la Recherche Médicale, U1086, Caen, France
Medical Oncology Department, Centre François Baclesse, Caen, France

Florence Joly
Cancer and Cognition Platform, Ligue Nationale Contre le Cancer, Caen, France
Institut National de la Santé et de la Recherche Médicale, U1086, Caen, France
Medical Oncology Department, Centre François Baclesse, Caen, France
Medical Oncology, University Hospital Center, Caen, France

Saúl Redondo-Blanco, Javier Fernández, Ignacio Gutiérrez-del-Río, Claudio J. Villar and Felipe Lombó
Departamento de Biología Funcional, Área de Microbiología, Facultad de Medicina, Instituto Universitario de Oncología del Principado de Asturias (IUOPA), Universidad de Oviedo, Oviedo, Spain

John A. Rudd
Emesis Research Group, School of Biomedical Sciences, Faculty of Medicine, The Chinese University of Hong Kong, Hong Kong, China
Brain and Mind Institute, The Chinese University of Hong Kong, Hong Kong, China

Man P. Ngan and Zengbing Lu
Emesis Research Group, School of Biomedical Sciences, Faculty of Medicine, The Chinese University of Hong Kong, Hong Kong, China

Guy A. Higgins
Intervivo Solutions Inc., Toronto, ON, Canada

Claudio Giuliano, Emanuela Lovati and Claudio Pietra
Research and Preclinical, Helsinn Healthcare SA., Lugano, Switzerland

Hee Kee Kim, Seon-Hee Hwang and Salahadin Abdi
Department of Pain Medicine, Division of Anesthesiology and Critical Care, The University of Texas MD Anderson Cancer Center, Houston, TX, USA

Nicolas Kerckhove and David Balayssac
INSERM U1107, NEURO-DOL, CHU Clermont-Ferrand, Délégation à la Recherche Clinique et à l'Innovation, Université Clermont Auvergne, Clermont-Ferrand, France

Aurore Collin
INSERM U1107, NEURO-DOL, Université Clermont Auvergne, Clermont-Ferrand, France

Sakahlé Condé
INSERM U1107, NEURO-DOL, CHU Clermont-Ferrand, Neurologie, Université Clermont Auvergne, Clermont-Ferrand, France

Carine Chaleteix
CHU Clermont-Ferrand, Hématologie Clinique Adulte, Clermont-Ferrand, France

Denis Pezet
INSERM U1071, CHU Clermont-Ferrand, Chirurgie et Oncologie Digestive, Université Clermont Auvergne, Clermont-Ferrand, France

Kouichi Yamamoto, Soichi Tatsutani and Takayuki Ishida
Division of Health Sciences, Department of Medical Science and Technology, Graduate School of Medicine, Osaka University, Osaka, Japan

Gema Vera, Rocío Girón, Ma Isabel Martín-Fontelles and Raquel Abalo
Área de Farmacología y Nutrición, Departamento de Ciencias Básicas de la Salud, Universidad Rey Juan Carlos, Alcorcón, Spain
Unidad Asociada ICDCi del Instituto de Química Médica, Consejo Superior de Investigaciones Científicas, Madrid, Spain
Unidad Asociada ICDCi del Instituto de Investigación en Ciencias de la Alimentación, Consejo Superior de Investigaciones Científicas, Madrid, Spain
Grupo de Excelencia Investigadora URJC-Banco de Santander-Grupo Multidisciplinar de Investigación y Tratamiento del Dolor (iCDOL), Alcorcón, Spain

Ana E. López-Pérez
Grupo de Excelencia Investigadora URJC-Banco de Santander-Grupo Multidisciplinar de Investigación y Tratamiento del Dolor (iCDOL), Alcorcón, Spain
Unidad del Dolor, Servicio de Anestesia, Hospital General Universitario Gregorio Marañón, Madrid, Spain

José A. Uranga
Unidad Asociada ICDCi del Instituto de Investigación en Ciencias de la Alimentación, Consejo Superior de Investigaciones Científicas, Madrid, Spain
Grupo de Excelencia Investigadora URJC-Banco de Santander-Grupo Multidisciplinar de Investigación y Tratamiento del Dolor (iCDOL), Alcorcón, Spain
Área de Histología Humana y Anatomía Patológica, Departamento de Ciencias Básicas de la Salud, Universidad Rey Juan Carlos, Alcorcón, Spain

Esperanza Herradón, Cristina González, Raquel Abalo, Ma I. Martín and Visitacion López-Miranda
Área de Farmacología, Nutrición y Bromatología, Facultad Ciencias de la Salud, Departamento de Ciencias Básicas de la Salud, Universidad Rey Juan Carlos, Alcorcón, Spain
Unidad Asociada ICDCi del Instituto de Química Médica, Consejo Superior de Investigaciones Científicas, Madrid, Spain
Grupo Interdisciplinar de Investigación en Dolor iCDol, Universidad Rey Juan Carlos-Banco de Santander, Alcorcón, Spain

José A. Uranga
Grupo Interdisciplinar de Investigación en Dolor iCDol, Universidad Rey Juan Carlos-Banco de Santander, Alcorcón, Spain
Área de Histología Humana y Anatomía Patológica, Departamento de Ciencias Básicas de la Salud, Universidad Rey Juan Carlos, Alcorcón, Spain

James C. Sorensen, Cara A. Timpani and Dean G. Campelj
Centre for Chronic Disease, College of Health & Biomedicine, Victoria University, Melbourne, VIC, Australia
Australian Institute for Musculoskeletal Science, Melbourne, VIC, Australia

Aaron C. Petersen and Adam J. Trewin
Institute of Sport, Exercise & Active Living, Victoria University, Melbourne, VIC, Australia

Jordan Cook and Vanesa Stojanovska
Centre for Chronic Disease, College of Health & Biomedicine, Victoria University, Melbourne, VIC, Australia

Mathew Stewart
Institute of Sustainability and Innovation, Victoria University, Melbourne, VIC, Australia

Alan Hayes and Emma Rybalka
Centre for Chronic Disease, College of Health & Biomedicine, Victoria University, Melbourne, VIC, Australia

Australian Institute for Musculoskeletal Science, Melbourne, VIC, Australia
Institute of Sport, Exercise & Active Living, Victoria University, Melbourne, VIC, Australia

Raghav Sundar, Nesaretnam Barr Kumarakulasinghe, Anand D. Jeyasekharan, Samuel Guan Wei Ow, Jingshan Ho, David Shao Peng Tan, Joline Si Jing Lim and Sally Ang
Department of Haematology-Oncology, National University Health System, Singapore, Singapore

Aishwarya Bandla
Singapore Institute for Neurotechnology, National University of Singapore, Singapore, Singapore
Department of Biomedical Engineering, National University of Singapore, Singapore, Singapore

Stacey Sze Hui Tan
Singapore Institute for Neurotechnology, National University of Singapore, Singapore, Singapore

Lun-De Liao
Singapore Institute for Neurotechnology, National University of Singapore, Singapore, Singapore
Institute of Biomedical Engineering and Nanomedicine, National Health Research Institutes, Zhunan Township, Taiwan

Joy Vijayan
Department of Medicine, National University Health System, Singapore, Singapore

Aravinda K. Therimadasamy
Neurology Diagnostic Laboratory, National University Hospital, Singapore, Singapore

Zarinah Hairom and Emily Ang
National University Cancer Institute, National University Health System, Singapore, Singapore

Nitish V. Thakor
Singapore Institute for Neurotechnology, National University of Singapore, Singapore, Singapore
Department of Biomedical Engineering, National University of Singapore, Singapore, Singapore
Department of Biomedical Engineering, Johns Hopkins University, Baltimore, MD, USA

Soo-Chin Lee
Department of Haematology-Oncology, National University Health System, Singapore, Singapore
Cancer Science Institute of Singapore, National University of Singapore, Singapore, Singapore

Einar P. V. Wilder-Smith
Singapore Institute for Neurotechnology, National University of Singapore, Singapore, Singapore
Department of Medicine, National University Health System, Singapore, Singapore
Department of Medicine, Yong Loo Lin School of Medicine, National University of Singapore, Singapore, Singapore

Salma Malik, Kapil Suchal, Jagriti Bhatia, Sana I. Khan, Swati Vasisth, Ameesha Tomar, Rajeev Kumar and Dharamvir S. Arya
Cardiovascular Research Laboratory, Department of Pharmacology, All India Institute of Medical Sciences, New Delhi, India

Sameer Goyal
Department of Pharmacology, R. C. Patel Institute of Pharmaceutical Education and Research, Shirpur, India

Shreesh K. Ojha
Department of Pharmacology and Therapeutics, College of Medicine and Health Sciences, United Arab Emirates University, Al Ain, UAE

Index

www.ingramcontent.com/pod-product-compliance
Lightning Source LLC
LaVergne TN
LVHW081034210926
848485LV00004B/1019